Advanced Topics in Gastroenterology

Advanced Topics in Gastroenterology

Edited by Cyrus Holt

hayle medical

New York

Hayle Medical,
750 Third Avenue, 9th Floor,
New York, NY 10017, USA

Visit us on the World Wide Web at:
www.haylemedical.com

ISBN: 978-1-63241-611-7

The publisher's policy is to use permanent paper from mills that operate a sustainable forestry policy. Furthermore, the publisher ensures that the text paper and cover boards used have met acceptable environmental accreditation standards.

Printed in China.

Cataloging-in-Publication Data

Advanced topics in gastroenterology / edited by Cyrus Holt.
p. cm.
Includes bibliographical references and index.
ISBN 978-1-63241-611-7
1. Gastroenterology. 2. Digestive organs--Diseases. I. Holt, Cyrus.
RC801 .A38 2019
616.33--dc23

Table of Contents

Preface

The branch of medicine that studies the functioning of the digestive system and its disorders is known as gastroenterology. It is mainly concerned with the disorders that affect the gastrointestinal tract, including organs from mouth to anus, along the alimentary canal. Hepatology is a subset of gastroenterology. It is concerned with the study of liver, gallbladder, bile ducts and pancreas. Physicians who are a specialist in the field of gastroenterology are known as gastroenterologists. They usually perform procedures like, endoscopy, colonoscopy, liver biopsy, endoscopic ultrasound and endoscopic retrograde cholangiancreatography to diagnose and treat gastrointestinal diseases. The topics included in this book on gastroenterology are of utmost significance and bound to provide incredible insights to readers. It explores all the important aspects of gastroenterology in the present day scenario. Doctors, researchers and students actively engaged in this field will find this book full of crucial and unexplored concepts.

The researches compiled throughout the book are authentic and of high quality, combining several disciplines and from very diverse regions from around the world. Drawing on the contributions of many researchers from diverse countries, the book's objective is to provide the readers with the latest achievements in the area of research. This book will surely be a source of knowledge to all interested and researching the field.

In the end, I would like to express my deep sense of gratitude to all the authors for meeting the set deadlines in completing and submitting their research chapters. I would also like to thank the publisher for the support offered to us throughout the course of the book. Finally, I extend my sincere thanks to my family for being a constant source of inspiration and encouragement.

Editor

Thickness of Subcutaneous Fat Is a Predictive Factor of Incisional Surgical Site Infection in Crohn's Disease Surgery: A Retrospective Study

Xingchen Cai,[1] Weisong Shen,[2] Zhen Guo,[2] Yi Li,[2] Lei Cao,[2] Jianfeng Gong,[2] and Weiming Zhu[2]

[1]*Department of General Surgery, Jinling Hospital, Nanjing Medical University, Nanjing, China*
[2]*Department of General Surgery, Jinling Hospital, Medical School of Nanjing University, Nanjing, China*

Correspondence should be addressed to Weiming Zhu; juwiming@nju.edu.cn

Academic Editor: Cristiano Pagnini

Background. Incisional surgical site infection (iSSI) is a frequent postoperative complication of abdominal surgeries in patients with Crohn's disease (CD). In this study, we investigated the association between thickness of subcutaneous fat (TSF) and iSSI in patients with CD undergoing intestinal resections. *Patients and Methods.* Patients with CD who had undergone abdominal surgery from January 2014 to January 2017 were included in this retrospective study. Patients' TSF and other possible predictors of iSSI, including clinical characteristics, preoperative medications, hematological index, surgery-related data, and postoperative outcomes, were collected. Univariate and multivariate statistical analyses were used to examine the potential factors. Receiver operating characteristic (ROC) curve analysis was used to evaluate the predictive value of factors. *Results.* The patient cohort comprised 246 patients (167 male (67.9%); mean age 35.7 ± 12.4 years; mean disease duration 69.6 ± 60.8 months). The incidence of iSSI was 24.8% (61/246). TSF was a significant predictor of iSSI (OR 1.079, 95% CIs (1.020, 1.142), $P = 0.008$), being 13.7 mm in patients with iSSI and 9.9 mm in those without iSSI ($P < 0.001$). Additionally, C-reactive protein (CRP) concentrations (OR 1.059, $P = 0.003$) were also possible predictors of iSSI, as indicated by both univariate and multivariate analysis. A model of iSSI comprising TSF and CRP concentrations was moderately accurate (AUC 0.827, CIs (0.766, 0.888)). *Conclusions.* Preoperative TSF and CRP independently affect iSSI in patients with CD undergoing intestinal resections.

1. Introduction

Crohn's disease (CD), a chronic inflammatory bowel disorder, involves the whole digestive tract. In recent years, there has been ongoing development of medical treatments, particularly immunosuppressant and biological agents [1, 2]. However, nearly 60% of patients with CD have to undergo at least one abdominal operation [3].

Surgical site infection (SSI) is the commonest infectious complication after abdominal surgery for colorectal cancer and diverticulitis, the incidence being 2%–5% [4]. Furthermore, it is responsible for the highest proportion of costs of hospital-acquired infections [4]. At 14%–24%, its incidence is much higher in patients with CD who have undergone abdominal surgery than in other patients [5–7]. Incisional SSI (iSSI) is a significant form of SSI. Therefore, identifying risk factors for iSSI could help to prevent this complication of surgery in patients with CD.

A range of risk factors contributes to iSSI, including preoperative malnutrition, obesity, intra-abdominal abscess, preoperative blood glucose concentration, and intraoperative blood transfusions [8]. Although patients with CD tend to have multiple risk factors for iSSI, such as malnutrition and immunosuppressive therapies, there have been few studies of risk factors in patients with CD undergoing surgery.

The thickness of subcutaneous fat (TSF) is a common index of nutritional status [9], and previous studies have reported that TSF is a strong risk factor for iSSI after open gastrectomy for gastric cancer and elective colorectal surgery for colorectal cancer [10, 11]. Because of the characteristics of their disease, TSF differs between patients with CD and those with other diseases. To our knowledge, no studies have investigated the relationship between TSF and rate of the iSSI in patients with CD.

The aim of the current study was therefore to focus on investigating any correlation between TSF and the iSSI in CD patients together with assessing other potential risk factors for iSSI, such as smoking, blood loss, and preoperative albumin and C-reactive protein (CRP) concentrations.

2. Materials and Methods

2.1. Patients. Data on patients with CD who had undergone intestinal resections from January 2014 to January 2017 in the Inflammatory Bowel Disease Center of Jinling Hospital were retrospectively collected. All study patients had undergone routine complete abdominal CT or MRI scans within the two weeks before surgery. This study was approved by the Jinling Hospital Ethics Committee.

Patients who were to undergo elective surgery received optimal therapy aimed at improving their nutritional status and reducing systematic inflammation for at least 3 weeks prior to surgery. The strategies included nutritional therapy, drainage of abscesses, weaning off steroids for >4 weeks in patients who had been taking > 20 mg prednisolone for >6 weeks, withdrawal of antitumor necrosis factor (TNF) for >3 months, antibiotics, and smoking cessation. Indications for emergency surgery included acute intestinal perforation and massive hemorrhage and prevented implementation of the full range of strategies listed above.

Preoperative nutritional support was provided as enteral nutrition (EN) (Nutrison Fibre, Enteral Nutrition Suspension; Nutricia Company, Amsterdam, the Netherlands) through a nasogastric tube in all patients who could tolerate it. Some patients initially received total parenteral nutrition (TPN) and then gradually transited to EN (Peptisorb Liquid, Enteral Nutrition Suspension; Nutricia Company, Amsterdam, the Netherlands). Patients with abdominal abscesses underwent preoperative percutaneous drainage if possible and antibiotic therapy. All operations were performed by the same surgical group, and perioperative management was in accordance with the principle of enhanced recovery after surgery (ERAS). All patients except for those undergoing emergency surgery were fed glucose and sodium chloride solution with nasogastric tube for 24 hours prior to surgery rather than undergoing preoperative mechanical bowel preparation. Incision protection sleeves were used in laparotomies. Prophylactic antibiotics (a single dose of second-generation cephalosporins) were typically administered 30 minutes preoperatively and by intravenous drip on the first and second postoperative days.

2.2. Definitions. Diagnoses of iSSI were made in accordance with the guidelines of the Centers for Disease Control and Prevention, Public Health Service, US Department of Health and Human Services [12]. Incisional SSIs were further subclassified as superficial or deep incisional SSI. Superficial incisional SSI was defined as occurring within 30 days of surgery, infection involving only skin or subcutaneous tissue of an incision, and at least one of the following: (1) purulent drainage; (2) organisms isolated from an aseptically obtained culture of fluid or tissue from the superficial part of an incision; or (3) signs or symptoms of infection, including pain, tenderness, localized swelling, redness, heat, and superficial part of an incision deliberately opened by the surgeon, unless the incision was culture-negative. Deep incisional SSI was defined as infection involving the fascia of the incision and at least one of the following: (1) purulent drainage deep in an incision; (2) spontaneous dehiscence or deliberate opening of a deep incision by a surgeon in a patient with the following signs or symptoms: fever (>38°C) and localized pain or tenderness, unless the site is culture-negative; (3) an abscess or other evidence of infection involving a deep incision is found on direct examination, during reoperation, or by histopathologic or radiologic examination. Diagnoses of an iSSI were made by a surgeon or attending physician.

The area selected for measurement of TSF by preoperative CT or MRI scans was one centimeter to the right of the umbilical plane, and the thickness was defined as the distance between the posterior lines of the dermis and the superficial fascia of musculus rectus abdominis [13]. Measurements were performed by two authors (Cai XC and Shen WS) using the Adobe Photoshop (version 16.0.0.88).

2.3. Data Collection. Specific variables recorded for each patient were as follows: age, gender, duration of disease, disease behavior, disease location, perianal disease, intra-abdominal septic complications (IASCs) including anastomotic leak, intra-abdominal abscess, or enterocutaneous fistula, previous abdominal surgery, BMI, smoking habits, preoperative hospitalizations, preoperative nutritional support and drug administration, surgical approach, length and class of incision, duration of operation, intraoperative blood loss, anastomosis position, postoperative IASCs, and stoma creation. Preoperative leukocyte counts and CRP, serum albumin, and blood glucose were all assessed within the 3 days before surgery.

2.4. Statistical Analysis. All data were analyzed using the SPSS version 22.0 (SPSS, Chicago, IL, USA). Continuous parametric variables are presented as the mean ± SD, whereas nonparametric data are presented as 5% to 95% confidence intervals. The series mean was chosen to replace missing values. Unpaired t-tests were used to compare parametric variables and the Mann–Whitney U test for nonparametric data. Categorical data were analyzed by the χ^2 tests and contingency tables. Univariate and multivariate logistic regression analyses were performed to identify possible predictors of postoperative iSSI. Backward Wald was selected to choose confounders, and only variables with $P < 0.10$ in univariate analysis were assessed by multivariate logistic regression analysis. Predictive accuracy was assessed by receiver operating characteristic (ROC) curve analysis. Multi-index combined ROC curve analysis was first performed with multivariate logistic regression analysis and output probabilities of predicted values, after which, probabilities were further assessed by constructing ROC curves. Overall, $P < 0.05$ was considered to denote statistical significance.

3. Results

3.1. Clinical Characteristics of Patients. The study cohort comprised 246 patients (167 men, 67.9%) of average age 35.7 years (8 to 71 years). The disease duration was 69.6 ± 60.8 months and the average TSF 10.87 mm (range 0.76–37.92 mm). The incidence of iSSI in this cohort was 24.8% (61/246).

Relevant patient data, preoperative medications, and operative data are summarized in Table 1 and hematological indexes in Table 2. TSF was 13.7 mm in patients who developed an iSSI and 9.9 mm in those who did not ($P < 0.001$). Univariate analysis showed that the potential risk factors for iSSI ($P < 0.1$) in patients with CD included previous abdominal surgery, length of incision, type of incision, preoperative CRP, hemoglobin, and blood glucose. To investigate associations between individual risk factors and development of iSSI, the factors were subjected to multivariate analysis, as shown in Table 3. TSF was a significant predictor of iSSI (OR 1.079, 95% CIs (1.020, 1.142), $P = 0.008$). Additionally, preoperative CRP concentrations were much higher in the iSSI group (OR 1.059, CIs (1.019, 1.100), $P = 0.003$).

3.2. ROC Curve Analysis. ROC curves were constructed to determine the predictive value of TSF for iSSI in patients with CD (Figure 1). The area under the curve (AUC) was 0.646 (CIs (0.583, 0.706)), the sensitivity of the cut-off value of 10.2 mm being 59.1% and the specificity 63.8%. Furthermore, the negative predictive value (NPV) was 82.5% and the positive predictive value (PPV) only 35.0%. An attempt was made to build a model for iSSI prediction comprising preoperative TSF and CRP concentrations. ROC curves were then constructed to analyze the predictive value, as shown in Figure 2. In this model, the cut-off point was 0.152 and AUC 0.827 (CIs (0.766, 0.888)). Cut-off point 0.152 was corresponding to TSF cut-off value 10.2 mm and CRP cut-off value 8.6 mg/L. The sensitivity was 90.2% and the specificity 63.2%. The NPV of the cut-off point was 95.1% and the PPV 44.7%, indicating that the model has a higher predictive value for iSSI than TSF or CRP alone.

3.3. Predictors of iSSI. Preoperative TSF and CRP concentrations were classified according to cut-off values of 10.2 mm and 8.6 mg/L, respectively. Multivariate analysis was performed to identify predictors significantly associated with iSSI; these are presented in Table 4. TSF (OR 2.519, CIs (1.350, 4.698), $P = 0.004$) and CRP (OR 4.556, CIs (2.378, 8.728), $P < 0.001$) were both associated with an increased risk of iSSI.

4. Discussion

Surgery for CD is challenging, often being accompanied by multiple postoperative complications. Infective complications are an important type of postoperative complication in these patients, previous studies having mainly focused on exploring risk factors for development of intra-abdominal sepsis [14–16]. Postoperative iSSI, the major form of infective complication, increases hospitalization costs, prolongs hospital stay, and negatively affects patients' quality of life. The incidence of iSSI is reportedly much higher in patients with CD than in those with other diseases [5, 17]; however, there are few studies on iSSI after abdominal surgery for CD. In the present retrospective study of patient data, our primary focus was on the relationship between postoperative iSSI and thickness of abdominal subcutaneous fat in patients with CD. First, the incidence of iSSI in our patients with CD who had undergone intestinal resection was 24.8% (61/246), this rate being quite close to that reported by Bhakta et al. [5]. Second, we found preoperative TSF to be an independent risk factor for iSSI after surgery for CD. Third, preoperative CRP concentrations were also predictors of iSSI, and a model including TSF and CRP concentrations had better predictive value (AUC 0.827) than these predictors alone.

The body fat distribution of patients with CD, especially those with aggressive disease, differs from that of other persons, this being mainly characterized by a higher ratio of visceral to subcutaneous fat [18]. TSF is associated with BMI, and several studies have shown that TSF is an independent risk factor for iSSI after elective colorectal surgeries [11, 19]. A relationship between iSSI and TSF makes intuitive sense and has long been proven. Soper and Bump [20] reported that only patients with depth of subcutaneous fat > 3 cm developed iSSI after undergoing abdominal hysterectomy. Fujii et al. [11] reported a cut-off value for TSF of 20 mm in Asian patients who developed iSSI after undergoing elective colorectal surgery. However, CD is a type of wasting disease, affecting individuals often having very thin abdominal subcutaneous fat, even as thin as a wafer. In our 246 patients, the minimum TSF was only 0.76 mm and the mean 10.87 mm. Therefore, previously demonstrated associations between TSF and iSSI cannot validly be assumed to apply to patients with CD. We found that TSF is an independent risk factor for iSSI in patients undergoing surgery for CD, the cut-off point being 10.2 mm. This cut-off value is markedly lower than the 20 mm reported by Fujii et al., indicating that CD differs from other diseases such that it is inappropriate to mechanically predict postoperative complications in patients using predictive models developed for other diseases.

CRP is synthesized in hepatocytes, and serum concentrations increase rapidly during inflammatory responses [21]; thus, serum CRP concentration often plays a role as a marker of inflammation in a clinical context. Given that peak CRP concentrations occur about 2 days after the initiation of an acute inflammatory response and facilitate detection of such responses, CRP concentrations can be used to predict postoperative infective complications [22]. Serum CRP concentration on the fourth postoperative day can be used to eliminate postoperative infectious complications [23]. Additionally, CRP concentration is reportedly the most frequently used noninvasive biomarker for evaluating the activity of CD. Furthermore, in a previous study, we found that preoperative CRP concentration is a practical predictor of intra-abdominal septic complications after performing primary anastomoses in patients with CD [14]. In the present study, we found that preoperative CRP concentration is a predictor of postoperative iSSI in patients with CD. This finding is in

TABLE 1: Clinical and operational characteristics of patients in the research group.

Variable	Incisional SSI Present ($n = 61$)	Incisional SSI Absent ($n = 185$)	P value
Gender (male/female)	41/20	126/59	0.507
Age (years)	36.5 ± 13.3	35.5 ± 12.7	0.593
Duration of disease (months)	65.6 ± 60.5	70.9 ± 61.1	0.554
Thickness of subcutaneous fat (mm)	13.7 ± 7.7	9.9 ± 6.1	<0.001
Disease behavior, n (%)			0.203
Stricture	38 (62.3)	87 (47.0)	—
Penetration	21 (34.4)	91 (49.2)	—
Others	2 (3.3)	7 (3.8)	—
Disease location, n (%)			0.373
Ileum	17 (27.9)	65 (35.1)	—
Colon	6 (9.8)	25 (13.5)	—
Ileocolon	38 (62.3)	93 (50.3)	—
Upper digestive tract	0 (0)	2 (1.1)	—
Perianal disease, n (%)	15 (24.6)	61 (33.0)	0.219
Abdominal abscess, n (%)	10 (16.4)	15 (8.1)	0.063
Previous abdominal surgery for CD, n (%)			0.119
0	25 (41.0)	102 (55.1)	—
1	26 (42.7)	65 (35.2)	—
>1	10 (16.3)	18 (9.7)	—
Smoking, n (%)	10 (16.3)	15 (8.1)	0.063
Length of preoperative hospitalization (days)	9.7 ± 16.5	8.1 ± 4.6	0.222
BMI (kg/m^2)	17.4 ± 5.5	16.7 ± 5.0	0.380
Preoperative PN, n (%)	13 (21.3)	34 (18.4)	0.613
Preoperative EN, n (%)	47 (77.0)	157 (84.9)	0.159
Preoperative drug administration, n (%)			
5-ASA	15 (24.6)	59 (31.9)	0.281
Steroids	5 (8.2)	12 (6.5)	0.771
Immunosuppressant	20 (32.8)	60 (32.4)	0.959
Anti-TNF α antibody	6 (9.8)	12 (6.5)	0.400
Emergency operation, n (%)	5 (8.2)	11 (5.9)	0.553
Surgical approach, n (%)			0.117
Laparotomy	52 (85.2)	140 (75.7)	—
Laparoscopic	9 (14.8)	45 (24.3)	—
Anastomosis position, n (%)			0.255
Nonanastomosis	11 (18.0)	39 (21.1)	—
Ileal anastomosis	15 (24.6)	62 (33.5)	—
Ileocolostomy	35 (57.4)	84 (45.4)	—
Stoma creation, n (%)			0.532
Ileostomy	13 (21.3)	44 (23.8)	—
Colostomy	4 (6.6)	3 (1.7)	—
Length of incision (cm)	12.2 ± 3.5	10.6 ± 4.2	0.009
Incision class, n (%)			0.011
Contaminated	51 (83.6)	174 (94.1)	—
Dirty	10 (16.4)	11 (5.9)	—
Duration of operation (min)	148.6 ± 49.5	141.2 ± 52.5	0.337
Intraoperative blood loss (mL)	218.2 ± 157.4	182.5 ± 116.2	0.059
Postoperative transferred to ICU, n (%)	10 (16.4)	19 (10.3)	0.189
Postoperative IASCs, n (%)			0.020

Table 1: Continued.

Variable	Incisional SSI		*P* value
	Present ($n = 61$)	Absent ($n = 185$)	
Anastomotic leak	3 (8.2)	2 (1.1)	—
Intra-abdominal abscess	3 (4.9)	1 (0.5)	—
Enterocutaneous fistula	1 (1.6)	1 (0.5)	—
Reoperation, *n* (%)	2 (3.3)	1 (0.5)	0.153

Data are reported as the number of patients (%) or mean ± SD. SSI: surgical site infection; CD: Crohn's disease; BMI: body mass index; PN: parenteral nutrition; EN: enteral nutrition; IASCs: intra-abdominal septic complications.

Table 2: Hematological index.

Variable	Incisional SSI		*P* value
	Present ($n = 61$)	Absent ($n = 185$)	
Preoperative leukocyte (10^9/L)	6.1 ± 3.9	5.4 ± 2.5	0.154
Preoperative CRP (mg/L)	32.0 ± 44.5	6.7 ± 18.9	<0.001
Preoperative albumin (g/L)	36.7 ± 7.5	37.0 ± 5.7	0.723
Preoperative hemoglobin (g/L)	112.0 ± 20.2	118.3 ± 16.3	0.014
Preoperative blood glucose (mmol/L)	5.8 ± 1.7	5.2 ± 1.2	0.029

Data are reported as mean ± SD. SSI: surgical site infection; CRP: C-reactive protein.

Table 3: Multivariable logistic regression analysis of predictors of iSSI in patients with CD after abdominal surgery.

Variable	95% CI	OR	*P* value
Thickness of subcutaneous fat	1.020–1.142	1.079	0.008
Abdominal abscess	0.236–4.500	1.030	0.969
Smoking	0.564–5.116	1.698	0.347
Length of incision	0.938–1.153	1.040	0.458
Incision class	0.113–6.450	0.854	0.878
Blood loss	0.998–1.004	1.001	0.497
Preoperative CRP	1.019–1.100	1.059	0.003
Preoperative hemoglobin	0.975–1.027	1.001	0.953
Preoperative blood glucose	0.924–1.597	1.215	0.164

OR: odds ratio; CI: confidence interval; CD: Crohn's disease; CRP: C-reactive protein; IASCs: intra-abdominal septic complications.

line with our hypothesis that preoperative CRP concentration reflects the activity and severity of CD.

Whether preoperative administration of infliximab influences the incidence of postoperative iSSI remains controversial. Some meta-analyses have indicated that preoperative infliximab is associated with increased risk of infectious complications in patients with CD who undergo surgeries [24, 25]. However, the findings of another meta-analysis suggested that infliximab does not increase the risks of postoperative infective complications [26]. Uchino et al. reported that preoperative administration of infliximab is not a risk factor for iSSI [27]. Thus, the relationship between such medications and postoperative iSSI is still under discussion. In our study, infliximab administration showed no correlation with postoperative iSSI in patients with CD.

The incidence of postoperative IASCs in this cohort was 4.5% (11/246), which is comparable to the 5%–20% reported by previous studies [15, 16, 28]. Only three patients with

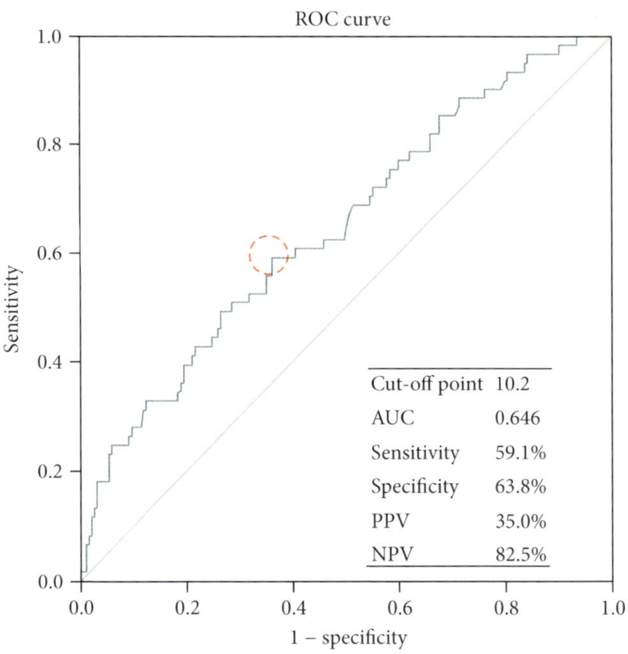

Figure 1: ROC curve showing preoperative TSF predictive value of postoperative iSSI. TSF: thickness of subcutaneous fat; ROC: receiver operating characteristic; AUC: area under the curve; PPV: positive predictive value; NPV: negative predictive value.

IASCs required revision surgery, the remaining IASCs resolved with percutaneous drainage. Though postoperative IASCs were strongly associated with iSSI, especially deep iSSI, we considered that IASCs have limited predictive value because they develop later than other indexes. We therefore did not include postoperative IASCs as a predictor of iSSI.

Our study had some limitations. First, it was a single-center retrospective study. However, it was relatively large,

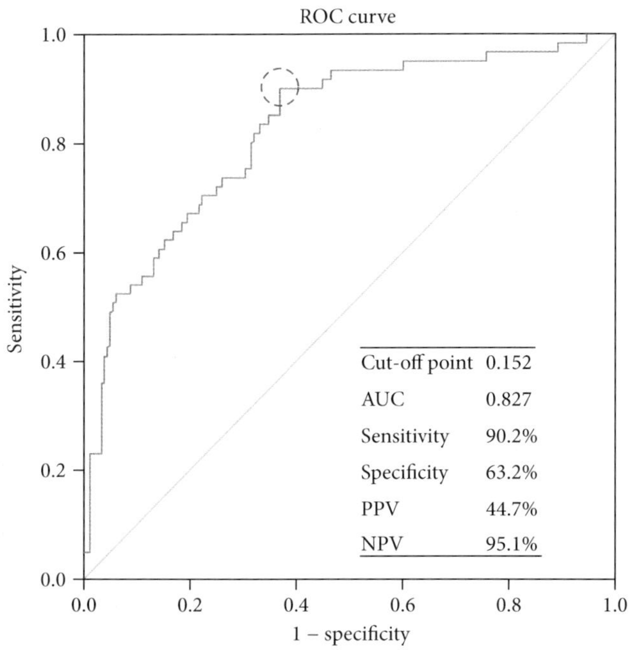

Figure 2: ROC curve showing the model within preoperative TSF and CRP levels predictive value of postoperative iSSI. CRP: C-reactive protein; ROC: receiver operating characteristic; AUC: area under the curve; PPV: positive predictive value; NPV: negative predictive value.

Table 4: Multivariable logistic regression analysis of iSSI predictors classified according to cut-off value.

Variable	95% CI	OR	*P* value
Thickness of subcutaneous fat	1.350–4.698	2.519	0.004
Preoperative CRP	2.378–8.728	4.556	<0.001

OR: odds ratio; CI: confidence interval: CRP: C-reactive protein.

including 246 patients. However, our findings are less persuasive than those of a prospective study would be and lack widespread applicability. Second, we found that TSF is a predictor of iSSI; we did not evaluate associations between iSSI severity and amount of TSF. Third, only 16 patients in our series had undergone emergency abdominal operation surgery, which may have influenced the accuracy of our data and the universality of our results. Despite these limitations, our findings indicate that TSF has predictive value for postoperative iSSI in patients with CD.

5. Conclusion

This study is the first to investigate the relationship between TSF and iSSI after abdominal surgery for CD. Our results suggest that preoperative TSF and CRP concentrations can predict development of postoperative iSSI. We therefore recommend the use of incision protection supplementary materials, more frequent checking of incisions, and prompt treatment to minimize the incidence of postoperative iSSI in patients with Crohn's disease, preoperative TSF >10.2 mm, and CRP > 8.6 mg/L.

Disclosure

The authors disclose that there is no financial and personal relationships with other people or organizations that could potentially and inappropriately influence (bias) their work and conclusions.

Authors' Contributions

Xingchen Cai, Weisong Shen, and Zhen Guo conceived and designed the study. Xingchen Cai collected the data and wrote the manuscript. Weisong Shen analyzed and interpreted the data. Yi Li, Lei Cao, and Jianfeng Gong provided critical revisions that were important for the intellectual content. Weiming Zhu approved the final version of the manuscript. Xingchen Cai and Weisong Shen contributed equally to this work.

Acknowledgments

The authors thank Dr. Trish Reynolds, MBBS, FRACP, from Liwen Bianji, Edanz Group China (http://www.liwenbianji.cn/ac), for editing the English text of a draft of this manuscript. This study was funded by the National Natural Science Foundation of China (81500429 and 81570500).

References

[1] D. C. Baumgart, "Crohn's disease," *The Lancet*, vol. 380, no. 9853, pp. 1590–1605, 2012.

[2] T. Dassopoulos, S. Sultan, Y. T. Falck-Ytter, J. M. Inadomi, and S. B. Hanauer, "American Gastroenterological Association Institute technical review on the use of thiopurines, methotrexate, and anti–TNF-α biologic drugs for the induction and maintenance of remission in inflammatory Crohn's disease," *Gastroenterology*, vol. 145, no. 6, pp. 1464–1478.e5, 2013.

[3] L. Peyrin-Biroulet, W. S. Harmsen, W. J. Tremaine, A. R. Zinsmeister, W. J. Sandborn, and E. V. Loftus, "Surgery in a population-based cohort of Crohn's disease from Olmsted County, Minnesota (1970–2004)," *The American Journal of Gastroenterology*, vol. 107, no. 11, pp. 1693–1701, 2012.

[4] K. A. Ban, J. P. Minei, C. Laronga et al., "American College of Surgeons and Surgical Infection Society: surgical site infection guidelines, 2016 update," *Journal of the American College of Surgeons*, vol. 224, no. 1, pp. 59–74, 2017.

[5] A. Bhakta, M. Tafen, O. Glotzer et al., "Increased incidence of surgical site infection in IBD patients," *Diseases of the Colon & Rectum*, vol. 59, no. 4, pp. 316–322, 2016.

[6] M. Uchino, H. Ikeuchi, T. Tsuchida, K. Nakajima, N. Tomita, and Y. Takesue, "Surgical site infection following surgery for inflammatory bowel disease in patients with clean-

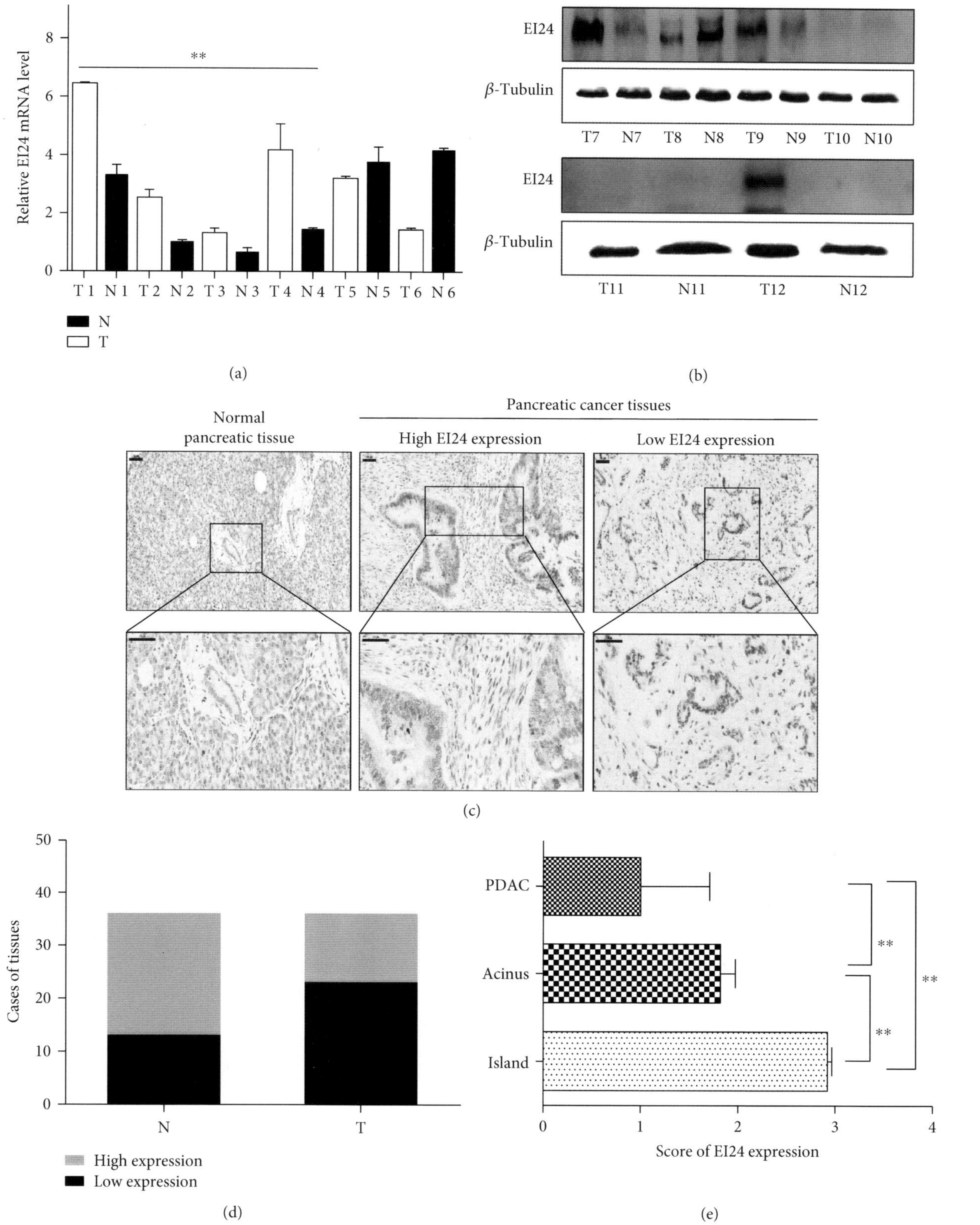

Figure 1: Expression levels of EI24 in PDAC tissues. (a, b) EI24 mRNA and protein expression levels in six pairs of PDAC tissues (T) and adjacent normal tissues (N) detected by RT-qPCR and Western blot analysis, respectively. (c) Immunohistochemical analysis of EI24 expression in pancreatic cancer tissues. Brown color represents positive cytoplasm and nucleus EI24 staining (scale bar represents 50 μm, 200x and 400x magnification). (d) Statistical gram shows that EI24 was downregulated in PDAC tissues (T) than in adjacent normal tissues (N). (e) Statistical analysis showed that EI24 expression was significantly lower in PDAC cells than in normal pancreatic acinus/islands. $^{*}P < 0.05$ and $^{**}P < 0.01$, compared with controls.

Table 1: Associations of EI24 expression with clinicopathological characteristics in PDAC patients.

Clinical parameters	Total (36)	EI24 expression Low ($n = 23$)	High ($n = 13$)	P value
Gender				0.2651
Male	21	15	6	
Female	15	8	7	
Age (years)				0.6359
≤60	10	7	3	
>60	26	16	10	
Histological differentiation				0.9685
Moderate/~well	22	14	8	
Poor/~moderate	14	9	5	
T classification				0.6436
T1 + T2	7	5	2	
T3 + T4	29	18	11	
N classification				0.3187
Absent	21	12	9	
Present	15	11	4	
Metastasis				0.6789
No	29	19	10	
Yes	7	4	3	

pancreatic cancer cell growth, induced cell cycle arrest in S phase, and attenuated cancer cell colony formation.

3.3. EI24 Suppresses Pancreatic Cancer Growth In Vivo. To examine the function of EI24 on pancreatic cancer tumorigenesis *in vivo*, we performed tumor formation assays in Balb/c nude mice. Mice subcutaneously implanted with CaPan-2-shEI cells showed a significant increase in tumor weight and volume compared with controls ($P < 0.05$ and $P < 0.01$) (Figures 3(a) and 3(b)). In contrast, the opposite results were shown in mice engrafted with PANC-1-EI cells compared with the control group ($P < 0.05$ and $P < 0.01$) (Figures 3(a) and 3(b)). There were no significant differences in body weight between the experimental groups and controls (data was not shown). These data indicated that EI24 overexpression suppressed pancreatic cancer tumorigenicity *in vivo*, while EI24 knockdown could promote pancreatic cancer tumorigenesis.

Immunohistochemical analysis of the tumors confirmed that Ki-67, a marker of cell proliferation, was marginally increased in tissues isolated from animals treated with CaPan-2-shEI cells compared with the controls ($P < 0.05$) (Figure 3(c)). Likewise, reduced expression of Ki-67 was detected in tumor samples from PANC-1-EI cells ($P < 0.05$) (Figure 3(d)). These data demonstrated that EI24 plays a key role in the proliferation and survival of tumor cells, in line with the *in vitro* results.

3.4. EI24 Attenuates Cell Proliferation by Downregulation of c-Myc Involving a Beclin-1/p62/c-Myc Signaling Pathway. Cleaved caspase-3 is an activated form of caspase-3 and functions as a marker of apoptosis. To examine whether the antitumor activity of EI24 involved induction of apoptosis, we examined caspase-3 expression levels in the stable cell lines with overexpression or downregulation of EI24 by Western blotting, but no apparent differences in protein levels were detected (Figure 4(a)). These results indicate that caspase-dependent apoptosis is not the mechanism by which EI24 affects cell viability. We also examined the effect of EI24 on the expression of several cell cycle regulators, including cyclinD1, p21, and c-Myc, in the stable pancreatic cancer cell lines using Western blotting assay (Figure 4(b)). Neither cyclinD1 nor p21 showed changes in expression in either the EI24 overexpressing or downregulated cell lines compared with controls. However, we observed a marked decline in the expression level of c-Myc in PANC-1-EI cells compared with controls, while an increase was observed in CaPan-2-shEI cells compared with controls. These results indicate that the overexpression of EI24 caused decreased c-Myc levels, resulting in growth suppression in pancreatic cancer cells. To validate the correlation between EI24 and c-Myc expression, we also examined the c-Myc level in human pancreatic tissues. Correlation studies showed that a high EI24 level correlated with low c-Myc expression in PDAC specimens. Conversely, a low EI24 level correlated with high c-Myc expression (Supplementary Figures 2A and B). Taken together, these results suggest that the absence of EI24 inversely correlates with c-Myc upregulation in PDAC and EI24 may exert its antitumor function partially through inhibiting c-Myc oncogenic function.

A previous study found that Beclin-1 accelerates the degradation of c-Myc and that the Beclin-1/p62/c-Myc signaling pathway functions in regulating tumor proliferation [11]. EI24 is an autophagy-associated transmembrane protein and an essential component of basal autophagy in mammals [12]. We wondered if the Beclin-1/p62/c-Myc signaling pathway is activated and functions in pancreatic cancer and whether EI24 plays a role in this pathway. To first clarify whether the suppression of pancreatic cancer tumorigenicity induced by EI24 was associated with autophagy, we examined Beclin-1, which is essential for autophagy upregulation, by immunofluorescence analysis in xenograft tissues. As shown in Figure 4(c), the expression of Beclin-1 increased by overexpression of EI24, while EI24 knockdown showed reduced levels compared with controls. Examination of the clearance of p62 (Figure 4(d)), another distinct feature of autophagy, was consistent with these results. Based on these findings, we concluded that EI24 overexpression in PDAC activates autophagy, and we speculated that this may be associated with the effects of EI24 on tumorigenesis *in vivo*. We next considered whether the autophagy induced by EI24 correlated with the deregulation of c-Myc. Overexpression of EI24 promoted conversion of LC3B-I to LC3B-II, and the opposite results were shown in cells with the knockdown of EI24 (Figure 4(e)). Ectopic expression of EI24 also caused induction of Beclin-1 (Figure 4(e)), and this paralleled the reduction of c-Myc. Together, these data suggested that EI24 suppresses tumor

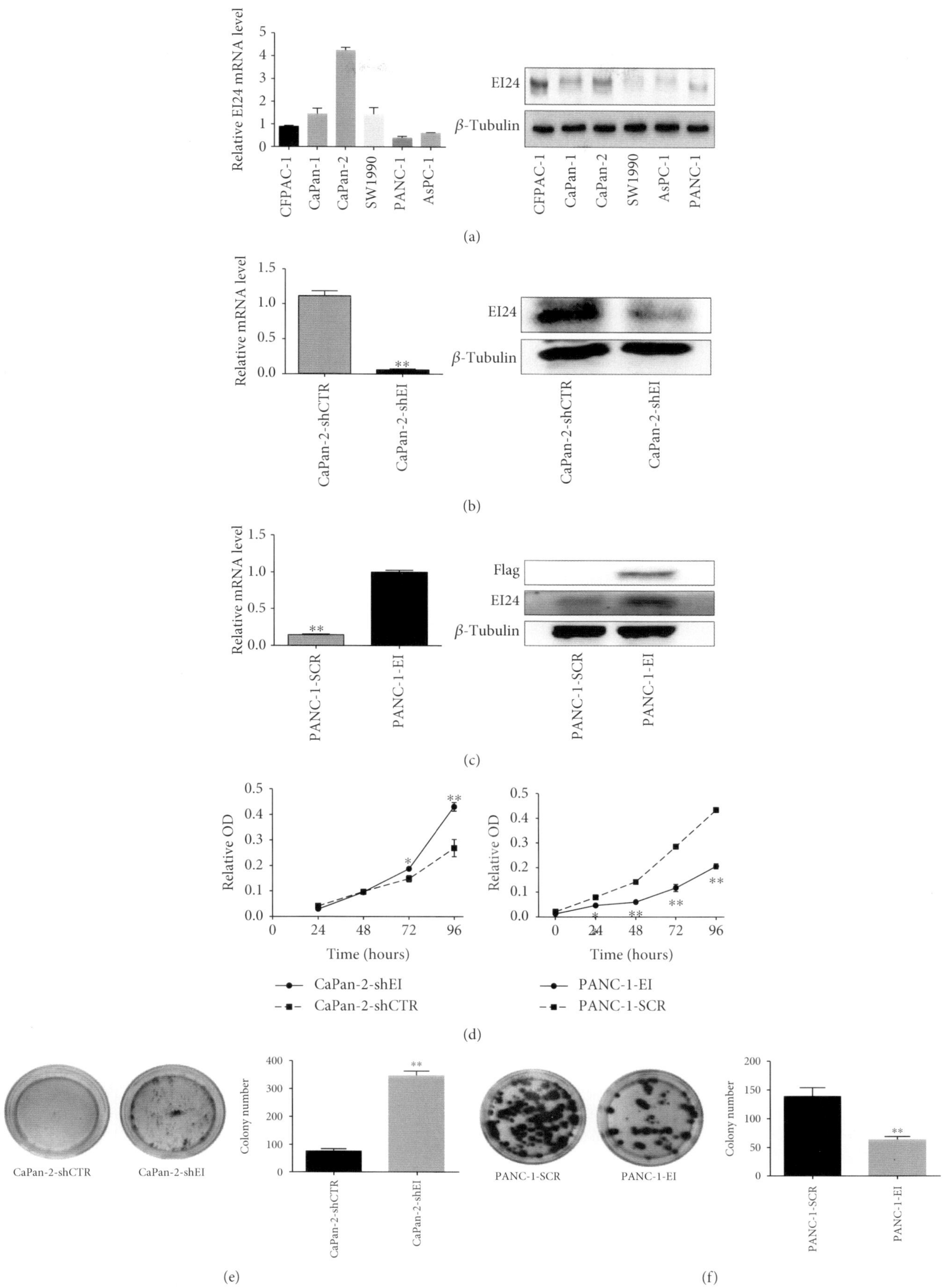

Figure 2: Continued.

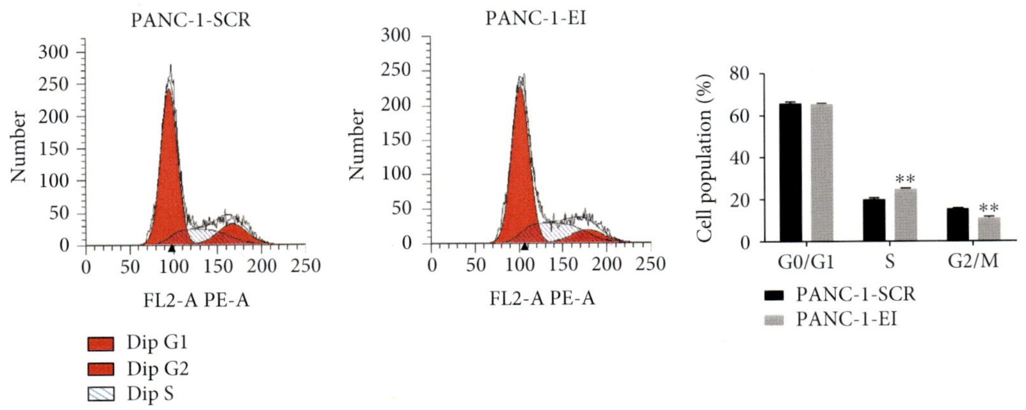

(g)

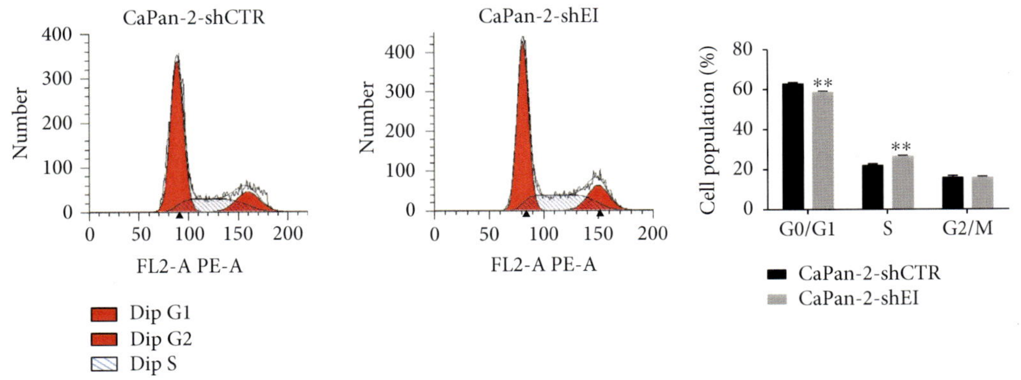

(h)

FIGURE 2: EI24 suppresses pancreatic cancer cell proliferation *in vitro*. (a) EI24 expression in different pancreatic cancer cell lines by qRT-PCR and Western blot analysis. (b, c) CaPan-2 and PANC-1 stable cells with either EI24 knockdown or overexpression, respectively, validated by qRT-PCR and Western blot. (d) CCK8 assays in EI24 knockdown and overexpressing cells. Growth curves of different cells were drawn. (e, f) Stably transfected cells were subjected to colony formation assays. (g, h) Stably transfected CaPan-2 and PANC-1 cells underwent cell cycle analysis by flow cytometry. $^{*}P < 0.05$ and $^{**}P < 0.01$, compared with controls.

proliferation possibly by the activation of autophagy to regulate the Beclin-1/p62/c-Myc signaling pathway.

4. Discussion

EI24 has been previously linked with inhibiting cancer cell growth and proapoptotic functions [7]. In the present study, we demonstrated decreased expression of EI24 in human PDAC compared with adjacent normal tissues and found higher EI24 expression in moderately to well-differentiated PDAC cells compared with poorly differentiated cells. We further clarified that EI24 acts as a tumor suppressor in PDAC cell lines by inhibiting cell proliferation, decreasing colony formation, and inducing cell cycle arrest. Furthermore, these effects were independent of caspase-dependent apoptosis. Because the induction of cell differentiation requires cell growth inhibition or cell cycle arrest [15], our results may give a reasonable explanation for the differential expressions of EI24 in differentiated cells. Notably, these findings could link the EI24 low expression level in PDAC with its tumor suppressor role. Downregulation of EI24 may result in a deregulated tumor suppression system and promoted tumorigenesis. Alternatively, EI24 was downregulated in PDAC than normal pancreatic acinus/islands. Considering acinar-to-ductal metaplasia in PDAC initiation [16], deficiency of EI24 may potentiate the initiation of tumors. Further studies will be conducted in pancreatic intraepithelial neoplasia (PanIN) cells and tissues to explore the effects of EI24 on tumor initiation.

c-Myc plays an important role in regulating cell proliferation, differentiation, and apoptosis [4]. Li et al. revealed that the PI3K/AKT signaling pathway was involved in PSCA-promoted cell proliferation and cell cycle progression by upregulating c-Myc in prostate cancer [17]. Moreover, the previous work demonstrated that c-Myc functions in pancreatic cancer as a central oncogene [4]. Our study found that the ectopic expression of EI24 reduced cell proliferation, impaired cell cycle progression, and reduced tumorigenesis. Furthermore, EI24 knockdown accelerated cell cycle transition from G1 phase to S phase, suggesting a promotion of cell proliferation in the absence of EI24; in contrast, EI24 overexpressing cells showed an increase in S phase cells accompanied with a decrease in G2 phase cells, indicating an S phase arrest. The Ki67 immunohistochemistry staining results were consistent with these data. To examine the mechanisms underlying EI24-mediated tumor suppression, we examined protein levels of several critical cell cycle and growth regulators and confirmed alterations in c-Myc in

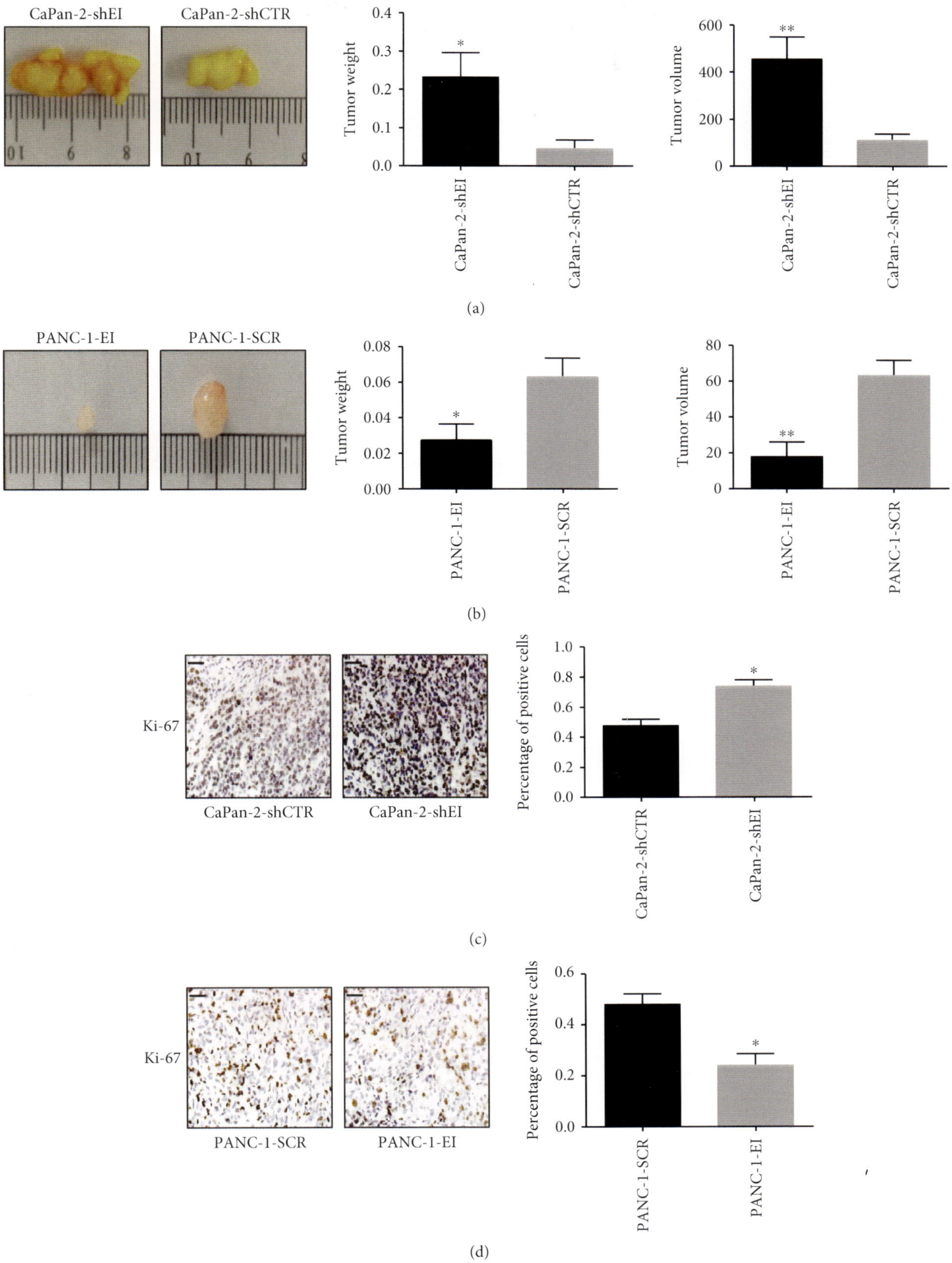

FIGURE 3: EI24 suppresses pancreatic cancer growth *in vivo*. (a) Representative images of tumors isolated from each group of mice. (b) Statistical gram shows relative changes of tumor weight and volume. (c, d) Immunohistochemical analysis of Ki-67 in tumor tissues (scale bar represents 50 μm, 400x magnification). Percentage of positive Ki-67 staining cells was counted. $^{*}P < 0.05$ and $^{**}P < 0.01$, compared with controls.

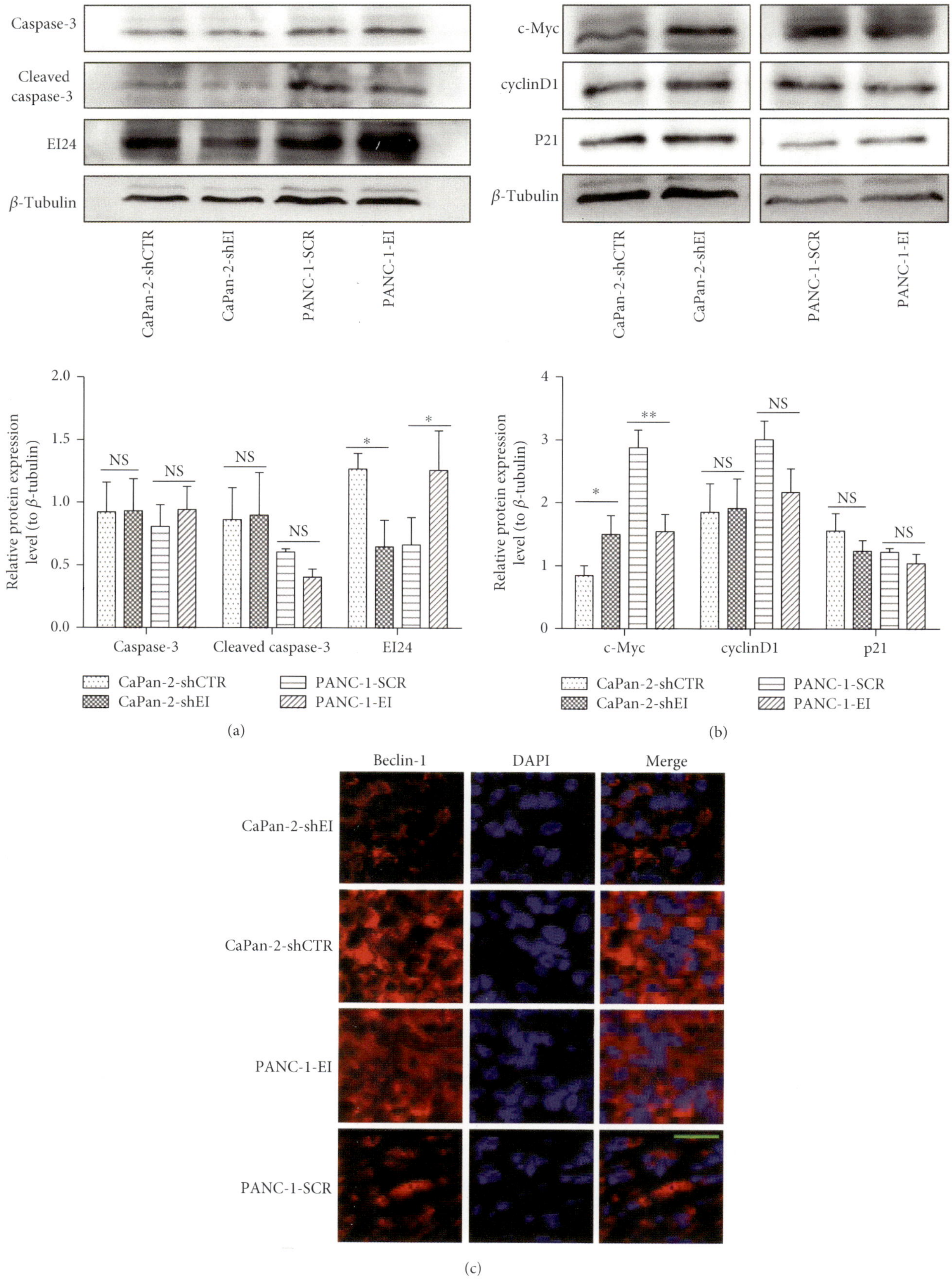

Figure 4: Continued.

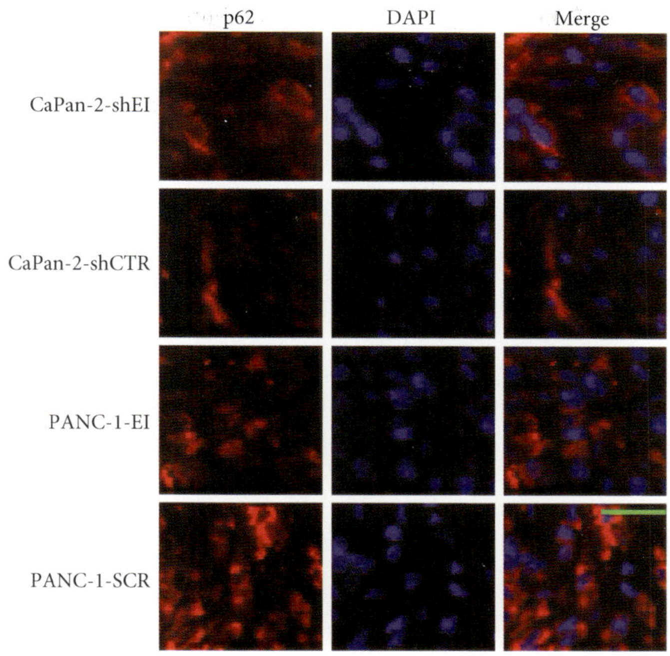

(d)

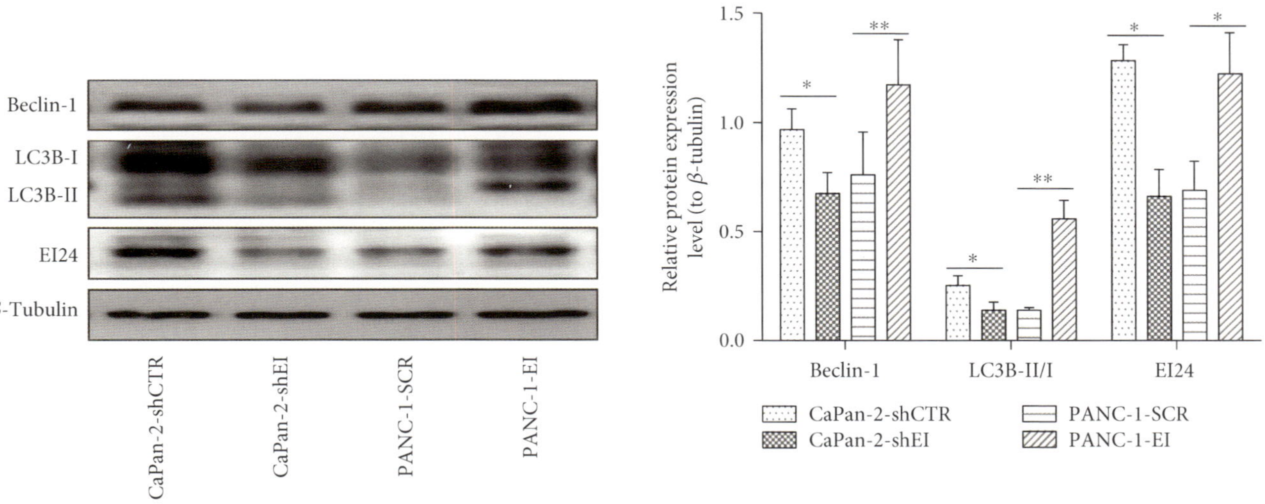

(e)

Figure 4: EI24 attenuates cell proliferation by inducing autophagy to regulate the Beclin-1/p62/c-Myc signaling pathway. (a) Expression level of caspase-3 and cleaved caspase-3 was detected by Western blot. (b) Western blot analysis shows cyclinD1, p21, and c-Myc protein levels in cancer cells. (c, d) Immunofluorescence analysis of Beclin-1 and p62 expression in xenograft tumor tissues. EI24 increased merged fluorescence image of Beclin-1 (red, Cy3 stained) with the nucleus (blue, DAPI staining) was observed, accompanied with a decrease of p62. Photos were telegraphed with 400x magnification. Scale bar represents 50 μm. (e) Expression levels of EI24-induced autophagy-related protein LC3B and Beclin-1 were detected by Western blot. $^{*}P < 0.05$, $^{**}P < 0.01$, and NS $P > 0.05$, compared with controls.

response to EI24. IHC staining of human pancreatic tissues also showed the inverse correlations between EI24 and c-Myc. The recent study confirmed that the activation of autophagy promotes the degradation of c-Myc, leading to reduced cell proliferation [11]. Thus, a similar degradation mechanism may occur in pancreatic cancer, in which the downregulation of c-Myc occurs in response to reinforced EI24 expression. Consistent with the demonstrated role for EI24 in autophagy, Beclin-1/p62 expression levels were altered in response to EI24, along with changes in c-Myc levels. Together, these findings reveal a possible EI24/Beclin-1/p62/c-Myc signal pathway. However, further studies are required to elucidate the mechanism underlying this pathway.

Previous studies demonstrated a function for EI24 in the ubiquitin-proteasome pathway-autophagy crosstalk [13], which further supports its potential link to c-Myc. Other studies have proven that c-Myc correlated with preacinar to acinar maturation and pancreatic homeostasis [18], providing insight into differentiation and carcinogenesis. In view of evidence that the induction of a dedifferentiated state caused by c-Myc overexpression contributes to pancreatic carcinogenesis [18] and our findings, this may help explain the downregulation of EI24 in PDAC compared with normal pancreatic acinus/islands and lower expression level in poorly differentiated cancer cells compared with well- and moderately differentiated cancer cells. This indicates that c-Myc is an important target of EI24 and essential to its role as a tumor suppressor. More studies are required to verify the functional interaction between EI24 and c-Myc and to investigate other molecular targets and mechanisms for EI24 to clarify its role in tumor initiation and progression.

Autophagy is required for maintaining cellular homeostasis and has been linked with both protumorigenic and tumor suppression functions [10]. The role of autophagy in PDAC is unclear, and the exact mechanisms have yet to be elucidated. Our study demonstrated that enhanced expression of EI24 activates autophagy *in vitro* and *in vivo* in pancreatic cancer cells. Our results suggest that the overexpression of EI24 affected tumorigenesis in pancreatic cancer by inducing autophagy, resulting in the downregulation of c-Myc and suppression of proliferation, as well as causing cell cycle arrest. Notably, in contrast with other findings, EI24 had no impact on apoptosis in the current study. Researchers have demonstrated autophagy-related cell death as an anticancer mechanism in PDAC [19], and induction of autophagy has become an emerging strategy for PDAC treatment [20]. Thus, autophagy may affect tumor progression by contributing to cell death independent of apoptosis. We plan to further examine the relation between EI24-induced autophagy and cell death and the mechanism underlying the crosstalk between EI24-mediated autophagy and apoptosis in pancreatic cancer in future studies.

In conclusion, our results not only indicate that EI24 is downregulated in PDAC tissues compared to the adjacent normal tissues but also provide evidence that EI24 exhibits a potent tumor suppressor effect on pancreatic cancer cells by inhibiting cell proliferation both *in vitro* and *in vivo* and inducing cell cycle arrest at S phase. The possible mechanism for this effect might involve EI24-mediated autophagy-related degradation of c-Myc, through regulating Beclin-1 and p62. Our present study provides insight into the crosstalk between autophagy and cell proliferation involving a possible EI24/Beclin-1/p62/c-Myc signaling pathway. These findings suggested that EI24, as a potential tumor suppressor, might serve as an effective therapeutic target against pancreatic cancer.

Disclosure

Yi Zang, Lei Zhu, and Tong Li share co-first authorship.

Acknowledgments

This work was supported by the National Natural Science Foundation of China (Grant nos. 81272263, 81672719, 81702740, and 81870385).

References

[1] R. L. Siegel, K. D. Miller, and A. Jemal, "Cancer statistics, 2018," *CA: A Cancer Journal for Clinicians*, vol. 68, no. 1, pp. 7–30, 2018.

[2] E. S. Knudsen, E. M. O'Reilly, J. R. Brody, and A. K. Witkiewicz, "Genetic diversity of pancreatic ductal adenocarcinoma and opportunities for precision medicine," *Gastroenterology*, vol. 150, no. 1, pp. 48–63, 2016.

[3] Q. Wang, J. Li, W. Wu et al., "Smad4-dependent suppressor pituitary homeobox 2 promotes PPP2R2A-mediated inhibition of Akt pathway in pancreatic cancer," *Oncotarget*, vol. 7, no. 10, pp. 11208–11222, 2016.

[4] E. Hessmann, G. Schneider, V. Ellenrieder, and J. T. Siveke, "MYC in pancreatic cancer: novel mechanistic insights and their translation into therapeutic strategies," *Oncogene*, vol. 35, no. 13, pp. 1609–1618, 2016.

[5] M. Gentile, M. Ahnstrom, F. Schon, and S. Wingren, "Candidate tumour suppressor genes at 11q23–q24 in breast cancer: evidence of alterations in PIG8, a gene involved in p53-induced apoptosis," *Oncogene*, vol. 20, no. 53, pp. 7753–7760, 2001.

[6] D. Mazumder Indra, S. Mitra, R. K. Singh et al., "Inactivation of *CHEK1* and *EI24* is associated with the development of invasive cervical carcinoma: clinical and prognostic implications," *International Journal of Cancer*, vol. 129, no. 8, pp. 1859–1871, 2011.

[7] Z. Gu, C. Flemington, T. Chittenden, and G. P. Zambetti, "*ei24*, a p53 response gene involved in growth suppression and apoptosis," *Molecular and Cellular Biology*, vol. 20, no. 1, pp. 233–241, 2000.

[8] X. Zhao, R. E. Ayer, S. L. Davis et al., "Apoptosis factor EI24/PIG8 is a novel endoplasmic reticulum–localized Bcl-2–binding protein which is associated with suppression of breast cancer invasiveness," *Cancer Research*, vol. 65, no. 6, pp. 2125–2129, 2005.

[9] S. Devkota, Y. H. Sung, J. M. Choi et al., "Ei24-deficiency attenuates protein kinase Cα signaling and skin carcinogenesis in mice," *The International Journal of Biochemistry & Cell Biology*, vol. 44, no. 11, pp. 1887–1896, 2012.

[10] S. Yang and A. C. Kimmelman, "A critical role for autophagy in pancreatic cancer," *Autophagy*, vol. 7, no. 8, pp. 912-913, 2011.

[11] H. Liu, W. L. Zhao, J. P. Wang, B. M. Xin, and R. G. Shao, "EBP50 suppresses the proliferation of MCF-7 human breast cancer cells via promoting Beclin-1/p62-mediated lysosomal degradation of c-Myc," *Acta Pharmacologica Sinica*, vol. 39, no. 8, pp. 1347–1358, 2018.

[12] Y. G. Zhao, H. Zhao, L. Miao, L. Wang, F. Sun, and H. Zhang, "The p53-induced gene *Ei24* is an essential component of the basal autophagy pathway," *Journal of Biological Chemistry*, vol. 287, no. 50, pp. 42053–42063, 2012.

[13] S. Devkota, H. Jeong, Y. Kim et al., "Functional characterization of EI24-induced autophagy in the degradation of RING-domain E3 ligases," *Autophagy*, vol. 12, no. 11, pp. 2038–2053, 2016.

[14] J. Li, D. Kong, Q. Wang et al., "Niacin ameliorates ulcerative colitis via prostaglandin D2-mediated D prostanoid receptor 1 activation," *EMBO Molecular Medicine*, vol. 9, no. 5, pp. 571–588, 2017.

[15] V. K. Xie, Z. Li, Y. Yan et al., "DNA-methyltransferase 1 induces dedifferentiation of pancreatic cancer cells through silencing of Krüppel-like factor 4 expression," *Clinical Cancer Research*, vol. 23, no. 18, pp. 5585–5597, 2017.

[16] D. Wei, L. Wang, Y. Yan et al., "KLF4 is essential for induction of cellular identity change and acinar-to-ductal reprogramming during early pancreatic carcinogenesis," *Cancer Cell*, vol. 29, no. 3, pp. 324–338, 2016.

[17] E. Li, L. Liu, F. Li et al., "PSCA promotes prostate cancer proliferation and cell-cycle progression by up-regulating c-Myc," *The Prostate*, vol. 77, no. 16, pp. 1563–1572, 2017.

[18] V. J. Sánchez-Arévalo Lobo, L. C. Fernández, E. Carrillo-de-Santa-Pau et al., "c-Myc downregulation is required for preacinar to acinar maturation and pancreatic homeostasis," *Gut*, vol. 67, no. 4, 2017.

[19] L. Sun, L. Hu, D. Cogdell et al., "*Mir506* induces autophagy-related cell death in pancreatic cancer cells by targeting the Stat3 pathway," *Autophagy*, vol. 13, no. 4, pp. 703–714, 2017.

[20] N. Mujumdar and A. K. Saluja, "Autophagy in pancreatic cancer: an emerging mechanism of cell death," *Autophagy*, vol. 6, no. 7, pp. 997-998, 2010.

3

Significance of Preoperative Systemic Immune Score for Stage I Gastric Cancer Patients

Jun Lu,[1,2,3,4] Long-long Cao,[1,2,3,4] Ping Li,[1,2,3,4] Jian-wei Xie,[1,2,3,4] Jia-bin Wang,[1,2,3,4] Jian-xian Lin,[1,2,3,4] Qi-yue Chen,[1,2,3,4] Mi Lin,[1,2,3,4] Ru-hong Tu,[1,2,3,4] Chang-ming Huang,[1,2,3,4] and Chao-hui Zheng[1,2,3,4]

[1]*Department of Gastric Surgery, Fujian Medical University Union Hospital, Fuzhou, China*
[2]*Department of General Surgery, Fujian Medical University Union Hospital, Fuzhou, China*
[3]*Key Laboratory of Ministry of Education of Gastrointestinal Cancer, Fujian Medical University, Fuzhou, China*
[4]*Fujian Key Laboratory of Tumor Microbiology, Fujian Medical University, Fuzhou, China*

Correspondence should be addressed to Chao-hui Zheng; wwkzch@163.com

Academic Editor: Fausto Rosa

Background. Determining preferences regarding the benefits of adjuvant chemotherapy (AC) for stage I GC is critical. *Methods.* We retrospectively reviewed 1069 patients with pathologically confirmed stage I GC who underwent R0 gastrectomy between 2006 and 2014. Univariate and multivariate survival analyses were conducted. Systemic inflammation factors were used to develop a scoring system for predicting AC benefits. *Results.* With a median follow-up of 47 months (range 3–113 months), the 5-year overall survival (OS) rate was 90.5%. The patient score was 1 for either a pretreatment hypoalbuminemia or elevated derived neutrophil-lymphocyte ratio (dNLR) and was 0 otherwise. The SIS served as an independent prognostic factor for reduced OS. AC was delivered to 13.5% (144/1069) of all patients. Compared to surgery alone, AC had no significant effect on survival in both the entire cohort and the IA/IB subgroup. However, in the high-risk group (SIS = 2), patients with AC had a significantly better OS than those undergoing surgery alone. *Conclusions.* Patients with SIS = 2 may benefit from AC and thus may be considered candidates for adjuvant treatment. However, to confirm our findings, future prospective studies are warranted.

1. Introduction

Gastric cancer (GC) is the fourth most common cancer and the second leading cause of cancer death worldwide [1]. Unlike the situation for stage II and stage III GC, there is no global agreement on adjuvant chemotherapy (AC) for stage I GC due to (1) the prognosis of stage I GC is relatively good, with over 90% of 5-year overall survival [2], (2) although the benefit of AC was established for patients with stage II and stage III GC, clinical trials included stage I population failed to show the benefit of AC over surgery alone [2–7]. However, relapse occurs in a small but definite number of patients, even those with stage I GC, after curative resection [8]. Moreover, recent studies showed that the prognosis and response to chemotherapy is different according to the molecular characteristics of gastric cancer [9–11]. Therefore, it is necessary to identify patients with stage I GC who might receive a therapeutic benefit from AC.

The role of the immune system in cancer has become increasingly prominent [12–17]. In addition to local inflammatory symptoms, cancer patients frequently present with systemic inflammation responses, including increased peripheral blood cell amounts and decreased serum albumin levels [18]. More recently, a study at the Memorial Sloan Kettering Cancer Center suggested that pretreatment neutrophil lymphocyte ratio (NLR) can be used to identify nonmetastatic melanoma patients who are more likely to benefit from adjuvant treatment [19]. In 2012, Proctor et al. [20] implemented a simplified index that is easier to apply to clinical data named the derived neutrophil-lymphocyte ratio (dNLR), and they were also able to demonstrate that the preoperative dNLR had similar prognostic value as the classical NLR.

Table 1: Demographic and clinical features.

Characteristics	Number	%	Characteristics	Number	%
Age, years (median, IQR)	60 (18–93)		ASA class		
Sex			1-2	1020	95.4
Male	795	74.4	≥3	49	4.6
Female	274	25.6	Type of surgery		
CEA level			Total gastrectomy	284	26.6
Normal	871	81.5	Subtotal gastrectomy	785	73.4
Above normal	116	10.9	Type of LN dissection		
Unknown	82	7.7	D1	11	1.0
CA 19–9 level			D1+	549	51.3
Normal	826	77.3	D2	509	47.7
Above normal	152	14.2	Lymphovascular invasion		
Unknown	91	8.5	No	945	88.4
Differentiation			Yes	93	8.6
Well or moderate	603	56.4	Unknown	31	2.9
Poor	466	43.6	T stage		
Tumor size, cm			T1	821	76.8
<3	590	55.2	T2	248	23.3
≥3	479	44.8	N stage		
Tumor location			N0	895	83.7
Lower	595	55.7	N1	174	16.3
Middle	138	12.9	TNM stage		
Upper	207	19.4	IA	635	59.4
Multiple	129	12.0	IB	434	40.6
Haemoglobin, g/l (median, IQR)	135 (53–174)		AC		
Albumin, g/l (median, IQR)	40 (20–52)		No (surgery alone)	925	86.5
WBC, 10^9/l (median, IQR)	6.0 (2.7–16.6)		Yes (surgery + AC)	144	13.5
Neutrophils, 10^9/l (median, IQR)	3.5 (0.7–14.6)		Pretreatment hypoalbuminemia		
Platelets, 10^9/l (median, IQR)	217 (80–523)		No	895	83.7
dNLR			Yes	174	16.3
<2	797	74.6			
≥2	272	25.4			

IQR = interquartile range; AC = adjuvant chemotherapy; dNLR = neutrophil count to (white cell count minus neutrophil count); ASA = American Society of Anesthesiologists. Pretreatment hypoalbuminemia: pretreatment serum albumin < 35 g/l.

Preoperative serum albumin levels are also reported as prognostic indicators for the prognosis of cancer patients [21, 22]. These markers are inexpensive to test and routinely performed in clinical setting and hence potentially provide readily available and objective information to help clinicians to estimate patient outcome.

To the best of our knowledge, the potential influence of the pretreatment dNLR and hypoalbuminemia has never been explored in large cohorts of stage I GC patient yet. The aim of the present study was to verify the hypothesis that the systemic immune score (SIS) based on preoperative dNLR and serum albumin is associated with worse survival in diagnosed stage I GC and more importantly to investigate whether SIS can distinguish subgroups of patients who would benefit from AC. If so, such commonly measured SIS could be used in developing a strategy for selecting stage I GC treatments.

2. Materials and Methods

2.1. Patients. A total of 1069 patients undergoing R0 resection for stage I GC at Fujian Medical University Union Hospital (FMUUH) from December 2006 to December 2016 were identified from a prospectively maintained database. The following exclusion criteria were then applied: (1) prior gastrectomy, (2) receiving neoadjuvant chemotherapy, (3) noncurative (R1/2) resection, (4) the presence of synchronous malignant disease, (5) autoimmune disorders and recent steroid therapy, and (6) incomplete medical records. Curative resection refers to R0 resection in Japanese Gastric Cancer Treatment Guidelines 2010 (version 3) [23]. Tumor stages were assessed according to the American Joint Committee on Cancer (AJCC) classification system, 7th edition [24]. Additional demographic and clinical data are summarized in Table 1. The study protocol was approved by the ethical committee of the FMUUH.

2.2. Adjuvant Chemotherapy. Since there is no established treatment strategy for stage I gastric cancer, decisions to administer AC in those patients were based on their surgeons' or oncologists' preference [25, 26]. According to the treatment protocol of our institute, stage I GC patients with lymph node metastasis, lymphovascular invasion, or other high risks [27, 28] are recommended for AC, unless contraindicated by a patient's condition or their refusal. All AC treatments were performed after individually obtaining written informed consent in accordance with the gastric cancer treatment program at the FMUUH that had been approved by its institutional review board. Finally, 144 (13.5%) patients with written informed consent received 5-fluorouracil plus cisplatin AC, at least one cycle [29]. The clinicopathological variables of both groups are summarized in Supplementary Table 1.

2.3. Systemic Immune Markers. Routine clinical laboratory analyses of peripheral blood samples collected within 1 week before the operation were used to ascertain white cell counts, neutrophil counts, and serum albumin. The pretreatment dNLR was calculated as follows: dNLR = neutrophil count to (white cell count-neutrophil count). The cutoff value (2.0) for the pretreatment dNLR was selected as described previously [20]. The cutoff value for the pretreatment hypoalbuminemia (35 g/l) was according to the normal value measured by the used test [22, 30]. All the measurements were performed in the central biochemical laboratory at the Department of Clinical Biochemistry and Hematology, FMUUH.

We combined the two risks to establish the SIS defined as follows: patients with both elevated dNLR and hypoalbuminemia ($dNLR \geq 2$ and albumin < 35 g/l, resp.) were assigned score 2, patients with either elevated dNLR or hypoalbuminemia were assigned score 1, and patients with both decreased dNLR and normal albumin ($dNLR < 2$ and albumin ≥ 35 g/l, resp.) were assigned score 0.

2.4. Follow-up. All patients were monitored postoperatively by physical examination and laboratory tests, including those for tumor markers (such as CEA and CA 19–9), every 3 months for the first 2 years, every 6 months for the next 3 years, and annually thereafter. In addition, examinations, including chest radiography, abdominopelvic computed tomography (CT), and endoscopy, were performed at least once a year. If necessary, further evaluation, such as positron emission tomography or magnetic resonance imaging, was initiated.

2.5. Statistical Analysis. Overall survival (OS) was defined as the time from the day of surgery to the death from any cause. Univariate survival trends were compared using Kaplan-Meier curves and significant differences determined via the log rank test, and those variables that achieved statistical significance in the univariate analysis were entered into the multivariable analysis. Multivariate analysis of prognostic factors was conducted with Cox's proportional hazards model. A p value < 0.05 was regarded statistically significant. Statistical analysis was performed using SPSS version 19.0 for Windows (SPSS Inc., Chicago, IL, USA).

Table 2: Patient baseline characteristics (adjuvant chemotherapy with surgery versus surgery alone).

Characteristics	AC group ($n = 144$)	Non-AC group ($n = 925$)	p value
Age, years (median, IQR)	58 (18–81)	60 (20–93)	0.402
Sex			0.474
Male	103	692	
Female	41	233	
CEA level			0.146
Normal	112	759	
Above normal	21	95	
Unknown	11	71	
CA 19–9 level			0.701
Normal	111	715	
Above normal	22	130	
Unknown	11	80	
Differentiation			
Well or moderate	78	525	
Poor	66	400	
Tumor size, cm			0.419
<3	84	506	
≥3	60	419	
Tumor location			0.591
Lower	76	519	
Middle	20	118	
Upper	31	176	
Multiple	17	112	
Type of surgery			0.522
Total gastrectomy	43	241	
Subtotal gastrectomy	101	684	
TNM stage			<0.001
IA	48	587	
IB	96	338	
Pretreatment dNLR			0.064
<2	116	681	
≥2	28	244	
Pretreatment hypoalbuminemia			0.260
No	121	774	
Yes	23	151	

3. Results

3.1. Patient Characteristics. A total of 1069 patients with pathologically documented stage I GC were included in this study. The study population comprised of 795 (74.4%) males and 274 (25.6%) females. The median age was 60 years (range 18–93). Descriptive clinicopathological and detailed

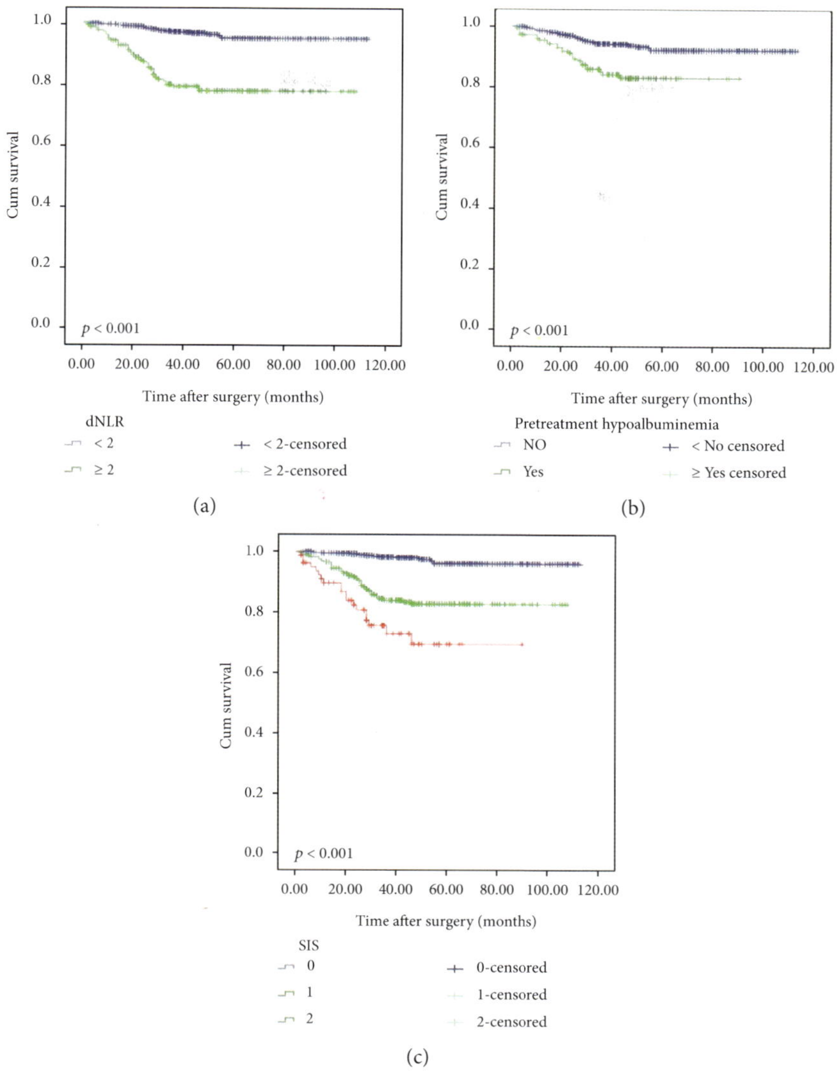

FIGURE 1: Kaplan-Meier curves for high versus low dNLR (a), with versus without pretreatment hypoalbuminemia (b), and patients according to different SIS (c) in the entire cohort.

blood count parameters of the study cohort are shown in Table 1. The percentage of patients with dNLR ≥ 2 was 25.4% (272/1069) in contrast to 74.6% (797/1069) for those with dNLR < 2. Pretreatment hypoalbuminemia (albumin < 35 g/l) occurred in 174 patients (16.3%). Overall, 925 (86.5%) patients received surgery alone (the non-AC group), and 144 (13.5%) received AC after surgery (the AC group). The baseline characteristics between the groups are shown in Table 2.

3.2. Survival. The 5-year OS rates in T1N0, T1N1, and T2N0 were 95.7%, 85.3%, and 80.0%, respectively ($p < 0.001$). There were significant differences in 5-year OS between patients with T1N0 and T1N1 ($p < 0.001$) or T2N0 tumors ($p < 0.001$). However, no difference was observed in OS between patients with T1N1 tumors and T2N0 tumors ($p = 0.461$) (Supplementary Figure 1a). The 5-year OS was significantly higher in stage IA patients than in stage IB patients (Supplementary Figure 1b).

The 5-year OS was significantly worse in high dNLR patients than in low dNLR patients (77.6% versus 94.7%, $p < 0.001$; Figure 1(a)). Patients with and without pretreatment hypoalbuminemia also differed significantly in 5-year OS (82.9% versus 92.1%, $p < 0.001$; Figure 1(b)).

3.3. Predictive Factors for Survival. The statistically significant prognostic factors identified by univariate analyses are shown in Table 3. Based on the multivariate analysis, the elevated pretreatment dNLR and hypoalbuminemia were independent prognostic factors for OS, together with TNM stage and lymphovascular invasion (Table 3).

3.4. Establishment and Prognostic Impact of the Novel Systemic Immune Score (SIS). Based on the systemic immune prognostic factors identified in the multivariate analysis, we combined the two factors to establish the SIS defined as follows: patients with both high dNLR and the pretreatment hypoalbuminemia were assigned a score of 2, patients with either high dNLR or the pretreatment hypoalbuminemia

Table 3: Univariate and multivariate Cox proportional analysis for survival.

Parameter	Categories	Univariate analysis HR (95% CI)	p	Multivariate analysis HR (95% CI)	p
Age	>65 versus <65	1.459 (0.974–2.186)	0.067		
Gender	Male versus female	1.408 (0.853–2.327)	0.181		
Tumor location	Upper versus other	1.254 (0.779–2.019)	0.351		
Tumor size	≥30 mm versus <30 mm	1.555 (1.041–2.324)	0.031	1.302 (0.731–1.816)	0.452
Lymphovascular invasion	Yes versus no	2.660 (1.509–4.689)	0.001	2.314 (1.419–4.417)	0.010
Tumor differentiation	Undifferentiated versus differentiated	1.392 (0.933–2.077)	0.105		
Extent of lymph node dissection	D1+/D1 versus D2	1.158 (0.643–1.391)	0.211		
AJCC TNM stage	IB versus IA	10.183 (5.765–17.987)	<0.001	8.098 (5.201–13.145)	<0.001
CEA level	Above normal versus normal	2.433 (1.440–4.110)	0.001	1.488 (0.873–2.426)	0.319
CA 19–9 level	Above normal versus normal	1.363 (0.789–2.356)	0.267		
Adjuvant chemotherapy	No versus yes	1.557 (0.784–3.092)	0.206		
dNLR	≥2 versus <2	4.357 (2.910–6.524)	<0.001	2.464 (1.301–4.312)	0.004
Pretreatment hypoalbuminemia	Yes versus no	2.181 (1.404–3.387)	0.001	2.102 (1.254–3.576)	0.028
SIS classification	2 versus ≤1	4.955 (3.175–7.733)	<0.001	3.023 (1.977–6.501)	0.002

CA: carbohydrate antigen; CEA: carcinoembryonic antigen; CI: confidence interval; HR: hazard ratio.

were assigned a score of 1, and patients with both low dNLR and normal albumin were assigned a score of 0. Namely, patients were given a total score of 0, 1, and 2 based on the sum of the points.

As mentioned above, we generate three subgroups based on the SIS. We found significant differences among the three subgroups. Thus, we combined the three subgroups to establish the SIS classification as follows: the low-risk group has no risk factor (SIS = 0), the medium-risk group has 1 risk factor (SIS = 1), and the high-risk group has two risk factors (SIS = 2) (Figure 1(c)). The SIS classification also was an independent prognostic factor for OS (Table 3). Supplementary Figure 2 depicts the association between the SIS and TNM as a bubble chart.

3.5. SIS Predicts the Benefits of Adjuvant Chemotherapy. Figure 2(a) shows the survival curves for patients with and without AC. In the entire cohort, there was no significant difference in 5-year OS between the groups with and without AC (93·4% versus 90.0%, $p = 0.109$). This lack of a difference was also apparent when the analysis was confined to stage IA (93.7 versus 96.0%, $p = 0.946$) and IB (83.7% versus 79.5%, $p = 0.426$) subgroup patients (Figures 2(b) and 2(c)). Moreover, the survival curves (Figure 3) show no difference between surgery alone versus surgery + AC according to pretreatment dNLR and hypoalbuminemia.

Surprisingly, for our original SIS system, Kaplan-Meier curves demonstrated that high-risk patients (SIS = 2) with AC had significantly better OS than their counterparts without AC (88.9% versus 69.4%, $p = 0.023$) (Figure 4(a)), while no significant difference was observed in the low-risk and medium-risk group (94.4% versus 97.6%, $p = 0.695$ and 91.6% versus 81.9%, $p = 0.130$) (Figures 4(b) and 4(c)). In other words, the survival benefit of AC was significant for patients with SIS = 2.

4. Discussion

With the increase in the detection of stage I GC, the number of stage I GC patients who experience recurrence has also increased, which may result in a large health problem in the real world [2, 8]. It is thus important to identify patients with apparent early-stage disease who will not be cured by surgery alone and should receive adjuvant chemotherapy (AC). To date, almost all of the data on AC are derived from large-scale clinical trials that included a large proportion of stages II and III patients but no or too few patients with stage I GC [3–6]. A prospective randomized clinical trial of AC versus surgery alone in stage I GC patients at high risk of recurrence or death is still ongoing (ClinicalTrials.gov identifier NCT01917552). Therefore, it will be clinically useful if a score system can be used to select candidates for AC.

A systemic inflammatory response has been determined to be an important tumor stage-independent predictor of prognosis in various malignances [31]. Pretreatment NLR values are associated with prognosis in various solid tumors, including gastric adenocarcinoma [15, 17, 32]. In 2012, Proctor et al. [20] reported the dNLR and NLR have similar prognostic value in a large cohort of unselected cancer patients. More recently, Dalpiaz [33] and his colleges found that the pretreatment dNLR was better than NLR in terms of acting as an independent prognostic factor for cancer patients. In this study, we also clearly demonstrate that dNLR was an independent predictor of long-term survival for stage I GC patients ($p < 0.001$).

In addition to pretreatment NLR, another systemic immune factor was predictive of prognosis in stage I GC in our cohort: pretreatment hypoalbuminemia. There is a growing appreciation that pretreatment hypoalbuminemia can influence the prognosis of cancer patients, possibly through

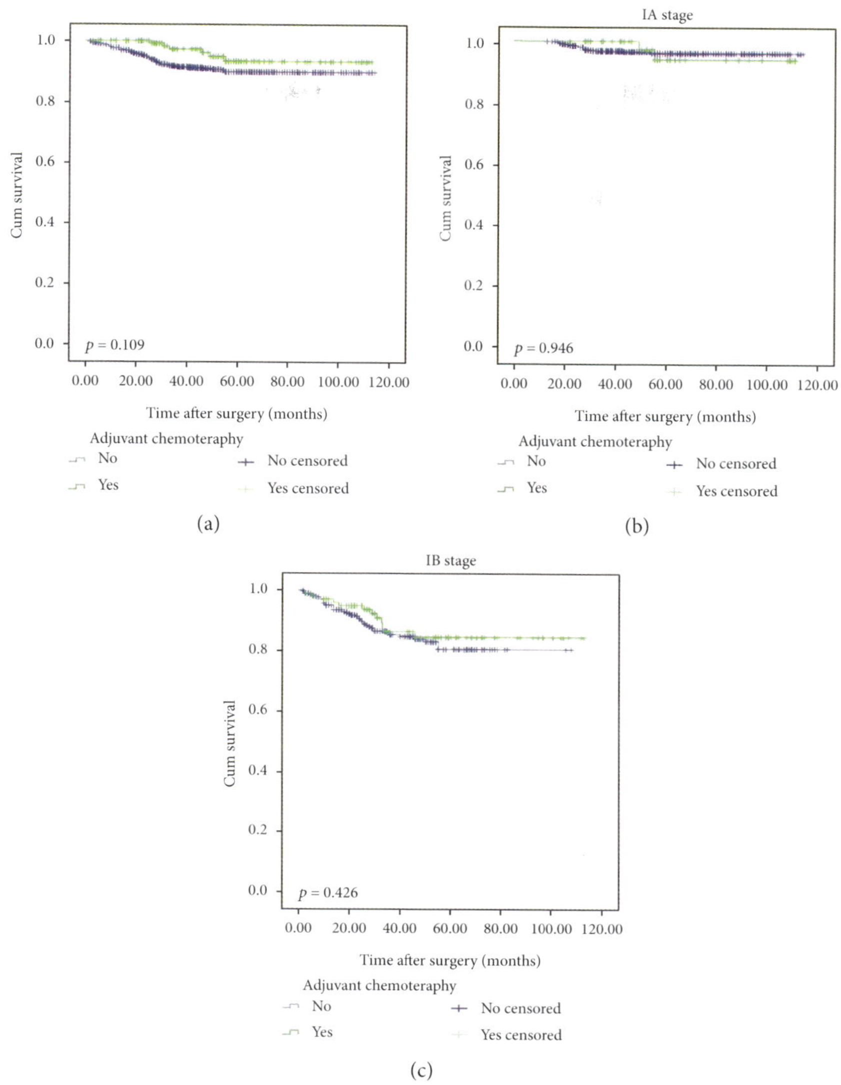

FIGURE 2: Comparison of OS between the adjuvant chemotherapy group and the surgery-only group. (a) Entire group, (b) IA stage subgroup, and (c) IB stage subgroup.

a systemic inflammatory response or impaired immunological response [34]. A recent meta-analysis of 29 studies on variety of gastrointestinal tract solid tumors reported that pretreatment serum albumin levels provide useful prognostic significance in cancer [30]. Several studies have found that low serum albumin level was an independent prognostic factor for worse outcomes in patients with gastric cancer [35, 36]. In line with previous studies, the results of the current study show an association between pretreatment hypoalbuminemia and decreased 5-year OS.

As stated above, dNLR and hypoalbuminemia were independent prognostic predictors of survival in patients with stage I GC. Consequently, we created a novel prognostic score named the SIS based on the combination of dNLR and hypoalbuminemia, and we hypothesize that the SIS may provide further information in addition to that from classical pathological prognostic factors for identifying patients who are at high risk for poor prognosis. By grouping the patients on the basis of SIS, we identified three risk groups with distinct survival outcomes, that is, a high-risk group (SIS = 2) with a 5-year OS rate of 71.2%, a medium-risk group (SIS = 1) with a 5-year OS rate of 83.1%, and a low-risk group (SIS = 0) with a 5-year OS rate of 96.1%. When the SIS is used for risk stratification, stage I GC patients could be categorized into three different risk groups displaying a 5-year OS rate difference of almost 25 percentage points.

Proceeding to the next step, NLR can be used to assist in risk stratification and potentially predicting immunotherapy treatment response of patients with nonmetastatic melanoma [19]. Another study from France found that pretreatment serum albumin level > 35 g/l was the only independent predictive factor of complete response to chemoradiotherapy (CRT) in esophageal cancer patients [37]. Therefore, we hypothesized that SIS may be used to detect patients who can benefit from AC in stage I GC. For stage I gastric cancer,

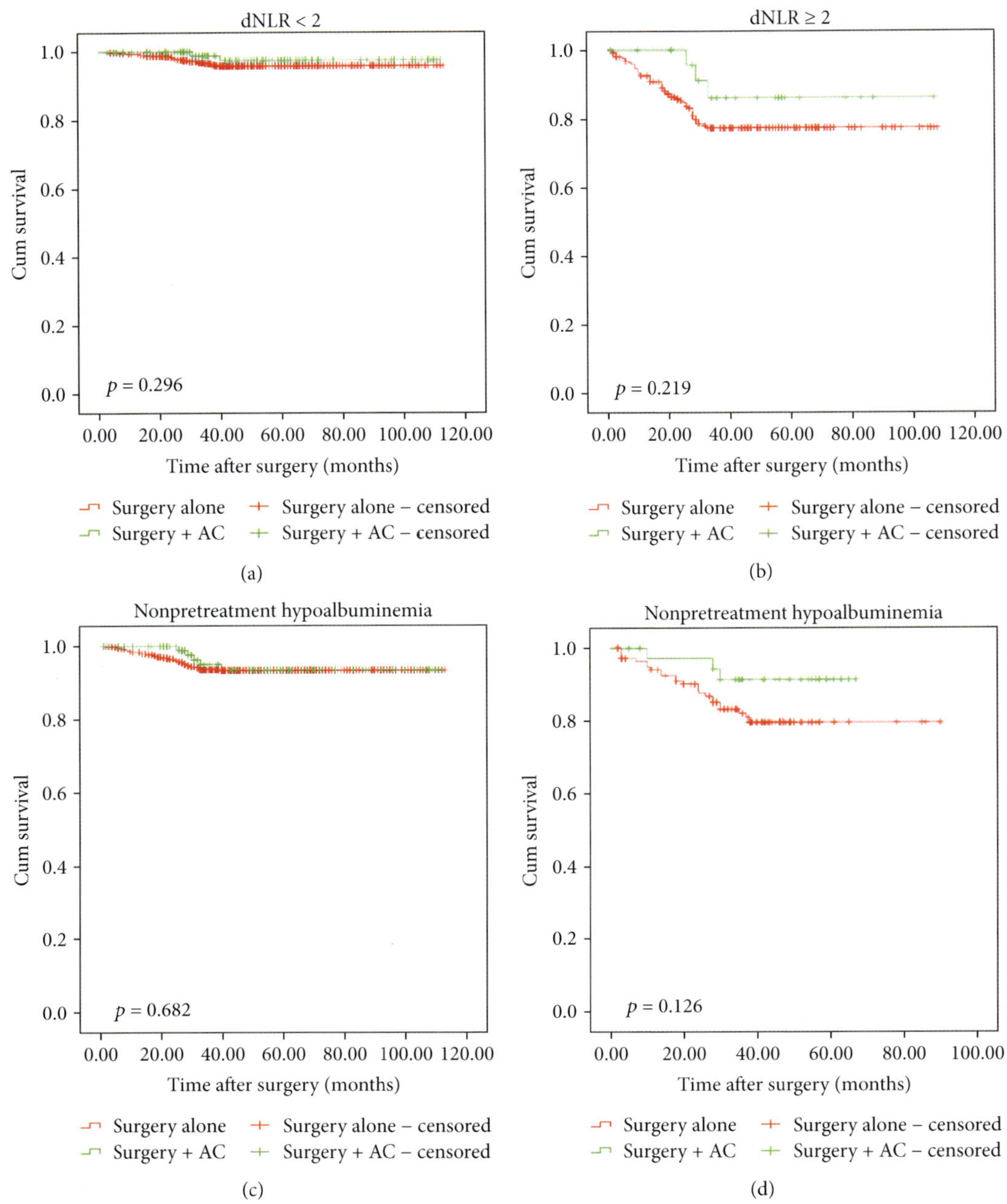

FIGURE 3: Comparison of OS between adjuvant chemotherapy group and surgery-only group. (a) dNLR < 2 subgroup, (b) dNLR ≥ 2 subgroup, (c) hypoalbuminemia subgroup, and (d) nonhypoalbuminemia subgroup.

poorly differentiated or higher-grade cancer, LBVI, PNI, or <50 years of age are considered high-risk features, and adjuvant therapy is recommended in these high-risk patients [27]. Kunisaki et al. [38] revealed that depth of invasion, lymph node metastasis, and LBVI independently influenced prognosis in stage I gastric cancer, and in their report, patients with stage I GC having lymphovascular invasion and stage II GC had similar survival outcomes; this finding suggests that adjuvant chemotherapy is suitable for stage I patients with moderate to severe lymphovascular invasion. However, none of the previous studies compared the prognosis between patients with AC and those without AC. Notably, distinct from the previous studies, we first directly compared the survival of stage I GC patients with or without AC in terms of differences in inflammation-immune status. The patients with an SIS = 2 could achieve significantly better prognosis if treated with AC and should thus be considered candidates for adjuvant treatment.

There were some limitations of the present study. First, it is a single-center retrospective study. Second, we did not perform external or internal validation of our risk model. However, it might be difficult to construct a dataset including a patient population as large as ours for external validation. Despite the large cohort size in this study, the number of events was considered not insufficient to divide patients into training and validation sets for internal validation, and the

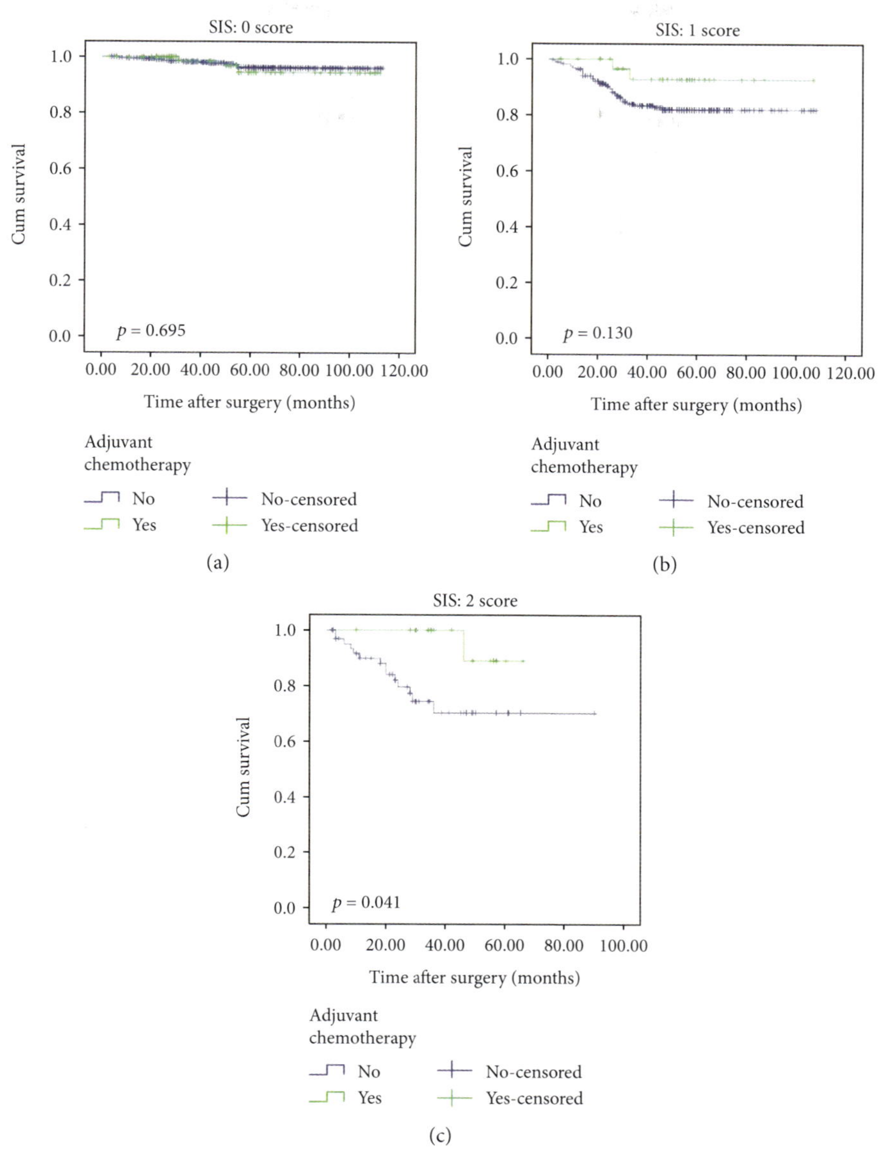

FIGURE 4: Comparison of OS between adjuvant chemotherapy group and surgery-only group. (a) 0 score subgroup, (b) 1 score subgroup, and (c) 2 score subgroup.

number of high-risk patients was relatively small. The prognostic significance of the SIS in GC patients remains to be investigated prospectively in other populations and larger cohorts in the future. Third, we did not compare the prognostic value of other SIS, such as PNI, PLR, NLR, and GPS. Finally, the optimal AC cycle for stage I patients had not yet been established.

5. Conclusions

The present study demonstrated that stage I GC patients with elevated pretreatment dNLR and pretreatment hypoalbuminemia were likely to receive a survival benefit from AC. In view of this, the SIS should be included in routine clinical assessments and might also be considered for risk stratification in future clinical trials of AC in early-stage GC. However, it is still necessary to conduct prospective clinical validation studies to confirm the findings of this study.

Ethical Approval

All procedures performed in studies involving human participants were in accordance with the ethical standards of the institutional and/or national research committee and with the 1964 Helsinki declaration and its later amendments or comparable ethical standards.

Disclosure

The funding source hand no role in the design of this article and will not have any role during its execution or publication.

Authors' Contributions

Jun Lu, Chao-hui Zheng, Chang-ming Huang designed this study. Jun Lu, Long-long Cao, Ping Li, Jian-wei Xie, Jia-bin Wang, and Jian-xian Lin collected the data. Jun Lu, Qi-yue

Chen, Mi Lin, and Ru-hong Tu carried out the statistical analysis. Jun Lu and Long-long Cao drafted the manuscript. Chao-hui Zheng and Chang-ming Huang revised the manuscript. All authors read and approved the final manuscript.

Acknowledgments

This study was supported by the Scientific and Technological Innovation Joint Capital Projects of Fujian Province (2016Y9031) and the Construction Project of Fujian Province Minimally Invasive Medical Center (no. [2017]171). The second batch of special support funds for the Fujian Province Innovation and Entrepreneurship Talents (2016B013), Youth Scientific Research Subject of Fujian Provincial Health and Family Planning Commission (no. 2015-1-37), and QIHANG Funds of Fujian Medical University (no. 2016QH025).

References

[1] J. Ferlay, H. R. Shin, F. Bray, D. Forman, C. Mathers, and D. M. Parkin, "Estimates of worldwide burden of cancer in 2008: GLOBOCAN," *International Journal of Cancer*, vol. 127, no. 12, pp. 2893–2917, 2010.

[2] J. H. Park, M. H. Ryu, H. J. Kim et al., "Risk factors for selection of patients at high risk of recurrence or death after complete surgical resection in stage I gastric cancer," *Gastric Cancer*, vol. 19, no. 1, pp. 226–233, 2016.

[3] S. H. Noh, S. R. Park, H. K. Yang et al., "Adjuvant capecitabine plus oxaliplatin for gastric cancer after D2 gastrectomy (CLASSIC): 5-year follow-up of an open-label, randomised phase 3 trial," *The Lancet Oncology*, vol. 15, no. 12, pp. 1389–1396, 2014.

[4] S. Sakuramoto, M. Sasako, T. Yamaguchi et al., "Adjuvant chemotherapy for gastric cancer with S-1, an oral fluoropyrimidine," *The New England Journal of Medicine*, vol. 357, no. 18, pp. 1810–1820, 2007.

[5] M. Sasako, S. Sakuramoto, H. Katai et al., "Five-year outcomes of a randomized phase III trial comparing adjuvant chemotherapy with S-1 versus surgery alone in stage II or III gastric cancer," *Journal of Clinical Oncology*, vol. 29, no. 33, pp. 4387–4393, 2011.

[6] Y. J. Bang, Y. W. Kim, H. K. Yang et al., "Adjuvant capecitabine and oxaliplatin for gastric cancer after D2 gastrectomy (CLASSIC): a phase 3 open-label, randomised controlled trial," *The Lancet*, vol. 379, no. 9813, pp. 315–321, 2012.

[7] H. Osumi, T. Yoshio, K. Chin et al., "Chemotherapy is effective for stage I gastric cancer in patients with synchronous esophageal cancer," *Gastric Cancer*, vol. 19, no. 2, pp. 625–630, 2016.

[8] H. G. Youn, J. Y. An, M. G. Choi, J. H. Noh, T. S. Sohn, and S. Kim, "Recurrence after curative resection of early gastric cancer," *Annals of Surgical Oncology*, vol. 17, no. 2, pp. 448–454, 2010.

[9] R. Cristescu, J. Lee, M. Nebozhyn et al., "Molecular analysis of gastric cancer identifies subtypes associated with distinct clinical outcomes," *Nature Medicine*, vol. 21, no. 5, pp. 449–456, 2015.

[10] Cancer Genome Atlas Research Network, "Comprehensive molecular characterization of gastric adenocarcinoma," *Nature*, vol. 513, no. 7517, pp. 202–209, 2014.

[11] J. H. Cheong, H. K. Yang, H. Kim et al., "Predictive test for chemotherapy response in resectable gastric cancer: a multicohort, retrospective analysis," *The Lancet Oncology*, vol. 19, no. 5, pp. 629–638, 2018.

[12] C. S. Roxburgh and D. C. McMillan, "Role of systemic inflammatory response in predicting survival in patients with primary operable cancer," *Future Oncology*, vol. 6, no. 1, pp. 149–163, 2010.

[13] M. Sierzega, M. Lenart, M. Rutkowska et al., "Preoperative neutrophil-lymphocyte and lymphocyte-monocyte ratios reflect immune cell population rearrangement in resectable pancreatic cancer," *Annals of Surgical Oncology*, vol. 24, no. 3, pp. 808–815, 2017.

[14] S. Hamada, A. Masamune, and T. Shimosegawa, "Inflammation and pancreatic cancer: disease promoter and new therapeutic target," *Journal of Gastroenterology*, vol. 49, no. 4, pp. 605–617, 2014.

[15] S. C. Wang, J. F. Chou, V. E. Strong, M. F. Brennan, M. Capanu, and D. G. Coit, "Pretreatment neutrophil to lymphocyte ratio independently predicts disease-specific survival in resectable gastroesophageal junction and gastric adenocarcinoma," *Annals of Surgery*, vol. 263, no. 2, pp. 292–297, 2016.

[16] Y. Asano, S. Kashiwagi, N. Onoda et al., "Predictive value of neutrophil/lymphocyte ratio for efficacy of preoperative chemotherapy in triple-negative breast cancer," *Annals of Surgical Oncology*, vol. 23, no. 4, pp. 1104–1110, 2016.

[17] G. Gemenetzis, F. Bagante, J. F. Griffin et al., "Neutrophil-to-lymphocyte ratio is a predictive marker for invasive malignancy in intraductal papillary mucinous neoplasms of the pancreas," *Annals of Surgery*, vol. 266, no. 2, pp. 339–345, 2016.

[18] M. Chechlinska, M. Kowalewska, and R. Nowak, "Systemic inflammation as a confounding factor in cancer biomarker discovery and validation," *Nature Reviews. Cancer*, vol. 10, no. 1, pp. 2-3, 2010.

[19] J. L. Davis, R. C. Langan, K. S. Panageas et al., "Elevated blood neutrophil-to-lymphocyte ratio: a readily available biomarker associated with death due to disease in high risk nonmetastatic melanoma," *Annals of Surgical Oncology*, vol. 24, no. 7, pp. 1989–1996, 2017.

[20] M. J. Proctor, D. C. McMillan, D. S. Morrison, C. D. Fletcher, P. G. Horgan, and S. J. Clarke, "A derived neutrophil to lymphocyte ratio predicts survival in patients with cancer," *British Journal of Cancer*, vol. 107, no. 4, pp. 695–699, 2012.

[21] D. C. McMillan, "The systemic inflammation-based Glasgow prognostic score: a decade of experience in patients with cancer," *Cancer Treatment Reviews*, vol. 39, no. 5, pp. 534–540, 2013.

[22] O. Fiala, M. Pesek, J. Finek et al., "Serum albumin is a strong predictor of survival in patients with advanced-stage non-small cell lung cancer treated with erlotinib," *Neoplasma*, vol. 63, no. 03, pp. 471–476, 2016.

[23] Japanese Gastric Cancer Association, "Japanese gastric cancer treatment guidelines 2010 (ver. 3)," *Gastric Cancer*, vol. 14, no. 2, pp. 113–123, 2011.

[24] K. Washington, "7th edition of the AJCC cancer staging manual: stomach," *Annals of Surgical Oncology*, vol. 17, no. 12, pp. 3077–3079, 2010.

[25] I. R. Cho, J. C. Park, C. H. Park et al., "Pre-treatment neutrophil to lymphocyte ratio as a prognostic marker to predict chemotherapeutic response and survival outcomes in metastatic advanced gastric cancer," *Gastric Cancer*, vol. 17, no. 4, pp. 703–710, 2014.

[26] H. B. Shin, J. Y. An, S. H. Lee et al., "Is adjuvant chemotherapy necessary in pT1N1 gastric cancer?," *BMC Cancer*, vol. 17, no. 1, p. 287, 2017.

[27] D. C1, Y. Zhou, H. Cai, G. Zhao, H. Fu, and Y. Q. Shi, "Poor prognostic factors in patients with stage I gastric cancer according to the seventh edition TNM classification: a comparative analysis of three subgroups," *Journal of Surgical Oncology*, vol. 105, no. 3, pp. 323–328, 2012.

[28] S. G. Barreto and J. A. Windsor, "Redefining early gastric cancer," *Surgical Endoscopy*, vol. 30, no. 1, pp. 24–37, 2016.

[29] H. Zhang, H. Liu, Z. Shen et al., "Tumor-infiltrating neutrophils is prognostic and predictive for postoperative adjuvant chemotherapy benefit in patients with gastric cancer," *Annals of Surgery*, vol. 267, no. 2, pp. 311–318, 2016.

[30] D. Gupta and C. G. Lis, "Pretreatment serum albumin as a predictor of cancer survival: a systematic review of the epidemiological literature," *Nutrition Journal*, vol. 22, no. 9, p. 69, 2010.

[31] S. Ghuman, M. Van Hemelrijck, H. Garmo et al., "Serum inflammatory markers and colorectal cancer risk and survival," *British Journal of Cancer*, vol. 116, no. 10, pp. 1358–1365, 2017.

[32] B. Bhindi, T. Hermanns, Y. Wei et al., "Identification of the best complete blood count-based predictors for bladder cancer outcomes in patients undergoing radical cystectomy," *British Journal of Cancer*, vol. 114, no. 2, pp. 207–212, 2016.

[33] O. Dalpiaz, T. Luef, M. Seles et al., "Critical evaluation of the potential prognostic value of the pretreatment-derived neutrophil–lymphocyte ratio under consideration of C-reactive protein levels in clear cell renal cell carcinoma," *British Journal of Cancer*, vol. 116, no. 1, pp. 85–90, 2017.

[34] D. C. McMillan, "Systemic inflammation, nutritional status and survival in patients with cancer," *Current Opinion in Clinical Nutrition and Metabolic Care*, vol. 12, no. 3, pp. 223–226, 2009.

[35] H. Sun, B. He, Z. Nie et al., "A nomogram based on serum bilirubin and albumin levels predicts survival in gastric cancer patients," *Oncotarget*, vol. 8, no. 25, pp. 41305–41318, 2017.

[36] L. F. Oñate-Ocaña, V. Aiello-Crocifoglio, D. Gallardo-Rincón et al., "Serum albumin as a significant prognostic factor for patients with gastric carcinoma," *Annals of Surgical Oncology*, vol. 14, no. 2, pp. 381–389, 2007.

[37] F. Di Fiore, S. Lecleire, D. Pop et al., "Baseline nutritional status is predictive of response to treatment and survival in patients treated by definitive chemoradiotherapy for a locally advanced esophageal cancer," *The American Journal of Gastroenterology*, vol. 102, no. 11, pp. 2557–2563, 2007.

[38] C. Kunisaki, H. Makino, J. Kimura et al., "Impact of lymphovascular invasion in patients with stage I gastric cancer," *Surgery*, vol. 147, no. 2, pp. 204–211, 2010.

4

Hemobilia: Perspective and Role of the Advanced Endoscopist

Rani Berry,[1] James Han,[2] Mohit Girotra,[3] and James H. Tabibian[4]

[1]*Department of Internal Medicine, Ronald Reagan UCLA Medical Center, Los Angeles, CA, USA*
[2]*Department of Internal Medicine, University of California, Irvine, CA, USA*
[3]*Division of Gastroenterology, University of Miami, Miller School of Medicine, Miami, FL, USA*
[4]*Division of Gastroenterology, Department of Medicine, Olive View-UCLA Medical Center, Sylmar, CA, USA*

Correspondence should be addressed to James H. Tabibian; jtabibian@dhs.lacounty.gov

Academic Editor: Andrea Casadei Gardini

Hemobilia refers to bleeding from and/or into the biliary tract and is an uncommon cause of gastrointestinal hemorrhage. Hemobilia has been documented since the 1600s, but due to its relative rarity, it has only been more critically examined in recent decades. Most cases of hemobilia are iatrogenic and caused by procedures involving the liver, pancreas, bile ducts, and/or the hepatopancreatobiliary vasculature, with trauma and malignancy representing the two other major causes. A classic triad of right upper quadrant pain, jaundice, and overt upper gastrointestinal bleeding has been described, but this is present in only 25–30% of patients with hemobilia. Historically, the gold standard for diagnosis and treatment has been angiography and interventional radiologic intervention, respectively. However, the paradigm is shifting, at least in select cases, towards first-line reliance on noninvasive imaging (e.g., computed tomography) and therapeutic endoscopy, owing to advances in and the less invasive nature of both, while saving interventional radiological and/or surgical intervention for refractory or imminently life-threatening cases.

1. Introduction

1.1. Overview. Hemobilia, in the most elemental sense, refers to the admixture of blood in bile or to blood in the biliary tract. The most common causes of hemobilia are surgical and nonsurgical trauma, malignancy, and/or cholangiovenous (or arterobiliary) fistulae. Though hemobilia remains an uncommon cause of digestive tract bleeding, its incidence has gradually increased as the arsenal of advanced endoscopic and other minimally invasive hepatopancreatobiliary procedures has expanded. Likewise, with more hepatopancreatobiliary procedures comes the advent of new therapeutic endoscopic and interventional radiologic approaches to diagnose and treat hemobilia [1].

1.2. Historic Background. The first known report of hemobilia was from Francis Glisson (Figure 1) in 1654, who described the clinical presentation of a nobleman whom in the midst of a sword fight suffered a fatal blow to the right upper quadrant, leading to massive (upper) gastrointestinal bleeding and death 1 week later. Post mortem, the source of bleeding was found to be from a liver laceration, which in turn led to the landmark description of hemobilia. Antonie Portal was the first to publish a case of hemobilia identified antemortem, reporting suspected hemobilia that was later confirmed on autopsy in 1777. Portal drew important attention to the difficulty in identifying the pinpoint source of bleed, a problem still faced today [2]. One hundred years later, Quincke identified the clinical triad of right upper quadrant pain, jaundice, and upper gastrointestinal tract bleeding, known as Quincke's triad [3]. By the 1900s, there were many scattered case reports of biliary tract hemorrhage, though the term hemobilia was not actually coined until 1948 in a paper entitled, "Hemorrhage into the Biliary Tract Following Trauma: Traumatic Hemobilia" [4].

2. Epidemiology

Though uncommon, hemobilia is an important cause of upper gastrointestinal hemorrhage. Published data on the topic is mainly in the form of case reports and three large case series. In 1973, Sandblom reported a series reviewing 355

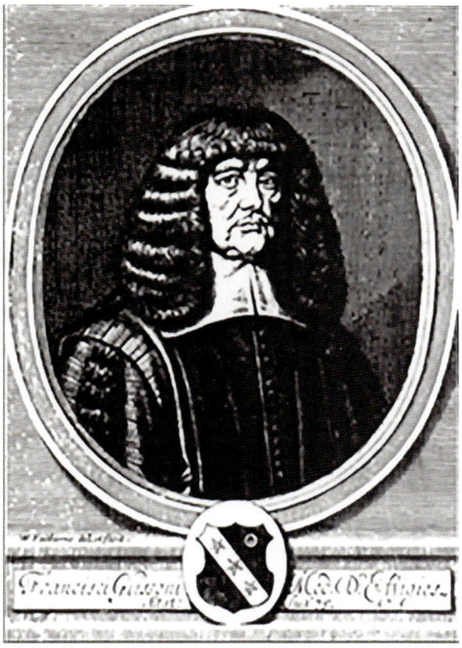

FIGURE 1: Francis Glisson, who recounted the first recorded case of hemobilia in his treatise *Anatomica Hepatis* [67].

cases and reporting 59 iatrogenic cases (16.6%) and 137 (38.6%) due to trauma [4]. Yoshida et al. published a series of 103 patients in 1987, of whom 41% of cases were iatrogenic and 19% were traumatic, thus reversing the incidence (compared to prior reports) to favor iatrogenic causes, citing increasing hepatobiliary interventional procedures as the primary contributing factor [5]. This sentiment was echoed later on by Green et al. in a series of 222 patients published in 2001, among whom 65% had an iatrogenic cause and only 6% had trauma (Figure 2) [6]. This is consistent with more recent reports indicating iatrogenic injury as the leading cause of hemobilia, accounting for over 50% of all cases.

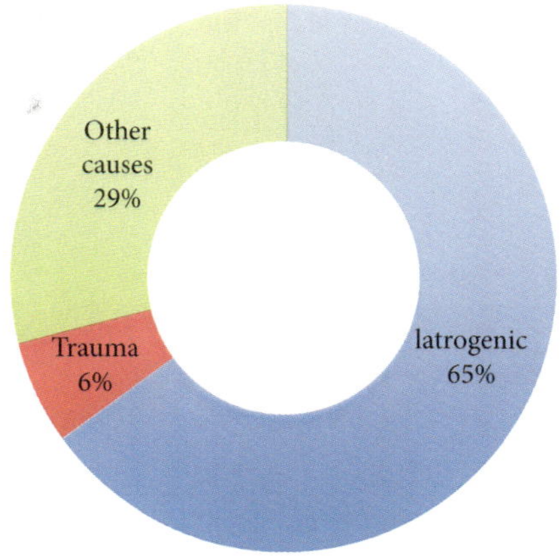

FIGURE 2: Common causes of hemobilia [6].

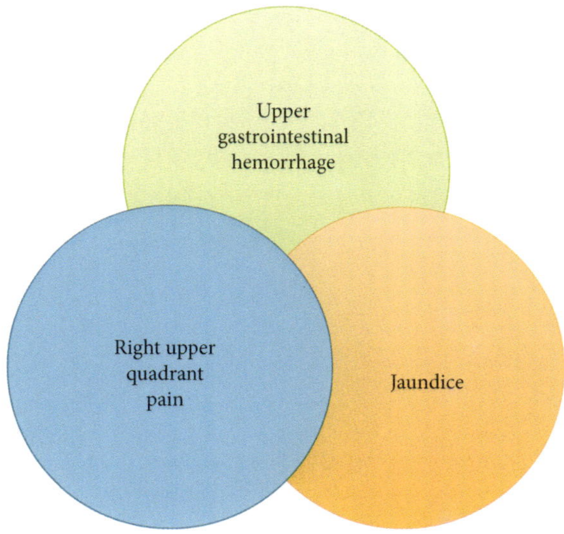

FIGURE 3: Quincke's triad of hemobilia. Notably, all three symptoms are only present in 22–35% of patients [6, 7].

3. Clinical Presentation and Pathophysiology

The classic presentation of hemobilia is formally known as Quincke's triad: jaundice, right upper quadrant abdominal pain, and upper gastrointestinal hemorrhage (Figure 3), but all three findings are only present in 22–35% of cases [6, 7]. The presentation of hemobilia often depends on the cause. For instance, patients with a percutaneous transhepatic biliary drain (PTBD) may present with bloody output from the biliary drain. The timing of presentation can also vary and possibly aid in diagnosis. Endoscopic retrograde cholangiopancreatography- (ERCP-) related hemobilia tends to present immediately or within a few days after the inciting biliary duct injury (e.g., sphincterotomy or biliary stricturoplasty) [8, 9]. In instances where the hepatic artery is ligated during surgery or interventional procedures, an environment for fistulization between a high-pressure arterial system and low-pressure biliary tract (i.e., arteriobilious fistula) is created. The difference in density between blood and bile causes the two to separate once joined within the biliary tree, and as the initial bleed stops, the blood that originally entered the biliary tract begins to clot, serving as a physical impediment to biliary outflow. These clots can cause symptomatic jaundice, biliary obstruction, and subsequent right upper quadrant pain. Clots also cause biliary stasis and hepatobiliary inflammation [8]. As clots travel through the hepatopancreatic ampulla, patients may preferentially complain of discomfort at the level of the right hypochondrium, extending to the epigastrum [8, 10]. Additionally, because of their similar echogenicity, clots can masquerade as biliary stones on imaging studies. Hemobilia can also emanate from venous blood flow, which in contrast tends to be of lower volume or self-limited (except in cases of portal hypertension, in which case it may be of larger volume and/or persistent).

Hemobilia presents on serum laboratory tests as (iron deficiency) anemia and/or as hyperbilirubinemia and elevated alkaline phosphatase and/or aminotransaminases, as seen with other causes of bleeding. Clinically, hemobilia can present as hematemesis, melena, or hematochezia, with or without choluria, depending on the rate of bleeding and anatomical factors (e.g., postbilioenteric surgical anatomy).

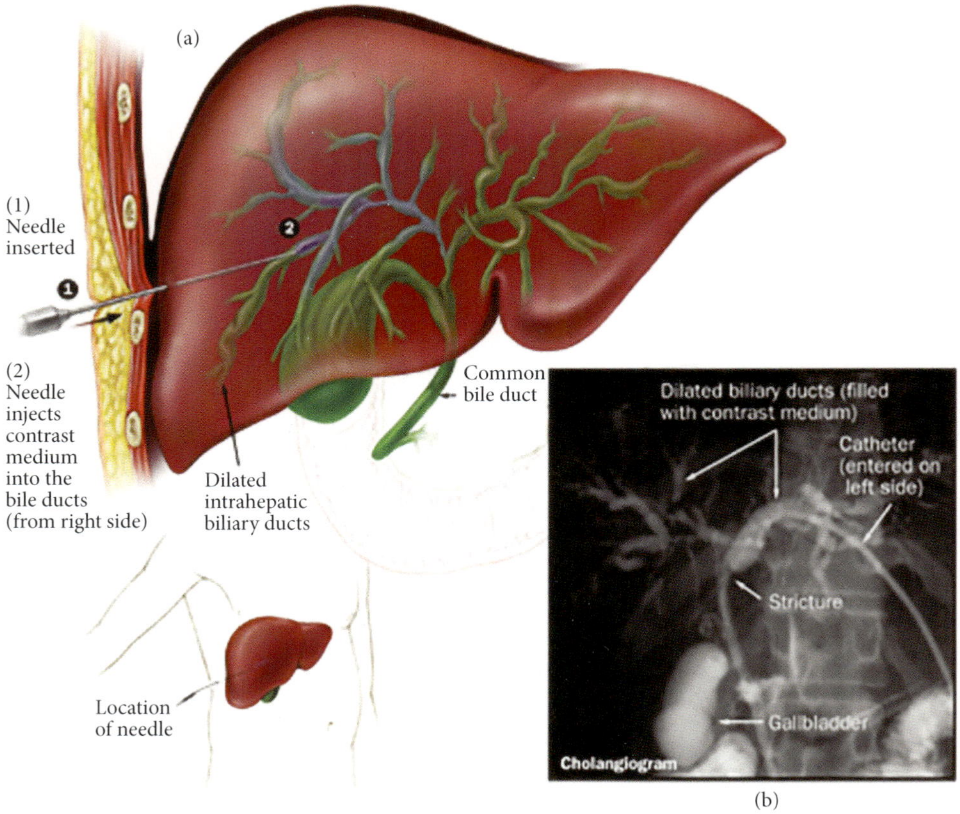

FIGURE 4: Percutaneous transhepatic cholangiography. This technique can be utilized to inject contrast directly into the biliary system and show, fluoroscopically, evidence of filling defects, which in the proper clinical context may be consistent with (clotted) hemobilia [68].

4. Causes of Hemobilia

The causes of hemobilia have evolved overtime, as alluded to earlier. Possible causes include iatrogenic, traumatic, neoplastic, inflammatory, infectious, and vascular. More recently, iatrogenic causes of hemobilia (though still relatively rare) have superseded other causes in most series/populations and can be categorized by procedural type.

4.1. Interventional Procedures

4.1.1. Percutaneous Hepatobiliary Interventions. Common causes of iatrogenic hemobilia include interventions including percutaneous and (to a lesser extent) transjugular liver biopsy, diagnostic percutaneous transhepatic cholangiography (PTC), (Figure 4), and percutaneous transhepatic cholangiography with biliary drain (PTBD) placement; percutaneous biliary therapies such as radiofrequency ablation can also cause hemobilia but collectively comprise a smaller proportion of cases due to their relative rarity [11].

(1) Percutaneous Liver Biopsy. The published literature shows some discrepancy in the risk of hemobilia due to liver biopsy; for example, a recent study by Zhou et al. found that "hemobilia accounts for 3% of all major percutaneous liver biopsy complications," whereas a larger retrospective study reported only 4 cases of hemobilia out of 68,276 liver biopsies (0.005% risk). The discrepancy between studies may suggest that either liver biopsies have become more risky overtime (e.g., due to detection and subsequent sampling of smaller or more central lesions), although another explanation could be that the difference is attributable to better detection and reporting of hemobilia over time, among other potential explanations [12, 13].

(2) Percutaneous Transhepatic Cholangiography with and without Biliary Drain. Percutaneous interventions run the risk of inadvertently nicking a vascular structure, resulting in hemobilia, with the risk being higher in the case of factors such as a nondilated biliary tree (i.e., a smaller target). Rivera et al. compared hemobilia caused by PTBD versus PTC and found that the risk of hemobilia is higher with PTBD (2.2%) versus the rate from PTC alone (0.7%) [14]. Thought varies as to the reason for this 3-fold increase in hemobilia with PTBD compared to PTC, but it is likely that at least some of this difference may be due to the greater size of the aperture made in the bile duct wall with PTBD and the presence of a foreign material remaining in the duct which can serve as cause of inflammation or erosion [8]. A retrospective cohort study had similar results, citing that the risk of hepatic artery injury was 2.6% with PTBD and 0.7% with PTC [15]. Less common interventional procedures which may result in hemobilia include ultrasound-guided radiofrequency ablation and transarterial chemoembolization as well as transjugular intrahepatic portosystemic shunt placement [16–20].

4.1.2. Endoscopic Hepatopancreatobiliary Interventions. The main endoscopic procedure associated with hemobilia is ERCP and, in particular, sphincterotomy. Though sphincterotomy-associated bleeding typically occurs at the level of cut papillary sphincter, as initially described by Sandblom, blood can occasionally flow into or reflux from the duodenum back into the biliary tree [4]. In general, the risk of hemobilia depends on the invasiveness of the maneuvers performed during ERCP (e.g., stricturoplasty and extraction of large stones) as well as patient-level variables such as coagulopathy or presence of malignant tissue. Additional risk factors for ERCP-related hemobilia which should be mentioned are variant anatomy, especially anomalous location of the ampulla, aggressive biliary balloon dilation or intraductal biopsying, vascular anomalies (e.g., associated with hereditary hemorrhagic telangiectasia), and transbiliary ductal drainage procedures (e.g., EUS-guided choledochoduodenostomy and hepaticogastrostomy) [8, 21–24].

4.2. Noniatrogenic Causes

4.2.1. Portal Biliopathy. Hemobilia can rarely occur due to portal biliopathy, with or without preceding biliary tract intervention. Portal biliopathy occurs as a result of hypertension of the peribiliary (e.g., choledochal) venous plexus, often in patients with portal vein thrombosis and ensuing portal cavernomas, and manifests radiographically or cholangiographically with multifocal biliary stenoses from tortuous venous structures encircling the bile duct. Hemobilia in this context often requires interventional radiologic or other endoscopic or nonendoscopic intervention as the bleeding is not from an abnormality of the biliary epithelium. Risk factors such as coagulopathy and biliary stenosis also increase the risk of ERCP-related hemobilia [25–27].

4.2.2. Chronic Ductal Obstruction. Obstruction of the hepatopancreatobiliary tract can potentially lead to inflammation, erosion, and fistulization with adjacent structures with resultant hemobilia [28]. As mentioned earlier, intrabiliary clots which form due to hemobilia are often mistaken as gallstones; however, even when gallstones are indeed present, there can still be concurrent hemobilia, especially in cases in which the stone erodes through the cystic artery or other vascular structures and cause bleeding, analogous to how a stone can erode and fistulize into the duodenum and cause outlet obstruction in Bouveret's syndrome [29]. It is worth mentioning here, although not classified as hemobilia, that hemosuccus pancreaticus (also referred to as Wirsungorrhagia) can occur via pathophysiologically similar mechanisms, for example, pancreatitis eroding into the splenic artery and causing bleeding into the main pancreatic duct [30, 31].

4.2.3. Malignancy. Arguably the most common natural cause of hemobilia is due to (primary or metastatic) hepatobiliary tumors [32]. The tumor tissue and vasculature both tend to be more friable leading to an increased risk of spontaneous hemorrhage [13]. As mentioned above, treatment of hepatobiliary tumors (e.g., with radiofrequency ablation) can also lead to hemobilia [29].

4.2.4. Infection. The most clinically significant cause of infectious hemobilia is "tropical hemobilia," a result of parasitic invasion of the biliary tract. Common instigators include the roundworm (*Ascaris lumbricoides*), the Chinese liver fluke (*Clonorchis sinensis*), and the sheep liver fluke (*Fasciola hepatica*). Echinococcal infections can indirectly cause hemobilia in that hydatid cysts may cause inflammation of perivascular tissue, weakening of vessel walls, and/or pseudoaneurysm formation with resultant bleeding into the biliary tract. Divided by region, China, Korea, and Vietnam carry the highest incidence of ascariasis and subsequently higher rates of hemobilia secondary to this infection [29].

4.3. Surgical Interventions. Though surgical intervention is now rarely needed in the treatment of hemobilia, it remains an important cause of hemobilia. Complications of both laparoscopic and laparotomic surgeries that are performed near the cystic and right hepatic artery are most prone to lacerating or otherwise manipulating nearby structures in a manner which can lead to hemobilia. Cholecystectomy, liver transplantation, and pancreaticoduodenectomy (Whipple procedure) are examples of surgeries which have been reported to cause hemobilia [29, 33].

5. Diagnosis

Hemobilia should be suspected in any patient with an unclear source of GI bleed, recent blunt force or penetrating trauma to the upper abdomen, or biliary instrumentation or manipulation, particularly in the context of contemporaneous signs or symptoms of biliary obstruction. The diagnosis of hemobilia requires radiographic or endoscopic findings such as direct visualization of blood emerging from the biliary tract or radiographic findings suggestive of intrabiliary hemorrhage (Figure 5).

5.1. Computed Tomography. Computed tomography (CT) of the abdomen (preferably angiography protocol) has become a first-choice diagnostic test for hemobilia due to its noninvasive nature, low radiation exposure compared to angiography, rapid results, and diagnostic performance characteristics. CT imaging has improved dramatically over the years such that even subtle salient abnormalities can be identified [30, 34, 35].

5.2. Upper Endoscopy and ERCP. Endoscopy is commonly used to evaluate upper gastrointestinal bleeding (with or without suspicion of hemobilia) and can, sometimes incidentally, find hemobilia as the cause/source of bleeding. Up to 60% of hemobilia cases can be diagnosed by endoscopy [35]. Depending on anatomical and other factors, a duodenoscope (i.e., side-viewing scope) may be needed to visualize the ampulla and assess clots or other evidence of bleeding. ERCP can be used to visualize the biliary tree or gallbladder and may offer therapeutic options in patients with hemobilia and/or associated biliary obstruction (Figure 6). Characteristic ERCP findings that suggest the presence of blood clots include amorphous, tubular, or cast-like filling defects; gallbladder filling defects, and otherwise unexplained common bile ductal dilation [36] (Figures 7 and 8).

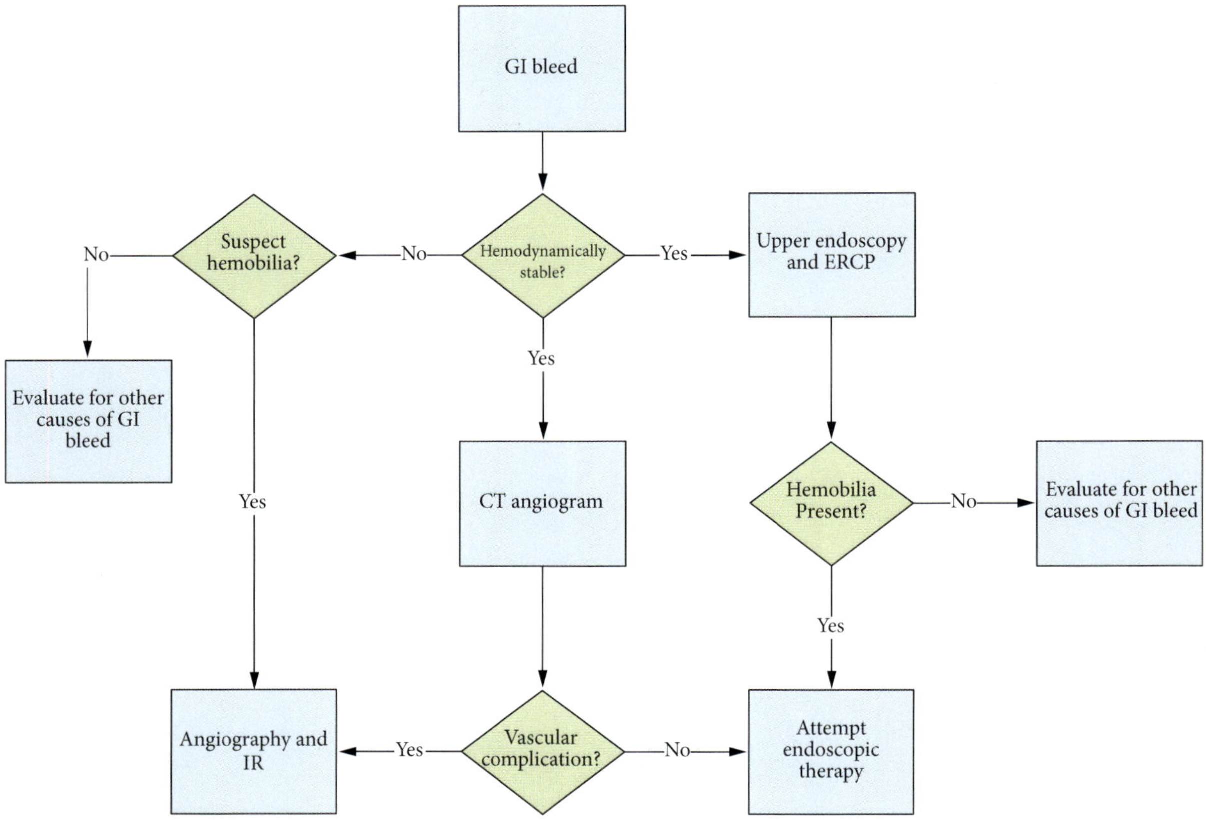

Figure 5: Proposed algorithm for the diagnosis of hemobilia. Vascular complications include hepatic artery aneurysms, pseudoaneurysms, and cholangiovenous or arterioductal fistulae.

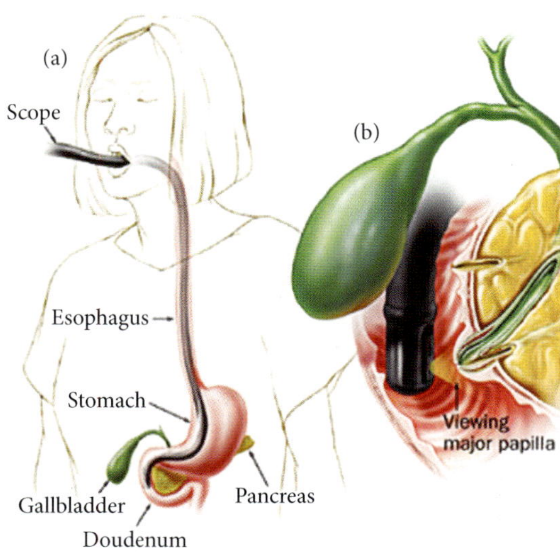

Figure 6: Endoscopic retrograde cholangiopancreatography (ERCP). (a) Schematic of duodenoscope trajectory to reach the major duodenal papilla. (b) Positioning and vantage point of duodenoscope viewing the major duodenal papilla [68].

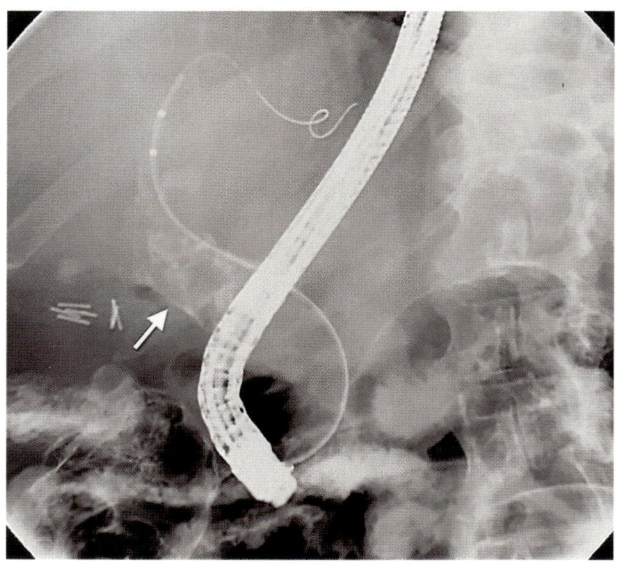

Figure 7: ERCP demonstrating radiolucent filling defects in a dilated CBD in a patient found to have hemobilia. This fluoroscopic image obtained during ERCP is from a patient with recent fine-needle aspiration (FNA) of a malignant-appearing pancreatic head mass one day prior. The radiolucent filling defects throughout the common hepatic duct and more proximal perihilar ducts in the context of recent FNA are consistent with hemobilia.

The presence of gallbladder filling defects does not necessary mean that the gallbladder is the source of bleeding, as blood can enter the gallbladder retrograde from the biliary ducts. If endoscopic ultrasound (EUS) is available, it may be used as an adjunctive noninvasive method to evaluate

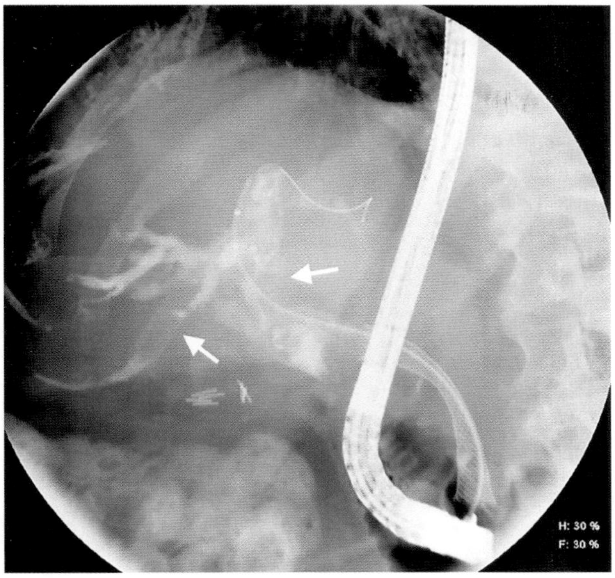

FIGURE 8: ERCP with therapeutic placement of self-expanding metallic stent (SEMS). A biliary SEMS has been placed during ERCP, which helps mitigate both bleeding and biliary obstruction (from large-volume hemobilia as well as the malignant pancreatic head mass).

vascular aneurysms and blood clots within the biliary ducts when ERCP findings are equivocal [36–38]. EUS can also be used to detect portal biliopathy-related bleeding (e.g., in the context of portal hypertension with intra- or paracholedochal varices [30].

5.3. Angiography. Although formal angiography is no longer used as first-line study, it remains the gold standard for both diagnosis and treatment of hemobilia in most settings. If the bleeding vessel has not already been identified on noninvasive imaging, the first angiographic study should be a celiac arteriogram with delayed phase imaging to visualize both the hepatic arteries and the portal vein. It is necessary to ensure that the portal vein is patent prior to hepatic artery embolization because the liver is supplied by both the hepatic artery and the portal vein; performing hepatic artery embolization when the portal vein is thrombosed or otherwise obstructed could potentially cause significant hepatic ischemia. This is especially important in patients who are liver transplant recipients as the transplanted liver does not receive as much blood from the portal vein as a native liver, thus making it more dependent on the hepatic artery for its blood supply. Patients with cirrhosis and hereditary hemorrhagic telangiectasia involving the liver are also at risk for hepatic ischemia for the same reason [39].

Any percutaneous drains should be removed over a guidewire (to maintain access) so as to disable the potential tamponade effect from the drain and allow for blood to flow and be visualized angiographically. Evaluation of the vasculature typically progresses in a stepwise fashion; if celiac arteriography does not reveal a clear source, then the catheter should be advanced and arteriographies of both the left and right hepatic arteries should be performed. If no branches of the celiac or hepatic arteries are identified as the source, then the superior mesenteric artery should be interrogated for potential accessory hepatic arteries. Contrast extravasation into the biliary tree, peripheral arterial truncation, arterial transection, pseudoaneurysms, and arterioportal fistula can all also suggest arterial injury [40].

5.4. Other Diagnostic Modalities. Lesser used methods include magnetic resonance cholangiopancreatography (MRCP), abdominal ultrasound (US), and surgical exploration. MRCP is a noninvasive alternative to ERCP but lacks the therapeutic options that ERCP offers and also requires more time for image acquisition. Abdominal US has been used to evaluate the presence of blood within the gallbladder, but its diagnostic effectiveness is limited due to its limited ability to visualize the biliary ducts, particular the distal CBD and in patients with truncal obesity. Surgical exploration is usually reserved as a final option in which other modalities are unable to identify or resolve the hemobilia [30].

6. Management

Management of hemobilia consists of two main objectives: (1) achieving hemostasis and (2) maintaining bile flow. The latter is important because the formation of blood clots within the biliary tract can cause complications such as obstructive jaundice, acute cholangitis, acute cholecystitis, and pancreatitis [8].

The approach to management depends on several factors, including the suspected source of bleeding (arterial versus venous bleeding), degree of hemodynamic instability, and etiology/cause (Figure 9). All patients should have a type and screen performed and be closely monitored for hemodynamic instability. Patients who present with minor hemobilia can potentially be addressed with conservative treatment, including intravenous fluids and correction of coagulopathy. Major hemobilia that causes significant hemoglobin drop or persistent bleeding typically requires endoscopic, radiologic, or, rarely, surgical intervention. Hemodynamically unstable patients should go directly to interventional radiology for hepatic angiogram and embolization or to surgery. Vasopressors may be necessary in cases of major hemobilia as part of resuscitative measures and as a bridge to therapeutic intervention.

6.1. Conservative Treatment. Minor hemobilia, which typically presents as blood-tinged output from a biliary drainage catheter, is often due to injury related to PTBD catheters and can often be treated conservatively. Exchanging a PTBD catheter with a larger sized one and adjusting its position such that the side holes of the tube are not in the same location as potential portal vein transgression sites can also help tamponade blood by increasing pressure on the walls of the bile ducts. Any underlying coagulopathies should be corrected as well. Minor hemobilia will often resolve with maturation of the surgically created tract. A tractogram or "tubogram", an imaging study where contrast is injected into the tract to visualize its course and patency, can be performed if bleeding persists or if there is impaired

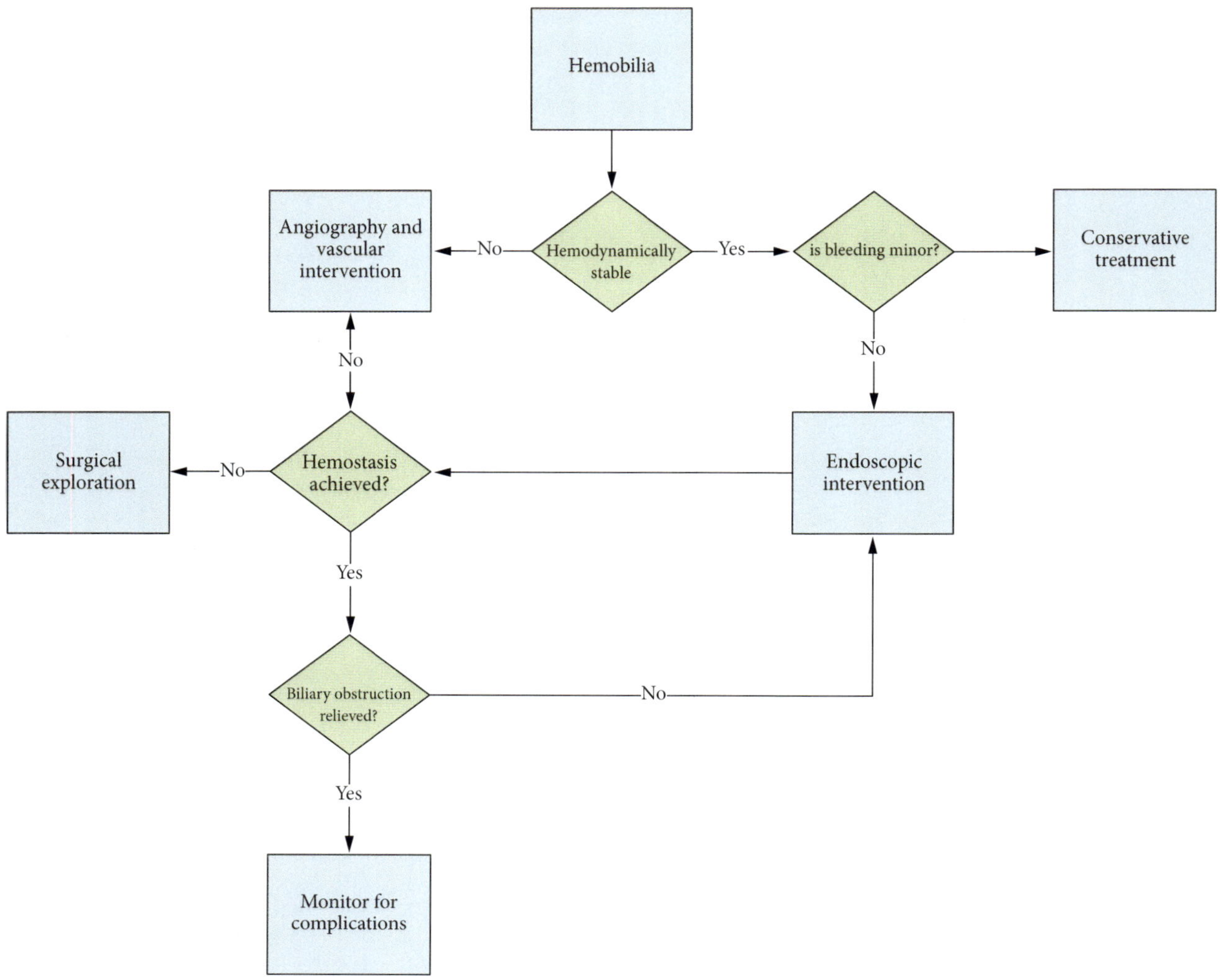

FIGURE 9: Proposed algorithm for management of hemobilia. Endoscopic intervention includes stenting, endonasal biliary drainage, and various techniques to achieve hemostasis at the ampulla.

drainage (e.g., due to obstruction from clot material). If hemobilia persists, options such as embolization of the existing percutaneous tract and creation of a new tract can be considered [39].

6.2. Advanced Endoscopic Techniques. For hemodynamically stable hemobilia without clear arterial sources of bleeding or significant vascular abnormalities on noninvasive imaging, upper endoscopy (with a duodenoscope or a clear endcap-outfitted gastroscope) and ERCP are typically the initial therapeutic procedure of choice because of its utility in concurrently managing both bleeding and biliary obstruction [41].

There are a wide variety of endoscopic techniques to achieve hemostasis; the choice of which to implement will depend on the cause (e.g., trauma), location (e.g., common hepatic duct), and source (e.g., paracholedochal vein) of hemobilia, for instance, postsphincterotomy hemobilia, which typically is a result of injury to the posterior branch of the superior pancreaticoduodenal artery (itself a branch of the gastroduodenal artery) during sphincterotomy. Management options for hemobilia in this context include spraying diluted epinephrine (1 : 10,000) over the area of hemorrhage, injection of epinephrine into the adjacent tissue, monopolar or bipolar coagulation, fibrin sealant injection, hemoclipping, balloon tamponading, and stent placement (Figure 10) [42–48]. These methods are most useful for postsphincterotomy hemobilia or in cases where the site of bleeding is distal, for example, located at the level of the papilla or ampulla. When hemobilia is from a more proximal (e.g., perihilar) bleeding source, the accessories and methods to treat the hemobilia tend to be different and include devices to extract intraductal clots, for example, extraction balloon catheters and retrieval baskets (Figures 10 and 11), followed by stent placement. One case report has also described the use of endobiliary radiofrequency ablation for hemorrhage secondary to malignant hemobilia [49].

6.2.1. Endoscopic Ultrasound-Guided Biliary Drainage Procedures (EUS-BD). ERCP-guided drainage using sphincterotomy, biliary stenting, and biliary drain placement is associated with over a 95% success rate and an adverse event rate of 5–10% [50]. The majority of complications arise to difficulties with biliary cannulation. In one study, biliary

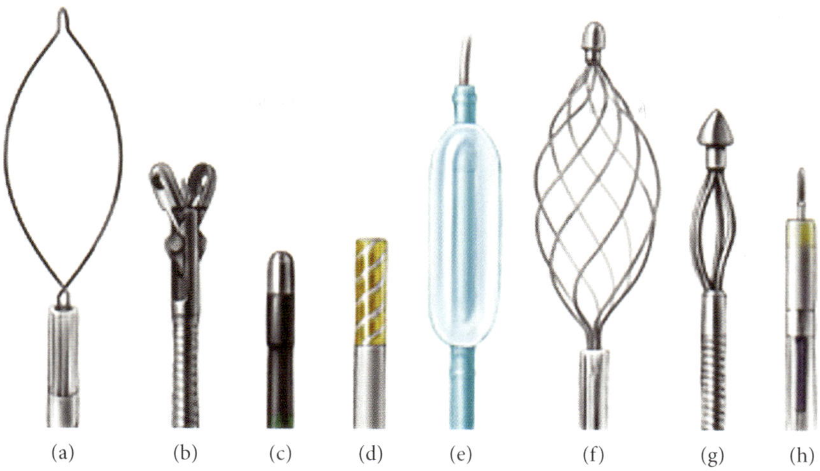

FIGURE 10: Accessory instruments relevant to hemobilia which may be used through a duodenoscope (or therapeutic gastroscope). (a) Snare, (b) biopsy forceps, (c) heater probe, (d) bipolar probe, (e) dilation balloon, (f) retrieval basket, (g) mechanical lithotriptor, and (h) sclerotherapy needle [68].

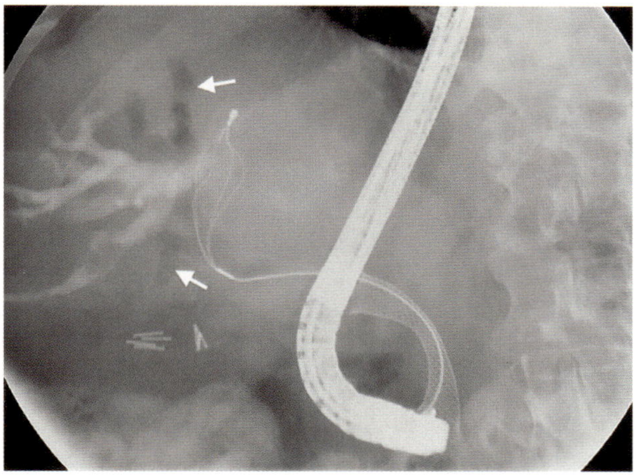

FIGURE 11: ERCP following several sweeps with flower basket demonstrating clearance of the hemobilia and resultant air cholangiogram. A self-expanding metallic stent is also noted in the biliary tree, which helps maintain luminal patency and flow. Arrows denote intraductal air, indicative of ductal patency (i.e., communication with the duodenum).

cannulation was rated as difficult in 15–22% of patients and not achievable in 7–13% of patients, mostly due to cancers of the pancreatic head causing obstruction [51]. Endoscopic drainage has similar rates of success and complications when compared to percutaneous drainage but is often preferred by patients due to its superior comfort [52].

When ERCP-guided drainage cannot be achieved, EUS-guided options for biliary drainage (EUS-BD) can be pursued as an alternative to percutaneous drainage. EUS-BD techniques include EUS-guided choledochoduodenostomy (EUS-CDS) and EUS-guided hepaticogastrostomy (EUS-HGS). When combined with stenting, these procedures are associated with a 90% success rate, and an adverse event rate of 8–25% [23, 24]. The procedure, however, is highly operator dependent and may require specialized training in EUS.

6.2.2. Biliary Stenting. The use of biliary stents merits additional discussion. Stents have been shown to achieve immediate hemostasis in certain cases and work by creating a tamponade effect on the bile wall while maintaining luminal patency and thus bile flow. It can act as salvage therapy when other methods fail and as a bridge to more permanent therapy through interventional radiology or surgery [53]. Both metal and plastic stents has been used successfully for hemobilia resulting from sphincterotomy, ductal dilation for biliary stenosis, fine-needle aspiration (e.g., pancreatic), bile duct biopsy, and malignancy, among other causes. Fully covered self-expanding metallic stents (FCSEMs) appear to have better tamponade and patency and have thus largely supplanted plastic stents when and where available [53–56]. Newer lumen-apposing biflanged FCSEMSs can be used to mitigate the risk of stent migration but at an increased risk of perforation during insertion [57].

Another type, the biodegradable biliary stent, has been proposed for use in hemobilia, but it has only been studied in patients with biliary strictures following hepaticojejunostomy procedures thus far (thereby potentially avoiding the need for cumbersome repeat ERCP); however, the long-term ductal patency after the use of biodegradable stents has not been studied yet [58]. Stenting can also be performed in conjunction with other methods; for example, balloon tamponade can be performed by inserting a biliary dilation balloon catheter into the common bile duct as a temporizing measure until blood flow has slowed adequately enough to permit stent placement as a more durable treatment [45]. In addition, endoscopic nasobiliary drainage can help treat hemobilia, though it is not commonly performed any longer (primarily due to the associated discomfort) and is mainly limited to postliver transplantation patients. An advantage to nasobiliary drainage is that it enables monitoring of bleeding, irrigation of the bile duct, and follow-up cholangiograms without a need for a repeat endoscopy; the same applies to percutaneous biliary drains [36, 59]. When drainage alone is inadequate, infusions of thrombolytic agents directly into the biliary tree via a drain have been described to dissolve biliary blood clots, though this technique requires validation before it can be widely recommended [44].

6.3. Transcatheter Arterial Embolization. As the cause of hemobilia has shifted away from traumatic to iatrogenic over the years, radiologic intervention has become the gold standard for both diagnosis and management of persistent or hemodynamically unstable hemobilia. Angiography with transcatheter arterial embolization (TAE) should be considered as the initial therapy of choice if noninvasive imaging shows significant arterial extravasation, the presence of large arterial aneurysms or pseudoaneurysms, presence of arteriobiliary fistulae, and/or intrahepatic or extrahepatic vascular lesions. The success rate of TAE has been reported to be as high as 80% to 100% [60, 61]. TAE should be avoided, however, in patients with liver allografts, cirrhosis with concurrent shock, and portal vein thrombosis given that these patients have compromised collateral blood flow from the portal vein, as a result of which TAE can lead to ischemic liver injury [30]. Such patients may benefit from arterial stenting (as a tamponading measure) instead.

Once the bleeding site has been identified angiographically, superselection of the injured artery via threading of a microcatheter to the target area is performed, followed by embolization using coils. Coiling should be deployed in a distal-to-proximal fashion to ensure that no back bleeding occurs via intrahepatic arterial collaterals [39]. Pseudoaneurysms should be embolized with coils from the two ends to reduce the risk of enlarging the aneurysm. Alternatives to coils include embolization with Gelfoam, PVA particles, and liquid embolic agents such as n-BCA, Onyx, or thrombin. There have also been case reports of percutaneous injection of thrombin into pseudoaneurysms under ultrasound guidance [62]. The method of embolization depends on the anatomy of the hepatic arteries, presence of vasospasms, tortuosity of vessels, and operator/center experience. For instance, liquid embolic agents may be helpful in patients with tortuous vessels or when there are several smaller feed into an aneurysm but require experienced radiologists due to the risk of spilling the agent and causing embolization of nontarget arteries or the biliary ducts [63].

If selective embolization of the bleeding artery cannot be performed, nonselective embolization of the left or right hepatic artery may be performed. In patients who are hemodynamically unstable, embolization of the main hepatic artery can be performed if the patient is a poor surgical candidate, though recognizing the increased risk of liver necrosis [39]. It is currently not recommended to empirically embolize any hepatic arteries if no bleeding source is detected due to this very risk, even with patent portal veins. Furthermore, because the bile ducts are supplied primary by the hepatic arteries rather than the portal vein, there is a risk of biliary ischemia and resultant multifocal strictures [7].

Complications of TAE include hepatic abscesses, postembolization syndrome, hyperaminotransaminasemia, hepatic ischemia, and hepatic infarction or rarely failure [35]. A study of 72 patients who underwent TAE showed that 55 experienced hepatic ischemia evidenced by transiently elevated serum liver enzymes, while 3 experienced focal hepatic infarcts in the areas corresponding to the embolized arterial branches [61].

6.4. Vascular Stenting. An alternative to embolization, as alluded to earlier, is the placement of a covered stent across the site of vascular injury. Stenting has the advantage of preserving flow through the artery, which may be beneficial if not crucial in patients with liver transplants or compromised portal vein flow. The diameter of most hepatic vessels is similar to the size of coronary vessels, making coronary stents ideal for this application. Stent diameter should be slightly oversized by about 10–20% of the diameter of the target vessel and extend approximately 10 mm to either side/end of the site of injury to ensure proper tamponade. There are also new flow-directing stents that reduces flow across the stents into pseudoaneurysms while preserving laminar flow [64, 65].

6.5. Surgery. Surgical intervention is rarely necessary and usually reserved for failed endoscopic, endovascular, and/or percutaneous therapies. However, it is a first line if pseudoaneurysms are infected or if they are compressing other vascular structures. Surgery may also be indicated if cholecystitis is present, among other uncommon scenarios. Options for surgery include hepatic artery ligation, pseudoaneurysm excision, or hepatic segmentectomy/lobectomy with the potential for concurrent cholecystectomy if cholecystitis is present or the gallbladder neck is involved. Although surgery has a high success rate of up to >90%, it is also associated with a high mortality of up to 10% [7].

6.6. Managing Complications. Complications that arise from hemobilia should be managed as they would be in any other scenario. For example, cholecystitis should be treated with early cholecystectomy, as it carries a high mortality rate with rates of gallbladder perforation between 2–15% [66]. Acute pancreatitis is another complication that can occur due to obstruction of the ampulla or more proximal main pancreatic duct by blood clots and reverse flow of blood into the pancreatic ducts and should be managed medically and in some instances by ERCP. Biliary strictures can form following hepatic artery embolization because the vascular supply for the biliary tree comes mostly from the hepatic artery and these will generally require treatment with endoscopic or percutaneous balloon dilation [7].

7. Conclusion

Hemobilia is an unusual but important cause of GI bleeding and most commonly due to hepatopancreatobiliary tract procedures, regional trauma, and malignancy. CT angiography and endoscopy/ERCP have become common initial diagnostic testing modalities due to their versatility in excluding other causes of bleeding, low contrast requirement, and relative safety. Most cases of minor hemobilia can be treated conservatively or with minimally invasive endoscopic management. Major hemobilia which is refractory to conservative measures or leading to hemodynamic instability should be managed by interventional radiology in conjunction with endoscopy/ERCP. While TAE is a mainstay, vascular stenting has gained traction as an alternative to arterial embolization due to the preservation of hepatic arterial blood supply. Surgery is typically reserved as a last resort due to its high mortality rate and invasive nature. Although the gold standard for management remains angiography, with new technologies and techniques such as advanced endoscopic procedures, endoscopy has become an attractive alternative for both the diagnosis and treatment of hemobilia.

Authors' Contributions

Rani Berry, James Han, and James H. Tabibian acquired the images; Rani Berry and James Han drafted the manuscript; James H. Tabibian provided supervision and critical revision of the manuscript.

References

[1] J. Parekh and C. U. Corvera, "Hemorrhagic cholecystitis," *Archives of Surgery*, vol. 145, no. 2, pp. 202–204, 2010.

[2] S. W. Merrell and P. D. Schneider, "Hemobilia–evolution of current diagnosis and treatment," *The Western Journal of Medicine*, vol. 155, no. 6, pp. 621–625, 1991.

[3] H. Quincke, "Ein Fall von Aneurysma der Leberarterie," *Berl Klin Wochenschr*, vol. 30, pp. 349–352, 1871.

[4] P. Sandblom, "Hemobilia," *The Surgical Clinics of North America*, vol. 53, no. 5, pp. 1191–1201, 1973.

[5] J. Yoshida, P. E. Donahue, and L. M. Nyhus, "Hemobilia: review of recent experience with a worldwide problem," *The American Journal of Gastroenterology*, vol. 82, no. 5, pp. 448–453, 1987.

[6] M. H. A. Green, R. M. Duell, C. D. Johnson, and N. V. Jamieson, "Haemobilia," *British Journal of Surgery*, vol. 88, no. 6, pp. 773–786, 2001.

[7] S. Devakumar Murugesan, J. Sathyanesan, A. Lakshmanan et al., "Massive hemobilia: a diagnostic and therapeutic challenge," *World Journal of Surgery*, vol. 38, no. 7, pp. 1755–1762, 2014.

[8] R. Navuluri, "Hemobilia," *Seminars in Interventional Radiology*, vol. 33, no. 4, pp. 324–331, 2016.

[9] P. P. Goffette and P.-F. Laterre, "Traumatic injuries: imaging and intervention in post-traumatic complications (delayed intervention)," *European Radiology*, vol. 12, no. 5, pp. 994–1021, 2002.

[10] H. Bismuth, "Hemobilia," *The New England Journal of Medicine*, vol. 288, no. 12, pp. 617–619, 1973.

[11] G. C. Gurakuqi, V. Stadlbauer, H. R. Portugaller, C. Högenauer, M. Trauner, and R. E. Stauber, "Fatal hemobilia resulting from an iatrogenic arteriobiliary fistula as a rare complication of transjugular liver biopsy," *European Journal of Gastroenterology & Hepatology*, vol. 20, no. 1, pp. 83–86, 2008.

[12] F. Piccinino, E. Sagnelli, G. Pasquale et al., "Complications following percutaneous liver biopsy: a multicentre retrospective study on 68 276 biopsies," *Journal of Hepatology*, vol. 2, no. 2, pp. 165–173, 1986.

[13] H.-B. Zhou, "Hemobilia and other complications caused by percutaneous ultrasound-guided liver biopsy," *World Journal of Gastroenterology*, vol. 20, no. 13, pp. 3712–3715, 2014.

[14] G. M. Rivera-Sanfeliz, O. S. A. Assar, J. M. LaBerge et al., "Incidence of important hemobilia following transhepatic biliary drainage: left-sided versus right-sided approaches," *Cardiovascular and Interventional Radiology*, vol. 27, no. 2, pp. 137–139, 2004.

[15] N. Fidelman, A. I. Bloom, R. K. Kerlan Jr. et al., "Hepatic arterial injuries after percutaneous biliary interventions in the era of laparoscopic surgery and liver transplantation: experience with 930 patients," *Radiology*, vol. 247, no. 3, pp. 880–886, 2008.

[16] W. Dolak, F. Schreiber, H. Schwaighofer et al., "Endoscopic radiofrequency ablation for malignant biliary obstruction: a nationwide retrospective study of 84 consecutive applications," *Surgical Endoscopy*, vol. 28, no. 3, pp. 854–860, 2014.

[17] H. Rhim, H. K. Lim, Y.-S. Kim, D. Choi, and K. T. Lee, "Hemobilia after radiofrequency ablation of hepatocellular carcinoma," *Abdominal Imaging*, vol. 32, no. 6, pp. 719–724, 2007.

[18] J. González-Abraldes, E. Moitinho, J. C. García-Pagán et al., "Selective arterial embolization for life threatening hemobilia after transjugular intrahepatic portosystemic shunt placement," *Journal of Hepatology*, vol. 34, no. 1, pp. 174–176, 2001.

[19] M. Rössle, V. Siegerstetter, M. Huber, and A. Ochs, "The first decade of the transjugular intrahepatic portosystemic shunt (TIPS): state of the art," *Liver*, vol. 18, no. 2, pp. 73–89, 1998.

[20] D. Kaswala, D. Gandhi, A. Moroianu et al., "Hemobilia secondary to transjugular intrahepatic portosystemic shunt procedure: a case report," *Journal of Clinical Medicine*, vol. 1, no. 1, pp. 15–21, 2012.

[21] Y.-K. Tsou, N.-J. Liu, and Y.-Y. Jan, "Biliary obstruction caused by hemobilia after endoscopic sphincterotomy in a patient with an anomalous location of papilla of Vater," *Gastrointestinal Endoscopy*, vol. 68, no. 6, pp. 1232–1234, 2008.

[22] T. Costa Macedo, R. Maldonado, A. Valente et al., "Hemobilia in hereditary hemorrhagic telangiectasia: an unusual complication of endoscopic retrograde cholangiopancreatography," *Endoscopy*, vol. 35, no. 6, pp. 531–533, 2003.

[23] M. A. Khan, A. Akbar, T. H. Baron et al., "Endoscopic ultrasound-guided biliary drainage: a systematic review and meta-analysis," *Digestive Diseases and Sciences*, vol. 61, no. 3, pp. 684–703, 2016.

[24] K. Wang, J. Zhu, L. Xing, Y. Wang, Z. Jin, and Z. Li, "Assessment of efficacy and safety of EUS-guided biliary drainage: a systematic review," *Gastrointestinal Endoscopy*, vol. 83, no. 6, pp. 1218–1227, 2016.

[25] R. K. Dhiman, A. Behera, Y. K. Chawla, J. B. Dilawari, and S. Suri, "Portal hypertensive biliopathy," *Gut*, vol. 56, no. 7, pp. 1001–1008, 2007.

[26] B. Schlansky, J. A. Kaufman, G. Bakis, and W. E. Naugler, "Portal biliopathy causing recurrent biliary obstruction and hemobilia," *ACG Case Reports Journal*, vol. 1, no. 1, pp. 44–46, 2013.

[27] V. A. Saraswat, P. Rai, T. Kumar, S. Mohindra, and R. K. Dhiman, "Endoscopic management of portal cavernoma cholangiopathy: practice, principles and strategy," *Journal of Clinical and Experimental Hepatology*, vol. 4, Supplement 1, pp. S67–S76, 2014.

[28] M. B. Luu and D. J. Deziel, "Unusual complications of gallstones," *The Surgical Clinics of North America*, vol. 94, no. 2, pp. 377–394, 2014.

[29] M. W. Chin and R. Enns, "Hemobilia," *Current Gastroenterology Reports*, vol. 12, no. 2, pp. 121–129, 2010.

[30] S. Cathcart, J. W. Birk, M. Tadros, and M. Schuster, "Hemobilia," *Journal of Clinical Gastroenterology*, vol. 51, no. 9, pp. 796–804, 2017.

[31] J. H. Tabibian, N. Tabibian, and J. C. Aguet, "Choledochal cyst complications presenting as duodenal obstruction in an 82-year-old patient with gallbladder agenesis," *Digestive Diseases and Sciences*, vol. 54, no. 1, pp. 184–187, 2009.

[32] D. Bates, "English manuscripts of Francis Glisson (1): from anatomia hepatis (the anatomy of the liver), 1654. Andrew Cunningham," *Isis*, vol. 87, no. 2, pp. 357-358, 1996.

[33] K. P. Balsara, C. Dubash, and C. R. Shah, "Pseudoaneurysm of the hepatic artery along with common bile duct injury following laparoscopic cholecystectomy," *Surgical Endoscopy*, vol. 12, no. 3, pp. 276-277, 1998.

[34] F. Wen, Y. Dong, Z. M. Lu, Z. Y. Liu, W. Li, and Q. Y. Guo, "Hemobilia after laparoscopic cholecystectomy: imaging features and management of an unusual complication," *Surgical Laparoscopy, Endoscopy & Percutaneous Techniques*, vol. 26, no. 1, pp. e18–e24, 2016.

[35] W. Feng, D. Yue, L. ZaiMing et al., "Iatrogenic hemobilia: imaging features and management with transcatheter arterial embolization in 30 patients," *Diagnostic and Interventional Radiology*, vol. 22, no. 4, pp. 371–377, 2016.

[36] K. H. Kim and T. N. Kim, "Etiology, clinical features, and endoscopic management of hemobilia: a retrospective analysis of 37 cases," *The Korean Journal of Gastroenterology*, vol. 59, no. 4, pp. 296–302, 2012.

[37] M. A. Konerman, Z. Zhang, and C. Piraka, "Endoscopic ultrasound as a diagnostic tool in a case of obscure hemobilia," *ACG Case Reports Journal*, vol. 3, no. 4, article e170, 2016.

[38] A. Trakarnsanga, T. Sriprayoon, T. Akaraviputh, and T. Tongdee, "Massive hemobilia from a ruptured hepatic artery aneurysm detected by endoscopic ultrasound (EUS) and successfully treated," *Endoscopy*, vol. 42, no. S 02, pp. E340–E341, 2010.

[39] W. E. A. Saad, M. G. Davies, and M. D. Darcy, "Management of bleeding after percutaneous transhepatic cholangiography or transhepatic biliary drain placement," *Techniques in Vascular and Interventional Radiology*, vol. 11, no. 1, pp. 60–71, 2008.

[40] D. N. Srivastava, S. Sharma, S. Pal et al., "Transcatheter arterial embolization in the management of hemobilia," *Abdominal Imaging*, vol. 31, no. 4, pp. 439–448, 2006.

[41] M. Abdelhafez, V. Phillip, A. Hapfelmeier et al., "Cap assisted upper endoscopy for examination of the major duodenal papilla: a randomized, blinded, controlled crossover study (CAPPA study)," *The American Journal of Gastroenterology*, vol. 112, no. 5, pp. 725–733, 2017.

[42] K. W. Sniderman, S. S. Morse, S. Rapoport, and G. R. Ross, "Hemobilia following transhepatic biliary drainage: occlusion of an hepatoportal fistula by balloon tamponade," *Radiology*, vol. 154, no. 3, p. 827, 1985.

[43] Y. Komaki, S. Kanmura, K. Funakawa et al., "A case of hereditary hemorrhagic telangiectasia with repeated hemobilia arrested by argon plasma coagulation under direct peroral cholangioscopy," *Gastrointestinal Endoscopy*, vol. 80, no. 3, pp. 528-529, 2014.

[44] R. K. Moparty, R. D. Brown, T. J. Layden, V. Chirravuri, T. Wiley, and R. P. Venu, "Dissolution of blood clots in the biliary ducts with a thrombolytic agent infused through nasobiliary catheter," *Gastrointestinal Endoscopy*, vol. 56, no. 3, pp. 436–438, 2002.

[45] P. Bagla, T. Erim, T. Berzin, and R. Chuttani, "Massive hemobilia during endoscopic retrograde cholangiopancreatography in a patient with cholangiocarcinoma: a case report," *Endoscopy*, vol. 44, no. S 02, p. E1, 2012.

[46] P. Katsinelos, G. Paroutoglou, A. Beltsis et al., "Endoscopic hemoclip placement for postsphincterotomy bleeding refractory to injection therapy: report of two cases," *Surgical Laparoscopy, Endoscopy & Percutaneous Techniques*, vol. 15, no. 4, pp. 238–240, 2005.

[47] P. Katsinelos, J. Kountouras, G. Chatzimavroudis et al., "Endoscopic hemostasis using monopolar coagulation for postendoscopic sphincterotomy bleeding refractory to injection treatment," *Surgical Laparoscopy, Endoscopy & Percutaneous Techniques*, vol. 20, no. 2, pp. 84–88, 2010.

[48] J. W. C. Leung, F. K. L. Chan, J. J. Y. Sung, and S. C. S. Chung, "Endoscopic sphincterotomy-induced hemorrhage: a study of risk factors and the role of epinephrine injection," *Gastrointestinal Endoscopy*, vol. 42, no. 6, pp. 550–554, 1995.

[49] C. M. Linz, R. M. Modi, and S. G. Krishna, "A dual-modality approach of endobiliary radiofrequency ablation and self-expandable metal stent placement to control malignant hemobilia," *Endoscopy*, vol. 49, no. S 01, pp. E21–E22, 2017.

[50] P. Rai, C. R. Lokesh, A. Goel, and R. Aggarwal, "Endoscopic ultrasound-guided choledochoduodenostomy using partially-covered self-expandable metal stent in patients with malignant distal biliary obstruction and unsuccessful ERCP," *Endoscopy International Open*, vol. 6, no. 1, pp. E67–E72, 2018.

[51] J. Halttunen, S. Meisner, L. Aabakken et al., "Difficult cannulation as defined by a prospective study of the Scandinavian Association for Digestive Endoscopy (SADE) in 907 ERCPs," *Scandinavian Journal of Gastroenterology*, vol. 49, no. 6, pp. 752–758, 2014.

[52] K. Quencer, A. Tadros, K. Marashi et al., "Bleeding after percutaneous transhepatic biliary drainage: incidence, causes and treatments," *Journal of Clinical Medicine*, vol. 7, no. 5, p. 94, 2018.

[53] M. K. Goenka, Y. Harwani, V. Rai, and U. Goenka, "Fully covered self-expandable metal biliary stent for hemobilia caused by portal biliopathy," *Gastrointestinal Endoscopy*, vol. 80, no. 6, p. 1175, 2014.

[54] K. Shinjo, H. Matsubayashi, T. Matsui et al., "Biliary hemostasis using an endoscopic plastic stent placement for uncontrolled hemobilia caused by transpapillary forceps biopsy (with video)," *Clinical Journal of Gastroenterology*, vol. 9, no. 2, pp. 86–88, 2016.

[55] J.-Y. Song, J. Moon, H. Choi et al., "Massive hemobilia following transpapillary bile duct biopsy treated by using a covered self-expandable metal stent," *Endoscopy*, vol. 46, no. S 01, pp. E161–E162, 2014.

[56] L. Barresi, I. Tarantino, D. Ligresti, G. Curcio, A. Granata, and M. Traina, "Fully covered self-expandable metal stent treatment of spurting bleeding into the biliary tract after endoscopic ultrasound-guided fine-needle aspiration of a solid lesion of the pancreatic head," *Endoscopy*, vol. 47, no. S 01, pp. E87–E88, 2015.

[57] R. Kunda, M. Pérez-Miranda, U. Will et al., "EUS-guided choledochoduodenostomy for malignant distal biliary obstruction

using a lumen-apposing fully covered metal stent after failed ERCP," *Surgical Endoscopy*, vol. 30, no. 11, pp. 5002–5008, 2016.

[58] M. E. Giménez, M. Palermo, E. Houghton et al., "Biodegradable biliary stents: a new approach for the management of hepaticojejunostomy strictures following bile duct injury. Prospective study," *ABCD. Arquivos Brasileiros de Cirurgia Digestiva (São Paulo)*, vol. 29, no. 2, pp. 112–116, 2016.

[59] T. Noro, N. Kawasaki, H. Ohdaira, R. Takizawa, N. Suzuki, and Y. Suzuki, "A new endoscopic method: percutaneous endoscopic trans-gastric biliary drainage as an option for biliary drainage," *Nihon Gekakei Rengo Gakkaishi (Journal of Japanese College of Surgeons)*, vol. 37, no. 5, pp. 937–940, 2012.

[60] T. Marynissen, G. Maleux, S. Heye et al., "Transcatheter arterial embolization for iatrogenic hemobilia is a safe and effective procedure: case series and review of the literature," *European Journal of Gastroenterology & Hepatology*, vol. 24, no. 8, pp. 905–909, 2012.

[61] S. H. Choi, D. I. Gwon, G.-Y. Ko et al., "Hepatic arterial injuries in 3110 patients following percutaneous transhepatic biliary drainage," *Radiology*, vol. 261, no. 3, pp. 969–975, 2011.

[62] A. Kumar, A. Sheikh, L. Partyka, and S. Contractor, "Cystic artery pseudoaneurysm presenting as a complication of laparoscopic cholecystectomy treated with percutaneous thrombin injection," *Clinical Imaging*, vol. 38, no. 4, pp. 522–525, 2014.

[63] B. Cagli, S. A. Tuncel, E. Sengul et al., "Hemobilia and occult cystic artery stump bleeding after a laparoscopic cholecystectomy: endovascular treatment with N-butyl cyanoacrylate," *Prague Medical Report*, vol. 112, no. 2, pp. 132–136, 2011.

[64] M. E. Krokidis and A. A. Hatzidakis, "Acute hemobilia after bilioplasty due to hepatic artery pseudoaneurysm: treatment with an ePTFE-covered stent," *Cardiovascular and Interventional Radiology*, vol. 32, no. 3, pp. 605–607, 2009.

[65] R. L. Hardman, P. Taussky, R. Kim, and R. G. O'Hara, "Post-transplant hepatic artery pseudoaneurysm treated with the pipeline flow-diverting stent," *Cardiovascular and Interventional Radiology*, vol. 38, no. 4, pp. 1043–1046, 2015.

[66] K. A. Suchniak-Mussari, B. A. Foreman, A. Sharma, T. Shah, and C. E. Dye, "Transjugular liver biopsy and the bloody mess that follows: a rare case of hemobilia and hemocholecystitis," *ACG Case Reports Journal*, vol. 3, no. 4, article e108, 2016.

[67] U. Themes, "Hemobilia and bilhemia," *Abdominal Key*May 2016. https://abdominalkey.com/hemobilia-and-bilhemia/.

[68] Johns Hopkins Department of Gastroenterology and Hepatology, "Primary sclerosing cholangitis," *Johns Hopkins Medicine*, February 2018 http://www.hopkinsmedicine.org/gastroenterology_hepatology/_pdfs/liver/primary_sclerosing_cholangitis.pdf.

5

Air Medical Transportation for Severe Acute Pancreatitis Patients over an Extra Long Distance: Is It Safe Enough?

Lin Gao,[1] Jingzhu Zhang,[1] Kun Gao,[1] Yiyuan Pan,[2] Xiaotao Qin,[3] Jie Zhang,[3] Jing Zhou,[1] Guotao Lu,[1,4] Weiqin Li,[1] and Zhihui Tong[1]

[1]*Surgical Intensive Care Unit (SICU), Department of General Surgery, Jinling Hospital, Medical School of Nanjing University, No. 305 Zhongshan East Road, Nanjing, 210002 Jiangsu, China*
[2]*Department of Intensive Care Unit, Suzhou Hospital Affiliated to Nanjing Medical University, No. 16 Baita West Road, Suzhou, 215002 Jiangsu, China*
[3]*Hope Assist Medical Assistance Service Company, No. 1111 Tower A, Chaoyang SOHO, Beijing 100020, China*
[4]*Department of Gastroenterology, Affiliated Hospital of Yangzhou University, No. 386 Hanjiang Media Road, Yangzhou, 225000 Jiangsu, China*

Correspondence should be addressed to Zhihui Tong; njzyantol@hotmail.com

Academic Editor: Piero Chirletti

Objective. Severe acute pancreatitis (SAP) patients usually develop persistent organ dysfunction which causes the majority of deaths. It is important for SAP patients to receive centralized diagnosis and treatment in an experienced tertiary center. China, as a vast country with uneven distribution of medical resources, should take advantage of air medical transportation to meet the challenge of patient transfer among different regions. The aim of this study was to evaluate the safety and effectiveness of air transport for SAP patients via extra long distance. *Methods.* This was a retrospective analysis of all air medical transportations for SAP patients admitted to Jinling Hospital from January 2010 to December 2016. The general characteristics, transportation process, and clinical outcomes of these patients were recorded, and the safety and effectiveness of air transport were evaluated. *Results.* All the 20 SAP patients were successfully transferred by chartered aircraft without any occurrence of severe transport-associated complications. The mean transport time was 5.86 hours and the average transport distance was 1530 kilometers. The majority of SAP patients got timely intervention and the ultimate mortality rate was 15%. *Conclusions.* Air medical transport appears to be safe and effective for SAP patients with vital organ dysfunctions during the extra long-distance transportation.

1. Introduction

Acute pancreatitis (AP) is a severe inflammatory disorder of the pancreas and one of the most fatal diseases of the gastrointestinal tract around the world. Recent studies showed that the annual incidence of AP varied between 13 and 45 cases per 100,000 people [1]. The majority of AP patients have a mild disease course and recover within several days; however, about 15%–20% of the patients will develop severe AP (SAP) [2–4]. Persistent organ failure poses the greatest threat and causes the majority of mortality cases in SAP patients [5]. In view of the low incidence and the complicated pathophysiological process of SAP, the Japanese guideline recommends that severe cases should be transferred immediately to a facility capable of providing treatment for SAP [6].

The Jinling Hospital SAP treatment center was established in 1997. In recent years, more than 300 SAP patients have been admitted each year and till now, more than 2000 cases have been admitted to our center of whom the mortality rate was below 5%. Our center is located in eastern China, and the extra long distance (in this study defined as over 1000 kilometers) between our center and the remote areas has hindered these remote SAP patients to get timely and effective treatment measures. Hence, it is of great challenge to transfer these SAP patients to our center safely and quickly. In the past, patients were mainly transported by ambulances which had the disadvantages of long travel time, limited onboard equipment and bumpy ride. These problems restricted the application of ambulances in SAP patient transportation over an extra long distance [7]. It usually took ambulances more than a whole day to transfer patients to our center which was extremely dangerous for SAP patients, hence most of them had to give up transportation. A few transferred patients had worsened disease conditions because of the lack of monitoring of close vital signs and lack of organ function support during the distant transport process.

The aforementioned dilemma had stimulated the growing need for air medical transport. Air medical transport in China had been put into practice for decades and experienced accelerating demand in the past few years [8]. There is no doubt that air transfer has created a new era for the transportation of SAP patients. However, controversy has existed for a long time regarding the safety, benefits, and potential risks of air transportation [9, 10]. Although SAP patients often benefit from transfer to tertiary care for services not available at the sending hospital, the risks of adverse clinical outcomes associated with transport and aviation accidents cannot be ignored [11]. Hence, it is of great importance to assess the safety and explore the benefits and risks of air transport for SAP patients over an extra long distance, considering the lack of relevant literature reported until now.

In the present study, we aimed to analyze cases that underwent air medical transport between 2010 and 2016 in terms of general characteristics, transportation process, transport-related data, and clinical outcomes, as well as to assess the safety of air transfer for SAP patients over an extra long distance.

2. Materials and Methods

This was a retrospective analysis of all air medical transportations for SAP patients admitted to Jinling Hospital, Medical School of Nanjing University from January 2010 to December 2016. Diagnosis and disease severity classification of AP were according to the Revised Atlanta Classification [12]. Inclusion criteria were SAP patients with single or multiple persistent organ failure (>48 h) and with transport distances over 1000 kilometers. It was important to note that all transport of patients was carried out by professional medical transfer organizations, after a request from the next of kin or legal guardian of the patient. This study was approved by the institutional review board of Jinling Hospital. Our study was carried out in accordance with the relevant guidelines and regulations of our hospital and oral informed consent was obtained from all participants. The disease-associated data before and during the transport were recorded and provided by the professional medical staff from Hope Assist Medical Assistance Service Company, and disease-associated data after the transport were recorded in our treatment center.

2.1. Definition

2.1.1. Systemic Complication. The definitions of organ dysfunction were based on a score of ≥2 in the sequential organ failure assessment (SOFA) scoring system. According to the Third International Consensus Definitions for Sepsis and Septic Shock (Sepsis-3), sepsis should be defined as a life-threatening organ dysfunction caused by a dysregulated host response to infection [13].

2.1.2. Local Complications. Apart from the common complications (acute peripancreatic fluid collection, pancreatic pseudocycts, acute necrotic collection, and walled-off necrosis) which involve the pancreas itself, in this study, we focused more on severe AP-induced complications, including intra-abdominal hemorrhage, gastrointestinal fistula and portal vein thrombosis [12].

2.1.3. Transfer Time and Transfer Distance. Transfer time was defined as time from actual delivery of the patient at the sending hospital to handing over to the primary medical team at our hospital. Transfer distance was defined as the sum of ground transportation distance from the sending hospital to the discharge disposition in the airport, intercity flight distance, and ground transportation distance from the admitting disposition in the airport to our hospital.

2.1.4. Vital Signs of Transferred SAP Patients before and after Transport. Vital signs of transferred SAP patients before and after transport (Table 1) refer to the vital signs and blood gas analysis recorded before departing from the sending hospital and the vital signs and blood gas analysis recorded immediately after arriving at our hospital.

2.1.5. The Definition of Abnormal Events of Vital Signs during Transfer (Table 2). The baseline values of vital signs refer to the values recorded for the first time during the transfer process. The heart rate, respiratory rate, blood pressure, and blood oxygen saturation were automatically measured by the ECG monitor, the axillary temperature was measured by the thermometer, and the urine volume per hour was collected by the sterile catheter and recorded by the nurse.

2.1.6. Increased Body Temperature. Axillary temperature was measured every half hour and if the temperature of a single measurement increased by 0.5 degrees compared to the baseline value, it was defined as an increased in body temperature.

2.1.7. Heart Rate Elevation. If the heart rate was elevated by 20% compared to the baseline value and lasted longer than 10 min, it was defined as heart rate elevation.

2.1.8. Tachypnea. If the respiratory rate was elevated by 5 times per minute compared to the baseline value and lasted longer than 10 min, it was defined as tachypnea.

2.1.9. Decreased Blood Pressure. Noninvasive blood pressure was measured every 10 minutes, and if the average arterial pressure dropped below 65 mmHg for two consecutive measurements, it was defined as decreased blood pressure.

2.1.10. Decreased Blood Oxygen Saturation. If oxygen saturation dropped by 5% compared to the baseline value and lasted longer than 5 minutes, it was defined as decreased blood oxygen saturation.

Table 1: Vital signs of transferred severe acute pancreatitis patients before and after transport.

Variables, number (%)	Before transfer	After transfer	P value
Heart rate			0.749
≤120 beats/min	12 (60)	11 (55)	
>120 beats/min	8 (40)	9 (45)	
Blood pressure			0.788
Without vasopressors	8 (40)	7 (35)	
Norepinephrine ≤ 0.1 μg/kg/min	7 (35)	6 (30)	
Norepinephrine > 0.1 μg/kg/min	5 (25)	7 (35)	
PaO_2/FiO_2 (mmHg)			0.746
>200	4 (20)	4 (20)	
100–200 and mechanically ventilated	12 (60)	10 (50)	
<100 and mechanically ventilated	4 (20)	6 (30)	
Urine volume			1
Anuria	12 (60)	12 (60)	
≤40 ml/h	6 (30)	6 (30)	
>40 ml/h	2 (10)	2 (10)	
pH			0.709
>7.45	4 (20)	3 (15)	
7.35–7.45	13 (65)	12 (60)	
<7.35	3 (15)	5 (25)	
Lactate			0.744
≤2	13 (65)	12 (60)	
>2	7 (35)	8 (40)	
$PaCO_2$			0.926
>45	4 (20)	5 (25)	
35–45	12 (60)	11 (55)	
<35	4 (20)	4 (20)	

Categorical variables were presented as absolute numbers and percentages.

Table 2: Transport-associated data of the severe acute pancreatitis patients transferred to our center.

Variables	All SAP patients
Transport time (hours)	5.86 (1.19)
Transport distance (kilometers)	1530 (433)
Alterations in vital signs	
Increased body temperature	4 (20)
Heart rate elevation	3 (15)
Decreased blood pressure	2 (10)
Tachypnea	4 (20)
Decreased blood oxygen saturation	1 (5)
Decreased urine volume	2 (10)

Data are presented as mean ± standard deviation for continuous variables and absolute numbers and percentages for categorical variables.

2.1.11. Decreased Urine Volume. If the urine volume was decreased by 10 ml/h compared to the baseline value for two consecutive measurements, it was defined as decreased urine volume (except for AKI patients with anuria).

2.2. Aircraft. Small fixed-wing and rotary aircraft (see Figure 1) available for the transfer of patients included the following types: HAWKER800, Alouette III; L-3; Astar; Twin Star; BO-105; AgustaWestland A109; BK-117; Bell 222; Dolphin; and S-76. Most of them can accommodate one doctor, one nurse, one accompanying person, and the patient on a stretcher (see Figure 2).

2.3. Equipment. Standard equipment for air medical transport includes transfer facilities (stretcher, air cushion, cervical collar, fracture-fixing apparatus, etc.), medical monitoring instruments (electrocardiogram monitor, pulse oximeter, etc.), airway management devices (oxygen supply equipment, medical ventilator, electric-drive phlegm-sucker, tracheal intubation kit, endotracheal tube, oropharyngeal airway, tracheotomy kit, atomization inhalation kit, etc.), vascular access devices (intravenous needle, bagged intravenous infusion, etc.), surgical treatment devices (bandage, dressing, gloves, masks, minor surgery kit, simple disinfection kit, etc.) and pregnancy- and delivery-associated devices (fetal Doppler monitor, delivery kit, neonatal rescue kit, etc.). An intra-aortic balloon pump (IABP), cardiac pacing device, and cardiac electric defibrillator are also prepared according to specific circumstances. A satellite phone is used to communicate with outside world while on the aircraft. All equipment is guaranteed to be compact, portable, and noninterfering with radio communications according to aviation standards.

2.4. Medicine in Storage. Standard medications for air medical transport include ATP-adenosine 20 mg/2 ml; adenosine 6 mg/2 ml; amiodarone 150 mg/3 ml; atropine 5 mg/10 ml; metoprolol 5 mg/5 ml; diltiazem 10 mg; dexamethasone 5 mg/1 ml; diazepam 10 mg/2 ml; diphenhydramine 50 mg/1 ml; dopamine 200 mg/5 ml; furosemide 20 mg/2 ml; 50% glucose 20 ml; heparin 1000 units/1 ml; hyoscine 20 mg/ml; KCL 1.5 g/10 ml; labetalol 25 mg/5 ml; lignocaine 100 mg/5 ml; metoclopramide 10 mg/2 ml; nitroglycerin 10 mg/10 ml; naloxone HCL 0.4 mg; normal saline 30 ml for injection; omeprazole 40 mg; paracetamol 250 mg/suppository; phenobarbital, 65 mg/ml or 130 mg/ml; salbutamol 0.5 mg/ml; sterile water, 30 ml for injection; tramadol 50 mg; terbutaline, 1 mg/1 ml; and verapamil, 5 mg/2 ml.

2.5. Procedure of Air Medical Transport. According to the flowchart developed by us to guide the transfer process of SAP patients (Figure 3), firstly, it is important to assess the patient condition and if the patient is in an unstable condition, necessary resuscitation measures should be provided. Then, the necessity for interhospital transfer needs to be assessed. When the resources at the current hospital are inadequate to address the patient's needs and the benefits of the transfer outweigh the risks, the patient had better be transferred to more capable hospitals. Afterwards, responsible doctors at the current hospital need to contact the receiving hospital and obtain informed consent from the family.

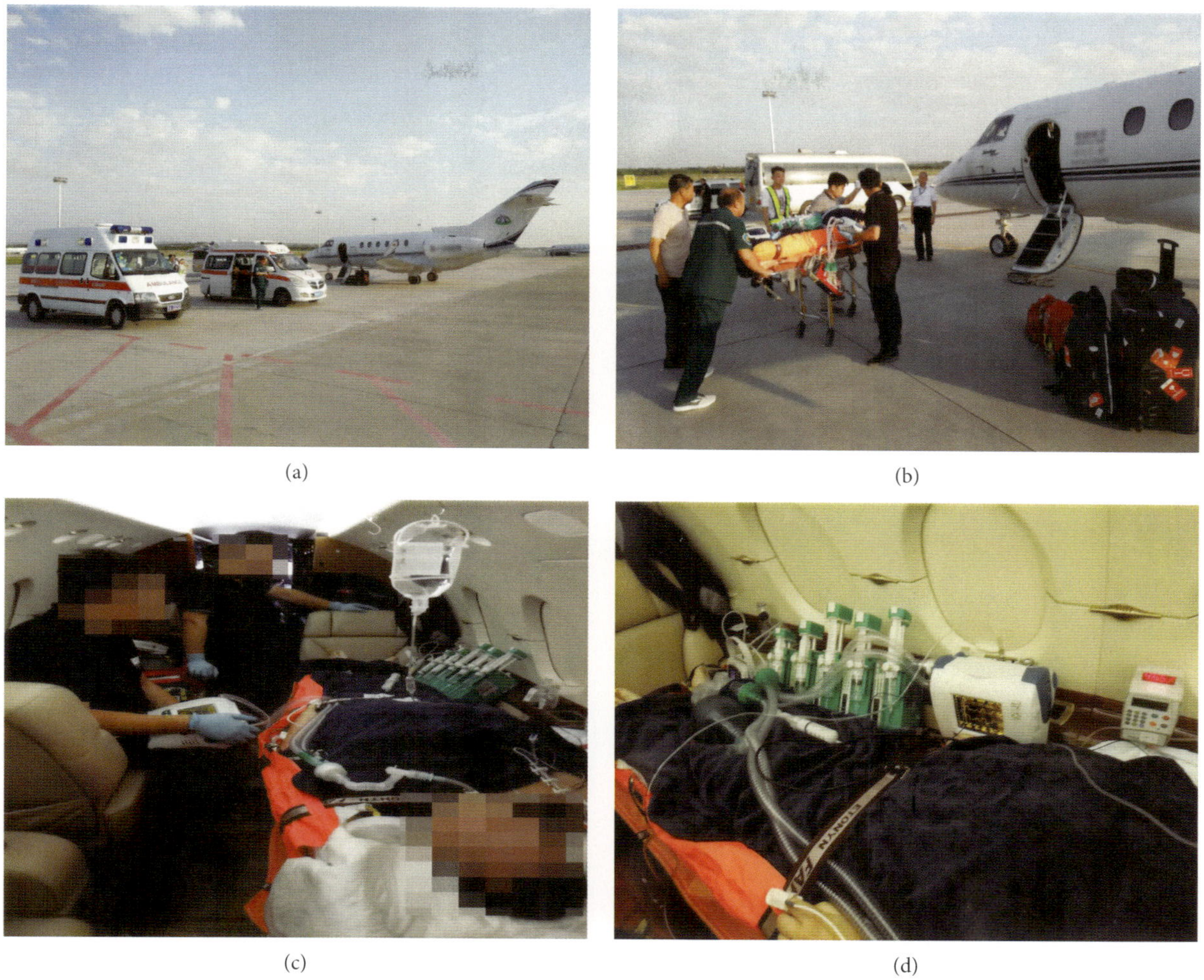

Figure 1: The emergency air medical transport of severe acute pancreatitis patients.

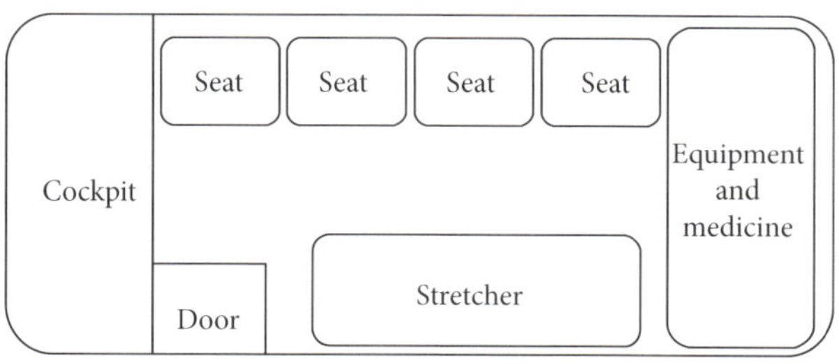

Figure 2: The general customized arrangement of an eight-seat chartered aircraft for medical transport. It can accommodate one doctor, one nurse, one accompanying person, and the patient on a stretcher.

What's more, inclusion into the flight line should be applied for in advance and approval from the China Air Force command should be obtained. If all goes according to plan, the transport process could be initiated as soon as possible and necessary medical records should be maintained among the transfer process.

2.6. Statistical Analysis. The SPSS 22.0 statistical software package (IBM Analytics, Armonk, NY) was used for statistical analyses. Data are presented as mean ± standard deviation (SD) for continuous variables and absolute numbers and percentages for categorical variables. Student's *t*-test or Mann–Whitney test was used for analyzing continuous variables and the Chi-square test was used for analyzing categorical variables.

3. Results

From January 2010 to December 2016, a total of 29 patients with SAP were transferred by air medical transportation to our SAP treatment center. They included 6 patients who were excluded for the utilization of air transport vehicles other than chartered aircraft (4 patients transferred by the stretchers in the commercial flights, 2 patients transferred by helicopters), 1 patient who was excluded because the transport distance was less than 1000 kilometers, and 2 other patients who were excluded due to the disease severity which was moderately severe AP. Finally, 20 SAP patients were included in our study. Their baseline characteristics and clinical features are shown in Table 3. The mean age of the patients was 42 years (range 23–72 years). 6 (30%) of these were women and 14 (70%) were men. The etiologies of AP are as follows: gallstone in 8 (40%) patients, hypertriglyceridemia in 10 (50%) patients,

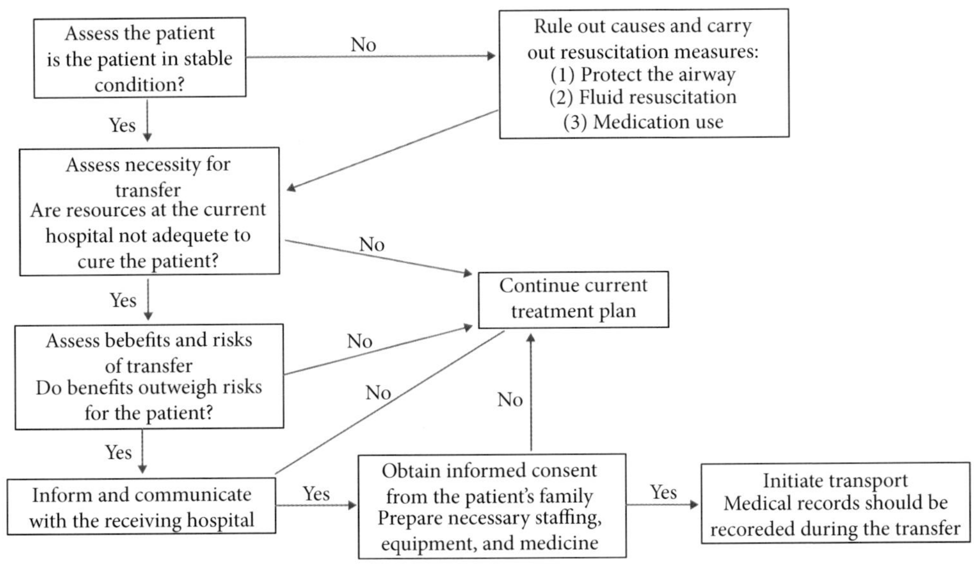

FIGURE 3: The flowchart to guide the transfer process of severe acute pancreatitis patients.

alcohol abuse in 1 (5%) patient, and trauma in 1 (5%) patient. The average body mass index was 26.8 (range 21.3–36.1), the average Acute Physiology and Chronic Health Evaluation II score was 17.1 (range 6–27), the average Sequential Organ Failure Assessment score was 6.2 (range 2–9), and the average Balthazar CT score was 8.5 (range 4–10). The mean time interval from pancreatitis onset to transportation was 27.6 days (range 8–66 days). All 20 (100%) patients were defined as severe AP on the basis of the severity of AP according to the Revised Atlanta Classification. All the 20 patients developed local or systemic complications before transportation. The most common systemic complications were acute respiratory distress syndrome (ARDS) and acute kidney injury (AKI). 16 (80%) patients suffered from ARDS and received mechanical ventilation, 18 (90%) patients developed AKI and needed renal replacement treatment, and 12 (60%) patients suffered from shock and were administrated vasoactive drugs. According to the updated Sepsis 3.0 definition, sepsis is defined as an infection plus a SOFA score ≥ 2; hence, the occurrence rate of sepsis in the 20 patients was 100%. As for severe AP-associated local complications, infected pancreatic necrosis was observed in all 20 (100%) patients, and intra-abdominal hemorrhage was observed in 6 (30%) patients. 2 (10%) patients were diagnosed with portal thrombosis and 3 (15%) patients developed gastrointestinal fistula during their disease course before transport. In terms of the treatment for infected pancreatic necrosis, 13 (65%) patients underwent invasive drainage, and 8 (40%) patients were performed with surgical operations. Sedative agents and analgesics were used in the majority of the transferred patients.

Transport-associated data and abnormal conditions that occurred during the transfer were recorded in Table 2. The average time spent for transport was 5.86 hours (range 3.5–8 hours) and the average transport distance was 1530 kilometers (range 1000–2300 kilometers). During the transport process, important medical records, for example, vital signs were monitored closely. Alterations in vital signs that occurred in the transfer process included the following: tachycardia, which happened in 3 (15%) patients and were handled with antiarrhythmic drugs discreetly; decreased blood pressure, which happened in 2 (10%) patients and vasoactive agents were applied to maintain steady blood pressure; fever, which happened in 4 (20%) patients and physical or drug cooling was used; SPO_2 reduction, which happened in 1 (5%) patient and was handled by adjusting the parameters of the mechanical ventilation; and 2 (10%) patients which showed decreased urine volume and were carefully observed.

Vital signs of transferred SAP patients before and after transport were recorded and compared in Table 1. It showed no significant alterations in vital signs between the two groups.

In terms of clinical course and outcomes (Table 4), the overall mortality rate was 15% in the 20 transferred SAP patients. The mean length of ICU stay and hospital stay were 46 days (range 8–116 days) and 65 days (range 15–175 days), respectively. During the hospitalization in our center, 20 (100%) patients developed MODS eventually and 17 (85%) patients received mechanical ventilation, 18 (90%) received renal replacement therapy, and 18 (90%) patients were managed with inotropic agents. In the management of infected pancreatic necrosis [14], 17 (85%) patients underwent percutaneous catheter drainage, then 8 (40%) patients underwent double-tube continuous negative-pressure suction, 3 (15%) patients underwent endoscopic necrosectomy, and 12 (60%) patients underwent open necrosectomy.

4. Discussion

The treatment of SAP patients is complicated and often requires multidisciplinary collaboration, which involves a gastroenterologist, general surgeon, ICU doctor, and an interventional radiologist. Furthermore, as to the SAP patients with organ dysfunction or infected pancreatic necrosis, it is vital to handle with organ function and conduct pancreatic necrotic tissue drainage or necrosectomy, which may

TABLE 3: Baseline characteristics and clinical features of the severe acute pancreatitis patients before transferred to our center.

Variables	All AP patients
Age (years)	42 (14)
Gender (male/female)	14/6
BMI	26.8 (4.11)
APACHE II score	17.1 (6.22)
SOFA score	6.2 (1.98)
CT severity index	8.5 (1.90)
Disease course when transfered (days)	27.6 (16.5)
Etiology of acute pancreatitis, number (%)	
Gallstone	8 (40)
Hypertriglyceridemia	10 (50)
Alcohol	1 (5)
Trauma	1 (5)
Other	0 (0)
Severity of AP, number (%)	
Mild	0 (0)
Moderately severe	0 (0)
Severe	20 (100)
Systemic complication, number (%)	
ARDS	16 (80)
AKI	18 (90)
Shock	12 (60)
Sepsis	20 (100)
Local complication, number (%)	
IPN	20 (100)
Intra-abdominal hemorrhage	6 (30)
Portal thrombosis	2 (10)
Gastrointestinal fistula	3 (15)
Treatment, number (%)	
Mechanical ventilation	16 (80)
CRRT	18 (90)
Vasoactive drugs	14 (70)
Sedative treatment	14 (70)
Analgesics	12 (60)
Invasive drainage	13 (65)
Operation	8 (40)

BMI—body mass index, APACHE II—acute physiology and chronic health enquiry II, SOFA—sequential organ failure assessment, CT—computed tomography, ARDS—acute respiratory distress syndrome, AKI—acute kidney injury, IPN—infected pancreatic necrosis, CRRT—continuous renal replacement therapy. Data are presented as mean ± standard deviation for continuous variables and absolute numbers and percentages for categorical variables.

not be that easy to operate for doctors from a single department [15, 16]. Hence, it is of great importance for SAP patients to be transferred to a professional and experienced treatment center to receive specialized care.

The decision to transport a critically ill patient to another medical facility is based on the careful assessment of the potential benefits of transport weighed against the risks [17, 18]. In this study, SAP patients were transported to our treatment center to obtain additional care which was not available at the sending hospital. All the 20 patients were diagnosed as IPN combined with a single or multiple persistent organ failure, as well as the presence of other severe complications, including hemorrhage and gastrointestinal fistula. After the timely and effective treatment in our center, the final in-hospital mortality rate of these patients was 15%. The transport most likely altered the management and the outcomes of the SAP patients, and there was no doubt that the majority of the patients obtained survival benefits from the transport.

TABLE 4: Clinical course and outcomes of severe acute pancreatitis patients transferred to our center.

Variables	All AP patients
IPN treatment	
PCD, number (%)	17 (85)
DCNP, number (%)	8 (40)
Endoscopic necrosectomy, number (%)	3 (15)
Open necrosectomy, number (%)	12 (60)
MODS treatment	
Mechanical ventilation	17 (85%)
Renal replacement therapy	18 (90%)
Inotropic agents	18 (90%)
Mortality, number (%)	3 (15)
Hospital duration (days)	65 (41.3)
ICU duration (days)	46 (30.6)
Cost (thousand CNY)	476 (267)

ICU—intensive care unit, IPN—infected pancreatic necrosis, PCD—percutaneous catheter drainage, DCNP—double-tube continuous negative pressure suction, MODS—multiple organ dysfunction syndrome. Data are presented as mean ± standard deviation for continuous variables and absolute numbers and percentages for categorical variables.

This was the first report to show that not only was there no air crash in 20 flights for SAP patients' transportation in six years over an extra long distance (≥1000 kilometers), but there was also no fatal transport-associated complications occurring during the transport. This demonstrated the effectiveness of patient safety and flight safety with a professional air medical transfer team. The transport of critical patients by air has become an integral part of healthcare systems [19]. Previous studies have stated that the development of effective time-critical interventions for acute disease patients, especially acute myocardial infarction and ischemic stroke, had improved the outcomes [20]. In our study, given the transport distance and the need for timely intervention, SAP patients with critical organ dysfunctions would undoubtedly benefit from the transport. There are several merits that ensure the safety and effectiveness of air transport: (1) the short time spent for the extra long-distance transport, (2) a chartered aircraft which has a relatively stable flight process compared to helicopters, (3) a mobile ICU with advanced medical equipment [21], (4) a professional transport team with experienced and high-quality personnel, and (5) a systemic and normative transport flowchart.

Critically ill patients are at increased risk of high morbidity and mortality during air transport. However, risks could be minimized and outcomes improved with careful planning, appropriate allocation of qualified personnel, and appropriate use of equipment and application of medication. During transport, it is of first priority to monitor and maintain the stability of patients' vital functions, for example, to ensure the effective ventilation of the airway and to keep blood pressure stable. Furthermore, the accompanying doctors and nurses are trained to handle emergency conditions and provide acute care needs for the patients [22].

The major risks of air transporting SAP patients are the low atmospheric pressure and gas expansion effect of flying altitude as well as the long-distance movement-related complications [23]. With the increase of flight height, the atmospheric pressure changes extremely and in the low-pressure environment, the gas stored in the gastrointestinal tract expands and causes gastrointestinal flatulence. This adverse consequence really becomes an added insult to SAP patients, which exacerbates the condition of their preexisting intra-abdominal hypertension. What make the things worse is the increase in intra-abdominal pressure that leads to limited breathing and even dyspnea, and into a vicious cycle in ARDS patients. In addition, the decrease in PiO_2 seems to be not easily tolerated by critically ill patients with limited reserves, which causes hyperventilation and tachycardia with an increase in cardiac output [24]. Hence, these adverse effects remind us to monitor and maintain the respiratory problem and intra-abdominal hypertension of SAP patients discreetly. Luckily, in our study, during the air transportation of SAP patients, none of them developed fatal transport-associated respiratory and cardiovascular complications; however, in a proportion of the patients, tachycardia, fluctuation of blood pressure, and SPO_2 reduction occurred which were handled discreetly.

Over the past decades, China has witnessed an explosive increase in interfacility air medical transport. However, despite that air transport is more likely to show its superiority in extra long-distance transfer, it has these limitations: (1) There must be airports near the hospitals involved in the transport process. (2) Inclusion into the flight line should be applied in advance. (3) It is money consuming and not covered by medical insurance in China. Despite the efficacy and safety of air medical transport, it is hard to satisfy the needs of the majority of SAP patients, hence, as for these extra long-distance transport patients, more transfer modes should be developed to complement the medical transport system.

In recent years, railway construction has been extremely rapid and complete, and China really ushered in the age of the high-speed railway system [25]. In view of the time spent for getting stuck in the airport and the super high speed of the modern railway, high-speed railway medical transport seems to be more stable, timesaving, and money saving than air transport. High-speed railway transport shows the following superior qualities of long-distance transport (>500 km): (1) Railway stations cover the majority of cities in China and is much more widespread than airports. (2) There are many trains going back and forth between two cities and it really saves a lot of time without complicated screening procedures. (3) The speed of a railway averages up to 300 km/h and it is timesaving. (4) The cost of the railway transport is extremely lower than airplanes, and is within the economical reach of most Chinese people. Hence, we have reasons to believe that the high-speed railway will be used for medical transport in the future and will undoubtedly play an important role in critically ill patients' transportation.

4.1. Limitations. Limitations of this study include the small number of SAP cases via air transport, a lack of a control group of AP patients transported by ground ambulance, as well as a lack of records and analyses of weather and traffic conditions at the time of each transfer.

In conclusion, during the extra long-distance transportation for SAP patients with vital organ dysfunctions, air medical transport appears to be an alternative choice to ensure that patients receive timely intervention and obtain better clinical outcomes.

Abbreviations

SAP: Severe acute pancreatitis
SOFA: Sequential organ failure assessment
IPN: Infected pancreatic necrosis
AKI: Acute kidney injury
ARDS: Acute respiratory distress syndrome
MODS: Multiple organ dysfunction syndrome
ICU: Intensive care unit.

Authors' Contributions

Zhihui Tong and Weiqin Li formulated the idea of the paper and supervised the research, and both authors reviewed and revised the manuscript. Lin Gao and Jingzhu Zhang performed the research and wrote the manuscript. Kun Gao and Yiyuan Pan provided comments and technical advice. Xiaotao Qin and Jie Zhang participated in preparing the figures and tables and in data analyzing. Jing Zhou and Guotao Lu revised the manuscript and provided comments. All authors reviewed the manuscript.

Acknowledgments

This work was supported by the National Natural Science Foundation of China (nos. 81570584 and 81670588) and the Key Research and Development Program Foundation of Jiangsu Province of China (nos. BE2015685 and BE2016749).

References

[1] M. M. Smits and E. J. M. van Geenen, "The clinical significance of pancreatic steatosis," *Nature Reviews Gastroenterology & Hepatology*, vol. 8, no. 3, pp. 169–177, 2011.

[2] P. G. Lankisch, M. Apte, and P. A. Banks, "Acute pancreatitis," *The Lancet*, vol. 386, no. 9988, pp. 85–96, 2015.

[3] E. Zerem, "Treatment of severe acute pancreatitis and its complications," *World Journal of Gastroenterology*, vol. 20, no. 38, pp. 13879–13892, 2014.

[4] H. G. Beger and B. M. Rau, "Severe acute pancreatitis: clinical course and management," *World Journal of Gastroenterology*, vol. 13, no. 38, pp. 5043–5051, 2007.

[5] V. A. Bendersky, M. K. Mallipeddi, A. Perez, and T. N. Pappas, "Necrotizing pancreatitis: challenges and solutions," *Clinical and Experimental Gastroenterology*, vol. Volume 9, pp. 345–350, 2016.

[6] M. Yokoe, T. Takada, T. Mayumi et al., "Japanese guidelines for the management of acute pancreatitis: Japanese guidelines 2015," *Journal of Hepato-Biliary-Pancreatic Sciences*, vol. 22, no. 6, pp. 405–432, 2015.

[7] J. Alvarado-Socarras, A. Bermon, N. Bernal, N. F. Naranjo-Estupinan, and A. J. Idrovo, "Intra-hospital mortality among neonates transported by ambulance in Colombia," *Pediatrics International*, vol. 56, no. 4, pp. 571–576, 2014.

[8] X. H. Li and J. C. Zheng, "Efficient post-disaster patient transportation and transfer: experiences and lessons learned in emergency medical rescue in Aceh after the 2004 Asian tsunami," *Military Medicine*, vol. 179, no. 8, pp. 913–919, 2014.

[9] U. Beckmann, D. M. Gillies, S. M. Berenholtz, A. W. Wu, and P. Pronovost, "Incidents relating to the intra-hospital transfer of critically ill patients. An analysis of the reports submitted to the Australian Incident Monitoring Study in Intensive Care," *Intensive Care Medicine*, vol. 30, no. 8, pp. 1579–1585, 2004.

[10] G. Bellingan, T. Olivier, S. Batson, and A. Webb, "Comparison of a specialist retrieval team with current United Kingdom practice for the transport of critically ill patients," *Intensive Care Medicine*, vol. 26, no. 6, pp. 740–744, 2000.

[11] H. G. Kreeftenberg Jr, J. J. Ligtenberg, L. G. Arnold, T. S. van der Werf, J. E. Tulleken, and J. G. Zijlstra, "Condition on arrival of transferred critically ill patients," *The Netherlands Journal of Medicine*, vol. 57, no. 5, pp. 180–184, 2000.

[12] P. A. Banks, T. L. Bollen, C. Dervenis et al., "Classification of acute pancreatitis—2012: revision of the Atlanta classification and definitions by international consensus," *Gut*, vol. 62, no. 1, pp. 102–111, 2013.

[13] M. Singer, C. S. Deutschman, C. W. Seymour et al., "The Third International Consensus Definitions for Sepsis and Septic Shock (Sepsis-3)," *JAMA*, vol. 315, no. 8, pp. 801–810, 2016.

[14] Z. Tong, L. Ke, B. Li et al., "Negative pressure irrigation and endoscopic necrosectomy through man-made sinus tract in infected necrotizing pancreatitis: a technical report," *BMC Surgery*, vol. 16, no. 1, p. 73, 2016.

[15] A. Rosenberg, E. A. Steensma, and L. M. Napolitano, "Necrotizing pancreatitis: new definitions and a new era in surgical management," *Surgical Infections*, vol. 16, no. 1, pp. 1–13, 2015.

[16] W. Jiang, Z. Tong, D. Yang et al., "Gastrointestinal fistulas in acute pancreatitis with infected pancreatic or peripancreatic necrosis: a 4-year single-center experience," *Medicine*, vol. 95, no. 14, article e3318, 2016.

[17] J. Warren, R. E. Fromm Jr., R. A. Orr, L. C. Rotello, and H. M. Horst, "Guidelines for the inter- and intrahospital transport of critically ill patients," *Critical Care Medicine*, vol. 32, no. 1, pp. 256–262, 2004.

[18] A. H. Brunsveld-Reinders, M. S. Arbous, S. G. Kuiper, and E. de Jonge, "A comprehensive method to develop a checklist to increase safety of intra-hospital transport of critically ill patients," *Critical Care*, vol. 19, no. 1, p. 214, 2015.

[19] W. L. Chen, H. P. Ma, C. H. Wu et al., "Clinical research of mortality in emergency air medical transport," *BioMed Research International*, vol. 2014, Article ID 767402, 5 pages, 2014.

[20] H. R. Andersen, T. T. Nielsen, K. Rasmussen et al., "A comparison of coronary angioplasty with fibrinolytic therapy in acute myocardial infarction," *The New England Journal of Medicine*, vol. 349, no. 8, pp. 733–742, 2003.

[21] J. M. Droogh, M. Smit, J. Hut, R. de Vos, J. J. M. Ligtenberg, and J. G. Zijlstra, "Inter-hospital transport of critically ill patients; expect surprises," *Critical Care*, vol. 16, no. 1, p. R26, 2012.

[22] J. M. Droogh, M. Smit, A. R. Absalom, J. J. Ligtenberg, and J. G. Zijlstra, "Transferring the critically ill patient: are we there yet?," *Critical Care*, vol. 19, no. 1, p. 62, 2015.

[23] "Medical aspects of transportation aboard commercial aircraft. AMA Commission on Emergency Medical Services," *JAMA*, vol. 247, no. 7, pp. 1007–1011, 1982.

[24] H. Gong Jr, "Air travel and oxygen therapy in cardiopulmonary patients," *Chest*, vol. 101, no. 4, pp. 1104–1113, 1992.

[25] Q. Hu, N. Gao, and B. Zhang, "High speed railway environment safety evaluation based on measurement attribute recognition model," vol. 2014, Article ID 470758, 10 pages, 2014.

6

Gastrointestinal Symptoms in Marfan Syndrome and Hypermobile Ehlers-Danlos Syndrome

N. Inayet,[1] J. O. Hayat,[1] A. Kaul,[2] M. Tome,[3] A. Child,[3] and A. Poullis[1]

[1]*Department of Gastroenterology, St. George's Hospital, London, UK*
[2]*Department of Rheumatology, St. George's Hospital, London, UK*
[3]*Department of Cardiology, St. George's Hospital, London, UK*

Correspondence should be addressed to N. Inayet; dr.nashiz@gmail.com

Academic Editor: Paul Enck

Objective. Marfan syndrome (MS) is a multisystem disorder caused by a mutation in FBN1 gene. It shares some phenotypic features with hypermobile Ehlers-Danlos syndrome (EDS) such as joint hypermobility. EDS is a group of inherited heterogenous multisystem disorders characterized by skin hyperextensibility, atrophic scarring, joint hypermobility, and generalized tissue fragility. Hypermobile EDS (hEDS) is thought to be the most common type. Recent studies have suggested an association between connective tissue hypermobility and functional gastrointestinal disorders (FGDs). The aim of this study is to determine the prevalence of gastrointestinal symptoms in patients with Marfan syndrome and hypermobile EDS. *Method.* Patients with a diagnosis of either MS or hEDS attending cardiology or rheumatology outpatients at our hospital were asked to complete SF36 RAND and Rome IV Diagnostic questionnaires. Questionnaires were also completed by patients who are members of Marfan Association UK. The same questionnaires were also completed by age- and gender-matched controls attending fracture clinic without existing diagnoses of MS or hEDS. *Results.* Data were collected from 45 MS patients (12 males and 33 females, age range 19–41 years, mean 28 years) and 45 hEDS patients (6 males and 39 females, age range 18–32 years, mean 24 years). None had a previous organic gastrointestinal diagnosis. The control group was matched for age and sex (18 males and 72 females, age range 18–45, mean 29 years). Both MS and hEDS groups showed a higher prevalence of abdominal symptoms compared to the control group; however, the hEDS group not only showed a higher prevalence but more frequent and severe symptoms meeting Rome IV criteria for diagnosis of FGIDs. Nearly half of the hEDS patients met the criteria for more than one FGID. The hEDS group also scored lower on quality of life (QOL) scores in comparison to either of the other groups with a mean score of 48.6 as compared to 54.2 in the Marfan group and 78.6 in the control group. *Conclusion.* FGIDs are reported in both Marfan syndrome and hypermobile Ehlers-Danlos syndrome but appear to be more common and severe in hEDS. These patients score lower on quality of life scores as well despite hypermobility being a common feature of both conditions. Further work is needed to understand the impact of connective tissue disorders on gastrointestinal symptoms.

1. Introduction

Marfan syndrome (MS) is a multisystem disorder caused by a mutation in FBN1 gene [1]. It shares some phenotypic features with hypermobile Ehlers-Danlos syndrome (EDS) such as joint hypermobility [2]. EDS is a group of inherited heterogenous multisystem disorders characterized by skin hyperextensibility, atrophic scarring, joint hypermobility, and generalized tissue fragility [3]. Hypermobile EDS (hEDS) is thought to be the most common type [4]. Recent studies have suggested an association between connective tissue hypermobility and functional gastrointestinal disorders (FGDs) [5–10].

Gastrointestinal symptoms are reported to be common in patients with hypermobility; however, much of the recent interest in this area is focused only on patients with hEDS. No previous study has compared the prevalence of gastrointestinal symptoms in patients with MS and compared to patients with hEDS. The aim of our study is to use standardised definitions for all gastrointestinal symptoms using

Diagnostic Rome IV questionnaire as well as look for the overall perception of health and well-being using RAND SF36 questionnaire. We have also investigated the use of the most commonly used medications which affect gastrointestinal function in these groups.

2. Method

Patients attending outpatients at St. George's Hospital who had an existing diagnosis of MS or hEDS were asked to complete SF36 RAND and Rome IV Diagnostic questionnaires. Some patients were recruited with the help of Marfan Association UK. All patients completed the questionnaires by themselves, either in the Outpatients Department or at home, and returned them by post.

Controls were recruited from outpatients attending the fracture clinic at St. George's Hospital, one control being recruited for each MS and hEDS patient, matched by gender and age (±10 years). Hypermobility was assessed in these controls using Beighton criteria, and scores of 4 or less were included. All patients completed the questionnaires themselves while attending clinic. No financial or other inducements were given.

All recruited subjects completed the SF36 RAND and Rome IV Diagnostic questionnaires. Additional questions regarding ethnicity, smoking and alcohol use, use of medicines, and other medical conditions were added using previously validated questionnaires. All participants were asked if they had used antisecretory/antacid therapy or laxatives, either regularly or on as required basis in the last six months. The scoring algorithm for Rome IV Diagnostic questionnaire for adults was used, and a functional gastrointestinal disorder was said to be present if the criteria were met. The presence of abdominal pain, constipation, and diarrhoea was investigated separately even if criteria for FGID were not met.

The Rome IV classification was followed for various gastrointestinal symptoms and diagnoses including the following:

(1) Oesophageal disorders (functional chest pain, functional heartburn, Globus, and functional dysphagia)

(2) Gastroduodenal disorders (functional dyspepsia, belching disorders, nausea and vomiting disorders, and rumination syndrome)

(3) Bowel disorders (irritable bowel syndrome (IBS), functional constipation, functional diarrhoea, functional abdominal bloating/distension, and unspecified functional bowel disorder)

(4) Centrally mediated abdominal pain syndrome

(5) Functional biliary pain

(6) Anorectal disorders (faecal incontinence and functional anorectal pain)

Functional chest pain was defined as retrosternal chest pain or discomfort at least weekly with no heartburn or dysphagia. Functional heartburn was defined as burning retrosternal discomfort or pain with no relief from antisecretory therapy. Globus was defined as persistent or intermittent, nonpainful sensation of a lump or foreign body in the throat with the absence of dysphagia or heartburn. Functional dysphagia was defined as sense of solid and/or liquid foods sticking, lodging, or passing abnormally through the oesophagus in the absence of organic disorders.

Functional dyspepsia was defined as postprandial fullness, early satiation, epigastric pain, or burning, severe enough to impact on usual activities or prevent finishing a regular size meal. Functional belching was defined as belching, severe enough to impact on usual activities, from the oesophagus or stomach more than 3 days a week. Nausea and vomiting disorders were defined as weekly nausea or vomiting episodes, severe enough to impact on usual activities. Rumination syndrome was defined as persistent or recurrent regurgitation of recently ingested food into the mouth with subsequent spitting or remastication and swallowing.

IBS was defined as recurrent abdominal pain related to defecation and associated with a change in frequency or form of stool. IBS subtypes (IBS-C, IBS-D, IBS-M, and IBS-U) were classified based on patient's perception of the usual consistency of abnormal stools, according to Bristol stool scale. Functional constipation was defined as bowel opening associated with two or more of straining, type 1-2 (Bristol stool scale) stools, sensation of incomplete evacuation, sensation of anorectal obstruction, manual manoeuvres to facilitate defecation, fewer than three spontaneous stools per week, and absence of loose stools. Functional diarrhoea was defined as the presence of loose, watery stools (type 5-6 Bristol stool scale) without predominant abdominal pain or bloating. Functional abdominal bloating/distension was defined as recurrent bloating or distension at least weekly where bloating predominates all other symptoms. Unspecified functional bowel disorder was defined as the presence of symptoms of abdominal pain, constipation, diarrhoea, or bloating which do not meet criteria for other conditions.

Centrally mediated abdominal pain syndrome was defined as continuous or nearly continuous abdominal pain with no (or occasional) relationship of pain to physiological events such as eating, defecation, or periods. Functional biliary pain was defined as pain in the epigastrium and/or right upper quadrant that builds up to a steady level, lasts 30 minutes or longer, occurring at different intervals, severe enough to interrupt usual activities and not related to bowel movements, posture change, or acid suppression.

Faecal incontinence was defined as recurrent uncontrolled passage of faecal material. Functional anorectal pain was defined as chronic or recurrent rectal pain or aching with episodes lasting 30 minutes or longer.

All participants completed the SF36 Quality of Life questionnaire. Mean scores out of 100 (where 0 was the worst outcome on the scale and 100 was the best) for all groups were calculated for each of the eight domains, that is, physical functioning, role limitations due to physical health, role limitations due to emotional problems, level of energy/fatigue, emotional well-being, social functioning, pain, and general health.

Table 1: Gastrointestinal symptoms in MS/hEDS patients compared with controls.

	Controls	MS/hEDS patients	P value (Fisher's exact test)
Number	90	90	
M : F	18 : 72	18 : 72	
Symptoms			
Abdominal pain	25	55	<0.0001***
Diarrhoea	8	30	<0.0001***
Constipation	15	49	<0.0001***
Medicines			
Antisecretory/antacids	17	48	<0.0001***
Laxatives	13	46	<0.0001***
Oesophageal disorders			
Functional chest pain	1	6	0.1177
Functional heartburn	11	30	0.0012**
Globus	1	3	0.6208
Functional dysphagia	3	13	0.016*
Gastroduodenal disorders			
Functional dyspepsia	7	25	0.0007***
Belching disorders	4	10	0.016*
Nausea and vomiting disorders	1	4	0.3680
Rumination syndrome	1	3	0.6208
Bowel disorders			
Irritable bowel syndrome	6	21	0.0029**
Functional constipation	11	32	0.0004***
Functional diarrhoea	5	19	0.0036**
Functional abdominal bloating/distension	6	23	0.0009***
Unspecified functional bowel disorder	22	50	<0.0001***
Centrally mediated abdominal pain syndrome	3	9	0.1324
Functional biliary pain	1	1	1
Anorectal disorders			
Faecal incontinence	1	2	1
Functional anorectal pain	2	4	0.6822

$^{*}P < 0.05$; $^{**}P < 0.01$; $^{***}P < 0.001$.

2.1. Statistical Analyses. Statistical analyses were performed using the IBM Statistical Package for the Social Science (SPSS) software version 25 (IBM SPSS Inc., Chicago, IL). The Fisher's exact test and Chi-squared test were used for comparing categorical variables. Independent sample t-test values were used to compare the mean scores in different modalities of SF36 questionnaire. As multiple comparisons were made, probability values of <0.05 were thought to be statistically significant.

2.2. Ethical Considerations. The study protocol was approved by the South West-Central Bristol Research Ethics Committee and NHS Health Research Authority UK.

3. Results

90 patients and 90 controls were included in this study. Data was collected from 45 MS patients (12 males and 33 females, age 19–41, mean 28 years) with no organic gastrointestinal diagnosis. Data was collected from 45 hEDS patients (6 males and 39 females, age 18–32, mean 24 years) with no organic gastrointestinal diagnosis.

3.1. Gastrointestinal Symptoms in MS/hEDS Patients. Combining the MS and hEDS patients together, these patients were more likely to report a wide range of gastrointestinal symptoms compared to controls (Table 1).

Abdominal pain, bowel symptoms, heartburn, dyspepsia, and dysphagia were all significantly more common in the combined hypermobile group compared with controls. Medication use was also significantly more common in this group.

3.2. Gastrointestinal Symptoms in MS. More Marfan patients reported abdominal pain, diarrhoea, and constipation than controls; however, only symptom of abdominal pain was thought to be statistically significant. The use of antisecretory

TABLE 2: Gastrointestinal symptoms in MS patients compared with controls.

	Control	MS	P value (Fisher's exact test)
Number	45	45	
M : F	12 : 33	12 : 33	
Symptoms			
Abdominal pain	13	24	0.0315*
Diarrhoea	4	9	0.2297
Constipation	8	16	0.0941
Medicines			
Antisecretory/antacids	9	11	0.8004
Laxatives	6	12	0.1868
Oesophageal disorders			
Functional chest pain	0	2	0.4944
Functional heartburn	5	9	0.3837
Globus	0	1	1
Functional dysphagia	1	4	1
Gastroduodenal disorders			
Functional dyspepsia	3	8	0.1966
Belching disorders	2	3	0.6766
Nausea and vomiting disorders	0	1	1
Rumination syndrome	0	1	—
Bowel disorders			
Irritable bowel syndrome	3	6	0.7136
Functional constipation	5	9	0.3837
Functional diarrhoea	2	7	1
Functional abdominal bloating/distension	3	9	0.1184
Unspecified functional bowel disorder	10	23	0.1760
Centrally mediated abdominal pain syndrome	1	2	0.6164
Functional biliary pain	0	0	
Anorectal disorders			
Faecal incontinence	0	1	
Functional anorectal pain	1	2	1

$^{*}P < 0.05$; $^{**}P < 0.01$; $^{***}P < 0.001$.

therapy and laxative was also reported in more MS patients than controls, but this did not reach statistical significance (Table 2).

3.3. Gastrointestinal Symptoms and Diagnoses in hEDS Patients (Table 3). All GI symptoms and use of medicines were considerably higher in the hEDS group meeting statistical significance for all three symptoms and use of medicines. FGIDs were also more frequently found in hEDS group meeting statistical significance for functional heartburn, functional dysphagia, functional dyspepsia, irritable bowel syndrome, functional constipation, functional diarrhoea, functional abdominal bloating, and unspecified bowel disorder (Table 3).

3.4. Perception of Health and Well-Being. The SF36 Quality of Life questionnaire generates a mean score out of 100 (where 0 was the worst outcome on the scale and 100 was the best) for eight domains: physical functioning, role limitations due to physical health, role limitations due to emotional problems, level of energy/fatigue, emotional well-being, social functioning, pain, and general health. The mean scores across all domains of MS patients were compared with controls showing statistical significance in most domains (Table 4). Similarly, the mean scores of hEDS patients showed statistical significance in almost all domains when compared to controls (Table 5). The hEDS group, however, scored the lowest on all domains of this questionnaire.

4. Discussion

This is the first study of its kind showing that connective tissue hypermobile syndromes are associated with a significant number of gastrointestinal symptoms compared to control patients. Despite the many phenotypic similarities, MS and hEDS exhibit different symptom complexes. The burden of functional gastrointestinal symptoms in MS in comparison with hEDS has never been studied and compared. Individuals with hEDS suffer a greater impairment to general well-being than MS patients.

TABLE 3: Gastrointestinal symptoms in hEDS patients compared with controls.

	Control	hEDS	*P* value (Fisher's exact test)
Number	45	45	
M : F	6 : 39	6 : 39	
Symptoms			
Abdominal pain	12	31	<0.0001***
Diarrhoea	4	21	<0.0001***
Constipation	7	33	<0.0001***
Medicines			
Antisecretory/antacids	8	37	<0.0001***
Laxatives	7	34	<0.0001***
Oesophageal disorders			
Functional chest pain	1	4	0.3607
Functional heartburn	6	21	0.0011**
Globus	1	2	1
Functional dysphagia	2	9	0.01*
Gastroduodenal disorders			
Functional dyspepsia	4	17	0.0291*
Belching disorders	2	7	0.2663
Nausea and vomiting disorders	1	3	0.6164
Rumination syndrome	1	2	0.6164
Bowel disorders			
Irritable bowel syndrome	3	15	0.0014**
Functional constipation	6	23	0.0002**
Functional diarrhoea	3	12	0.0014**
Functional abdominal bloating/distension	3	14	0.0059**
Unspecified functional bowel disorder	12	27	<0.0001***
Centrally mediated abdominal pain syndrome	2	7	0.2663
Functional biliary pain	1	1	1
Anorectal disorders			
Faecal incontinence	1	1	1
Functional anorectal pain	1	2	0.6164

*$P < 0.05$; **$P < 0.01$; ***$P < 0.001$.

TABLE 4: Quality of life scores in MS patients.

	Controls (mean scores)	MS (mean scores)	Independent sample *t*-test
Physical functioning	100.0	80.0	0.0012**
Role limitations due to physical health	100.0	50.0	<0.0001***
Role limitations due to emotional problems	100.0	100.0	1
Level of energy/fatigue	95.0	45.0	<0.0001***
Emotional well-being	100.0	68.0	<0.0001***
Social functioning	87.5	50.0	<0.0001***
Pain	77.5	67.5	0.1732
General health	100	30.0	<0.0001***

*$P < 0.05$; **$P < 0.01$; ***$P < 0.001$.

Table 5: Quality of life scores in hEDS patients.

	Controls (mean scores)	hEDS (mean scores)	Independent sample t-test
Physical functioning	100.0	60.0	<0.0001***
Role limitations due to physical health	100.0	50.0	<0.0001***
Role limitations due to emotional problems	100.0	50.0	<0.0001***
Level of energy/fatigue	95.0	30.0	<0.0001***
Emotional well-being	100.0	50.0	<0.0001***
Social functioning	87.5	50.0	<0.0001***
Pain	77.5	50.0	0.0251*
General health	100	45.0	<0.0001***

*$P < 0.05$; **$P < 0.01$; ***$P < 0.001$.

Marfan syndrome is a spectrum of heritable disorders of connective tissue with a high degree of clinical variability. It has an autosomal dominant mode of transmission mainly affecting the connective tissue protein fibrillin. The defect itself has been isolated to the FBN1 gene on chromosome 15, which codes for the connective tissue protein fibrillin [11]. The most serious and common complications of Marfan syndrome are usually cardiovascular, skeletal, pulmonary, and ocular. Aortic root dilatation and dissection [12] are perhaps the most serious manifestations whereas skeletal deformities [13] including thoracolumbar scoliosis, thoracic lordosis, and pectus excavatum can lead to pulmonary problems [14] if left untreated. In addition, ocular problems such as superior dislocation of the lens, retinal detachment, myopia, glaucoma, and cataracts are common findings and can lead to blindness if remain unrecognized [15–17]. The diagnosis of Marfan syndrome is based on family history, the presence of certain clinical features such as aortic root dilatation and ectopia lentis, and genetic testing for FBN1. The revised Ghent criteria for diagnosing Marfan syndrome were published in 2010 [18, 19].

A variety of large surgical publications have highlighted the anatomical or structural complications involving the gastrointestinal tract in patients with Marfan syndrome [20–32]; however, there have not been many studies looking at GI symptoms in these patients.

Ehlers-Danlos syndrome is described as a group of inherited noninflammatory connective tissue disorders primarily caused by a defect in the synthesis of collagen. The syndrome derives its name from clinical case reports presented by 2 physicians: Edvard Ehlers, a Danish dermatologist in 1901, and Henri-Alexandre Danlos, a French physician in 1908. The types of EDS have traditionally been classified according to the Revised Villefranche Nosology presented in 1997 [33].

The current classification of EDS is based on the 2017 international classification of Ehlers-Danlos syndrome which includes the traditional six types as well as other rarer types [34]. All these types share some clinical manifestations such as joint laxity, soft skin, and easy bruising; however, each type is thought to involve a unique defect in connective tissue, although not all the genes responsible for causing EDS have been found. The hypermobile and classical types are thought to be much more common than the other types. Diagnosis is mainly clinical using Beighton criteria for joint hypermobility in the presence of symptoms of skin elasticity and easy bruising. Skin histopathology and molecular genetics can be helpful in diagnosis.

One of the first descriptions of gastrointestinal involvement in EDS was an observational study published in 1969 [35]. However, more recently, several published studies have shown that there is a high prevalence of functional gastrointestinal symptoms in Ehlers-Danlos syndrome whereas more catastrophic gastrointestinal complications remain relatively rare. Structural abnormalities have been reported in up to 20% of individuals and functional gastrointestinal symptoms in up to 75% [10, 36]. A retrospective study from Mayo Clinic including all Ehlers-Danlos syndrome subtypes reported gastrointestinal symptoms in 66 percent of patients over a 20-year period. The most commonly reported GI symptoms were abdominal pain (56.1%), nausea (42.3%), constipation (38.6%), heartburn (37.6%), and irritable bowel syndrome-like symptoms (27.5%); however, all gastrointestinal symptoms were more common in the hypermobility subtype. A review of investigations carried out in this cohort showed nearly 40 percent of patients had either hiatus hernia, erosive reflux oesophagitis, or gastritis identified on OGD. Gastrointestinal motility was affected with abnormal gastric emptying in 25 percent and abnormal colonic transit in 30 percent of their patients. The use of medicines was also higher as compared to the general population with 38 percent of their group using PPI on a regular basis and another 23 percent using laxatives [36]. Some studies have shown the prevalence of functional gastrointestinal disorders to be much higher up to 84 percent with nearly half of the studied population reporting irritable bowel syndrome and nearly two-thirds of the population reporting symptoms of gastro-oesophageal reflux [37].

Symptoms of functional gastrointestinal disorders appear to be more prevalent in the hypermobility subtype of Ehlers-Danlos syndrome. A comparison of patients affected by joint hypermobility syndrome/hypermobile Ehlers-Danlos syndrome with matched controls showed that all gastrointestinal symptoms were more common in this group and affected the quality of life adversely [38]. The association between joint hypermobility and functional gastrointestinal is increasingly being recognized although the reasons for that remain unclear [7]. Joint hypermobility appears to be commoner in patients attending gastroenterology clinics for functional disorders than in patients attending for organic disorders [6].

In this study, patients with hypermobility reported a wide range of gastrointestinal symptoms, frequently met the criteria for the diagnosis of functional gastrointestinal disorders, and showed increased use of medications for gastrointestinal symptoms. These appear to be more common in hypermobile Ehlers-Danlos syndrome patients than in Marfan syndrome patients. Both groups scored lower than controls on quality of life indicators; however, hEDS patients had lower mean scores as compared to MS patients.

However, our study does have some limitations. The sample size is small, and although individuals with a known organic gastrointestinal diagnosis were excluded, undiagnosed conditions may have been present. Finally, although it would be expected that all MS patients are under secondary or tertiary care, it is likely that only the severe hEDS would be under rheumatology specialist care. This selection bias might explain the more severe symptoms in this group compared to the MS group.

A greater understanding of functional gastrointestinal symptoms in patients with connective tissue disorders may give further understanding to the aetiology of gastrointestinal symptoms in individuals not formally diagnosed with connective tissue abnormalities and may give insight into the causes of functional gastrointestinal disorders and irritable bowel syndrome.

Disclosure

This research is part of a postgraduate degree.

Acknowledgments

This research is supported by Gastroenterology Department, St. George's Hospital.

References

[1] H. Dietz, "Marfan syndrome. 2001 Apr 18 [Updated 2017 Oct 12]," in *Gene Reviews® [Internet]*, M. P. Adam, H. H. Ardinger, R. A. Pagon, and N. Inayet, Eds., University of Washington, Seattle, WA, USA, 1993-2018, Available from: https://www.ncbi.nlm.nih.gov/books/NBK1335/.

[2] D. P. Judge and H. C. Dietz, "Marfan's syndrome," *The Lancet*, vol. 366, no. 9501, pp. 1965–1976, 2005.

[3] B. Callewaert, F. Malfait, B. Loeys, and A. De Paepe, "Ehlers-Danlos syndromes and Marfan syndrome," *Best Practice & Research. Clinical Rheumatology*, vol. 22, no. 1, pp. 165–189, 2008.

[4] B. Tinkle, M. Castori, B. Berglund et al., "Hypermobile Ehlers-Danlos syndrome (a.k.a. Ehlers-Danlos syndrome type III and Ehlers-Danlos syndrome hypermobility type): clinical description and natural history," *American Journal of Medical Genetics Part C: Seminars in Medical Genetics*, vol. 175, no. 1, pp. 48–69, 2017.

[5] A. B. Beckers, D. Keszthelyi, A. Fikree et al., "Gastrointestinal disorders in joint hypermobility syndrome/Ehlers-Danlos syndrome hypermobility type: a review for the gastroenterologist," *Neurogastroenterology and Motility*, vol. 29, no. 8, 2017.

[6] A. Fikree, R. Grahame, R. Aktar et al., "A prospective evaluation of undiagnosed joint hypermobility syndrome in patients with gastrointestinal symptoms," *Clinical Gastroenterology and Hepatology*, vol. 12, no. 10, pp. 1680–1687.e2, 2014.

[7] A. Fikree, R. Aktar, R. Grahame et al., "Functional gastrointestinal disorders are associated with the joint hypermobility syndrome in secondary care: a case-control study," *Neurogastroenterology and Motility*, vol. 27, no. 4, pp. 569–579, 2015.

[8] N. Zarate, A. D. Farmer, R. Grahame et al., "Unexplained gastrointestinal symptoms and joint hypermobility: is connective tissue the missing link?," *Neurogastroenterology and Motility*, vol. 22, no. 3, pp. 252–e78, 2010.

[9] K. Kovacic, T. C. Chelimsky, M. R. Sood, P. Simpson, M. Nugent, and G. Chelimsky, "Joint hypermobility: a common association with complex functional gastrointestinal disorders," *The Journal of Pediatrics*, vol. 165, no. 5, pp. 973–978, 2014.

[10] M. Castori, S. Morlino, G. Pascolini, C. Blundo, and P. Grammatico, "Gastrointestinal and nutritional issues in joint hypermobility syndrome/Ehlers-Danlos syndrome, hypermobility type," *American Journal of Medical Genetics Part C: Seminars in Medical Genetics*, vol. 169, no. 1, pp. 54–75, 2015.

[11] K. Kainulainen, L. Pulkkinen, A. Savolainen, I. Kaitila, and L. Peltonen, "Location on chromosome 15 of the gene defect causing Marfan syndrome," *The New England Journal of Medicine*, vol. 323, no. 14, pp. 935–939, 1990.

[12] N. M. Ammash, T. M. Sundt, and H. M. Connolly, "Marfan syndrome-diagnosis and management," *Current Problems in Cardiology*, vol. 33, no. 1, pp. 7–39, 2008.

[13] H. I. Wilner and N. Finby, "Skeletal manifestations in the Marfan syndrome," *JAMA*, vol. 187, no. 7, pp. 490–495, 1964.

[14] J. R. Wood, D. Bellamy, A. H. Child, and K. M. Citron, "Pulmonary disease in patients with Marfan syndrome," *Thorax*, vol. 39, no. 10, pp. 780–784, 1984.

[15] A. Y. Nemet, E. I. Assia, D. J. Apple, and I. S. Barequet, "Current concepts of ocular manifestations in Marfan syndrome," *Survey of Ophthalmology*, vol. 51, no. 6, pp. 561–575, 2006.

[16] H. E. Cross and A. D. Jensen, "Ocular manifestations in the Marfan syndrome and homocystinuria," *American Journal of Ophthalmology*, vol. 75, no. 3, pp. 405–420, 1973.

[17] R. A. Allen, B. R. Straatsma, L. Apt, and M. O. Hall, "Ocular manifestations of the Marfan syndrome," *Transactions-American Academy of Ophthalmology and Otolaryngology*, vol. 71, no. 1, pp. 18–38, 1967.

[18] B. L. Loeys, H. C. Dietz, A. C. Braverman et al., "The revised Ghent nosology for the Marfan syndrome," *Journal of Medical Genetics*, vol. 47, no. 7, pp. 476–485, 2010.

[19] Y. von Kodolitsch, J. de Backer, H. Schüler et al., "Perspectives on the revised Ghent criteria for the diagnosis of Marfan syndrome," *The Application of Clinical Genetics*, vol. 8, p. 137, 2015.

[20] S. M. Suster, M. Ronnen, and J. J. Bubis, "Diverticulosis coli in association with Marfan's syndrome," *Archives of Internal Medicine*, vol. 144, no. 1, p. 203, 1984.

[21] R. N. Keswani, V. N. Prachand, and H. S. Te, "Paraesophageal hernia: a rare presentation of Marfan syndrome in adults," *Gastrointestinal Endoscopy*, vol. 66, no. 5, pp. 1050–1052, 2007.

[22] R. Eliashar, J. Y. Sichel, A. Biron, and I. Dano, "Multiple gastrointestinal complications in Marfan syndrome," *Postgraduate Medical Journal*, vol. 74, no. 874, pp. 495–497, 1998.

[23] J. Kothari, M. Hinduja, K. Baria, and H. Pandya, "Ascending aortic aneurysm and diaphragmatic hernia in a case of Marfan syndrome," *Asian Cardiovascular and Thoracic Annals*, vol. 25, no. 5, pp. 378–380, 2017.

[24] S. Thakur, A. Jhobta, B. Sharma, A. Chauhan, and C. S. Thakur, "Unusual presentation of adult Marfan syndrome as a complex diaphragmatic hiatus hernia," *Asian Journal of Surgery*, vol. 40, no. 4, pp. 313–316, 2017.

[25] L. Leci-Tahiri, A. Tahiri, R. Bajrami, and M. Maxhuni, "Acute abdomen due to torsion of the wandering spleen in a patient with Marfan syndrome," *World Journal of Emergency Surgery*, vol. 8, no. 1, p. 30, 2013.

[26] F. Inayat, A. Hurairah, and F. Shaikh, "Imaging, endoscopic and genetic assessment of Marfan syndrome presenting with sigmoid volvulus: a review," *Cureus*, vol. 8, no. 5, article e619, 2016.

[27] P. Junpaparp, M. Chayanupatkul, S. Buppajarntham, and P. Phowthongkum, "Sigmoid volvulus: is it related to Marfan syndrome?," *International Journal of Colorectal Disease*, vol. 29, no. 6, pp. 771-772, 2014.

[28] K. Chow, R. E. Pyeritz, and H. I. Litt, "Abdominal visceral findings in patients with Marfan syndrome," *Genetics in Medicine*, vol. 9, no. 4, pp. 208–212, 2007.

[29] S. K. Parida, V. M. Kriss, and B. D. Hall, "Hiatus/paraesophageal hernias in neonatal Marfan syndrome," *American Journal of Medical Genetics*, vol. 72, no. 2, pp. 156–158, 1997.

[30] P. Laumonerie, S. Mouttalib, T. Edouard, and P. Galinier, "Hernie de la fente de Larrey chez un nourrisson de trois mois atteint du syndrome de Marfan," *Archives de Pédiatrie*, vol. 22, no. 11, pp. 1151–1153, 2015.

[31] T. F. Beck, P. M. Campeau, S. N. Jhangiani et al., "*FBN1* contributing to familial congenital diaphragmatic hernia," *American Journal of Medical Genetics Part A*, vol. 167, no. 4, pp. 831–836, 2015.

[32] T. E. Herman, M. J. Siegel, A. Mathur, and A. Vachharajani, "Neonatal marfan syndrome with hiatus hernia and intrathoracic stomach," *Journal of Perinatology*, vol. 33, no. 8, pp. 652-653, 2013.

[33] P. Beighton, A. D. Paepe, B. Steinmann, P. Tsipouras, and R. J. Wenstrup, "Ehlers-Danlos syndromes: revised nosology, Villefranche, 1997," *American Journal of Medical Genetics*, vol. 77, no. 1, pp. 31–37, 1998.

[34] F. Malfait, C. Francomano, P. Byers et al., "The 2017 international classification of the Ehlers-Danlos syndromes," *American Journal of Medical Genetics Part C: Seminars in Medical Genetics*, vol. 175, no. 1, pp. 8–26, 2017.

[35] P. H. Beighton, J. L. Murdoch, and T. Votteler, "Gastrointestinal complications of the Ehlers-Danlos syndrome," *Gut*, vol. 10, no. 12, pp. 1004–1008, 1969.

[36] A. D. Nelson, M. A. Mouchli, N. Valentin et al., "Ehlers Danlos syndrome and gastrointestinal manifestations: a 20-year experience at Mayo Clinic," *Neurogastroenterology and Motility*, vol. 27, no. 11, pp. 1657–1666, 2015.

[37] J.-D. Zeitoun, J. H. Lefèvre, V. de Parades et al., "Functional digestive symptoms and quality of life in patients with Ehlers-Danlos syndromes: results of a National Cohort Study on 134 patients," *PLoS One*, vol. 8, no. 11, article e80321, 2013.

[38] G. Bolasco, C. Celletti, F. Camerota, I. Biviano, E. S. Corazziari, and D. Badiali, "PP-5 joint hypermobility syndrome/Ehlers-Danlos syndrome hypermobility type and gastrointestinal symptoms," *Journal of Pediatric Gastroenterology and Nutrition*, vol. 61, no. 4, p. 522, 2015.

7

Additional Thirty Seconds Observation with Linked Color Imaging Improves Detection of Missed Polyps in the Right-Sided Colon

Naohisa Yoshida,[1] Yutaka Inada,[2] Ritsu Yasuda,[1] Takaaki Murakami,[1] Ryohei Hirose,[1] Ken Inoue,[1] Osamu Dohi,[1] Yuji Naito,[1] Kiyoshi Ogiso,[3] Yukiko Morinaga,[4] Mitsuo Kishimoto,[4] Eiichi Konishi,[4] and Yoshito Itoh[1]

[1]*Department of Molecular Gastroenterology and Hepatology, Kyoto Prefectural University of Medicine, Graduate School of Medical Science, Kyoto, Japan*
[2]*Department of Gastroenterology, Fukuchiyama City Hospital, Kyoto, Japan*
[3]*Department of Gastroenterology, Osaka General Hospital of West Japan Railway Company, Osaka, Japan*
[4]*Department of Surgical Pathology, Kyoto Prefectural University of Medicine, Graduate School of Medical Science, Kyoto, Japan*

Correspondence should be addressed to Naohisa Yoshida; naohisa@koto.kpu-m.ac.jp

Academic Editor: Jean F. Rey

Background and Aims. Missed polyps are a pitfall of colonoscopy. In this study, we analyzed the efficacy of an additional 30 seconds observation using linked color imaging (LCI) for detecting adenoma and sessile serrated adenoma/polyp (SSA/P). *Materials and Methods.* We enrolled patients undergoing colonoscopy from February to October 2017 in two institutions. In all patients, the cecum and ascending colon were observed with white light imaging (WLI) first. The colonoscope was inserted again, and the cecum and ascending colon were observed for an additional 30 seconds using either LCI or WLI. The method for the 30 sec observation was to insufflate the cecum and ascending colon sufficiently and observe them in a distant view, because the length of the second observation was determined to be precisely 30 sec. For the second observation, LCI was performed for the first 65 patients and WLI for the next 65. Adenoma and SSA/P detection rate (ASDR) in the second observation were examined in both groups. According to a pilot study, the sample size was estimated 65. *Results.* In the first observation, ASDR were 30.7% in the LCI group and 32.2% in the WLI group ($p = 0.85$). For the second observation, 13 polyps were detected in the LCI group and 5 polyps in the WLI group ($p = 0.04$). Additionally, ASDR for the second observation were 18.5% and 6.1%, respectively ($p = 0.03$). There were no significant differences between the LCI and WLI groups with respect to morphology (ratio of polypoid) (38.5% versus 60.0%, $p = 0.52$) and histology (ratio of adenoma) (92.3% versus 100.0%, $p = 0.91$). Total adenoma and SSA/P number were 48 in the LCI group and 36 in the WLI group ($p = 0.02$). *Conclusion.* The 30 seconds additional observation with LCI improved the detection of adenoma and SSA/P in the right-sided colon.

1. Introduction

Removal of adenomatous polyps by colonoscopy has been proven to prevent colorectal cancer and associated with the reduction in the incidence of proximal and distal colorectal cancers [1–3]. Colonoscopy is the most effective tool for detecting colorectal adenomas. However, the rate of missed polyps by white light imaging (WLI) observation was reported at 20–27% [4, 5]. There are some risk factors for missed polyps, such as flat morphology, smaller size, presence in the ascending colon, male sex, patients with multiple polyps at their first colonoscopy, and patients with a history of polyps [6, 7].

A LASER endoscopic system (LASEREO: Fujifilm Co., Tokyo, Japan) was developed in 2012. It allows blue laser imaging (BLI), BLI-bright, and linked color imaging (LCI)

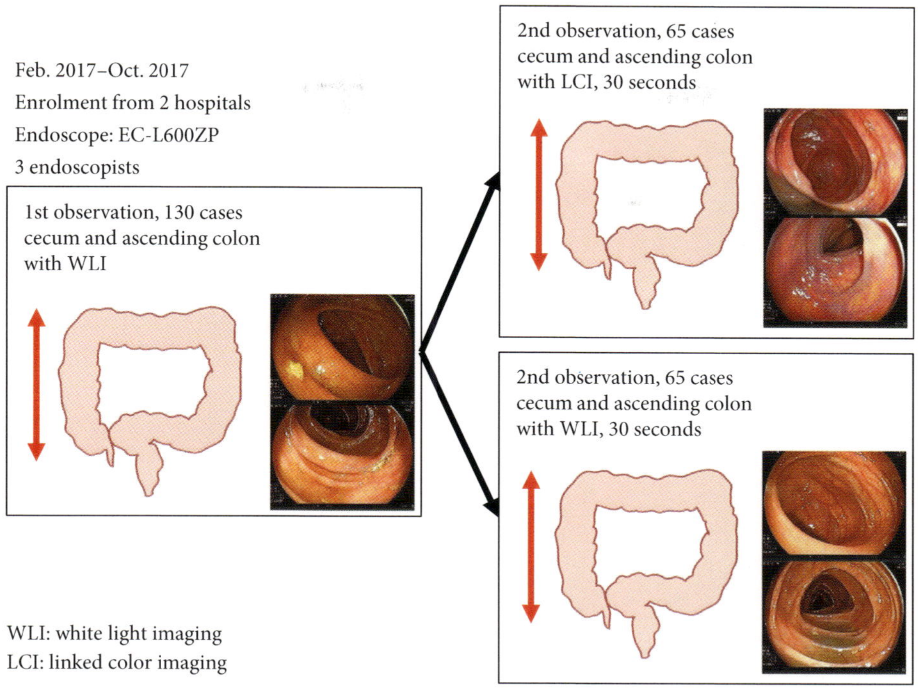

Figure 1: Study flow of the first observation and the second observation.

as narrow band light observation [8–11]. BLI is used with magnification and is useful for diagnosing various gastrointestinal cancers. BLI-bright is brighter than BLI and is expected to improve tumor detection. For colorectal tumors, BLI-bright makes a neoplastic lesion appear brownish in color and makes it easier to detect. Previously, we reported that BLI-bright improved numbers of polyps and adenomas more significantly than WLI did in a multicenter study [12]. However, there are several limitations in the use of BLI and BLI-bright. One of the limitations is that the residual liquid becomes reddish, which worsens the endoscopic view. Narrow band imaging (NBI) also has this limitation. The other limitation is that the endoscopic view using BLI and BLI-bright is darker than in WLI. However, LCI is brighter than BLI and BLI-bright and differentiates a lesion from the surrounding mucosa by making it appear reddish and the surrounding mucosa appears whitish, making the lesion easy to visualize. Moreover, residual liquid becomes yellowish with LCI. We previously reported that LCI improved polyp visibility using endoscopic figures and movies [13, 14]. However, there are no previous reports about whether LCI can decrease missed polyps.

In this study, we developed an additional 30 seconds (sec) observation as a second observation with LCI for decreasing missed adenoma and sessile serrated adenoma and polyp (SSA/P) and analyzed the efficacy of this method.

2. Materials and Methods

This was an observational study and was conducted at two affiliated hospitals: the Department of Molecular Gastroenterology and Hepatology, Kyoto Prefectural University of Medicine, and the Department of Gastroenterology, North Medical Center, Kyoto Prefectural University of Medicine. We examined 130 consecutive patients who received total colonoscopy using LCI and WLI with the LASER endoscopic system (LL-4450 light source, the VP-4450HD, Fujifilm Co., Tokyo, Japan) and the LASER endoscope (EC-L600ZP) from February 2017 to October 2017. We divided all patients into a LCI or a WLI group. First, in all patients, the cecum and ascending colon were observed with WLI as the first observation (Figure 1). Next, we inserted the colonoscope in the cecum again, and the cecum and ascending colon were observed for an additional 30 sec using either LCI or WLI as the second observation. In the first 65 cases, LCI was performed, and in the next 65 cases, WLI was used. The method for the 30 sec observation was to insufflate the cecum and the ascending colon sufficiently and observe them not in a close view, but in a distant view, because the length of the second observation was determined to be precisely 30 sec. Thus, even if the observation of the cecum and ascending colon had not finished during the 30 sec, the second observation would have finished. In this study, the number of adenoma and SSA/P detected in the first observation and the second observation was examined. The diagnosis of adenoma and SSA/P was performed with BLI magnification according to previous reports and local protocols based on the Preservation and Incorporation of Valuable Endoscopic Innovations (PIVI) statements, and all polyps diagnosed as either adenoma or SSA/P were resected using polypectomy, endoscopic mucosal resection (EMR), and endoscopic submucosal dissection (ESD) according to size and morphology [9, 15, 16]. Polyps diagnosed as hyperplastic polyps and inflammatory polyps were diagnosed with biopsy.

As the main purpose of this study, the number of adenoma and SSA/P in the second observation was analyzed

Table 1: Clinical characteristics in the LCI and WLI groups.

	LCI	WLI	*p* value
Case number	65	65	
Age, years, mean ± SD	63.5 ± 13.0	68.1 ± 14.3	0.10
Sex, %, *n* men : women	60.0 : 40.0 34 : 31	62.3 : 37.7 38 : 27	0.48
Insertion time, sec	284 ± 151	328 ± 202	0.33
First WLII observation time, sec	162 ± 80	169 ± 112	0.77
BBPS ≥ 2, %, *n*	84.6, 55	87.6, 57	0.61
Antispasm drug, %, *n*	80.0, 57	71.5, 58	0.78
Sedation, %, *n*	23.1, 15	12.3, 8	0.11

LCI: linked color imaging; WLI: white light; BBPS: Boston Bowel Preparation Score; SD: standard deviation.

in the LCI group compared to that in the WLI group. The number of adenoma and SSA/P in the first observation was also analyzed both in the LCI and WLI groups, respectively. Moreover, adenoma detection rates (ADR) and adenoma and SSA/P detection rates (ASDR) both in the first and second observations were calculated. Polyp characteristics such as size, location, morphology, and histology were examined in each group. Additionally, patient characteristics such as mean age, sex, insertion time, first observation time, local Boston bowel preparation score (BBPS) for the cecum and ascending colon, usage of antispasm drugs, and sedation were examined. Overall, adenoma and SSS/P numbers, adenoma numbers, ASDR, and ADR in the first and second observations in each group were analyzed. Removal time for detected polyps was not included for either the 1st observation or the 2nd observation. Moreover, polyps detected during removal were not included in this study.

The inclusion criteria were as follows: patients receiving total colonoscopies for follow-up of polyps, surveillance after polyp or cancer resection, and positive fecal occult blood performed by three experts (N.Y., Y.I., and T.M.). We excluded patients with recurrent lesions after a previous EMR and polypectomy, and T1–T4 colorectal cancers. We also excluded patients who underwent surgical operations of the cecum or the ascending colon. Of the three endoscopists, all had performed more than 1000 colonoscopies and 50 withdrawing colonoscopies with LCI prior to this study. The size of a polyp was defined by its maximum diameter and was calculated in accordance with the size of the snares and biopsy forceps. Polyps were divided into polypoid and nonpolypoid types, according to the Paris classification [17]. Histological diagnosis was performed according to the World Health Organization classification, and intramucosal cancer was categorized as adenoma in this study [18].

Regarding bowel preparation, patients followed a low-residue diet and took 10 mL of sodium picosulfate with 200 mL of water one day before the examination. All patients also received a total of 1.0 L of a highly concentrated polyethylene glycol solution with ascorbic acid (MOVIPREP; Ajinomoto Pharma Co., Ltd., Tokyo, Japan) and more than 0.5 L of water in the morning on the day of the examination according to our previous report [19].

Table 2: Results of first observation in the LCI and WLI groups.

	LCI 65 cases	WLI 65 cases	*p* value
First observation Ad and SSA/P number, *n*	35	31	0.29
Polyp size, mm, mean ± SD (range)	4.8 ± 3.6 (2–20)	4.0 ± 2.8 (2–15)	0.30
Location, %, *n* C : A	14.3 : 85.7 5 : 30	29.0 : 71.0 9 : 22	0.14
Morphology, %, *n* Polypoid: nonpolypoid	48.6 : 51.4 17 : 18	64.5 : 35.5 20 : 11	0.19
Histology Ad : SSA/P	88.6 : 11.4 31 : 4	80.6 : 19.4 25 : 6	0.37
First observation ASDR, %, *n*	30.7 20	32.3 21	0.85
First observation ADR, %, *n*	26.2 17	26.2 17	1.00

LCI: linked color imaging; WLI: white light; Ad: adenoma; SSA/P: sessile serrated adenoma and polyp; C: cecum; A: ascending colon; ASDR: adenoma and SSA/P detection rate; ADR: adenoma detection rate; SD: standard deviation.

Table 3: Results of the second observation in the LCI and WLI groups.

	LCI 65 cases	WLI 65 cases	*p* value
Second observation Ad and SSA/P number, *n*	13	5	0.04
Polyp number in cases with BBPS 0 or 1 in first observation	1	1	0.92
Polyp size, mm, mean ± SD (range)	5.6 ± 4.1 (2.0–15.0)	2.2 ± 0.4 (2.0–3.0)	0.33
Location, %, *n* C : A	23.1 : 76.9 3 : 10	40.0 : 60.0 2 : 3	0.37
Morphology, %, *n* Polypoid : nonpolypoid	38.5 : 61.5 5 : 8	60.0 : 40.0 3 : 2	0.52
Histology Ad : SSA/P	92.3 : 7.7 12 : 1	100.0 : 0 5 : 0	0.91
Second observation ASDR, %, *n*	18.5 12	6.1 4	0.03
Second observation ADR, %, *n*	16.9 11	6.1 4	0.05

LCI: linked color imaging; WLI: white light; Ad: adenoma; SSA/P: sessile serrated adenoma and polyp; C: cecum; A: ascending colon; ASDR: adenoma and SSA/P detection rate; ADR: adenoma detection rate; SD: standard deviation.

All patients provided written informed consent to participate in this study. This study was conducted in accordance with the World Medical Association Helsinki Declaration. This study was also approved by the institutional review board and the ethics committees of Kyoto Prefectural University of Medicine.

2.1. Statistical Assessment. Regarding the sample size, we hypothesized that LCI improves the number of adenoma and SSAP by 20% in the second observation according to

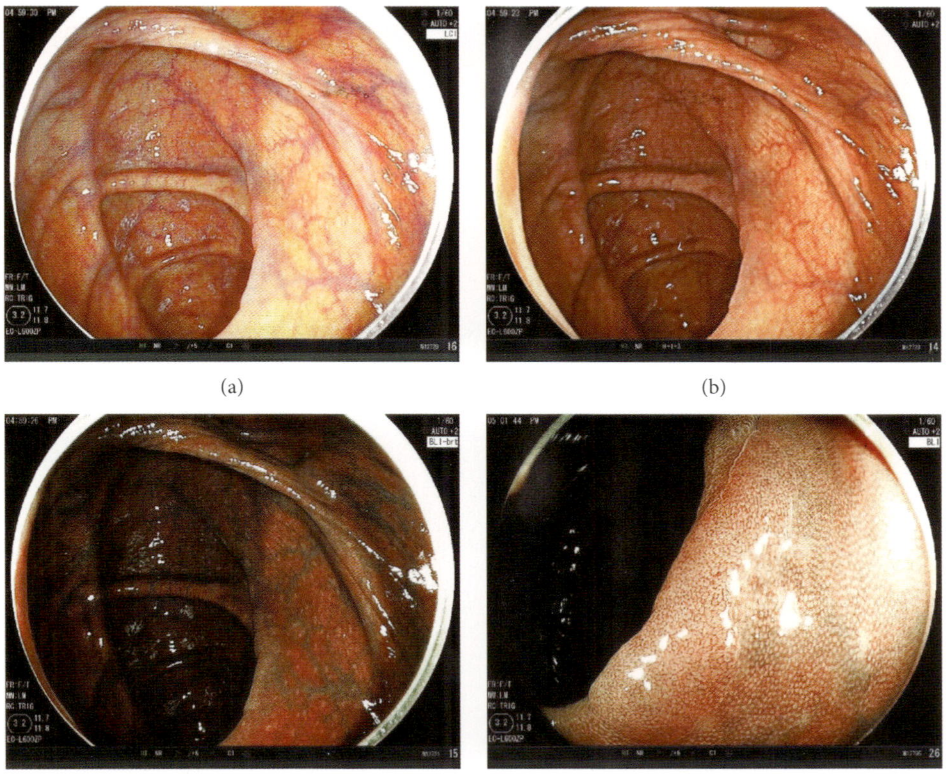

(a) (b) (c) (d)

FIGURE 2: Case presentation. (a) A nonpolypoid adenomatous polyp 10 mm in size on the ascending colon. The first WLI observation could not detect this tumor. LCI could detect the tumor in a distant view. The endoscopic view was bright, and the tumor was on the fold. It was well-visualized as a little pinkish lesion under LCI compared to the surrounding mucosa. (b) WLI image of this tumor was taken afterwards. The color of it was almost similar to the surrounding tumor. (c) The BLI-bright image of it was also taken. The endoscopic view was a little dark, but the color of the tumor became brownish. (d) BLI magnification showed an adenomatous vessel pattern and surface pattern.

our pilot study of 20 cases by a single expert endoscopist (N.Y.). Using the sign test, the α error was calculated at 5% and the β error at 20%. The calculated minimum sample size was 47. We considered the exclusion cases and finally determined the sample size to be 65. The Mann–Whitney U test, Wilcoxon signed-rank test with Bonferroni correction, and chi-squared test (SPSS version 22.0 for Windows, IBM Japan, Ltd., Tokyo, Japan) were used in this study. Continuous variables such as patient age and tumor size were analyzed using the Mann–Whitney U test. A p value of < 0.05 was considered statistically significant.

3. Results

The patients' characteristics in the LCI group and the WLI group are shown in Table 1. The first observation times (sec) for each group were 162 ± 80 in the LCI group and 169 ± 112 in the WLI group ($p = 0.77$). There was no significant difference in the ratio of local BBPS ≥ 2 for the cecum and the ascending colon (LCI versus WLI: 84.6 versus 87.6, $p = 0.61$). On the contrary, regarding poor preparation cases showing BBPS 0 or 1, there were 10 in the LCI group and 8 in the WLI group.

The results of the first observation using WLI in the LCI and WLI groups are shown in Table 2. The numbers of adenoma and SSA/P in the LCI group and the WLI group were 35 and 31, respectively ($p = 0.29$). Regarding polyp location, the ratios of cecal location were 14.3% in the LCI group and 29.0% in the WLI group ($p = 0.14$). The ratios of polypoid morphology were 48.6% in the LCI group and 64.5% in the WLI group ($p = 0.19$). Histology showed that the ratios of adenomas were 88.6% in the LCI group and 80.6% in the WLI group ($p = 0.37$). ASDRs of the LCI and WLI groups were 30.7% and 32.3%, respectively ($p = 0.85$), and ADRs of the LCI and WLI groups were 26.2% and 26.2%, respectively ($p = 1.0$).

The results of the 30 sec second observation using LCI or WLI are shown in Table 3. The numbers of adenoma and SSA/P in the LCI and WLI groups were 13 and 5, respectively ($p = 0.04$) (Figures 2 and 3). Polyp numbers in cases with BBPS 0 or 1 were 1 in the LCI group and 1 in the WLI group ($p = 0.92$). Regarding the comparison between LCI and WLI, there were no differences between polyp sizes (mm) (5.6 ± 4.1 versus 2.2 ± 0.4, $p = 0.33$), the ratio of cecal location (23.1% versus 40.0%, $p = 0.37$), the ratio of polypoid morphology (38.5% versus 60.0%, $p = 0.52$), and the ratio of adenoma histology (92.3% versus 100.0%, $p = 0.91$). ASDRs of LCI and WLI were 18.5% and 6.1%, respectively ($p = 0.03$), and ADRs of LCI and WLI were 16.9% and 6.1%, respectively ($p = 0.05$).

The overall results of the first and second observations are shown in Table 4. The overall adenoma and SSA/P

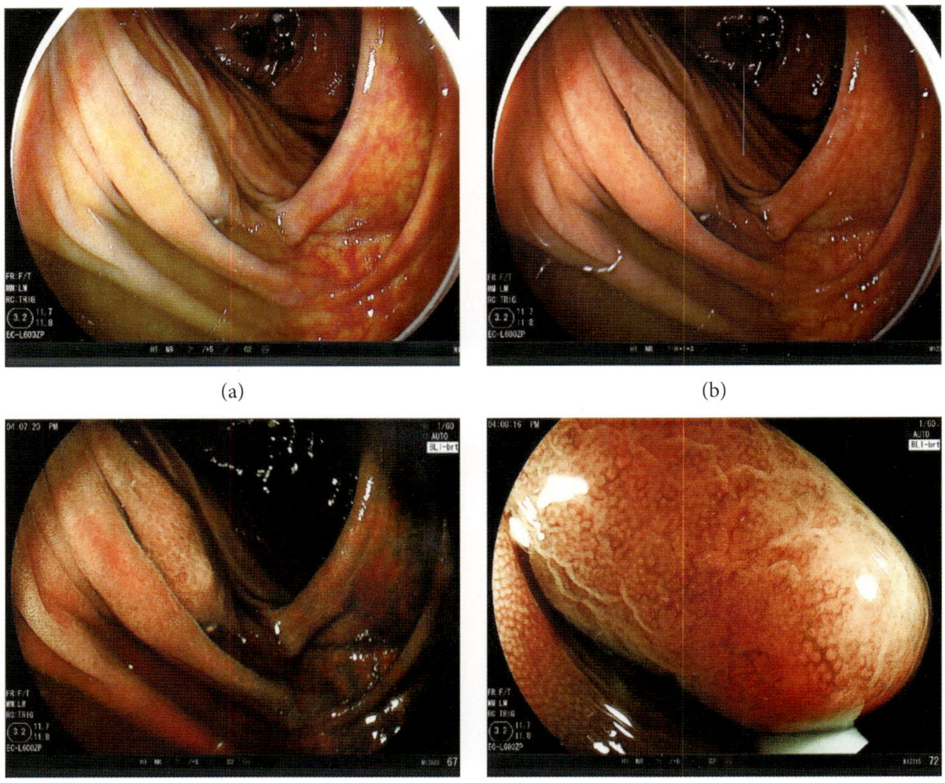

(a) (b) (c) (d)

Figure 3: Case presentation. (a) A nonpolypoid polyp (SSA/P) 15 mm in size on the ascending colon under poor preparation. The first WLI observation could not detect this tumor. There were two other polyps which the first observation with WLI could detect in this patient. LCI could detect the tumor in a distant view. The endoscopic view was bright, and the tumor was on the fold. The color of it was more whitish under LCI compared to the surrounding mucosa. Residual liquid became still yellowish in LCI. (b) WLI image of this tumor was taken afterwards. The color of it was almost similar to the surrounding tumor. (c) The BLI-bright image of it was also taken. The endoscopic view was a little dark, and the residual liquid became reddish. The color of the tumor became brownish. (d) BLI magnification showed a dilated vessel pattern and a dilated surface pattern, consistent with typical SSA/P findings.

Table 4: Overall results of the first and second observations.

	LCI 65 cases	WLI 65 cases	p value
Overall Ad and SSA/P numbers in the first and second observations	48	36	0.02
Overall Ad numbers in the first and second observations	43	30	0.02
Overall ASDR, %, n	43.1 28	35.4 23	0.36
Overall ADR, %, n	36.9 24	30.8 20	0.45

LCI: linked color imaging; WLI: white light; Ad: adenoma; SSA/P: sessile serrated adenoma and polyp; ASDR: adenoma and SSA/P detection rate; ADR: adenoma detection rate.

numbers in the first and second observations were 48 in the LCI group and 36 in the WLI group, respectively ($p = 0.02$). Additionally, the overall adenoma numbers of the first and second observations were 43 in the LCI group and 30 in the WLI group, respectively ($p = 0.02$). The overall ASDRs of the LCI and WLI groups were 43.1 and 35.4, respectively ($p = 0.36$), and the overall ADRs of the LCI and WLI groups were 36.9 and 30.8 ($p = 0.45$), respectively. Regarding the LCI group, the numbers of adenoma and SSA/P in the first and second observations were significantly higher than in the first observation (48 versus 35, $p = 0.017$) though there was no significant difference about that in the WLI group (36 versus 31, $p = 0.38$). The second observation with LCI also increased ASDR from 30.7% to 43.1% and increased ADR from 26.2% to 36.9%, but there were no significant differences between the first observation and the first + second observations ($p = 0.14$, $p = 0.18$).

4. Discussion

In our study, a 30 sec additional observation with LCI could improve overall adenoma and SSA/P numbers and overall adenoma numbers significantly more than those detected with WLI. Additionally, it significantly increased the adenoma and SSA/P numbers than the numbers in the first observation.

Our previous randomized controlled multicenter study conducted at 8 Japanese academic institutions showed that BLI-bright (489 cases) improved the mean number of adenomatous polyps detected per patient in comparison to WLI (474 cases) (1.27 ± 1.73 versus 1.01 ± 1.36, $p = 0.008$) and also improved the mean number of total polyps per patient in comparison to WLI (1.84 ± 2.09 versus 1.43 ± 1.64, $p = 0.001$) [11]. However, an observation using BLI-bright is not widely accepted. One of the reasons is that BLI-bright required longer observation times than WLI did (9.5 ± 3.8 min versus 8.4 ± 2.9 min, $p < 0.001$). The other reason is that BLI-bright is less bright than WLI and the reddish residual liquid in BLI-bright may become a disadvantage. Generally, poor preparation is detected in 20–25% of all colonoscopies [20, 21]. In those cases, BLI-bright is no more useful than WLI. As our case presentation showed, residual liquid disturbed the observation in BLI-bright. Additionally, NBI is not useful in poor preparations due to the same reasons, although current NBI systems and endoscopes showed positive results for polyp detection compared to the previous ones [22–24]. However, residual liquid is not reddish in LCI compared to BLI-bright. Thus, we suspect that LCI may be more useful for polyp detection than BLI-bright. In fact, a multicenter study from China proved that LCI increased ADR (LCI versus WLI: 37% versus 28%; 95% confidence interval, 2.3%–19.4%) [25]. The study also revealed that LCI significantly improved the rate of adenoma and SSA/P detected, more than WLI did (91% versus 73%, $p < 0.001$).

Our previous study showed that LCI improved polyp visibility more than WLI and BLI-bright did [13]. In brief, we used our original polyp visibility score (score 1: poor visibility, score 4: excellent visibility) and evaluated recorded short movies using LCI, BLI-bright, and WLI in 101 colorectal polyps. The mean polyp visibility scores of LCI were higher than those of WLI (2.86 ± 1.08 versus 2.54 ± 1.15, $p < 0.001$) and were also higher than those of BLI-bright (2.86 ± 1.08 versus 2.73 ± 1.47, $p < 0.001$). Additionally, LCI decreased the number of polyps detected showing poorer polyp visibility scores (score 1 or 2) than WLI did (experts: 35.6% versus 49.6%, $p < 0.015$; nonexperts: 33.6% versus 50.5%, $p = 0.046$). A similar study using polyp visibility scores showed that LCI improved the endoscopic visualization of nongranular colorectal lesions [26]. It also showed the efficacy of LCI for SSA/P. Moreover, our previous study showed the efficacies of LCI for nonpolypoid tumors and SSA/P [13]. Another study of ours showed the efficacy of LCI for diminutive polyps less than 5 mm in size [14]. In the study, color difference values between the tumor and the surrounding mucosa were calculated among endoscopic figures of 54 colorectal polyps taken by WLI and LCI for evaluating polyp visibility. Color difference value is thought as an objective indicator for polyp visibility. The study showed that LCI improved color difference values more than WLI did (33.6 ± 13.9 versus 20.7 ± 13.6, $p < 0.001$).

LCI presents the problem of halation in the endoscopic view due to its powerful brightness, which could lead to missed polyps, although it did not affect the results in the current study. The multicenter crossover study using LCI and WLI from China showed that there were 12 adenomas which were not detected in LCI, but were detected in WLI among 150 total adenomas [25]. Additionally, there were 29 polyps which were not detected in LCI, but were detected in WLI among 308 total polyps. We suggested that these outcomes were partially due to the powerful brightness of LCI. Missed polyps due to LCI should be examined in detail. However, the additional 30-second 2nd observation proposed in our study did not confer any additional risk of missed polyps due to LCI, because LCI is only used for second observations. In spite of this short 2nd observation time with LCI, it significantly increased the adenoma and SSA/P numbers than the numbers in the first observation. It also increased ASDR from 30.7% to 43.1% and increased ADR from 26.2% to 36.9% though it did not show significant difference ($p = 0.14$, $p = 0.18$).

Regarding serrated polyps, there are three types of polyps such as hyperplastic polyp, traditional serrated adenoma (TSA), and SSA/P [27]. TSA and SSA/P have an increased risk of progression to colorectal cancer [28, 29]. Thus, we analyzed not hyperplastic polyps but SSA/Ps in this study. Because of that, we could not calculate the polyp detection rate including hyperplastic polyps though most of previous similar studies did so.

There were some limitations in our study. This study was a parallel design without formal randomization, and a small number of patients were enrolled in two hospitals though the sample number was calculated statistically. Only three endoscopists performed all colonoscopies. There was a slight difference in the sedation rate between the WLI group and the LCI group though it was not significant. It might affect polyp detection. Though our study showed significant improvement in LCI about polyp detection in the study setting, more studies are needed to show whether this improvement is achieved in real-life settings.

5. Conclusions

Our study showed that a 30 sec additional observation with LCI significantly improved the number of adenoma and SSA/P in comparison to WLI. We think that our method will be easily accepted and is a less risky way for improving missed polyps.

Acknowledgments

The authors thank all the members of the Department of Molecular Gastroenterology and Hepatology, Kyoto Prefectural University of Medicine, for their assistance with this study.

References

[1] R. Nishihara, K. Wu, P. Lochhead et al., "Long-term colorectal-cancer incidence and mortality after lower endoscopy," *The New England Journal of Medicine*, vol. 369, no. 12, pp. 1095–1105, 2013.

[2] S. J. Winawer, A. G. Zauber, M. N. Ho et al., "Prevention of colorectal cancer by colonoscopic polypectomy," *The New England Journal of Medicine*, vol. 329, no. 27, pp. 1977–1981, 1993.

[3] A. G. Zauber, S. J. Winawer, M. J. O'Brien et al., "Colonoscopic polypectomy and long-term prevention of colorectal-cancer deaths," *The New England Journal of Medicine*, vol. 366, no. 8, pp. 687–696, 2012.

[4] D. Heresbach, T. Barrioz, M. G. Lapalus et al., "Miss rate for colorectal neoplastic polyps: a prospective multicenter study of back-to-back video colonoscopies," *Endoscopy*, vol. 40, no. 4, pp. 284–290, 2008.

[5] D. K. Rex, C. S. Cutler, G. T. Lemmel et al., "Colonoscopic miss rates of adenomas determined by back-to-back colonoscopies," *Gastroenterology*, vol. 112, no. 1, pp. 24–28, 1997.

[6] N. H. Kim, Y. S. Jung, W. S. Jeong et al., "Miss rate of colorectal neoplastic polyps and risk factors for missed polyps in consecutive colonoscopies," *Intestinal Research*, vol. 15, no. 3, pp. 411–418, 2017.

[7] J. Lee, S. W. Park, Y. S. Kim et al., "Risk factors of missed colorectal lesions after colonoscopy," *Medicine*, vol. 96, no. 27, article e7468, 2017.

[8] H. Osawa and H. Yamamoto, "Present and future status of flexible spectral imaging color enhancement and blue laser imaging technology," *Digestive Endoscopy*, vol. 26, pp. 105–115, 2014.

[9] N. Yoshida, T. Hisabe, Y. Inada et al., "The ability of a novel blue laser imaging system for the diagnosis of invasion depth of colorectal neoplasms," *Journal of Gastroenterology*, vol. 49, no. 1, pp. 73–80, 2014.

[10] N. Yoshida, T. Hisabe, R. Hirose et al., "Improvement in the visibility of colorectal polyps by using blue laser imaging (with video)," *Gastrointestinal Endoscopy*, vol. 82, no. 3, pp. 542–549, 2015.

[11] H. Kanzaki, R. Takenaka, Y. Kawahara et al., "Linked color imaging (LCI), a novel image-enhanced endoscopy technology, emphasizes the color of early gastric cancer," *Endoscopy International Open*, vol. 5, no. 10, pp. E1005–E1013, 2017.

[12] H. Ikematsu, T. Sakamoto, K. Togashi et al., "Detectability of colorectal neoplastic lesions using a novel endoscopic system with blue laser imaging: a multicenter randomized controlled trial," *Gastrointestinal Endoscopy*, vol. 86, no. 2, pp. 386–394, 2017.

[13] N. Yoshida, Y. Naito, T. Murakami et al., "Linked color imaging improves the visibility of colorectal polyps: a video study," *Endoscopy International Open*, vol. 5, no. 6, pp. E518–E525, 2017.

[14] N. Yoshida, Y. Naito, R. Yasuda et al., "Linked color imaging improves the visibility of various featured colorectal polyps in an endoscopist's visibility and color difference value," *International Journal of Colorectal Disease*, vol. 32, no. 9, pp. 1253–1260, 2017.

[15] T. Yamashina, Y. Takeuchi, N. Uedo et al., "Diagnostic features of sessile serrated adenoma/polyps on magnifying narrow band imaging: a prospective study of diagnostic accuracy," *Journal of Gastroenterology and Hepatology*, vol. 30, no. 1, pp. 117–123, 2015.

[16] D. K. Rex, C. Kahi, M. O'Brien et al., "The American Society for Gastrointestinal Endoscopy PIVI (Preservation and Incorporation of Valuable Endoscopic Innovations) on real-time endoscopic assessment of the histology of diminutive colorectal polyps," *Gastrointestinal Endoscopy*, vol. 73, no. 3, pp. 419–422, 2011.

[17] Participants in the Paris Workshop, "The Paris endoscopic classification of superficial neoplastic lesions: esophagus, stomach, and colon," *Gastrointestinal Endoscopy*, vol. 58, no. 6, pp. S3–S43, 2003.

[18] S. R. Hamilton and L. A. Aaltonen, Eds., *World Health Organization Classification of Tumors. Pathology and Genetics of Tumours of the Digestive System*, IARC Press, Lyon, France, 2010.

[19] N. Yoshida, Y. Naito, T. Murakami et al., "Safety and efficacy of a same-day low-volume 1 L PEG bowel preparation in colonoscopy for the elderly people and people with renal dysfunction," *Digestive Diseases and Sciences*, vol. 61, no. 11, pp. 3229–3235, 2016.

[20] F. Froehlich, V. Wietlisbach, J. J. Gonvers, B. Burnand, and J. P. Vader, "Impact of colonic cleansing on quality and diagnostic yield of colonoscopy: the European Panel of Appropriateness of Gastrointestinal Endoscopy European multicenter study," *Gastrointestinal Endoscopy*, vol. 61, no. 3, pp. 378–384, 2005.

[21] G. C. Harewood, V. K. Sharma, and P. de Garmo, "Impact of colonoscopy preparation quality on detection of suspected colonic neoplasia," *Gastrointestinal Endoscopy*, vol. 58, no. 1, pp. 76–79, 2003.

[22] T. Horimatsu, Y. Sano, S. Tanaka et al., "Next-generation narrow band imaging system for colonic polyp detection: a prospective multicenter randomized trial," *International Journal of Colorectal Disease*, vol. 30, no. 7, pp. 947–954, 2015.

[23] A. Adler, H. Pohl, I. S. Papanikolaou et al., "A prospective randomised study on narrow-band imaging versus conventional colonoscopy for adenoma detection: does narrow-band imaging induce a learning effect?," *Gut*, vol. 57, no. 1, pp. 59–64, 2008.

[24] D. K. Rex and C. C. Helbig, "High yields of small and flat adenomas with high-definition colonoscopes using either white light or narrow band imaging," *Gastroenterology*, vol. 133, no. 1, pp. 42–47, 2007.

[25] M. Min, P. Deng, W. Zhang, X. Sun, Y. Liu, and B. Nong, "Comparison of linked color imaging and white-light colonoscopy for detection of colorectal polyps: a multicenter, randomized, crossover trial," *Gastrointestinal Endoscopy*, vol. 86, no. 4, pp. 724–730, 2017.

[26] T. Suzuki, T. Hara, Y. Kitagawa et al., "Linked-color imaging improves endoscopic visibility of colorectal nongranular flat lesions," *Gastrointestinal Endoscopy*, vol. 86, no. 4, pp. 692–697, 2017.

[27] D. Snover, D. Ahnen, R. Burt, and R. D. Odze, "Serrated polyps of the colon and rectum and serrated polyposis," in *World Health Organization Classification of Tumours. Tumors of the Digestive System*, F. Bosman, F. Cameiro, R. Hruban, and N. D. Theise, Eds., pp. 160–165, International Agency for Research on Cancer (IARC) Press, Lyon, France, 4th edition, 2010.

[28] D. C. Snover, "Update on the serrated pathway to colorectal carcinoma," *Human Pathology*, vol. 42, no. 1, pp. 1–10, 2011.

[29] D. K. Rex, D. J. Ahnen, J. A. Baron et al., "Serrated lesions of the colorectum: review and recommendations from an expert panel," *The American Journal of Gastroenterology*, vol. 107, no. 9, pp. 1315–1329, 2012.

8

Diagnosis of Superficial Gastric Lesions Together with Six Gastric Lymphoma Cases via Probe-Based Confocal Laser Endomicroscopy: A Retrospective Observational Study

Qian Chen,[1] Heng-Hui Cheng,[2] Shuang Deng,[3] Dong Kuang,[2] Chang Shu,[4] Li Cao,[1] Guang-Quan Liao,[1] Qiao-Zhen Guo,[1] and Qi Zhou[1]

[1]*Endoscopic Unit, Department of Gastroenterology and Hepatology at Tongji Hospital, Tongji Medical College, Huazhong University of Science and Technology (HUST), Wuhan, China*
[2]*Department of Pathology at Tongji Hospital, Tongji Medical College, HUST, Wuhan, China*
[3]*Tongji Medical College, HUST, Wuhan, China*
[4]*Department of Epidemiology and Biostatistics, School of Public Health, Tongji Medical College, HUST, Wuhan, China*

Correspondence should be addressed to Qi Zhou; zhouqi1973@hotmail.com

Academic Editor: Francesco Selvaggi

Objective. To evaluate the performance of probe-based confocal laser endomicroscopy (pCLE) in diagnosis of gastric lesions. *Methods.* An outpatient department- (OPD-) based retrospective study was conducted for patients with suspected upper gastrointestinal (GI) tract lesions who underwent pCLE between 2014 and 2016 at a tertiary hospital in China. Final diagnosis was based on the histopathological reports. CLE reports were compared to histopathological reports to evaluate the diagnostic ability, including sensitivity, specificity, positive predictive value (PPV), negative predictive value (NPV), and diagnostic accuracy. *Results.* 322 of 380 patients were diagnosed with gastric lesions via pCLE, including inflammation and benign ulcers ($n = 110$), atrophy and intestinal metaplasia ($n = 152$), intraepithelial neoplasia ($n = 27$), adenocarcinoma ($n = 27$), and lymphoma ($n = 6$). In total, the diagnostic ability of CLE in evaluation of gastric lesions showed sensitivity 72.4% (95% confidence interval (CI): 67.1–77.2%); specificity 93.1% (95% CI: 5.6–8.4%); PPV 72.4% (95% CI: 67.1–77.2%); NPV 93.1% (95% CI: 5.6–8.4%); and accuracy 88.9% (95% CI: 87.3–90.4%), respectively. We further observed the capability of pCLE in diagnosing six gastric lymphoma showing those affected mucosa densely infiltrated with identical and round-shaped abnormal cells. Immunohistochemistry analysis confirmed one patient with diffuse large B-cell non-Hodgkin's lymphoma (DLBCL) and five with mucosa-associated lymphoid tissue (MALT) lymphoma. *Conclusion.* pCLE is an accurate tool for the detection of gastric lesions and shows optimal values of sensitivity and negative predictivity. Moreover, combining pCLE with white light endoscopy (WLE) may be a promising adjunct to conventional biopsy sampling in evaluating GI tract with suspected lymphoma.

1. Introduction

CLE technology is an emerging technology and enables endoscopists to collect real-time *in vivo* histological images or "virtual biopsies" of the gastrointestinal (GI) mucosa at high resolution [1]. With 1000x magnification of the mucosal layer, the epithelial cells, connective tissue, and changes in vascular patterns of GI tract can be assessed during endoscopy [2]. At present, the potential role of CLE in revealing premalignant and malignant lesions has been of extreme relevance to different pathologic conditions. Accordingly, many studies demonstrate a high correlation between CLE and histopathology results with accuracy ranging from 86% to 96% [3].

Two CLE-based systems are used in routine clinical practice and research. One is an endoscope-integrated CLE (eCLE) system that collects images at a manually adjustable scan rate of 1.6 frames per second. The optical slices of this specialized endoscope are parallel with the mucosal surface with a lateral resolution of 0.7 μm, and the scanning depth can be dynamically adjusted from 0 to 250 μm [2, 4]. In contrast to the eCLE system, pCLE has a fixed scanning depth of 55–65 μm. Nevertheless, pCLE image data are collected at 12 frames per second, enabling real-time video quality and direct visualization of blood on a single erythrocyte scale [5]. Depending on the probe used, the field of view ranges from 240 μm to 600 μm, whereas fixed 475 μm in diameter for eCLE [6]. Thus, the advantage of eCLE system is its high resolution whereas pCLE probe denotes greater flexibility to be introduced through the working channels of any kinds of endoscopes [3, 4, 6].

Currently, CLE technique is not yet routinely used in the clinical practice although it has the prospective impact to improve diagnosis and treatment approach for patients. Many factors, including the cost of the procedure, no clear indications for standard of care, and also the lack of image interpretation training for physician, limit its application in clinics. Furthermore, lack of cross talk between pathologist and physician but relying on histopathology for the final diagnosis of diseases could lead to a 20 to 30% misdiagnosis rate [3]. On the basis of these considerations, we retrospectively analyzed 380 patients who underwent OPD-based pCLE procedures from October 13, 2014, the first day when it became available at our hospital, to December 30, 2016. We aimed to evaluate its diagnostic accuracy and furthermore to validate the use of pCLE in managing selected diseases with diagnostic uncertainties, of which may result in the improvement of therapeutic decisions and/or follow-up procedures in these patients.

2. Materials and Methods

2.1. Single Endoscopy Unit Study. A database of all patients examined by pCLE procedure from October 13, 2014, to December 30, 2016, at the OPD-based endoscopy unit of Tongji Hospital, HUST, was accessed. Tongji Hospital is a state-owned teaching hospital. The endoscopy unit has availability of all endoscopic facilities and treatment modalities for diagnostic, therapeutic, and palliative endoscopies, including narrow band imaging (NBI) and pCLE examination. To detect and localize suspicious areas in GI tact, physicians at Tongji Hospital initially referred these patients for either NBI or pCLE examination. However, patients made final decisions after being informed between the two procedures, based on their financial status and also health insurance policy. In the study period, about 362 patients with 386 lesions chose pCLE at this unit, including 55 esophageal-cardia, 327 gastric, and 4 duodenal lesions.

2.2. Retrospective Analysis. For the purposes of this study, the records of the endoscopy unit were retrospectively reviewed, as well as hospital medical records. All authors had access to information that could identify individual participants during data collection. Approval for the study was given by the Institutional Ethics Committee.

2.3. CLE Criteria for Gastric Superficial Lesions. The pCLE criteria were based on the 2011 Miami classification [5] and Qilu classification for gastric superficial lesions [7–9]. Four pCLE diagnoses were given through evaluating architecture of glands, cells, and microvessels as follows: (1) normal gastric mucosa or benign inflammatory lesions were defined as regularly ranged glands with good polarity, and when inflammation occurred in gastric body, noncontinuous short rod-like glands with short thread-like opening could be seen or when inflammation occurred in antral mucosa, elongated and tortuous branch-like glands could be seen, with honeycomb-like microvessels (gastric body) or coil-shaped microvessels (gastric antrum); (2) atrophy and/or intestinal metaplasia (IM) was defined as the number of glands decreasing with dilating appearance for atrophy and uniform villiform architecture for IM cases, with characteristic black goblet seen in IM, with normal caliber, honeycomb-like or coil-shaped microvessels; (3) intraepithelial neoplasia (IEN) was defined as impaired gland polarity with irregularity in size and epithelial heights, with abnormal cell polarity and increased stratification and hyperdense epithelial cells, and with dilated and distorted microvessel appearance; (4) cancer was defined as the appearance of destroyed gland architecture and loss of gland polarity, absence of cell polarity with disordered appearance, and increased calibre microvessels with irregularity in size and shape, respectively, [5, 7–9].

CLE criteria for gastric lymphoma were based on recent established findings as follows [10–12]: (1) darkened areas made up of small roundish cells of similar size and morphology for the mucosa-associated lymphoid tissue (MALT) lymphoma or larger roundish cells for diffuse large B-cell lymphoma (DLBCL); abnormal cells in a dense arrangement; (2) cellular infiltrates typically affecting but not limited to the lamina propria; (3) cellular invasion of various epithelial structures; (4) altered tissue morphology to complete loss of structural integrity of the epithelium.

2.4. Endoscopy Equipment and Procedure. All procedures were performed using an Evis Lucera Spectrum system (Olympus Medical Systems Co., Tokyo, Japan) with a high-resolution upper GI zoom endoscopy (GIF-Q260, Olympus). After a mucosal lesion was visualized by WLE, fluorescein-aided pCLE was performed with the GastroFlex UHD miniprobe (Cellvizio; Mauna Kea Technologies, Paris, France). To obtain control pCLE images, the probe was first gently contacted to normal mucosa around the lesion, ideally showing regular round or oval glands with homogeneous epithelial cells. The probe was subsequently moved to suspicious lesion to obtain pCLE image, and following it, biopsies were obtained from the area. The diagnosing of gastric lymphoma was based on endoscopic appearance (varying from slight mucosal irregularities to large ulcers) and CLE findings followed by the histopathological examination of 8–10 biopsies taken from suspicious GI lesions [13]. The pCLE images used in the study were taken by two endoscopists (Q.C. and Q.Z.), each with at least a three-year experience in performing endoscopy procedures.

2.5. Histopathology Assessment for Gastric Lymphoma. The lymphomas were categorized in accordance with the 2008 World Health Organization classification of hemopoietic malignancies [14]. A histopathological diagnosis of MALT lymphoma was made when a Wotherspoon histologic score of any one specimen was 5, indicating the presence of dense, diffuse infiltrate of centrocyte-like cells in the lamina propria with prominent lymphoepithelial lesions [15]. In all patients of suspicious lymphoma, paraffin sections were processed with immunochemical techniques for the demonstration of light chain restriction and the phenotypes CD20, CD79, CD10, BCL-6, c-myc, MUM1, CD3, CD43, CD5, BCL-2, cyclin D1, Ki-67, CD21 and CD23, and so on. DLBCL is characterized by expression of B-cell-associated antigens (CD19, CD20, and CD79), with high-Ki-67 proliferation index [16]. Accordingly, BCL-6 expresses in approximately 80% of DLBCL and expression of CD10 and multiple myeloma oncogene (MUM-1) is associated with poor prognosis [17, 18]. The immunophenotype of a MALT lymphoma cell recapitulates that of the marginal zone B-cell. Typically, tumors express pan-B antigens (CD19, CD20, CD22, and CD79a), but they lack CD5, CD10, CD23, and BCL-1 expression. In rare cases, MALT lymphomas exhibit aberrant CD5 expression, which may be associated with a more aggressive clinical course [13, 19, 20].

2.6. Statistical Analysis. Categorical variables were summarized with number and percentage. The diagnostic accuracy of CLE and the prediction of gastric lesions in comparison to standard histology were assessed by using StatsDirect statistical software. Sensitivity and specificity were estimated for pCLE, along with exact bionormal 95% confidence intervals (95% CI), with standard histopathology diagnosis serving as gold standards. PPV = (number who have disease and screened positive) × 100%/[(number who have disease and screened positive) + (number who have no disease and screened positive)]. NPV = (number who have disease and screened negative) × 100%/[(number who have disease and screened negative) + (number who have no disease and screened negative)].

3. Results

3.1. Demographic Baseline Data. Between October 13, 2014, and December 30, 2016, a total of 327 gastric lesions from 327 patients using WLE and pCLE procedures were retrospectively assessed at OPD-based endoscopy unit in HUST. Five patients were excluded from the investigation due to missing histopathological diagnosis, and overall, 322 patients (225 males, 102 females) were analyzed. Thus, median age of patients at the time of pCLE was 53 years (range, 22–78 years) among 322 patients (Table 1). The final diagnosis was given based on standard histology results, leading to a diagnosis of benign inflammatory lesions such as gastritis or benign gastric ulcers in 110 cases (34.1%), atrophy and/or IM in 152 cases (47.2%), IEN in 27 cases (8.4%), adenocarcinoma in 27 cases (8.4%), and lymphoma in 6 cases (1.9%), respectively.

3.2. Diagnosis Accuracy of pCLE Compared to Histopathology. Final diagnosis was categorized based on pathology reports. Except the inflammation or benign ulcerative lesions, for

TABLE 1: Demographic characteristic of 322 patients with gastric lesions.

Variable	Summary ($n = 322$)
*Age, Y	53 (22, 78)
Gender, n (%)	
Male	223 (69.3)
Female	99 (30.7)
Histopathology diagnosis	
Inflammation or benign ulcer, n (%)	110 (34.1)
Atrophy and/or IM, n (%)	152 (47.2)
IEN, n (%)	27 (8.4)
Adenocarcinoma, n (%)	27 (8.4)
Lymphoma, n (%)	6 (1.9)

*Age was summarized as median (minimum and maximum). IM: intestinal metaplasia; IEN: intraepithelial neoplasia.

those suspected with precancerous or malignant lesions, their individual-linked IHC reports were extracted to confirm the diagnosis. pCLE images in combination of WLE revealed abnormalities that led to a suspicion of inflammation or benign ulcer in 45 lesions compared to 110 diagnosed by histopathology; a suspicion of 132 atrophy and/or IM among 152 lesions; and 26 IEN among 27 lesions, 24 cancer among 27 lesions, and 6 lymphoma, respectively. In total, 233 pCLE findings matched the histopathology results. Thus, the sensitivity, specificity, PPV, NPV, and accuracy in diagnosing inflammation or benign ulcer compared to histopathology ($n = 110$) were 40.9%, 94.8%, 80.4%, 75.6%, and 76.4%, respectively. The sensitivity, specificity, PPV, NPV, and accuracy for diagnosing atrophy and/or IM were 86.8%, 81.8%, 81%, 87.4%, and 84.2%; 96.3%, 87.1%, 40.6%, 99.6%, and 87.9% for diagnosing IEN; and 88.9%, 97%, 72.7%, 99%, and 96.3% for diagnosing cancer, respectively (Table 2). In addition, six lymphoma cases were able to be correctively diagnosed following CLE criteria [10–12]. Together, pCLE showed sensitivity of 72.4% (95% CI: 67.1–77.2%), specificity of 93.1% (95% CI: 5.6–8.4%), PPV of 72.4% (95% CI: 67.1–77.2%), NPV of 93.1% (95% CI: 5.6–8.4%), and diagnostic accuracy of 88.9% (95% CI: 87.3–90.4%), respectively (Table 2).

3.3. pCLE in Diagnosing Gastric Lymphoma Compared to Histopathology. In our retrospective study, we reviewed the pCLE imaging of those lymphomas (Table 3) and observed the affected mucosa infiltrated with densely identical and round-shaped abnormal cells (Figure 1). In DLBCL case, pCLE revealed many dark and large roundish cells infiltrated widely in the exiting glands in a sheet-like fashion (Figures 1(b) and 1(c)). In MALT lymphoma, pCLE revealed lymphoepithelial lesions (Figure 1(e)) and massive infiltrate of small roundish cells with similar size and morphology in a dense arrangement (Figures 1(f) and 1(i)).

Histology staining further showed massive large cell infiltration with vesicular nuclei, prominent nucleoli, and basophilic cytoplasm in DLBCL (Figure 2(a)), and dense diffuse infiltrate of centrocyte-like cells and the presence of

Table 2: Sensitivity, specificity, PPV, NPV, and diagnostic accuracy of pCLE for gastric lesions ($n = 322$).

	Inflammation or benign ulcer ($n = 110$)	Atrophy and/or IM ($n = 152$)	IEN ($n = 27$)	Adenocarcinoma ($n = 27$)	Lymphoma ($n = 6$)	Total ($n = 322$)
Sensitivity (%) (95% CI)	40.9 (31.6–50.7%)	86.8 (80.4–91.8%)	96.3 (81.0–99.9%)	88.9 (70.8–97.7%)	100 (54.1–100%)	72.4 (67.1–77.2%)
Specificity (%) (95% CI)	94.8 (2.6–9.1%)	81.8 (12.7–24.9%)	87.1 (9.3–17.3%)	97.0 (1.4–5.7%)	100 (98.8–100%)	93.1 (5.6–8.4%)
PPV (%) (95% CI)	80.4 (67.6–89.8%)	81.0 (74.1–86.7%)	40.6 (28.5–53.6%)	72.7 (54.5–86.7%)	100 (54.1–100%)	72.4 (67.1–77.2%)
NPV (%) (95% CI)	75.6 (19.4–30.1%)	87.4 (7.9–18.8%)	99.6 (0.1–2.1%)	99.0 (0.2–3%)	100 (98.8–100%)	93.1 (5.6–8.4%)
Accuracy (%) (95% CI)	76.4 (71.4–80.9%)	84.2 (79.7–88.0%)	87.9 (83.9–91.2%)	96.3 (94.0–98.1%)	100 (98.9–100%)	88.9 (87.3–90.4%)

CI: confidential interval; PPV: positive predictive value; NPV: negative predictive value; IM: intestinal metaplasia; IEN: intraepithelial neoplasia.

Table 3: Gastric lymphoma patients' clinical characteristics.

Case number	Age (Y)	Gender	Lymphoma	Macroscopic findings	Tumor location
1	56	Male	DLBCL	Single nodule with depressed surface	Body
2	49	Male	MALT lymphoma	Fold thickening and erosions	Body
3	50	Female	MALT lymphoma	Ulcers	Angular and antrum
4	20	Female	MALT lymphoma	Ulcers	Body
5	63	Male	MALT lymphoma	Fold thickening and erosions	Body
6	26	Male	MALT lymphoma	Erosions and erythema	Angular and antrum

MALT: mucosa-associated lymphoid tissue; DLBCL: diffuse large B-cell lymphoma.

lymphoepithelial lesions in MALT lymphoma (Figures 2(d) and 2(g)). IHC analysis confirmed that tumors express pan-B antigens (CD20, CD79), but lack CD5 expression (Table 4 and Figure 2). DLBCL was focally positive for BCL-6, with high Ki-67 proliferation index. In contrast, the five MALTs were BCL-6$^-$ and CD10$^-$, indicating no transformation of follicular lymphoma occurred. Except case 6, MALT lymphomas expressed MUM-1, indicating its origin of postgerminal center B-cells, but may be associated with a more aggressive clinical course (Table 4) [17, 18].

4. Discussion

The present study retrospectively evaluated patients who have been performed pCLE procedures based on a single-center experience. We demonstrated that a pCLE system could be a useful tool to examine patients with gastric lesions ($n = 322$) with sensitivity of 72.4%, specificity of 93.1%, PPV of 72.4%, NPV of 93.1%, and diagnostic accuracy of 88.9%, respectively (Table 2). Accordingly, many studies have demonstrated a high correlation between CLE and histopathology results with accuracy ranging from 86% to 96% [3]. In particular, several studies indicate that the pCLE system has an advantage in predicting IEN with a high level of accuracy of 99%, 97.4% of sensitivity, and 97.4% of specificity [21]. However, we show that the sensitivity, specificity, PPV, NPV, and accuracy in diagnosing IEN compared to histopathology ($n = 27$) were 96.3%, 87.1%, 40.6%, 99.6%, and 87.9% (Table 2); it is currently difficult to make direct comparisons of our study to others. It is possible that our group with less experience is still "on the learning curve." Further study on the learning curve of pCLE imaging is warranted and underway.

Gastrointestinal lymphoma is the most common form of primary extranodal non-Hodgkin's lymphoma (PE-NHL) referring to lymphomas originated from any organ or tissue other than lymph nodes or spleen [13]. For gastric NHL, the majority is B-cell lymphoma with two main histological subtypes (>90% of cases), including MALT lymphoma and DLBCL [13, 22, 23]. Currently, the diagnostic approach for patients with gastric lymphoma is based on thorough upper gastrointestinal endoscopy [24]. When gastric lymphoma is suspected, the most frequent problem in the diagnosis is its differentiation from *H. pylori*-associated gastritis. Particularly at OPD settings, those cases arise in patients in whom standard WLE showed nonspecific macroscopic features such as inflammation, thicken folds, superficial erosions, or ulceration [25]. The histological features favoring MALT lymphoma have been previously reported, including a dense lymphoid infiltrate dominating most of the biopsy specimens, prominent lymphoepithelial lesions, Dutcher bodies in plasma cells, and infiltration of muscularis mucosae and centrocyte-like cells, which are small to medium-sized cells with small irregular nuclei [19, 20]. For DLBCL, lesions are characterized by an intense cellular infiltration of the lamina propria and the predominant cells resemble either centroblasts (large noncleaved cells) or immunoblasts [16]. Nevertheless, many endoscopic biopsy specimens lack several of

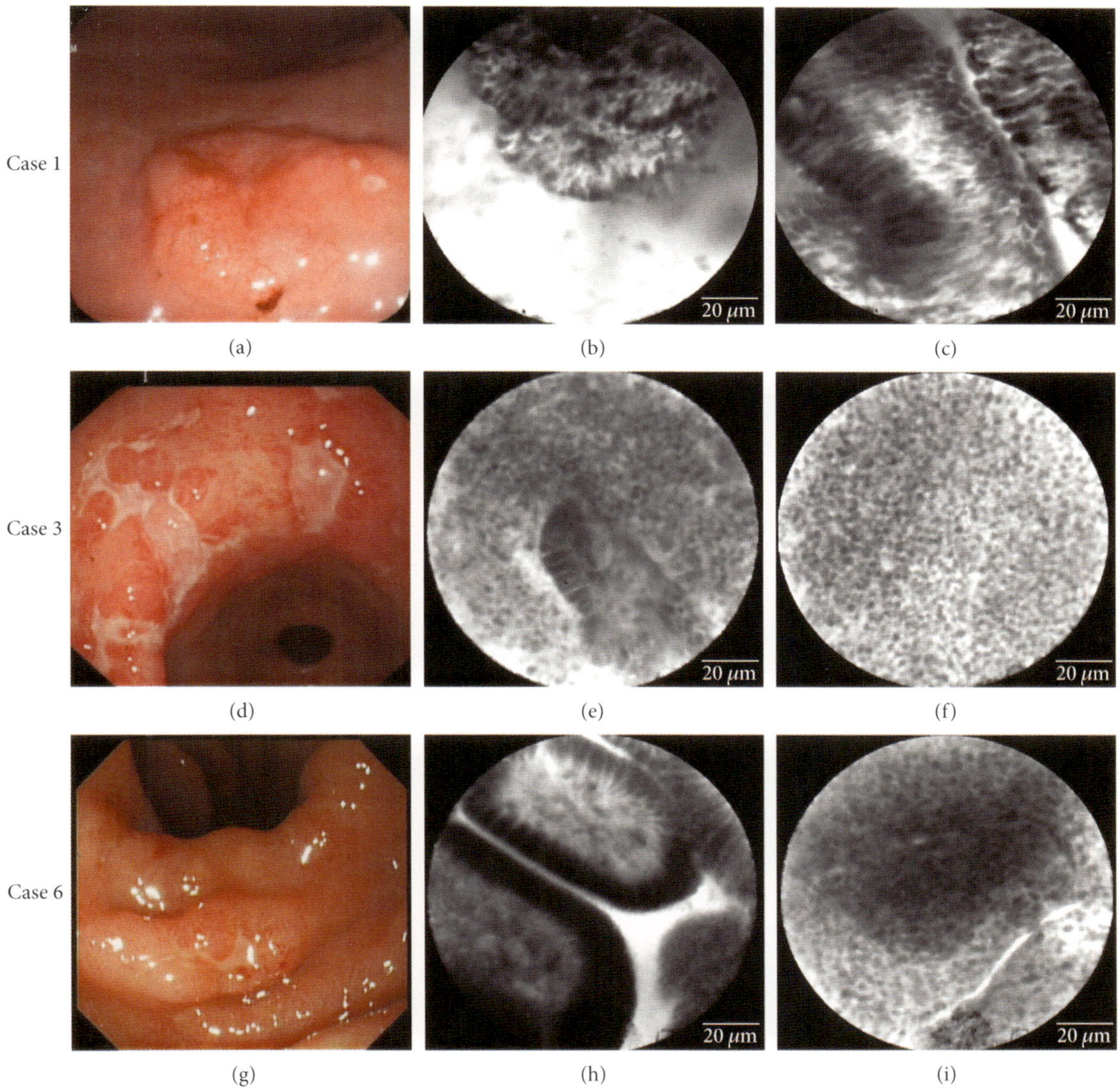

FIGURE 1: WLE and pCLE imaging of gastric lymphoma for case 1 (a–c, DLBCL), case 3 (d–f, MALT lymphoma), and case 6 (g–i, MALT lymphoma). The conventional endoscopic imaging revealed a single-nodule lesion with depressed surface in gastric body (a), multiple ulcerative lesions in gastric angular and antrum (d), and erosions and erythematous lesions in gastric angular (g). In the DLBCL case, pCLE revealed many dark and large roundish cells infiltrated widely in the exiting glands in a sheet-like fashion (b, c). In a MALT lymphoma case, pCLE revealed a massive infiltrate of small roundish cells with similar size and morphology, and in a dense arrangement (f, i), lymphoepithelial lesions could be observed (e, f, i). In (e), most pylorus glands were replaced by lymphocytic infiltrate except one gland showing the impaired structure infiltrated with small and roundish cells. In contrast, normal angular glands in the mucosa around the lesion in case 6 (h) showed regular oval or short rod-like pit pattern with homogenous epithelial cells.

these features. Therefore, at present, repeated biopsy and pathology play important roles in diagnosis and management of the diseases. Occasionally, gastric lymphoma can present as a multifocal stomach disease with numerous clonally identical foci in macroscopically unaffected tissue [13]. Overall, extensive biopsy sampling and gastric mapping of those macroscopically unaffected mucosa are crucially recommended in order to establish diagnosis. In terms of determination of the depth of invasion and the sensitive detection of affected regional lymph nodes, endoscopic ultrasonography (EUS) has the great impact in locoregional staging of the disease [24].

Our study confirms two previous findings, which demonstrate the applicability of CLE in diagnosing of gastric lymphoma [11, 12]. The first study by Dolak and colleagues used a pCLE system with a fixed scanning depth of 55–65 μm and characterized that a dense infiltration of small cells with a size of approximately 5 μm was a special finding for gastric MALT lymphoma [11]. Recently, a pilot study by Nonaka and colleagues set up descriptive criteria for MALT lymphoma by using integrated CLE, which in contrast to pCLE is a confocal scanner integrated into the distal tip of endoscope and the scanning depth can be dynamically adjusted from 0 to 250 μm [12]. The evaluation of 24 patients

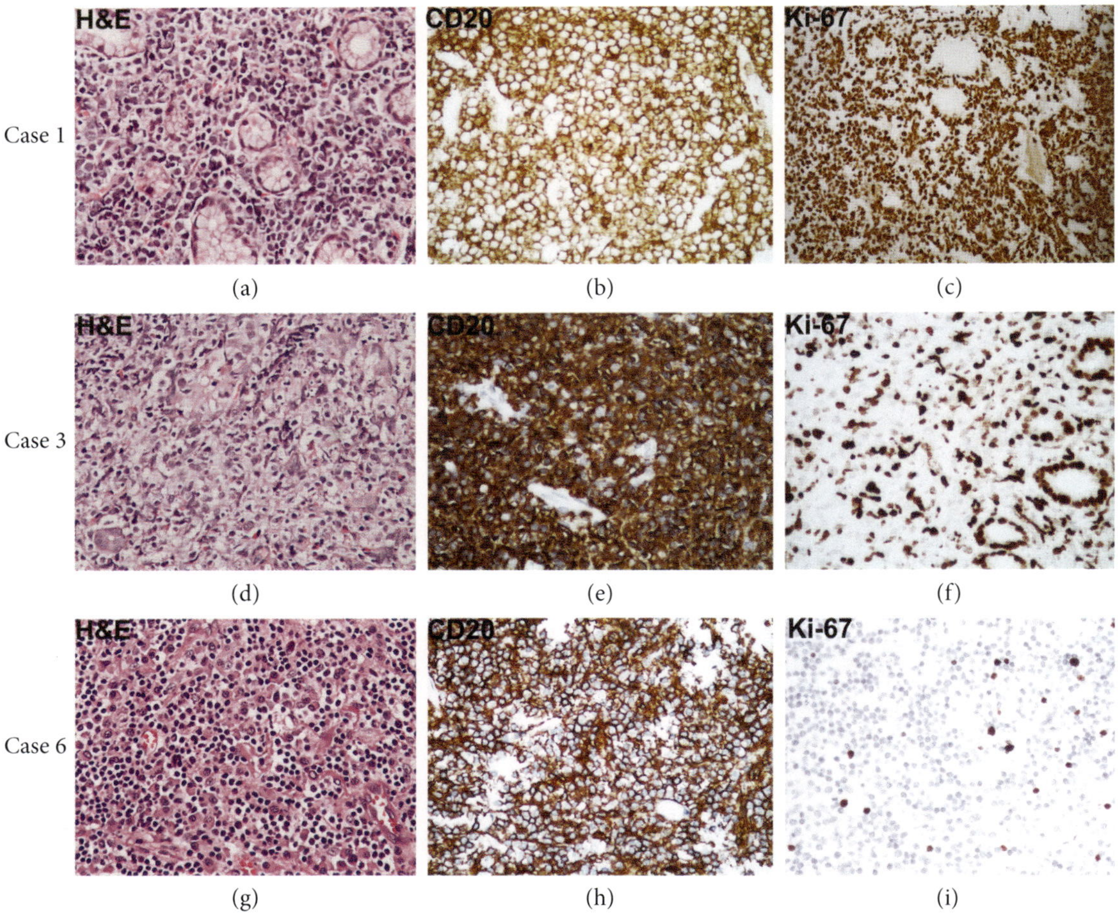

FIGURE 2: Histopathological examination for case 1 (a–c, DLBCL), case 3 (d–f, MALT lymphoma), and case 6 (g–i, MALT lymphoma). For DLBCL, hematoxylin and eosin (H&E) staining shows massive large cell infiltration with vesicular nuclei, prominent nucleoli, and basophilic cytoplasm (a, ×40). For MALT lymphoma, H&E staining shows dense diffuse infiltrate of centrocyte-like cells and the presence of lymphoepithelial lesions (d, g; ×40). Immunohistochemistry (IHC) sections showing infiltrating lymphoma cells express strong positivity with anti-CD20 stain, confirming their B-cell origin (b, e, h; ×400). (c, f, i) indicate the IHC staining for Ki-67 (×400). Positive staining is indicated by the brown color. In the DLBCL case (c), the neoplastic cells show prominent immunoreactivity to Ki-67.

with gastrointestinal MALT lymphoma by comparing EUS, WLE, and CLE suggested that their sensitivity was 80%, 100%, and 93%, whereas the specificity was 67%, 23%, and 100%, respectively. It is also highlighted that identification of darkened areas made up of small roundish cells of similar size and morphology is the criteria together with the cellular infiltration patterns as well as altered tissue morphology of which are actually quite close to conventional histology and immunohistochemistry findings. Although pCLE has a fixed scanning depth of 55–65 μm, in clinical practice, we are able to visualize varying depths of mucosa, including the lamina propria by increasing or decreasing the pressure of the probe against the GI wall. Thus, those infiltrated lymphoid cells and lymphoepithelial lesions, we observed by pCLE lesions in lamina propria and epithelium. Accordingly, our current study confirms the effectiveness of pCLE in diagnosing lymphoma and thus suggests that CLE may serve as a promising adjunct to conventional biopsy sampling. However, the limited sample size is regarded as a shortcoming, and thus, a controlled, blinded prospective clinical trial should be initiated in a large cohort in the future study.

Till now, the characteristics of DLBCL have not clearly been addressed by CLE approach, although several reports have valued CLE in diagnosing DLBCL [10, 26]. This may be due to the fact that such deep diagnostic tools have not been routinely used in GI lymphoma staging and follow-up. At our endoscopy unit, we offer patient options including EUS and narrow-band imaging in combination with magnification endoscopy (NBI-ME), as well as pCLE when lesions were suspected and required further assessment. Many patients preferred NBI-ME over pCLE because of lack of sufficient health care reimbursement. Previous studies have showed the application of NBI-ME in diagnosis of gastric lymphoma through observing the destroyed glandular structures and presence of branching abnormal blood vessels [25, 27–29]. Nevertheless, the absence of gastric pit pattern or a nonstructural mucosal pattern is frequently appeared in gastric cancer, and therefore, the distinction between gastric cancer and lymphomas might be difficult by magnifying endoscopy alone in certain cases. In our retrospective study, we showed that pCLE revealed DLBCL with many dark and large roundish cells infiltrated widely in the exiting glands

TABLE 4: Immunohistochemistry features for the 6 gastric lymphoma patients.

Case number	1	2	3	4	5	6
CD20	+	+	+	+	+	+
CD79α	+	+	+	+	+	+
PAX-5	+	+	+	+	+	+
CD10	+	–	–	–	–	–
BCL-6	+		–	–	–	–
c-myc	+	–	–	–	–	–
Kappa	+	–	(Weak) +	(Weak) +	–	(Weak) +
Lambda	+	–	+	(Weak) +	–	+
MUM1	–	–	–	–	–	+
CD3	–	–	–	–	–	–
CD43	–	–	+	–	+	–
CD5	–	–	–	–	–	–
BCL-2	–	N/A	+	–	+	+
Cyclin D1	–	–	–	–	–	–
*Ki-67	>95%	7%	30%	2%	5%	15%
CD21	–	N/A	N/A	+	+	+
CD23	–	N/A	N/A	N/A	+	+
Histology grades	High	Low	Low	Low	Low	Low

∗ indicates Ki-67 labeling.

and this finding served as the major feature. However, given that for example, those abnormal cells in a sheet-like fashion (Figures 1(b) and 1(c)) could also be shared by gastric cancer; biopsy is needed at present to distinguish them. One of the limitations of the current study was that the pathology or IHC data was from the previous horizontal-sectional histologic examination. Given that pCLE provides the cross-sectional virtual histologic images *in vivo* are obviously different from those found by horizontal pathological examination [7], in the current retrospective study, the relation between pCLE scanning depth and resultant pathological findings could not be addressed. Applying the cross-sectional pathological examination demonstrated by Zhang et al. [7] will be guaranteed in future study in order to further understand pCLE images. Another limitation of this study was those patients were OPD-based, and we could not check the rearrangement of BCL-2, BCL-6, or MYC gene arrangement to further confirm our diagnosis. Thus, in the future, more DLBCL patients should be monitored under pCLE system and followed up at our endoscopy unit in order to develop diagnostic criteria. It may help us in managing selected diseases with diagnostic uncertainties, of which may result in the improvement of therapeutic decisions and/or follow-up procedures in these patients.

In summary, the prediction of gastric lesions based on pCLE has a relatively high diagnostic accuracy as compared to histology analysis. Regarding gastric lymphoma, this novel technique maps the affected mucosa and aids biopsy sampling during endoscopic procedure and thus may reduce the number of unnecessary biopsy in order to establish diagnosis. Given that combining pCLE with WLE may be a promising alternative to evaluate GI tract with suspected lymphoma, new clinical trials on pCLE are warranted and ongoing.

Authors' Contributions

Qi Zhou and Qian Chen were involved in the study design. Heng-hui Cheng and Dong Kuang provided histopathology analysis. Chang Shu provided statistical analysis. Shuang Deng, Qiao-Zhen Guo, and Guang-Quan Liao collected the clinical data and subsequently provided the assessment and interpretation of the data. Qian Chen wrote the manuscript. All authors read and approved the manuscript.

Acknowledgments

The authors thank all the staffs at the endoscopy unit of Tongji Hospital for their contributions and Mrs. Lian-jun Chen, Mrs. Lan Chen, and Mrs. Qing Zhou for collecting the clinical data for this manuscript. This work was supported by grants of the National Natural Science Foundation of China (81471612).

References

[1] J. E. East, J. L. Vleugels, P. Roelandt et al., "Advanced endoscopic imaging: European Society of Gastrointestinal Endoscopy (ESGE) Technology Review," *Endoscopy*, vol. 48, no. 11, pp. 1029–1045, 2016.

[2] D. I. Gheonea, T. Cartana, T. Ciurea, C. Popescu, A. Badarau, and A. Saftoiu, "Confocal laser endomicroscopy and immunoendoscopy for real-time assessment of vascularization in gastrointestinal malignancies," *World Journal of Gastroenterology*, vol. 17, no. 1, pp. 21–27, 2011.

[3] C. Robles-Medranda, "Confocal endomicroscopy: is it time to move on?," *World Journal of Gastrointestinal Endoscopy*, vol. 8, no. 1, pp. 1–3, 2016.

[4] G. D. D. Palma, "Confocal laser endomicroscopy in the "in vivo" histological diagnosis of the gastrointestinal tract," *World Journal of Gastroenterology*, vol. 15, no. 46, pp. 5770–5775, 2009.

[5] M. Wallace, G. Y. Lauwers, Y. Chen et al., "Miami classification for probe-based confocal laser endomicroscopy," *Endoscopy*, vol. 43, no. 10, pp. 882–891, 2011.

[6] M. B. Wallace and P. Fockens, "Probe-based confocal laser endomicroscopy," *Gastroenterology*, vol. 136, no. 5, pp. 1509–1513, 2009.

[7] J. N. Zhang, Y. Q. Li, Y. A. Zhao et al., "Classification of gastric pit patterns by confocal endomicroscopy," *Gastrointestinal Endoscopy*, vol. 67, no. 6, pp. 843–853, 2008.

[8] Z. Li, T. Yu, X. L. Zuo et al., "Confocal laser endomicroscopy for in vivo diagnosis of gastric intraepithelial neoplasia: a feasibility study," *Gastrointestinal Endoscopy*, vol. 72, no. 6, pp. 1146–1153, 2010.

[9] W. B. Li, X. L. Zuo, C. Q. Li et al., "Diagnostic value of confocal laser endomicroscopy for gastric superficial cancerous lesions," *Gut*, vol. 60, no. 3, pp. 299–306, 2011.

[10] T. Kav, M. Ozen, A. Uner, S. Abdullazade, B. Ozseker, and Y. Bayraktar, "How confocal laser endomicroscopy can help us in diagnosing gastric lymphomas?," *Bratislava Medical Journal*, vol. 113, no. 11, pp. 680–682, 2012.

[11] W. Dolak, B. Kiesewetter, L. Mullauer et al., "A pilot study of confocal laser endomicroscopy for diagnosing gastrointestinal mucosa-associated lymphoid tissue (MALT) lymphoma," *Surgical Endoscopy*, vol. 30, no. 7, pp. 2879–2885, 2016.

[12] K. Nonaka, K. Ohata, S. Ban, M. Takita, Y. Minato, and N. Matsuhashi, "Confocal laser endomicroscopic and magnifying narrow-band imaging findings of gastric mucosa-associated lymphoid tissue lymphoma," *Endoscopy*, vol. 47, Supplement 1, pp. E641–E642, 2015.

[13] A. Psyrri, S. Papageorgiou, and T. Economopoulos, "Primary extranodal lymphomas of stomach: clinical presentation, diagnostic pitfalls and management," *Annals of Oncology*, vol. 19, no. 12, pp. 1992–1999, 2008.

[14] J. W. Vardiman, J. Thiele, D. A. Arber et al., "The 2008 revision of the World Health Organization (WHO) classification of myeloid neoplasms and acute leukemia: rationale and important changes," *Blood*, vol. 114, no. 5, pp. 937–951, 2009.

[15] A. C. Wotherspoon, T. C. Diss, L. Pan et al., "Regression of primary low-grade B-cell gastric lymphoma of mucosa-associated lymphoid tissue type after eradication of helicobacter pylori," *The Lancet*, vol. 342, no. 8871, pp. 575–577, 1993.

[16] A. J. M. Ferreri and C. Montalbán, "Primary diffuse large B-cell lymphoma of the stomach," *Critical Reviews in Oncology/Hematology*, vol. 63, no. 1, pp. 65–71, 2007.

[17] C. A. L. de Mello, V. P. de Andrade, V. C. C. de Lima, A. L. Carvalho, and F. A. Soares, "Prognostic impact of MUM1 expression by immunohistochemistry on primary mediastinal large B-cell lymphoma," *Leukemia & Lymphoma*, vol. 52, no. 8, pp. 1495–1503, 2011.

[18] P. Uherova, C. W. Ross, B. Schnitzer, T. P. Singleton, and W. G. Finn, "The clinical significance of CD10 antigen expression in diffuse large B-cell lymphoma," *American Journal of Clinical Pathology*, vol. 115, no. 4, pp. 582–588, 2001.

[19] C. M. Bacon, M. Q. Du, and A. Dogan, "Mucosa-associated lymphoid tissue (MALT) lymphoma: a practical guide for pathologists," *Journal of Clinical Pathology*, vol. 60, no. 4, pp. 361–372, 2007.

[20] S. M. Cohen, M. Petryk, M. Varma, P. S. Kozuch, E. D. Ames, and M. L. Grossbard, "Non-Hodgkin's lymphoma of mucosa-associated lymphoid tissue," *The Oncologist*, vol. 11, no. 10, pp. 1100–1117, 2006.

[21] A. M. Buchner, M. W. Shahid, M. G. Heckman et al., "Comparison of probe-based confocal laser endomicroscopy with virtual chromoendoscopy for classification of colon polyps," *Gastroenterology*, vol. 138, no. 3, pp. 834–842, 2010.

[22] "A clinical evaluation of the International Lymphoma Study Group classification of non-Hodgkin's lymphoma. The non-Hodgkin's lymphoma classification project," *Blood*, vol. 89, no. 11, pp. 3909–3918, 1997.

[23] P. G. Isaacson and M. Q. Du, "MALT lymphoma: from morphology to molecules," *Nature Reviews Cancer*, vol. 4, no. 8, pp. 644–653, 2004.

[24] J. Janssen, "The impact of EUS in primary gastric lymphoma," *Best Practice & Research. Clinical Gastroenterology*, vol. 23, no. 5, pp. 671–678, 2009.

[25] H. Isomoto, K. Matsushima, T. Hayashi et al., "Endocytoscopic findings of lymphomas of the stomach," *BMC Gastroenterology*, vol. 13, no. 1, 2013.

[26] K. Dunbar and M. Canto, "Confocal endomicroscopy," *Current Opinion in Gastroenterology*, vol. 24, no. 5, pp. 631–637, 2008.

[27] K. Nonaka, K. Ishikawa, M. Shimizu et al., "Gastrointestinal: Gastric mucosa-associated lymphoma presented with unique vascular features on magnified endoscopy combined with narrow-band imaging," *Journal of Gastroenterology and Hepatology*, vol. 24, no. 10, p. 1697, 2009.

[28] K. Nonaka, K. Ishikawa, S. Arai et al., "A case of gastric mucosa-associated lymphoid tissue lymphoma in which magnified endoscopy with narrow band imaging was useful in the diagnosis," *World Journal of Gastrointestinal Endoscopy*, vol. 4, no. 4, pp. 151–156, 2012.

[29] K. Nonaka, K. Ohata, N. Matsuhashi et al., "Is narrow-band imaging useful for histological evaluation of gastric mucosa-associated lymphoid tissue lymphoma after treatment?," *Digestive Endoscopy*, vol. 26, no. 3, pp. 358–364, 2014.

Radiological Patterns of Lung Involvement in Inflammatory Bowel Disease

Diletta Cozzi,[1] Chiara Moroni,[1] Gloria Addeo,[1] Ginevra Danti,[1] Monica Marina Lanzetta,[1] Edoardo Cavigli,[1] Massimo Falchini,[2] Fabio Marra,[3] Claudia Lucia Piccolo,[4] Luca Brunese,[4] and Vittorio Miele[1]

[1]*Department of Radiology, Careggi University Hospital, Florence, Italy*
[2]*Department of Experimental and Clinical Biomedical Sciences, Radiodiagnostic Unit No. 2, University of Florence-Careggi University Hospital, Florence, Italy*
[3]*Department of Clinical and Experimental Medicine, Internal Medicine and Hepatology, University of Florence, Florence, Italy*
[4]*Department of Medicine and Health Sciences, University of Molise, Campobasso, Italy*

Correspondence should be addressed to Vittorio Miele; vmiele@sirm.org

Academic Editor: Fabiana Zingone

Inflammatory bowel disease (IBD) is a form of chronic inflammation of the gastrointestinal tract, including two major entities: ulcerative colitis and Crohn's disease. Although intestinal imaging of IBD is well known, imaging of extraintestinal manifestations is not extensively covered. In particular, the spectrum of IBD-associated or related changes in the chest is broad and may mimic other conditions. The common embryonic origin of intestine and lungs from the foregut, autoimmunity, smoking, and bacterial translocation from the colon may all be involved in the pathogenesis of these manifestations in IBD patients. Chest involvement in IBD can present concomitant with or years after the onset of the bowel disease even postcolectomy and can affect more than one thoracic structure. The purpose of the present paper is to present the different radiological spectrum of IBD-related chest manifestations, including lung parenchyma, airways, serosal surfaces, and pulmonary vasculature. The most prevalent and distinctive pattern of respiratory involvement is large airway inflammation, followed by lung alterations. Pulmonary manifestations are mainly detected by pulmonary function tests and high-resolution computed tomography (HRCT). It is desirable that radiologists know the various radiological patterns of possible respiratory involvement in such patients, especially at HRCT. It is essential for radiologists to work in multidisciplinary teams in order to establish the correct diagnosis and treatment, which rests on corticosteroids at variance with any other form of bronchiectasis.

1. Introduction

Inflammatory bowel disease (IBD) is a broad term that describes miscellaneous inflammatory diseases of the gastrointestinal tract. The principal pathological entities are Crohn's disease (CD) and ulcerative colitis (UC) [1]. From a pathophysiological point of view, these two conditions are distinct. CD is a relapsing inflammatory disease involving any site of the gastrointestinal tract manifesting with transmural and noncontiguous lesions. UC is an inflammation of the rectum and colon only, characterized by continuous, ascendant alterations that involves only the mucosa, leaving the rest of the colorectal wall unscathed [1–3]. The increasing incidence of IBD in industrialized countries has permitted a better knowledge of these diseases in the last few decades [4]. Extraintestinal manifestations commonly occur in IBD with a prevalence between 21% and 47% [5, 6]. The most common extraintestinal manifestations are cutaneous (*erythema nodosum*, *pyoderma gangrenosum*, and enterocutaneous fistulas), hepatobiliary (primary sclerosing cholangitis, hepatitis, pancreatitis, and portal vein thrombosis), musculoskeletal (arthritis), genitourinary (renal stones, obstructive uropathy), ocular (uveitis, conjunctivitis, and episcleritis), and respiratory (progressive airway and lung involvement, pulmonary vasculature alterations). Radiological imaging plays a fundamental contributory role in detection, characterization, and surveillance of IBD, thanks to computed tomography (CT) and magnetic resonance (MR). Some of the extraintestinal manifestations of IBD can be detected with imaging examinations optimized for the bowel study: these include hepatobiliary, pancreatic, and genitourinary disorders. Further radiological investigations must be warranted if an extraintestinal manifestation is suspected, and it is not possible to study it well with a bowel-targeted examination. In this article, we reviewed the different radiological patterns at high-resolution computed tomography (HRCT) related to respiratory involvement in patients with IBD. Radiologists should be aware of these potential extraintestinal alterations and collaborate with clinicians and reach an accurate diagnosis.

2. Respiratory System Involvement in IBD

Respiratory involvement in IBD was first described by Lopez Botet and Rosalem Archer in 1962, and since then, the association has been relentlessly reported [7–10]. The association is rare (prevalence < 1%) and the spectrum of manifestations is broad [5, 6, 9–12]. Current estimates for the prevalence of respiratory abnormality in patients with IBD are around 40%, many of these being subclinical presentations and of uncertain clinical significance, and overall they may be underestimated [8]. Furthermore, in up to 10% patients with IBD, respiratory involvement may be underdiagnosed because their manifestations may precede presentation of bowel disease by months or years [10, 12, 13]. In their review, Black et al. found that IBD patients experience respiratory symptoms with a greater frequency than the general population [8]. Respiratory symptoms may occur more commonly in UC than in CD [10]. Camus et al. noticed that symptoms may develop or worsen after total colectomy in patients with UC [10]. The reason is unknown: the shift of the inflammatory process from the bowel to the lung is often possibly because of the common ancestry of the bowel and the bronchial tree from the primitive gut [10]. Furthermore, additional evidences have to be considered: the parallel flares of bowel and lung symptoms seen in some patients, the steroid sensitivity of the airway disease seen in many patients, and the fact that the biliary tract (which originates from the primitive gut) can also be involved in IBD [10]. Papanikolaou et al. in their study showed a genetic predisposition for various extraintestinal manifestations: haplotypes HLA-A2 and HLA-DR1 in CD and HLA-B27, HLA-B58, and HLA-B8/D3 in UC are more related to joint, skin, and eye disorders [5]. A specific genetic predisposition for respiratory involvement has not been demonstrated yet [5]. The pathogenesis of lung involvement is not yet perfectly known but may relate to a common embryologic origin of respiratory and intestinal mucosa (both derived from the primitive foregut): both the colonic and respiratory epithelia possess goblet cells and submucosal glands. In addition, they both contain submucosal lymphoid tissue and play crucial roles in host mucosal defence. Hypothetically, intestinal and respiratory alterations in these patients could result from epithelial exposure to common antigens by inhalation/ingestion, leading to a sensitization of lymphoid tissue and inflammation. Another physiopathologic theory is that respiratory involvement may be due to inflammatory mediators released by the bowel mucosa [8, 14]. Clinically, patients may present nonspecific respiratory symptoms, such as cough, wheezing, and shortness of breath. Songür et al. found that 16 of 36 IBD patients (44%) in a gastroenterology department had symptoms of wheeze, cough, sputum production, and breathlessness without any evidence of pulmonary infections [15]. Pulmonary function tests (PFTs) are usually suboptimal in patients with IBD in comparison with nonaffected subjects. Furthermore, PFTs may not generally correlate with IBD activity [8, 16]. A number of reports have demonstrated a decrease in diffusion capacity of the lung of carbon monoxide (DLCO) between asymptomatic affected patients and control subjects [15, 17, 18]. Respiratory system involvement includes the airways, lung parenchyma, lung vasculature, and pleural/pericardial serosa (Table 1). The airways may be involved at any level with a wide spectrum of alterations including bronchiectasis, tracheal stenosis, chronic bronchitis, asthma, bronchiolitis, and COPD [8]. Lung involvement patterns in IBD are mainly related to opportunistic infections (which are the main cause, also due to the immunosuppression after IBD-related therapy) and drug-induced toxicity or directly related to primary IBD inflammation [12]. Occasionally, there are concomitant diseases involving the respiratory system in IBD patients, such as asthma, sarcoidosis, chronic obstructive pulmonary disease (COPD), and emphysema related to A1-antitrypsin deficiency (AATD). After arthritis, asthma is the most common comorbidity in both UC and CD, affecting especially males, while sarcoidosis is more common in CD. COPD in IBD patients should be investigated and recognized promptly because it increases the mortality in CD patients, even if it is known that cigarette smoke is a protecting factor against UC (but promotes CD progression) [19]. Furthermore, AATD must be suspected in young patients with IBD and emphysema [5]. Anyway, a clinically oriented approach is necessary, accompanied by targeted radiological diagnostic procedures.

3. Role of Imaging

High-resolution computed tomography (HRCT) has been shown to be the imaging modality of choice for the detection and assessment of adult pulmonary involvement in IBD [6, 8]. HRCT alterations have a prevalence range between 22% and 89%, and radiological findings may be independent of symptoms, pulmonary function tests, and the activity of intestinal inflammation [5, 9]. On the other hand, Songür et al. showed that HRCT abnormalities are present in a large proportion of patients with IBD and approximately 80% of these had active bowel disease [15]. The most common HRCT findings in respiratory involvement include bronchial wall thickening (that may decrease following corticosteroids), bronchiectasis, lung opacities, emphysema, and ground-glass alterations. Recently, HRCT scans at suspended full expiration have been used to study air trapping mainly in patients with asthma, emphysema, bronchiectasis, and constrictive bronchiolitis [15, 20]. Expiratory scans may be also

TABLE 1: Respiratory and heart involvement in IBD: sites and patterns. –: not described; ±: unusual; +: occasionally observed; ++: relatively common.

Site of involvement	Pattern	UC	CD
Upper airway	Glottic and subglottic edema/stenosis	++	+
	Isolated tracheal inflammation/bulging	++	+
Large airways	Bronchiectasis	++	+
	Suppurative airway disease	++	±
	Acute bronchitis	+	±
	Chronic bronchitis	++	±
Small airways	Diffuse panbronchiolitis	+	–
	Granulomatous bronchiolitis	–	+
	Bronchiolitis obliterans syndrome	+	–
	Necrotizing bronchiolitis	+	++
Lung parenchyma	OP	++	±
	Eosinophilic pneumonia	+	±
	NSIP cellular	+	++
	DIP	+	–
	Fibrosing alveolitis	±	±
	Sterile necrobiotic nodules	+	+
Pulmonary vasculature	Pulmonary embolism	±	±
	Granulomatosis with polyangiitis (GPA)	+	+
	Eosinophilic GPA (EGPA)	±	+
	"Pulmonary vasculitis"	+	+
Serosal surface	Pleural effusion	+	+
	Pericardial effusion	+	+
Concomitant diseases involving lung/airways	Sarcoidosis-like	+	+
	A1-antitrypsin deficiency	+	+
	COPD	+	+
	Amyloidosis	±	±
Various patterns	Pneumomediastinum	±	±
	Pulmonary interstitial emphysema	+	+
Heart/pericardial involvement	Myocarditis	+	+
	Atrioventricular block	+	+
	Pericardial tamponade	+	+

useful for detecting the main causes of mosaic pattern (infiltrative lung disease, small airway disease, and pulmonary vascular disease) [21, 22]. Due to radiation exposure and young age of most IBD patients, HRCT should be used in symptomatic patients in which clinicians have high suspicion of respiratory involvement (Figure 1). Usually, findings at chest X-ray are insensitive and not specific [23]. As chest X-ray is often normal in patients with respiratory symptoms, the radiological patterns remain poorly characterized [10, 23, 24]. The prevalence of pulmonary involvement in children with IBD is low and pulmonary HRCT changes are not common. Therefore, it is not recommended to perform HRCT in children except in those cases with severe clinical respiratory manifestations [25].

4. Imaging Features

4.1. Airway Disease. The most prevalent and distinctive pattern of respiratory involvement in IBD is airway inflammation representing 40–63% of the total of clinically significant respiratory complaints [10]. A wide range of airway abnormalities have been identified in UC patients or less commonly in CD, including subglottic stenosis, chronic bronchitis, and chronic suppurative inflammation of both large and small airways [8, 22]. If left untreated, airway disease can lead to irreversible stenosis in the airway. Upper airway involvement (UAI) in IBD is a rare entity that may involve the pharynx, larynx, trachea, and mainstream bronchi. It may occur up to years after the diagnosis of intestinal bowel disease and in UC can occur after total colectomy [5]. In patients with UC, edema, ulceration, and haemorrhage within the trachea and large airways may mimic the mucosal alterations seen in the colon wall. Instead, tracheobronchitis related to CD has noncaseating and epithelioid granulomas, which may manifest as nodular thickening (Figure 2) [26–28]. Upper airway involvement in IBD may present with cough, hoarseness, stridor, and respiratory distress. Imaging can help in the diagnosis. Chest X-ray is not helpful but sometimes it is possible to show a tracheal narrowing. On the other side, HRCT is able to show definite circumferential or nodular thickening of the tracheobronchial wall. The main differential diagnosis of UAI in IBD includes granulomatosis with polyangiitis (GPA), infections, burns, sarcoidosis, and amyloidosis [29]. Supraglottic, laryngeal, and glottic involvement in patients with sarcoidosis are well recognized, and traction bronchiectasis is often visible in sarcoidosis patients, together with typical mediastinal lymphadenopathy [30]. Respiratory involvement in patients with amyloidosis may occur as part of multisystemic disease or isolated, in case of localized amyloidosis, and the tracheal wall is a frequent site of involvement. Large airways are the most common anatomic site of respiratory involvement in IBD, estimated for about 50% of total respiratory manifestations [5, 26]. Large airway involvement (LAI) is often associated with other extraintestinal manifestations, and it is more common in nonsmoking female with UC. Patients may present with acute/chronic bronchitis, suppurative bronchitis, and bronchiectasis: chronic suppurative airway disease may precede (10%–15%), coexist with (5%–10%), or follow the development of inflammatory bowel disease (8%–85%) [5, 8, 10]. Of particular interest is the fact that, unlike other causes of bronchiectasis, chronic suppurative airway disease associated with UC frequently responds to treatment with inhaled steroids. Chest X-ray may show increased interstitial markings, a reticular pattern, or may appear normal (Figure 3). HRCT classical pattern is characterized by diffuse or sporadic concentric bronchial wall thickening (with or without mucoid impaction) and bronchiectasis (cylindric, varicose, or cystic) (Figures 4 and 5) [12, 31]. Mahadeva et al. demonstrated that 13 out of 17 patients (76%) had bronchiectasis on HRCT [23]. Small airway involvement (SAI)

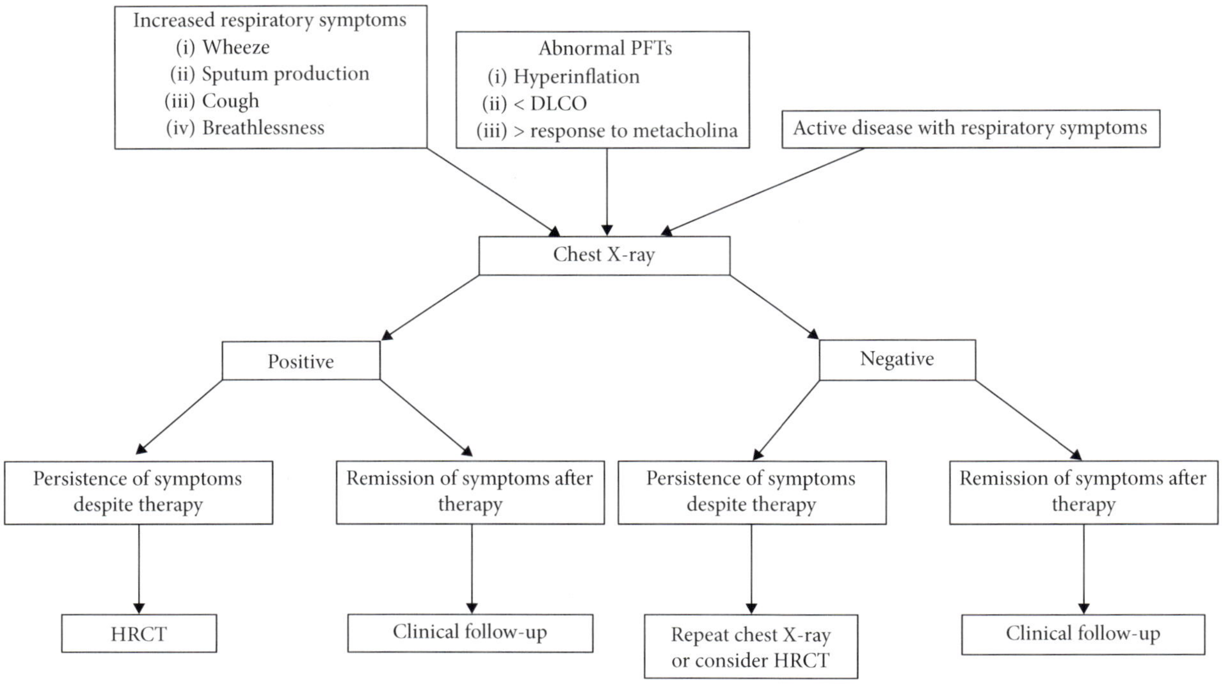

FIGURE 1: The flowchart indicates when to perform chest X-ray and HRCT in IBD patients.

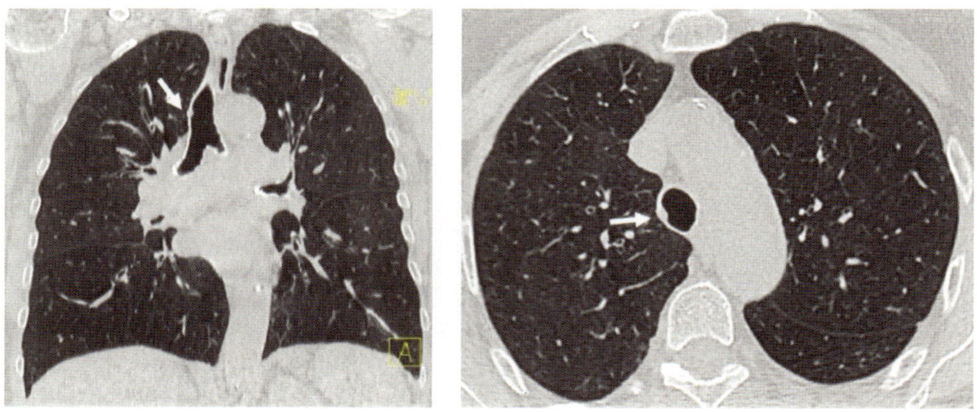

(a) (b)

FIGURE 2: A 77-year-old woman with old history of CD. These HRCT coronal (a) and axial (b) reconstructions show a small nodule in the tracheal wall, most likely referring to a granuloma (arrows).

is rarely encountered clinically (3%–10%). It occurs at younger age and tends to present at an earlier point in the disease course than LAI [32–34]. However, with more widespread HRCT use, the detection of SAI in IBD patients is increasing [8]. Chest X-ray can be normal or shows increased lung volumes consistent with air trapping and/or reticulonodular or ground-glass opacities. The typical pattern on HRCT is bronchitis/bronchiolitis characterized by bronchiolar wall thickening, mucoid impaction, centrilobular ground-glass nodules, tree in bud, and mosaic due to air trapping (Figure 6). Chronic bronchiolitis may lead to the progressive bronchiectasis and bronchiolectasis (Figure 7). Inhaled/systemic steroids are the therapy of choice in large and small airway disease in patients with IBD; rarely, immunomodulators, such as TNF-alpha, have been used, because of their limited clinical evidence for efficacy [32, 35–41]. Details of therapy are available in the article by Camus and Colby [42]. At times, bronchial thickness may decrease while steroids are given [43].

4.2. Lung Parenchymal Involvement. Lung parenchymal involvement in IBD can be due to nonspecific infection, while true IBD-related interstitial lung disease is rare [8, 10, 12]. Not infrequently in patients who are not postcolectomy, the IBD drug toxicity is involved. Many of the HRCT patterns found in these patients are not pathognomonic for IBD and can be present in more than one context: infection, drug toxicity, or IBD-related changes [44].

It may be difficult for the radiologist alone to differentiate the exact aetiology, and a multidisciplinary approach to lung alterations in IBD is recommended. Ulcerative colitis is more often reported to be related with parenchymal involvement

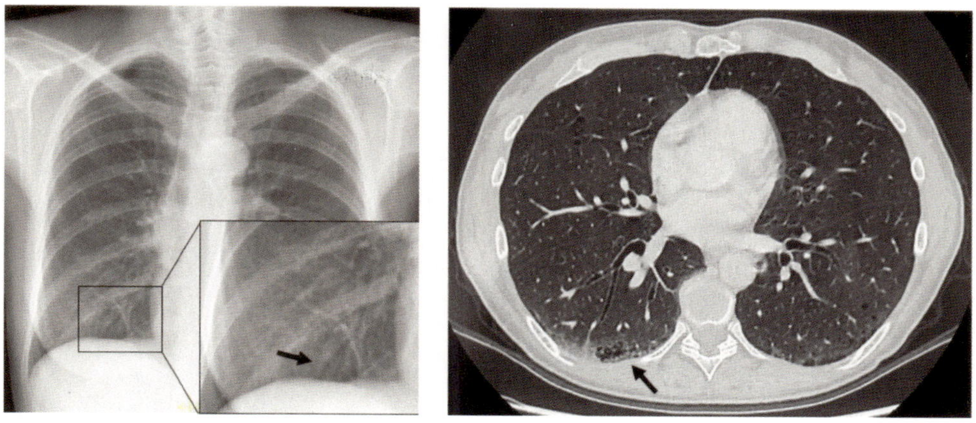

FIGURE 3: A 55-year-old woman with CD. Chest X-ray shows right basal bronchial wall thickening suggesting bronchitis (a). Axial HRCT study shows peribronchial wall thickening associated with bronchiolectasis (arrow) and signs of subpleural emphysema (b).

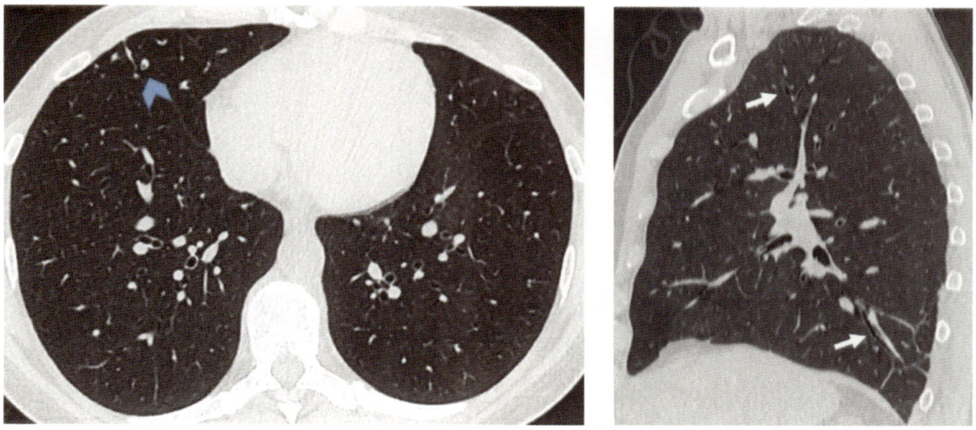

FIGURE 4: Axial HRCT scan (a) and sagittal reconstruction (b) show bilateral bronchiectasis (arrows) and some small mucoid impactions (blue arrowhead).

as opposed to Crohn's. Age of onset is variable and there is a female predominance. Parenchymal disease usually manifests with consolidations consistent with an organizing pneumonia (OP) patterns: although an OP pattern may also develop with infection or occur as a manifestation of drug toxicity, some authors attributed cases related to IBD itself [8, 10, 45]. Chest X-ray shows focal or diffuse peripheral predominant opacities and air bronchograms. HRCT shows patchy, asymmetric, unilateral, or bilateral foci of consolidation in a peripheral or peribronchovascular distribution, large irregular nodules, or ill-defined centrilobular nodules; ground-glass opacities and crazy paving are other characteristics. A "reverse-halo sign" (or "atoll sign") is considered to be suggestive, although it is seen only in 20% of patients with OP (mainly seen during the OP healing/recovery phase) (Figure 8) [46]. Another parenchymal disease in IBD is cellular nonspecific interstitial pneumonia (cellular NSIP) that has different prognostic values compared to fibrotic NSIP (the former responds to treatment and has a better prognosis). Typical cellular NSIP findings at HRCT are ground-glass opacity with tiny reticulation and a subpleural and basal distribution. A sparing of the immediate subpleural lung is particularly suggestive of NSIP (Figure 9). Honeycombing is typically absent. Except for the colectomized UC patient who is tacking no medication, any discussion regarding interstitial lung disease in IBD should include the patient's drug history. In fact, NSIP is a common pattern of lung drug toxicity (Figure 10) [46]. In particular, sulfasalazine and mesalazine are used in the management of IBD and both can produce pulmonary toxicity that is usually expressed as NSIP, OP, or eosinophilic pneumonia [10, 47, 48]. Patients with a eosinophilic reaction show a combination of lung abnormalities on imaging and increased serum eosinophils. HRCT may show a peripheral, upper lobe predominant consolidation associated with patchy bilateral-nodular or oval mass-like consolidation. These characteristics may closely resemble or mimic OP, but eosinophilic pneumonia often shows an upper lobe predominance instead of OP, where lung bases are most involved.

Pulmonary necrobiotic nodules have also been seen in patients with IBD and should be differentiated from malignancies and an infection. Histologically, these lesions have

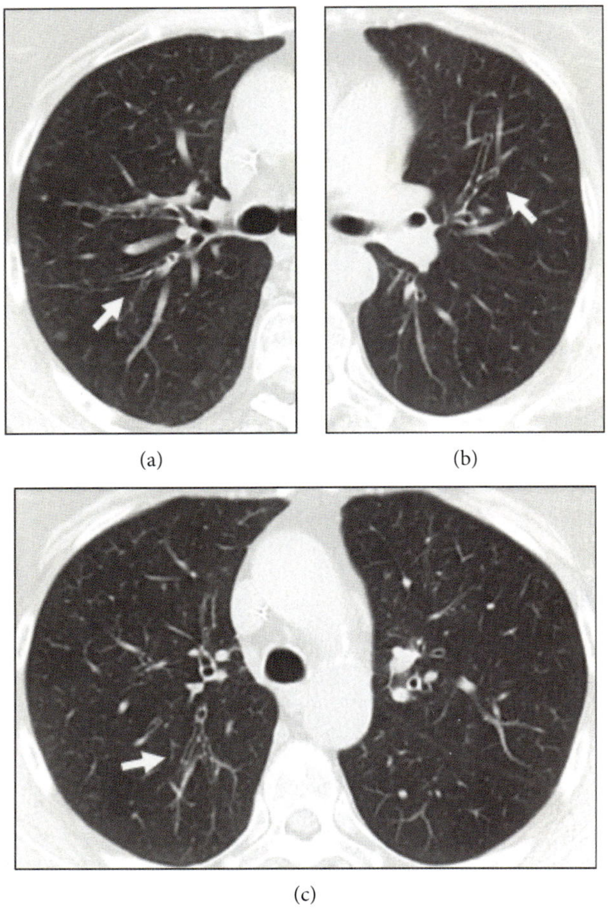

Figure 5: Multiple bilateral bronchiectasis in a 72-year-old woman with CD (arrows). Axial HRCT scans (a, b, c).

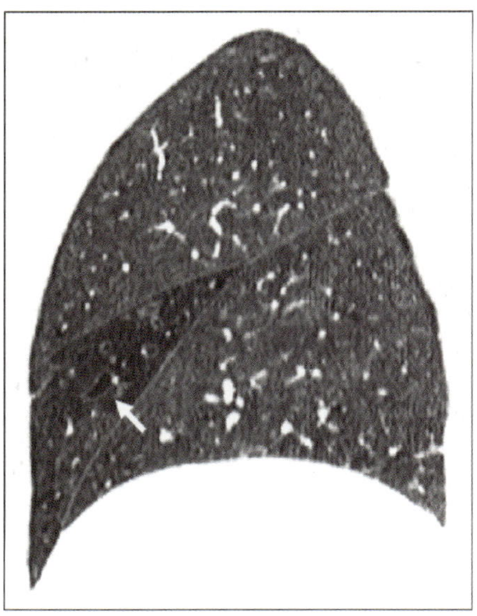

Figure 6: HRCT sagittal reconstruction. Cylindrical and varicose bronchiectasis (arrow) in the middle lobe in a 62-year-old woman with CD. A mosaic pattern due to air trapping is present.

been reported to be mainly necrobiotic (25%) or granulomatous (12.5%) [8]. On imaging, these nodules are round and well-defined, sometimes cavitated, and can measure up to a

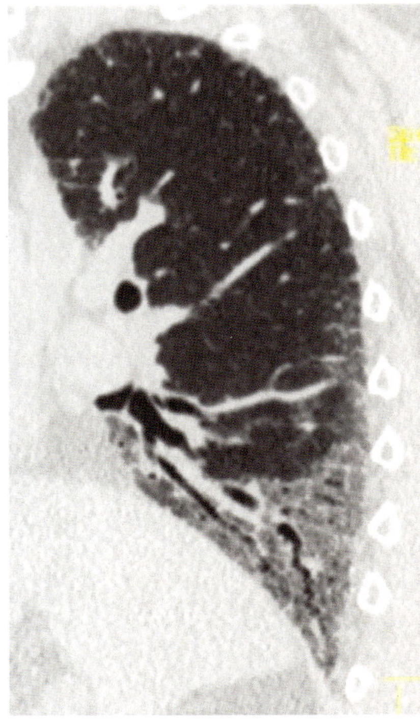

Figure 7: Sagittal HRCT of a 52-year-old male patient with CD shows lower bronchiectasis and bronchiolectasis, associated with diffuse basal parenchymal opacities (ground glass pattern) and interstitial septal thickening.

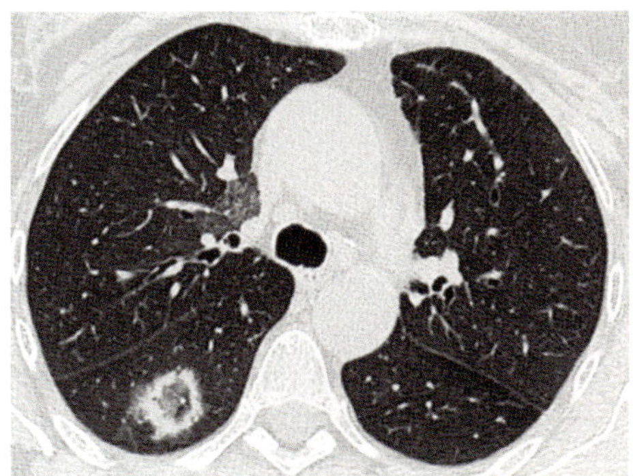

Figure 8: Reverse halo or atoll sign in a patient with UC and possible OP.

few centimetres in diameter (Figure 11). An infection should be excluded because these nodules respond to steroids but not to antibiotics [10, 12]. Any patient on anti-TNF therapy may develop opportunistic infections or tuberculosis [47]. As for the airways, it is also important to remember that occasionally there are concomitant diseases involving lung parenchyma, such as sarcoidosis and emphysema related to AATD [30]. Further investigations are still needed to better elucidate these connections.

4.3. Vascular Manifestation. Vascular disease rarely occurs in IBD. They may be represented by granulomatosis with polyangiitis (GPA), microscopic polyangiitis, eosinophilic granulomatosis with polyangiitis (EGPA), and other pulmonary vasculitis non-ANCA+ that have been reported by some

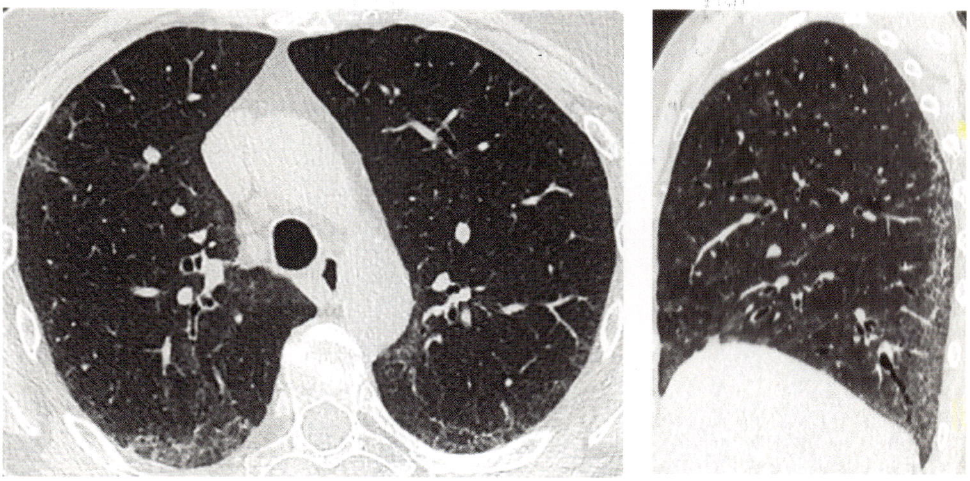

(a) (b)

Figure 9: A 67-year-old woman with CD. In both basal posterior segments of the lower lobes, an interlobular-intralobular interstitial thickening associated with ground glass opacities and some traction bronchiectasis and bronchiolectasis is appreciable. A subpleural sparing is associated. These findings are compatible with NSIP. Axial HRCT study (a) and sagittal reconstruction (b).

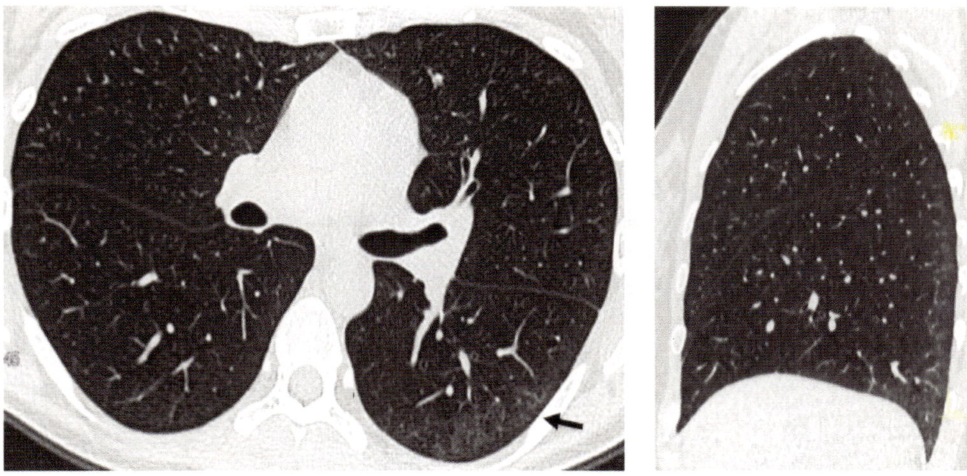

(a) (b)

Figure 10: A 36-year-old woman with UC and previous total colectomy. In the basal posterolateral segment of lower lobes (more evident in the left), a fine interstitial thickening associated with ground glass opacities and some traction bronchiolectasis is appreciable. A subpleural sparing is associated (arrow). These findings are consistent with NSIP. Axial HRCT study (a) and sagittal reconstruction (b).

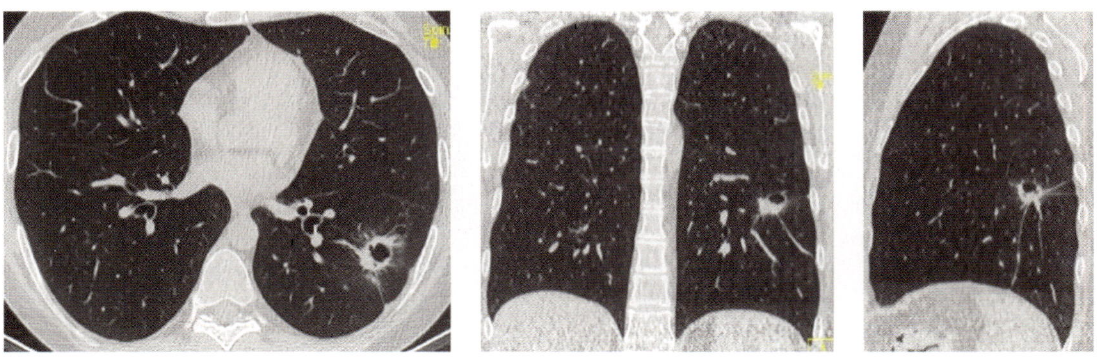

(a) (b) (c)

Figure 11: A 55-year-old woman with coexisting CD and GPA disease. These HRCT images (axial (a), coronal (b), sagittal (c)) show a pulmonary necrotic nodule in the lower left lobe: it is possible to notice the necrotic cavity inside. Whether this is due to CD of GPA was unclear.

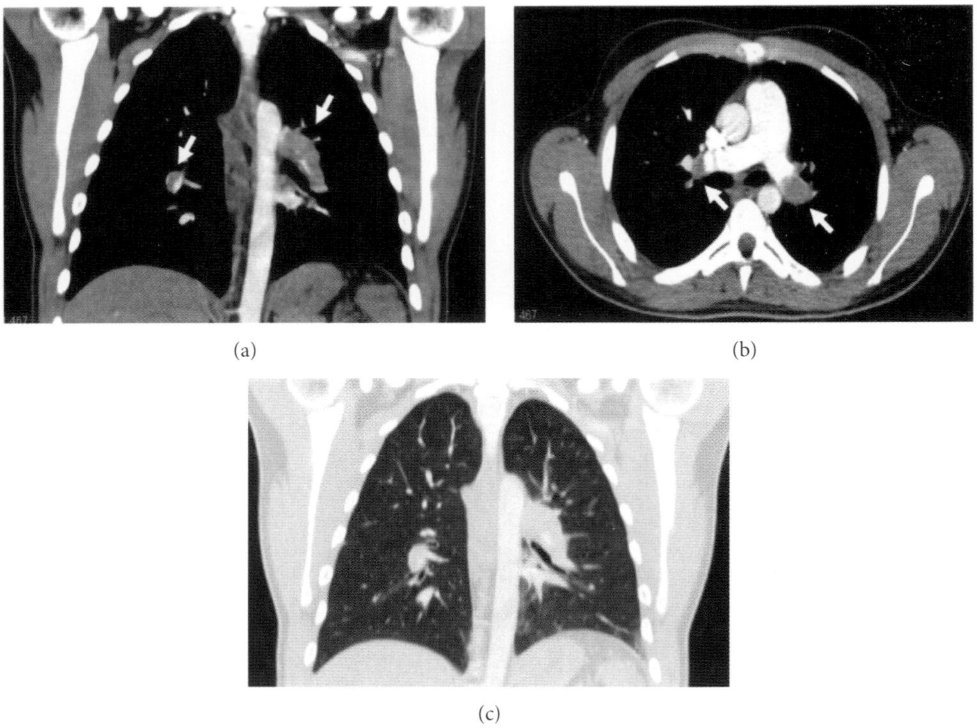

FIGURE 12: An 18-year-old male with Crohn's disease in the acute phase and no additional comorbidities, who presented with mild shortness of breath. Coronal and axial reconstruction of contrast-enhanced chest CT reveals bilateral pulmonary embolism in both main pulmonary arteries (arrows, a-b). Coronal reconstruction for lung parenchyma (c).

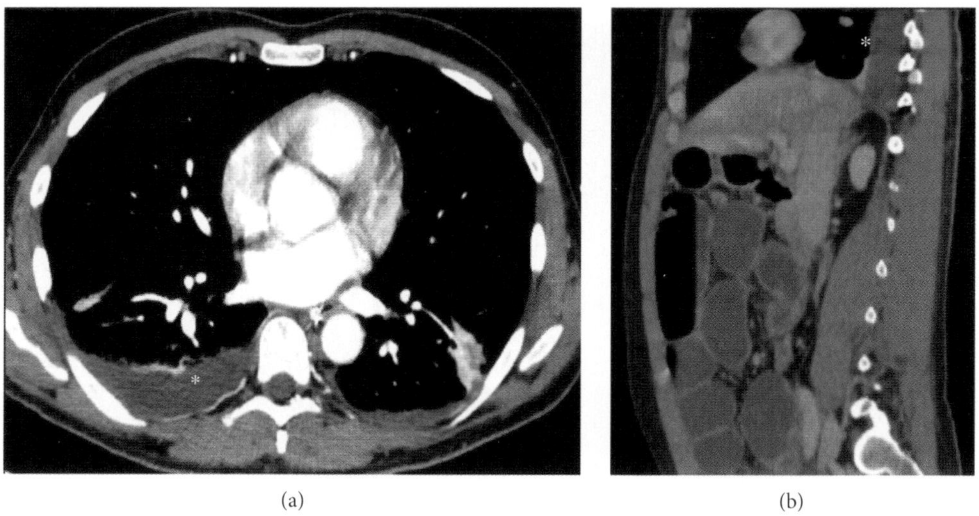

FIGURE 13: A 43-year-old man with Crohn's disease subjected to previous surgical ileal resection. Asterisks (*) show unilateral pleural effusion during acute abdomen due to intestinal obstruction. Axial CT study (a) and sagittal reconstruction (b).

authors [49–52]. As venous thromboembolism occurs frequently in IBD patients, acute pulmonary embolism remains the most clinically important pulmonary vascular manifestation in these patients (Figure 12) [6, 8]. In fact, it is known that these patients have increased risk of thromboembolic disease: Bernstein et al. argued that the risk is three times higher compared with age-matched control subjects [53]. Thromboembolic risk in IBD patients may be due to the pathology itself and its related conditions such as abdominal surgery, immobility, drugs, and frequent central venous catheterization [8]. Risk may be further increased during the activity phases of IBD, but up to one-third of thrombotic events occur while the disease is quiescent, suggesting ongoing thrombotic risk unrelated to disease activity or to eventual therapy [54].

4.4. Serosal Involvement. Pleural and pericardial involvement is rare in IBD [6, 8, 10, 12]. Pleural effusion is nearly always unilateral and exudative in nature (Figure 13). When the pericardium is involved, it is usually not accompanied by pleural effusion: concomitant pleural and pericardial involvement is rare [8, 10, 12, 55]. Serositis may be associated with intense chest pain and the association with myocarditis is possible [10].

5. Conclusions

Nowadays, increasing evidence suggests that IBD and extraintestinal manifestations are not isolated diseases but may have common pathophysiological pathways. With the increased use of HRCT, pulmonary manifestations of IBD are more commonly encountered. Bronchiectasis is the most common alteration seen among patients with IBD but the spectrum of respiratory involvement is wide, from organ to specific manifestation. Pulmonary involvement in inflammatory bowel disease should be considered in all patients, even when gastrointestinal symptoms are minimal or well-controlled. Radiologists must be aware that they have the key role to optimize clinical management of IBD patients, escaping from errors and vain therapies, in order to avoid destructive airway changes or irreversible pulmonary fibrosis.

References

[1] D. C. Baumgart and S. R. Carding, "Inflammatory bowel disease: cause and immunobiology," *The Lancet*, vol. 369, no. 9573, pp. 1627–1640, 2007.

[2] R. Rodriguez-Roisin, S. D. Bartolome, G. Huchon, and M. J. Krowka, "Inflammatory bowel diseases, chronic liver diseases and the lung," *European Respiratory Journal*, vol. 47, no. 2, pp. 638–650, 2016.

[3] S. Danese and C. Fiocchi, "Ulcerative colitis," *The New England Journal of Medicine*, vol. 365, no. 18, pp. 1713–1725, 2011.

[4] E. V. Loftus Jr., "Clinical epidemiology of inflammatory bowel disease: incidence, prevalence and environmental influences," *Gastroenterology*, vol. 126, no. 6, pp. 1504–1517, 2004.

[5] I. Papanikolaou, K. Kagouridis, and S. A. Papiris, "Patterns of airway involvement in inflammatory bowel diseases," *World Journal of Gastrointestinal Pathophysiology*, vol. 5, no. 4, pp. 560–569, 2014.

[6] J. D. Olpin, B. P. Sjoberg, S. E. Stilwill, L. E. Jensen, M. Rezvani, and A. M. Shaaban, "Beyond the bowel: extraintestinal manifestations of inflammatory bowel disease," *RadioGraphics*, vol. 37, no. 4, pp. 1135–1160, 2017.

[7] E. Lopez Botet and R. Rosalem Archer, "Severe ulcerous colitis and ulcerous bronchitis in the same patient," *Revista Clinica Espanola*, vol. 84, pp. 190–193, 1962.

[8] H. Black, M. Mendoza, and S. Murin, "Thoracic manifestations of inflammatory bowel disease," *Chest*, vol. 131, no. 2, pp. 524–532, 2007.

[9] D. Desai, S. Patil, Z. Udwadia, S. Maheshwari, P. Abraham, and A. Joshi, "Pulmonary manifestations in inflammatory bowel disease: a prospective study," *Indian Journal of Gastroenterology*, vol. 30, no. 5, pp. 225–228, 2011.

[10] P. Camus, F. Piard, T. Ashcroft, A. A. Gal, and T. V. Colby, "The lung in inflammatory bowel disease," *Medicine*, vol. 72, no. 3, pp. 151–183, 1993.

[11] R. M. Hoffmann and W. Kruis, "Rare extraintestinal manifestations of inflammatory bowel disease," *Inflammatory Bowel Diseases*, vol. 10, no. 2, pp. 140–147, 2004.

[12] S. L. Betancourt, D. Palacio, C. A. Jimenez, S. Martinez, and E. M. Marom, "Thoracic manifestations of inflammatory bowel disease," *American Journal of Roentgenology*, vol. 197, no. 3, pp. W452–W456, 2011.

[13] T. Higenbottam, G. M. Cochrane, T. J. Clark, D. Turner, R. Millis, and W. Seymour, "Bronchial disease in ulcerative colitis," *Thorax*, vol. 35, no. 8, pp. 581–585, 1980.

[14] J. G. Douglas, C. F. McDonald, M. J. Leslie, J. Gillon, G. K. Crompton, and G. J. R. McHardy, "Respiratory impairment in inflammatory bowel disease: does it vary with disease activity?," *Respiratory Medicine*, vol. 83, no. 5, pp. 389–394, 1989.

[15] N. Songür, Y. Songür, M. Tüzün et al., "Pulmonary function tests and high-resolution CT in the detection of pulmonary involvement in inflammatory bowel disease," *Journal of Clinical Gastroenterology*, vol. 37, no. 4, pp. 292–298, 2003.

[16] L. Kuzela, A. Vavrecka, M. Prikazska et al., "Pulmonary complications in patients with inflammatory bowel disease," *Hepato-Gastroenterology*, vol. 46, no. 27, pp. 1714–1719, 1999.

[17] M. Marvisi, P. D. Borrello, M. Brianti, G. Fornarsari, G. Marani, and A. Guariglia, "Changes in the carbon monoxide diffusing capacity of the lung in ulcerative colitis," *European Respiratory Journal*, vol. 16, no. 5, pp. 965–968, 2000.

[18] K. R. Herrlinger, M. K. Noftz, K. Dalhoff, D. Ludwig, E. F. Stange, and K. Fellermann, "Alterations in pulmonary function in inflammatory bowel disease are frequent and persist during remission," *The American Journal of Gastroenterology*, vol. 97, no. 2, pp. 377–381, 2002.

[19] D. Duricova, N. Pedersen, M. Elkjaer, M. Gamborg, P. Munkholm, and T. Jess, "Overall and cause-specific mortality in Crohn's disease: a meta-analysis of population-based studies," *Inflammatory Bowel Diseases*, vol. 16, no. 2, pp. 347–353, 2010.

[20] E. J. Stern and M. S. Frank, "Small-airway diseases of the lungs: findings at expiratory CT," *American Journal of Roentgenology*, vol. 163, no. 1, pp. 37–41, 1994.

[21] E. J. Stern, S. J. Swensen, T. E. Hartman, and M. S. Frank, "CT mosaic pattern of lung attenuation: distinguishing different causes," *American Journal of Roentgenology*, vol. 165, no. 4, pp. 813–816, 1995.

[22] M. Remy-Jardin, J. Remy, F. Giraud, L. Wattinne, and B. Gosselin, "Computed tomography assessment of ground-glass opacity: semiology and significance," *Journal of Thoracic Imaging*, vol. 8, no. 4, pp. 249–264, 1993.

[23] R. Mahadeva, G. Walsh, C. D. R. Flower, and J. M. Shneerson, "Clinical and radiological characteristics of lung disease in inflammatory bowel disease," *European Respiratory Journal*, vol. 15, no. 1, pp. 41–48, 2000.

[24] A. Yilmaz, N. Yilmaz Demirci, D. Hoşgün et al., "Pulmonary involvement in inflammatory bowel disease," *World Journal of Gastroenterology*, vol. 16, no. 39, pp. 4952–4957, 2010.

[25] J. Peradzyńska, K. Krenke, J. Lange et al., "Low prevalence of pulmonary involvement in children with inflammatory bowel disease," *Respiratory Medicine*, vol. 106, no. 7, pp. 1048–1054, 2012.

[26] A. K. Yamamoto and J. L. Babar, "Case 184: ulcerative tracheobronchitis," *Radiology*, vol. 264, no. 2, pp. 609–613, 2012.

[27] T. Kuźniar, C. Sleiman, O. Brugière et al., "Severe tracheobronchial stenosis in a patient with Crohn's disease," *European Respiratory Journal*, vol. 15, no. 1, pp. 209–212, 2000.

[28] C. Lamblin, M. C. Copin, C. Billaut et al., "Acute respiratory failure due to tracheobronchial involvement in Crohn's disease," *European Respiratory Journal*, vol. 9, no. 10, pp. 2176-2177, 1996.

[29] J. S. Prince, D. R. Duhamel, D. L. Levin, J. H. Harrell, and P. J. Friedman, "Nonneoplastic lesions of the tracheobronchial wall: radiologic findings with bronchoscopic correlation," *RadioGraphics*, vol. 22, Supplement 1, pp. S215–S230, 2002.

[30] D. Cozzi, E. Bargagli, A. G. Calabrò et al., "Atypical HRCT manifestations of pulmonary sarcoidosis," *La Radiologia Medica*, vol. 123, no. 3, pp. 174–184, 2018.

[31] K. Garg, D. A. Lynch, and J. D. Newell, "Inflammatory airways disease in ulcerative colitis: CT and high resolution CT features," *Journal of Thoracic Imaging*, vol. 8, no. 2, pp. 159–163, 1993.

[32] H. Ward, K. L. Fisher, R. Waghray, J. L. Wright, S. E. Card, and D. W. Cockcroft, "Constrictive bronchiolitis and ulcerative colitis," *Canadian Respiratory Journal*, vol. 6, no. 2, p. 200, 1999.

[33] O. Vandenplas, S. Casel, M. Delos, J. P. Trigaux, M. Melange, and E. Marchand, "Granulomatous bronchiolitis associated with Crohn's disease," *American Journal of Respiratory and Critical Care Medicine*, vol. 158, no. 5, pp. 1676–1679, 1998.

[34] M. B. Casey, H. D. Tazelaar, J. L. Myers et al., "Noninfectious lung pathology in patients with Crohn's disease," *The American Journal of Surgical Pathology*, vol. 27, no. 2, pp. 213–219, 2003.

[35] A. I. Alrashid, R. D. Brown, M. L. Mihalov, M. Sekosan, B. J. Pastika, and R. P. Venu, "Crohn's disease involving the lung: resolution with infliximab," *Digestive Diseases and Sciences*, vol. 46, no. 8, pp. 1736–1739, 2001.

[36] M. S. Cappell, A. Saad, J. S. Bortman, and M. Amin, "Ileocolonic tuberculosis clinically, endoscopically, and radiologically mimicking Crohn's disease: disseminated infection after treatment with infliximab," *Journal of Crohn's and Colitis*, vol. 8, no. 6, pp. 560–562, 2014.

[37] S. H. Wong, M. Ip, W. Tang et al., "Performance of interferon-gamma release assay for tuberculosis screening in inflammatory bowel disease patients," *Inflammatory Bowel Diseases*, vol. 20, no. 11, pp. 2067–2072, 2014.

[38] G. Van Assche, S. Vermeire, and P. Rutgeerts, "Treatment of severe steroid refractory ulcerative colitis," *World Journal of Gastroenterology*, vol. 14, no. 36, pp. 5508–5511, 2008.

[39] I. Uthman and A. Sharara, "The usefulness of PPD testing in inflammatory bowel disease patients before infliximab therapy," *Clinical Gastroenterology and Hepatology*, vol. 2, no. 9, article A22, 2004.

[40] T. K. Kim, S. H. Kang, H. S. Moon, J. K. Sung, H. Y. Jeong, and H. S. Eun, "Pulmonary sarcoidosis that developed during the treatment of a patient with Crohn disease by using infliximab," *Annals of Coloproctology*, vol. 33, no. 2, pp. 74–77, 2017.

[41] A. Obrador, A. López San Román, P. Muñoz, J. Fortún, M. A. Gassull, and Grupo Español de Trabajo de Enfermedad de Crohn y Colitis Ulcerosa (GETECCU), "Guía de consenso sobre tuberculosis y tratamiento de la enfermedad inflamatoria intestinal con infliximab," *Gastroenterología y Hepatología*, vol. 26, no. 1, pp. 29–33, 2003.

[42] P. Camus and T. V. Colby, "The lung in inflammatory bowel disease," *European Respiratory Journal*, vol. 15, no. 1, pp. 5–10, 2000.

[43] M. Hiyoshi, K. Kawai, M. Shibuya et al., "Tracheobronchitis with dyspnea in a patient with ulcerative colitis," *Internal Medicine*, vol. 54, no. 7, pp. 749–753, 2015.

[44] P. Camus, "Pneumotox II (V2.1)," 2017, February 2018, https://www.pneumotox.com.

[45] I. Storch, D. Sachar, and S. Katz, "Pulmonary manifestations of inflammatory bowel disease," *Inflammatory Bowel Diseases*, vol. 9, no. 2, pp. 104–115, 2003.

[46] S. J. Kim, K. S. Lee, Y. H. Ryu et al., "Reversed halo sign on high-resolution CT of cryptogenic organizing pneumonia: diagnostic implications," *American Journal of Roentgenology*, vol. 180, no. 5, pp. 1251–1254, 2003.

[47] S. D. Parry, C. Barbatzas, E. T. Peel, and J. R. Barton, "Sulphasalazine and lung toxicity," *European Respiratory Journal*, vol. 19, no. 4, pp. 756–764, 2002.

[48] S. Cappabianca, V. Granata, G. Di Grezia et al., "The role of nasoenteric intubation in the MR study of patients with Crohn's disease: our experience and literature review," *La Radiologia Medica*, vol. 116, no. 3, pp. 389–406, 2011.

[49] S. Yano, K. Kobayashi, K. Kato, and K. Nishimura, "A limited form of Wegener's granulomatosis with bronchiolitis obliterans organizing pneumonitis-like variant in an ulcerative colitis patient," *Internal Medicine*, vol. 41, no. 11, pp. 1013–1015, 2002.

[50] J. Stebbing, F. Askin, E. Fishman, and J. Stone, "Pulmonary manifestations of ulcerative colitis mimicking Wegener's granulomatosis," *The Journal of Rheumatology*, vol. 26, no. 7, pp. 1617–1621, 1999.

[51] A. A. Prekates, S. E. Orfanos, C. J. Routsi, A. C. Pantelidaki, and C. S. Roussos, "Churg-Strauss syndrome occurring 30 years after the onset of ulcerative colitis," *Respiratory Care*, vol. 47, no. 2, pp. 167–170, 2002.

[52] F. Martinez, J. H. Chung, S. R. Digumarthy et al., "Common and uncommon manifestations of Wegener granulomatosis at chest CT: radiologic-pathologic correlation," *RadioGraphics*, vol. 32, no. 1, pp. 51–69, 2012.

[53] C. N. Bernstein, J. F. Blanchard, D. S. Houston, and A. Wajda, "The incidence of deep venous thrombosis and pulmonary embolism among patients with inflammatory bowel disease: a population-based cohort study," *Thrombosis and Haemostasis*, vol. 85, no. 3, pp. 430–434, 2001.

[54] A. Papa, S. Danese, A. Grillo, G. Gasbarrini, and A. Gasbarrini, "Review article: inherited thrombophilia in inflammatory bowel disease," *The American Journal of Gastroenterology*, vol. 98, no. 6, pp. 1247–1251, 2003.

[55] M. Faller, B. Gasser, G. Massard, G. Pauli, and E. Quoix, "Pulmonary migratory infiltrates and pachypleuritis in a patient with Crohn's disease," *Respiration*, vol. 67, no. 4, pp. 459–463, 2000.

10

Endoscopic Dilation with Bougies versus Balloon Dilation in Esophageal Benign Strictures

Iatagan R. Josino, Antônio C. Madruga-Neto, Igor B. Ribeiro, Hugo G. Guedes, Vitor O. Brunaldi, Diogo T. H. de Moura, Wanderley M. Bernardo, and Eduardo G. H. de Moura

Gastrointestinal Endoscopy Unit, University of São Paulo Medical School, Dr. Arnaldo Av 455, São Paulo 01246-903, Brazil

Correspondence should be addressed to Iatagan R. Josino; iataganjosino@gmail.com

Academic Editor: Amosy M'Koma

Background. The use of bougies and balloons to dilate benign esophageal strictures (BES) is a consolidated procedure. However, the amount of evidence available in scientific literature supporting which is the best technique is very low, despite the great prevalence and importance of such pathology. This systematic review with meta-analysis aims at comparing both techniques, providing good quality of evidence. *Methods.* We searched for randomized clinical trials (RCTs) published from insertion to November 2017, using MEDLINE, EMBASE, Cochrane Central Register of Controlled Trials, LILACS, and grey literature. After the data extraction, a meta-analysis was performed. The main outcomes were symptomatic relief and recurrence rate. The secondary outcomes were bleeding, perforation, and postprocedure pain. *Results.* We included 5 randomized clinical trials (RCTs), totalizing 461 patients. Among them, 151 were treated with bougie dilation and 225 underwent balloon dilation. Regarding symptomatic relief, recurrence, bleeding, and perforation rates, there were no differences between the methods. Concerning postprocedure pain, patients submitted to balloon dilation had less intense pain (RD 0.27, 95% IC −0.42 to −0.07, $P = 0.007$). *Conclusion.* We conclude that there is no difference between bougie and balloon dilation of BESs regarding symptomatic relief, recurrence rate at 12 months, bleeding, and perforation. Patients undergoing balloon dilation present less severe postprocedure pain.

1. Introduction

Benign esophageal strictures (BESs) are defined as any type of nonmalignant narrowing of the esophageal lumen. The physiopathological mechanisms of BESs are diverse and may entail embryonary defects, inflammatory injuries, and iatrogenesis. Also, there are several etiologic causes that may result from the combination of different mechanisms [1]. The most common clinical presentation is dysphagia, but others as retrosternal pain, regurgitation, and odynophagia might be present [1]. The impact on quality of life is usually remarkable since the patient frequently suffers from weight loss and aspiration pneumonia [2].

Modern bougies are made of polyvinyl chloride. The dilation procedure consists in passing a guidewire through the narrowing of the esophagus (fluoroscopy-guided or not) followed by bougination with gradually thicker dilators. This process generates an axial pressure on the stricture ring and theoretically poses a higher risk of esophageal perforation compared to the balloon dilation [3].

Balloon dilatation catheters were traditionally designed to treat patients with achalasia. In the early 1980s, they were introduced for the treatment of BESs. To dilate, the balloon should stand exactly at the stricture, in most cases secured by a guidewire. Then, it applies a radial pressure on the ring and ideally carries a lower risk of perforation. Other hypothetical advantages of the balloons are a greater precision (since it dilates only the exact narrowing) and the possibility to visualize the dilation process endoscopically as it occurs [4].

Despite all these theoretical advantages, there is no consensus in the available scientific literature to favor balloons over bougies [5, 6]. Also, there is no systematic review comparing both methods in patients with BES. Therefore, we developed this study to comprehensively search and compile all available data regarding this topic and ultimately provide practitioners with the most reliable evidence.

2. Objectives

The objective of this study is to compare the safety and efficacy of bougie and balloon endoscopic dilation in patients with BES.

3. Methods

This systematic review and meta-analysis was performed according to the PRISMA guidelines (Preferred Reporting Items for Systematic Reviews and Meta-Analyses) and was registered in PROSPERO (International Prospective Register of Systematic Reviews) under the registry number CRD42018085541.

4. Search

We searched MEDLINE, EMBASE, Cochrane Central Register of Controlled Trials, LILACS, and grey literature from inception to August 2017.

Our search strategy for MEDLINE (PubMed) was (Esophageal stenosis OR Esophageal Stenoses OR Esophageal Stricture) AND (Balloon OR dilatation OR savary OR bougie OR pneumodiltation OR pneumodilation). For other databases, we employed a simpler strategy: (Esophag* AND (Balloon OR dilatation OR savary OR savary-gilliard OR bougie OR bougienage OR pneumodilatation OR pneumodilation).

4.1. Inclusion Criteria/Eligibility. We considered a study eligible if it fulfilled the following criteria:

(a) Types of study: full-text randomized controlled trials (RCTs) with no language or publication date restrictions

(b) Types of participants: patients with benign esophageal strictures and no history of previous dilation

(c) Types of intervention: balloon and bougie dilation

(d) Types of outcomes:

  (i) Primary outcomes: symptomatic relief after dilation and recurrence rate at 12-month follow-up

  (ii) Secondary outcomes: adverse event rates (bleeding, perforation and postprocedure pain)

4.2. Exclusion Criteria

(a) Patients with malignant esophageal strictures or previous esophageal dilation

(b) Studies that did not report the outcomes assessed in this review

(c) Studies with no extractable data

4.3. Study Selection. We combined studies identified in different databases and removed the duplicates. The first screening assessed titles and abstracts for eligibility. Then, a full-text analysis confirmed eligibility or excluded them from analysis.

In our meta-analysis, we included only studies providing complete data in the text, tables, or figures. If necessary, we assessed supplementary data available in online platforms (e.g., Clinical Trials or PROSPERO) or tried to contact the authors by email.

Study selection was performed by two independent researchers. In case of disagreement, it was resolved by consensus with a third researcher.

4.4. Methodology Quality and Risk of Bias Assessment. The studies were assessed using Cochrane's risk of bias tool [7], which classifies the risk of bias as low, high, or unclear.

4.5. Data Extraction. Two independent researchers extracted data using a standard Excel spreadsheet detailing the absolute numbers reported in the articles. We extracted data regarding the following dichotomous outcomes: symptomatic relief, recurrence, bleeding, perforation, and postprocedure pain.

4.6. Analysis. We used the RevMan software version 5.3 to perform all analyses and employed mean or absolute risk difference. We applied the Mantel-Haenszel test for categorical variables and considered statistically significant results with 95% confidence interval (CI) and $P < 0.05$.

We used the method of inverse variance and fixed effect model to provide the forest plots. Heterogeneity was assessed with the Higgins test [8](I^2), and values higher than 50% were considered highly heterogeneous. Funnel plot analyses were also employed to assess publication bias across studies.

If I [2] was higher than 50%, we searched for outlier studies through the funnel plot. Articles outside the limits of the funnel were excluded, and heterogeneity was reassessed. If the sample became homogenous ($I^2 < 50\%$), the excluded studies were considered true outliers and were permanently removed. If we did not find an outlier, we considered true heterogeneity and switched from fixed to random effect analysis.

5. Results

Initially, we identified 23,672 studies. After the title/abstract assessment, we selected 12 articles for full-text evaluation. Finally, 5 RCTs [9–13] fulfilled eligibility criteria and were included in our analysis. Figure 1 summarizes the selection process.

The 5 RCTs included in our review enrolled a total of 461 patients, including 197 bougie and 264 balloon dilations.

The selected trials were developed in several countries from different continents and enrolled a great variety of patients and clinical presentations. However, all patients

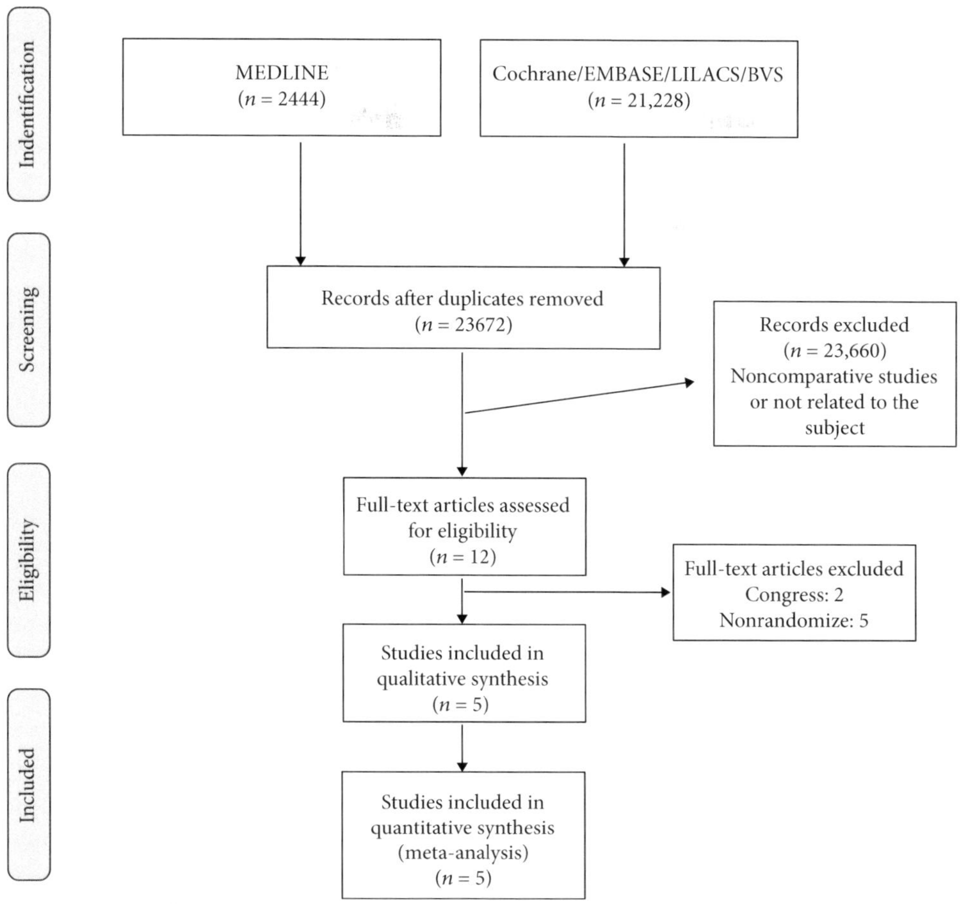

FIGURE 1: Flow diagram summarizing the selection process.

underwent esophageal dilation at least up to 15 mm. Table 1 summarizes the studies' characteristics.

6. Risk of Bias

Assessing risk of bias, we identified issues during randomization and blinding processes but adequate intention to treat analysis in most of the included trials. Therefore, we assigned fair quality to all studies. Figures 2 and 3 synthesize the risk of bias assessment.

7. Outcomes

7.1. Symptomatic Relief. Four studies [10–13] enrolling 376 patients were included. Among them, 151 underwent bougination while 225 underwent balloon dilation. Regarding postprocedure symptomatic relief, the meta-analysis found no difference between the groups with $I^2 = 0\%$ (95% CI [−0.08, 0.08]). Figure 4 shows the forest plot for symptomatic relief.

7.2. Recurrence Rate. Four studies [10–13] reported the recurrence rate at 12 months. The risk difference was 0.03 (95% CI [−0.05, 0.10]) with $I^2 = 59\%$ (Figure 5). After the funnel plot analysis, we identified and removed an outlier (Saeed et al.) (Figure 6). Then, we pooled data again and found a decrease in heterogeneity ($I^2 = 20$), but still no difference between the methods (Figure 7).

7.3. Bleeding. Two RCTs [11, 13] enrolling a total of 282 patients reported bleeding rates. Among them, 104 patients were allocated for the bougie group and 178 for the balloon group. This analysis was highly homogenous ($I^2 = 0\%$), and the risk difference was −0.02 (95% CI [−0.06, 0.02]). Therefore, we found equivalence of methods regarding bleeding rates (Figure 8).

7.4. Perforation. For this analysis, we included five RCTs [9–13]. A total of 461 patients were enrolled, 190 treated with bougie and 271 with balloon dilation. Again, the meta-analysis identified highly homogenous data ($I^2 = 0\%$) with risk difference between groups of −0.01 (95% CI [−0.03, 0.02]). Therefore, we found no difference concerning perforation rates (Figure 9).

7.5. Postprocedure Pain. Two trials [10, 13] reported postprocedure pain incidence. A total of 65 patients were enrolled (33 in the bougie group and 32 in the balloon dilation group). This analysis was highly homogenous ($I^2 = 0\%$). The balloon group had a significantly lower incidence of pain after the procedure (RD 0.27, 95% CI 0.08–0.47, $P = 0.007$). Figure 10 shows the forest plot regarding postprocedure pain incidence.

Table 1: Characteristic of the included studies. Yamamoto et al. and Saeed et al. did not specify the etiology of the BESs.

Study	Control (*n*)	Intervention (*n*)	Population
Shemesh, 90	Savary-Gilliard (30) *Dilation with bougies up to 17 mm*	Microvasive (30) *Dilation with balloons up to 18 mm*	Peptic stricture (39) Caustic stricture (11) Postoperative (10)
Yamamoto, 92	Eder-Puestow (16) *Dilation with bougies up to 15 mm*	Medi-Tech (15) *Dilation with balloons up to 20 mm*	n/a
Cox, 94	Celestin + Eder-Puestow (39) *Dilation with Celestin bougies up to 18 mm, followed by Eder-Puestow bougies up to 19.3 mm*	Rigiflex Microvasive (46) *Dilation with balloons up to 20 mm*	Peptic stricture (61) Barrett's esophagus (8) Postoperative (11) Postesclerotherapy (1) Postcricoid (1) Systemic sclerosis (2) Caustic stricture (1)
Saeed, 95	Savary-Gilliard (17) *Dilation with bougies up to 15 mm*	Rigiflex Microvasive (17) *Dilation with balloons up to 15 mm*	n/a
Scolapio, 99	Savary-Gilliard (88) *Dilation with bougies up to 17 mm*	Bard (82) + Microvasive (81) *Dilation with balloons up to 15 mm*	Peptic stricture (114) Schatzki ring (139)

n/a: not applicable.

8. Discussion

Systematic reviews and meta-analyses are statistic tools used to pool data from different studies, aiming at improving the level of evidence available. Regarding the treatment of BESs, we identified the absence of high-quality randomized clinical trials, particularly in the last 20 years. Most published articles are case series, which are fairly reliable in terms of level of evidence. Therefore, this is the most trustworthy study available concerning the endoscopic treatment of BESs [14].

This systematic review included all 5 RCTs [9–13] available in the literature, which were all published before the 2000s. This fact demonstrates the lack of current evidence, which is necessary to guide treatment and management of such complex disease. Usually, the scientific community stops researching about a specific theme when steady data is found and we achieve a consensus. However, our systematic review clearly found conflicting results when comparing techniques, and therefore refuses any kind of consensus. In 2015, the World Society of Emergency Surgery published a consensus [15] observing that there was no clear advantage of any of the methods in peptic esophageal strictures, but Savary dilators would be more reliable and effective due to the possibility to "feel the resistance to dilation under the operators hands". However, such statement was not supported by any good quality study, being rated as level 4 recommendation.

Our meta-analysis included 461 patients with different etiologies for the BESs, such as peptic, Schatzki ring, postradiation, postanastomotic, and caustic. Also, different kinds of bougies (e.g., Savary-Gilliard and Puestow) and balloons (e.g., CRE, Rigiflex, and Bard) were used for dilation in the studies. These factors probably explain the high heterogeneity found in the recurrence rate analysis. Particularly, Saeed et al. was the main cause for the high heterogeneity and therefore was excluded as an outlier. The remainder were homogenous, but the result still showed equivalence of methods.

The employment of different bougies, each with particular physicochemical characteristics, may also be a confounding factor. To date, no randomized clinical trial compared thermoplastic (Savary-Miller) to metallic (Eder-Puestow) bougies. In our personal experience, the metallic ones carry higher perforation rates while handling is more challenging. Thus, we no longer employ such dilator in our daily practice.

Similarly, there are no high-quality studies comparing high- to low-complacency balloons. Theoretically, the highly complacent ones pose a higher risk of perforation due to their capacity to mold according to the shape of the stricture. This mechanism results in overpressure beyond the narrowing, which might result in esophageal perforation. However, there is no concrete literature supporting this hypothesis.

Regarding the cause of BESs, the lack of literature is even more impressive. Some etiologies such as peptic present a better response to dilation because the inflammatory process is usually limited to superficial layers and spares the *muscularis propria* [16]. Moreover, the efficacy of PPI treatment decreased the number of patients suffering from peptic strictures. Controversially, other etiologies such as postradiation and caustic carry full-thickness inflammation and fibrosis. In these cases, the symptomatic relief after dilation is usually shorter [16]. Therefore, it is always imperative to consider not only the technique but also the etiology of the BES when analyzing outcomes.

Concerning the interval between sessions, some authors advise early redilation regardless of symptoms, while others recommend dilation according to the patient's complaints [17]. Again, there is no current consensus regarding this topic, and each trial included in our meta-analysis may have employed a different interval between sessions. This fact might be considered another confounding factor.

The consistency of the diet is also central. The included RCTs did not specify if the patients were kept on a liquid, soft, or solid diet. This information is essential since the failure of treatment should be determined based

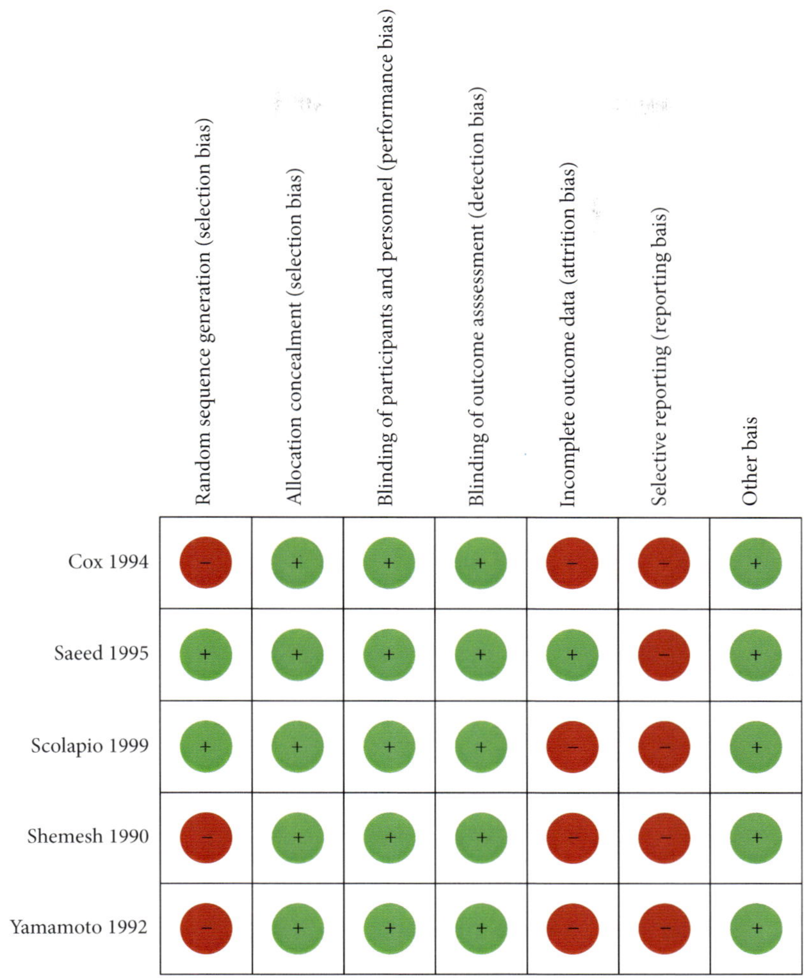

FIGURE 2: Risk of bias within studies.

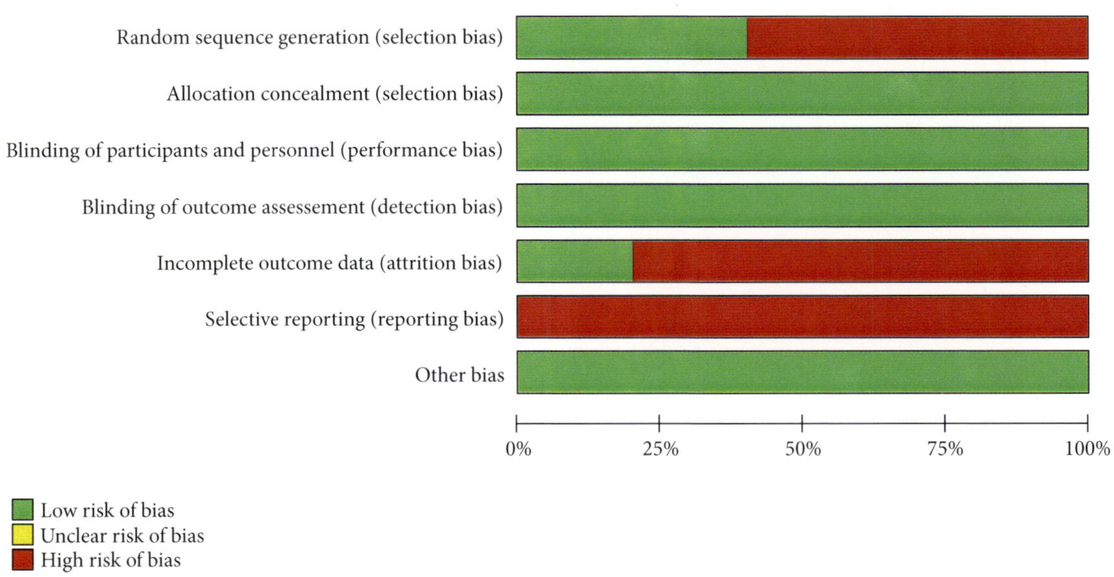

FIGURE 3: Risk of bias across studies.

on symptoms, especially dysphagia and weight loss. It is not uncommon to find patients with severe strictures but only mild or none dysphagia. Those cases should not be deemed failure of treatment because the patient is able to eat the minimum nutrients and calories needed with an acceptable quality of life.

Study or subgroup	Balloon Events	Balloon Total	Bougie Events	Bougie Total	Weight	Risk difference M-H, fixed, 95% CI	Risk of bias A B C D E F G
Yamamoto 1992	15	15	16	16	8.8%	0.00 [−0.12, 0.12]	− + + + − − +
Saeed 1995	17	17	17	17	9.6%	0.00 [−0.11, 0.11]	+ + + + + − +
Shemesh 1990	30	30	30	30	17.0%	0.00 [−0.06, 0.06]	− + + + − − +
Scolaplo 1999	112	163	61	88	64.7%	−0.01 [−0.13, 0.11]	+ + + + − − +
Total (95% CI)		225		151	100.0%	−0.00 [−0.08, 0.08]	
Total events	174		124				

Heterogeneity. chi^2 = 0.03, df = 3 (P = 1.00); I^2 = 0%
Test for overall effect: Z = 0.10 (P = 0.92)

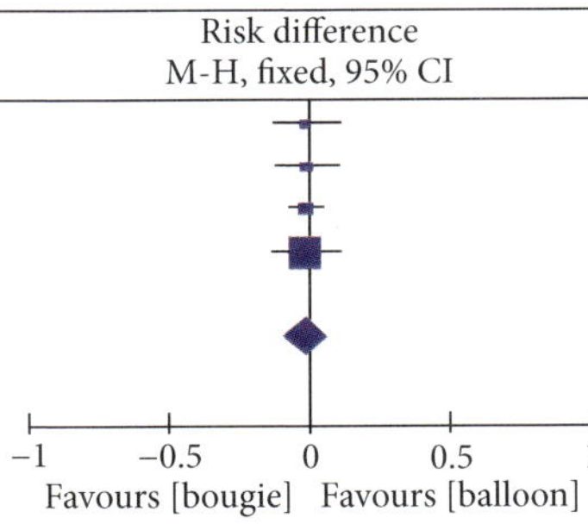

Risk of bias legend
(A) Random sequence generation (selection bias)
(B) Allocation concealment (selection bias)
(C) Blinding of participants and personnel (performance bias)
(D) Blinding of outcome assessment (detection bias)
(E) Incomplete outcome data (attrition bias)
(F) Selective reporting (reporting bias)
(G) Other bias

FIGURE 4: Symptomatic relief: forest plot.

Study or subgroup	Balloon Events	Balloon Total	Bougie Events	Bougie Total	Weight	Risk difference M-H, fixed, 95% CI	Risk of bias A B C D E F G
Saeed 1995	10	17	15	17	9.6%	−0.29 [−0.57, −0.01]	+ + + + + − +
Scolapio 1999	18	163	8	88	64.7%	0.02 [−0.06, 0.10]	+ + + + − − +
Shemesh 1990	17	30	11	30	17.0%	0.20 [−0.05, 0.45]	− + + + − − +
Yamamoto 1992	12	15	11	16	8.8%	0.11 [−0.19, 0.42]	− + + + − − +
Total (95% CI)		225		151	100.0%	0.03 [−0.05, 0.10]	
Total events	57		45				

Heterogeneity. chi^2 = 7.30, df = 3 (P = 0.06); I^2 = 59%
Test for overall effect: Z = 0.73 (P = 0. 46)

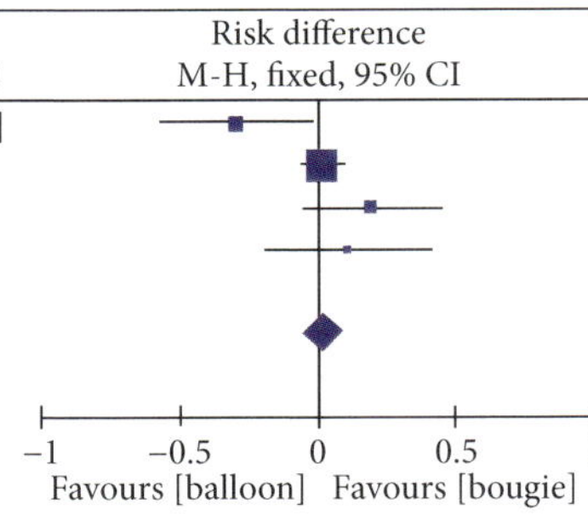

Risk of bias legend
(A) Random sequence generation (selection bias)
(B) Allocation concealment (selection bias)
(C) Blinding of participants and personnel (performance bias)
(D) Blinding of outcome assessment (detection bias)
(E) Incomplete outcome data (attrition bias)
(F) Selective reporting (reporting bias)
(G) Other bias

FIGURE 5: Recurrence rate: forest plot.

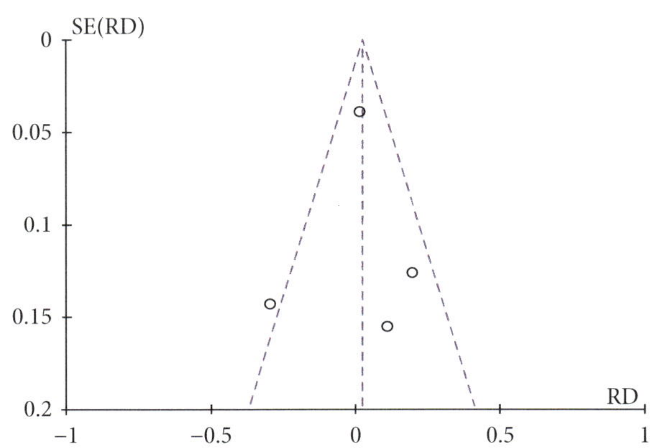

FIGURE 6: Recurrence rate: funnel plot demonstrating an outlier.

Considering all aforementioned limitations and confounding factors, our systematic review was the first to show that patients treated with bougie dilation suffered more frequent episodes of postprocedure pain than those treated with the balloon. In the meantime, we found no difference regarding symptomatic relief, recurrence rate, bleeding, and perforation. Progressive dilation sessions and particular orientation of diet possibly explain our results. Moreover, the short follow-up (12 months) may also have contributed to this result, since it is insufficient to adequately assess the response of complex and refractory esophageal strictures.

The postprocedure pain was more present in the bougie dilation group. The two trials included in this analysis did not mention which scales were used to measure the symptoms. Thus, we used this data as postprocedure pain incidence, regardless of its intensity. The endoscopic dilation with a TTS (through the scope) balloon allows the endoscopist to see the dilation process as it occurs. Opposingly, the bougie dilation is performed blindly or fluoroscopy-guided,

Study or subgroup	Balloon Events	Balloon Total	Bougie Events	Bougie Total	Weight	Risk difference M-H, fixed, 95% CI
Saeed 1995	10	17	15	17	0.0%	−0.29 [−0.57, −0.01]
Scolapio 1999	18	163	8	88	71.5%	0.02 [−0.06, 0.10]
Shemesh 1990	17	30	11	30	18.8%	0.20 [−0.05, 0.45]
Yamamoto 1992	12	15	11	15	9.7%	0.11 [−0.59, 0.42]
Total (95% CI)		208		134	100.0%	0.06 [−0.02, 0.14]
Total events	47		30			

Heterogeneity. chi^2 = 2.49, df = 2 (P = 0.29); I^2 = 20%
Test for overall effect: Z = 1.57 (P = 0. 12)

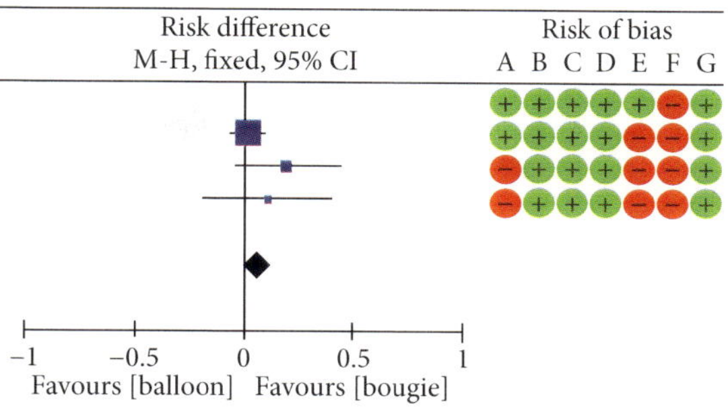

Risk of bias legend
(A) Random sequence generation (selection bias)
(B) Allocation concealment (selection bias)
(C) Blinding of participants and personnel (performance bias)
(D) Blinding of outcome assessment (detection bias)
(E) Incomplete outcome data (attrition bias)
(F) Selective reporting (reporting bias)
(G) Other bias

FIGURE 7: Recurrent rate: forest plot after outlier exclusion.

Study or subgroup	Balloon Events	Balloon Total	Bougie Events	Bougie Total	Weight	Risk difference M-H, fixed, 95% CI
Scolapio 1999	2	163	3	88	88.1%	−0.02 [−0.06, 0.02]
Yamamoto 1992	1	15	1	16	11.9%	0.00 [−0.17, 0.18]
Total (95% CI)		178		104	100.0%	−0.02 [−0.06, 0.02]
Total events	3		4			

Heterogeneity. chi^2 = 0.09, df = 1 (P = 0.77); I^2 = 0%
Test for overall effect: Z = 0.87 (P = 0. 38)

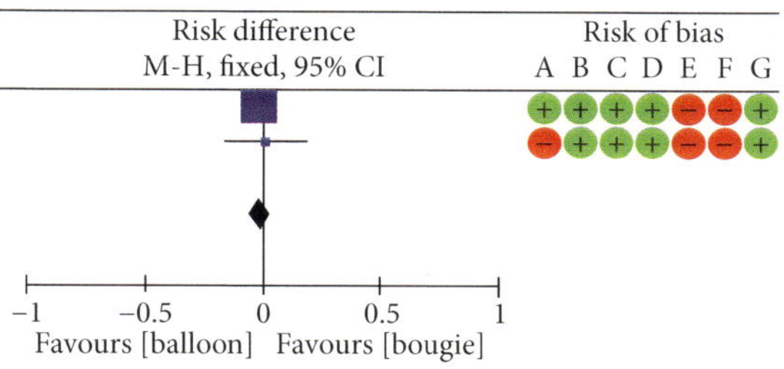

Risk of bias legend
(A) Random sequence generation (selection bias)
(B) Allocation concealment (selection bias)
(C) Blinding of participants and personnel (performance bias)
(D) Blinding of outcome assessment (detection bias)
(E) Incomplete outcome data (attrition bias)
(F) Selective reporting (reporting bias)
(G) Other bias

FIGURE 8: Bleeding: forest plot.

Study or subgroup	Balloon Events	Balloon Total	Bougie Events	Bougie Total	Weight	Risk difference M-H, fixed, 95% CI
Cox 1994	1	46	1	39	19.3%	−0.00 [−0.07, 0.06]
Saeed 1995	0	17	0	17	7.8%	0.00 [−0.11, 0.11]
Scolapio 1999	0	163	0	88	52.2%	0.00 [−0.02, 0.02]
Shemesh 1990	0	30	0	30	13.7%	0.00 [−0.06, 0.06]
Yamamoto 1992	0	15	1	16	7.1%	−0.00 [−0.22, 0.10]
Total (95% CI)		271		190	100.0%	−0.01 [−0.03, 0.02]
Total events	1		2			

Heterogeneity. chi^2 = 0.86, df = 4 (P = 0.93); I^2 = 0%
Test for overall effect: Z = 0.43 (P = 0.66)

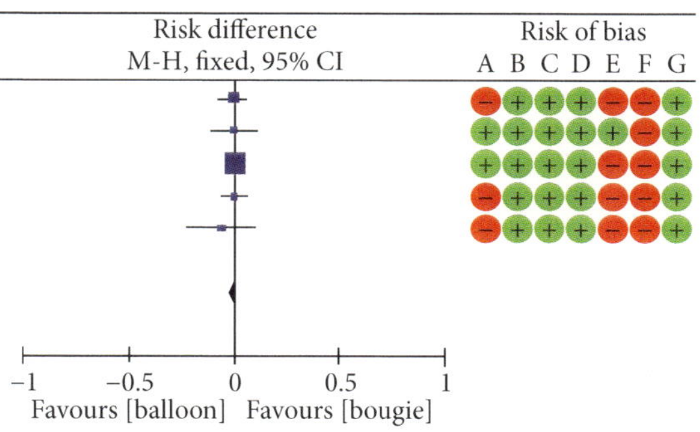

Risk of bias legend
(A) Random sequence generation (selection bias)
(B) Allocation concealment (selection bias)
(C) Blinding of participants and personnel (performance bias)
(D) Blinding of outcome assessment (detection bias)
(E) Incomplete outcome data (attrition bias)
(F) Selective reporting (reporting bias)
(G) Other bias

FIGURE 9: Perforation rate: forest plot.

Study or subgroup	Balloon Events	Balloon Total	Bougie Events	Bougie Total	Weight	Risk difference M-H, fixed, 95% CI	Risk of bias A B C D E F G
Saeed 1995	8	17	13	17	52.3%	−0.29 [−0.61, 0.02]	+ + + + + − +
Yamamoto 1992	0	15	4	16	47.7%	−0.25 [−0.48, −0.02]	− + + + − − +
Total (95% CI)		32		33	100.0%	−0.27 [−0.47, −0.07]	
Total events	8		17				

Heterogeneity. chi^2 = 0.06, df = 1 (P = 0.81); I^2 = 0%
Test for overall effect: Z = 0.63 (P = 0.007)

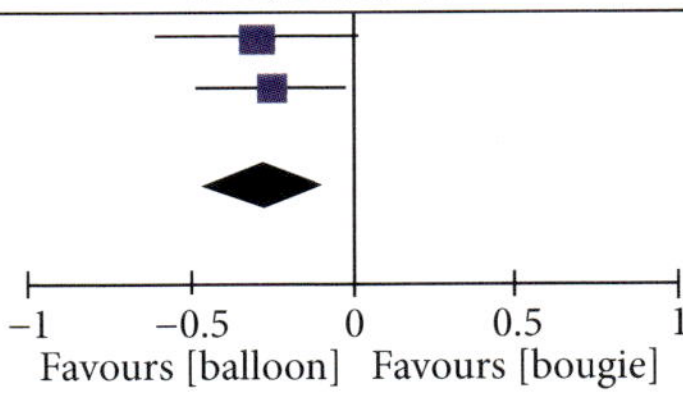

Risk of bias legend
(A) Random sequence generation (selection bias)
(B) Allocation concealment (selection bias)
(C) Blinding of participants and personnel (performance bias)
(D) Blinding of outcome assessment (detection bias)
(E) Incomplete outcome data (attrition bias)
(F) Selective reporting (reporting bias)
(G) Other bias

FIGURE 10: Postprocedure pain incidence: forest plot.

theoretically increasing the risk of deep laceration and postprocedure pain. Another plausible explanation for this finding is that the bougie passes through the soft palate and crosses the upper esophageal sphincter, while the balloon is inflated in a distal position, after those structures. However, there is no literature supporting these theories.

In summary, the efficacy and complication rates of bougie and dilation are similar. Considering this level of evidence 1A study, we can state that there is no significant difference between methods to recommend one over the other. However, all the confounding factors and limitations should be considered. The difficult to perform good quality trials in this field is very clear, so we hope our study is able to guide and encourage the development of new randomized clinical trials, aiming to fulfill all the remaining gaps in the literature.

9. Conclusion

We conclude that there is no difference between bougie and balloon dilation of BESs regarding symptomatic relief, recurrence rate at 12 months, bleeding, and perforation. Patients undergoing balloon dilation experience less severe postprocedure pain. In addition, we have identified many confounding factors and limitations that should be addressed by specifically designed trials.

Authors' Contributions

Iatagan R. Josino and Wanderley M. Bernardo performed the systematic review and meta-analysis. Iatagan R. Josino, Igor B. Ribeiro, and Antonio C. M. Neto wrote the article. Hugo G. Guedes, Vitor O. Brunaldi, Diogo T. H. de Moura, and Eduardo G. H. de Moura revised the manuscript. The final version of the manuscript was approved by all authors.

References

[1] A. Ruigómez, L. Alberto García Rodríguez, M.-A. Wallander, S. Johansson, and S. Eklund, "Esophageal stricture: incidence, treatment patterns, and recurrence rate," *The American Journal of Gastroenterology*, vol. 101, no. 12, pp. 2685–2692, 2006.

[2] L. Poincloux, O. Rouquette, and A. Abergel, "Endoscopic treatment of benign esophageal strictures: a literature review," *Expert Review of Gastroenterology & Hepatology*, vol. 11, no. 1, pp. 53–64, 2016.

[3] W. J. Ravich, "Endoscopic management of benign esophageal strictures," *Current Gastroenterology Reports*, vol. 19, no. 10, p. 50, 2017.

[4] G. W. Dryden and S. A. McClave, "Methods of treating dysphagia caused by benign esophageal strictures," *Techniques in Gastrointestinal Endoscopy*, vol. 3, no. 3, pp. 135–143, 2001.

[5] E. G. Hourneaux de Moura, K. Toma, K. L. Goh et al., "Stents for benign and malignant esophageal strictures," *Annals of the New York Academy of Sciences*, vol. 1300, no. 1, pp. 119–143, 2013.

[6] Y. Vandenplas, "Management of benign esophageal strictures in children," *Pediatric Gastroenterology, Hepatology & Nutrition*, vol. 20, no. 4, pp. 211–215, 2017.

[7] Cochrane, *Cochrane Handbook for Systematic Reviews of Interventions*, J. P. Higgins and S. Green, Eds., vol. 4, John Wiley & Sons, 2011.

[8] J. P. T. Higgins and S. Green, *Cochrane Handbook for Systematic Reviews of Interventions Version 5.1.0 [updated March 2011]*, The Cochrane Collaboration, 2011.

[9] J. G. C. Cox, R. K. Winter, S. C. Maslin et al., "Balloon or Bougie for dilatation of benign esophageal stricture," *Digestive Diseases and Sciences*, vol. 39, no. 4, pp. 776–781, 1994.

[10] Z. A. Saeed, C. B. Winchester, P. S. Ferro, P. A. Michaletz, J. T. Schwartz, and D. Y. Graham, "Prospective randomized comparison of polyvinyl bougies and through-the-scope balloons for dilation of peptic strictures of the esophagus," *Gastrointestinal Endoscopy*, vol. 41, no. 3, pp. 189–195, 1995.

[11] J. S. Scolapio, T. M. Pasha, C. J. Gostout et al., "A randomized prospective study comparing rigid to balloon dilators for benign esophageal strictures and rings," *Gastrointestinal Endoscopy*, vol. 50, no. 1, pp. 13–17, 1999.

[12] E. Shemesh and A. Czerniak, "Comparison between Savary-Gilliard and balloon dilatation of benign esophageal strictures," *World Journal of Surgery*, vol. 14, no. 4, pp. 518–521, 1990.

[13] H. Yamamoto, R. W. Hughes Jr., K. W. Schroeder, T. R. Viggiano, and E. P. DiMagno, "Treatment of benign esophageal stricture by Eder-Puestow or balloon dilators: a comparison between randomized and prospective nonrandomized trials," *Mayo Clinic Proceedings*, vol. 67, no. 3, pp. 228–236, 1992.

[14] B. Phillips, C. Ball, D. Sackett, D. Badenoch, S. Straus, and B. Haynes, *Centre for Evidence-Based Medicine—Levels of Evidence—CEBM*, Centre for Evidence-Based Medicine , M. D. Oxford, 2009.

[15] L. Bonavina, M. Chirica, O. Skrobic et al., "Foregut caustic injuries: results of the world society of emergency surgery consensus conference," *World Journal of Emergency Surgery*, vol. 10, no. 1, p. 44, 2015.

[16] S. L. Broor, A. Kumar, S. T. Chari et al., "Corrosive oesophageal strictures following acid ingestion: clinical profile and results of endoscopic dilatation," *Journal of Gastroenterology and Hepatology*, vol. 4, no. 1, pp. 55–61, 1989.

[17] S. Contini, M. Garatti, A. Swarray-Deen, N. Depetris, S. Cecchini, and C. Scarpignato, "Corrosive oesophageal strictures in children: outcomes after timely or delayed dilatation," *Digestive and Liver Disease*, vol. 41, no. 4, pp. 263–268, 2009.

Systematic Review with Network Meta-Analysis: Efficacy of Induction Therapy with a Second Biological Agent in Anti-TNF-Experienced Crohn's Disease Patients

Cristiano Pagnini[1], **Spyros I. Siakavellas**[2] **and Giorgos Bamias**[3]

[1]*Digestive and Liver Disease Department, S. Andrea Hospital, Rome, Italy*
[2]*Academic Department of Gastroenterology, Laiko General Hospital, University of Athens Medical School, Athens, Greece*
[3]*Gastroenterology Unit, Third Depatment of Internal Medicine, Sotiria General Hospital, University of Athens Medical School, Athens, Greece*

Correspondence should be addressed to Giorgos Bamias; gbamias@gmail.com

Academic Editor: Paolo Gionchetti

Background and Aim. Crohn's disease (CD) is a chronic inflammatory condition of the gastrointestinal tract with the potential to progress to a severe debilitating state. Treatment with biological agents is highly efficient, improving both short-term outcomes and long-term prognosis. Nonetheless, up to 60% of patients receiving biological therapy will exhibit nonresponse at some point. The optimal management of such patients is not clearly defined. Besides traditional anti-TNF agents (infliximab, adalimumab, and certolizumab), alternative biological therapies (natalizumab, vedolizumab, and ustekinumab) are currently available for the treatment of CD. Our aim was to analyze all available evidence regarding efficacy of a second biological in "biological-treatment-experienced" patients. *Methods.* A systematic review of the literature was conducted using specific criteria for selecting relevant randomized clinical trials evaluating response to administration of secondary biological therapy in "anti-TNF-experienced" CD patients. Data from these studies was used to perform (a) traditional meta-analysis to ascertain the effect of secondary treatment versus placebo and (b) network meta-analysis to compare indirectly the efficacy of available biological agents. *Results.* Out of initially 977 studies, only eight were included for analysis, providing a total of 1281 treated and 733 placebo-receiving CD patients. Treatment with a second biological was found to be superior to placebo for both induction of remission (OR 2.2, 95% CI 1.7 to 3) and response (OR 1.9, 95% CI 1.5 to 2.5), with global rates of 24% and 42%, respectively (placebo rate: 11% and 27%, $p < 0.0001$ for both). Indirect comparisons performed with network meta-analysis suggest no specific agent is clearly superior to others, with relatively better results observed for adalimumab in inducing disease remission. *Conclusion.* In anti-TNF-experienced CD patients, secondary biological administration may be efficient, while no specific agent seems to outperform the others. Further research is needed to identify optimal management strategies for this challenging subset of patients.

1. Introduction

Crohn's disease (CD) is a pathologic condition of unknown etiology that is characterized by dysregulated mucosal immunity, resulting in recurrent-remittent inflammation of the bowel [1]. Its clinical course consists of an early inflammatory phenotype, which tends to progress towards stenotic or fistulizing complications, thus resulting in a gradually debilitating disease [2]. In line with this, it has been suggested that potent and aggressive treatment interventions during the early phase of CD may hopefully arrest disease progression and preclude a degenerative course. Such favorable outcomes have been possible in recent years with the development and application of biological agents in the treatment of CD. Those target-specific immunological therapies have shown significant efficacy in the induction and maintenance of remission in CD patients. In fact, they may affect not only short-term outcomes (i.e., symptoms relief, corticosteroids withdrawal, and mucosal healing) but also long-term disease prognosis (hospitalization, surgery, and quality of life) [3, 4].

Monoclonal antibodies that neutralize TNF were pioneer drugs and have been the first biological agents that were used in CD. Those include the recombinant chimeric human-murine antibody infliximab and the recombinant human antibody adalimumab which are marketed in US and Europe for almost two decades. A third antibody, the recombinant humanized Fab' fragment certolizumab pegol, is currently approved only by the FDA. Due to their well-established efficacy, anti-TNF antibodies have been increasingly chosen as rescue therapies for conventional-treatment-refractory CD as well as early treatment for CD patients with features of severe disease and/or prognostic factors for poor prognosis [5, 6]. Notwithstanding their aforementioned efficacy, almost one third of patients will not respond ab initio (primary failure), and probably more than one-third exhibit loss of response during the next months/years (secondary failure) or may not be able to tolerate this particular treatment regimen [7–9]. Therefore, about 60% of patients who start anti-TNF therapy will be classified as "treatment-failures" at some point, representing a particularly challenging subgroup of patients for future treatment. Considering the increasing use of anti-TNF drugs and the fact that for many years anti-TNF inhibitors have been the only available option for biological treatment (except for natalizumab that had been of limited availability [10]), it is easy to infer that the number of the patients in this subgroup of anti-TNF-experienced patients is rapidly increasing, and guidance about the management of such patients is urgently needed.

In the last few years, novel molecules have become available with mechanisms of action different from anti-TNF blockade, and many more are tested in the therapeutic pipeline for CD [11]. Consequently, therapeutic options for anti-TNF-experienced CD patients are constantly expanding, creating new opportunities for the management of those difficult-to-treat patients. Biological drugs with alternative mechanism of action currently available include natalizumab (a recombinant humanized monoclonal IgG4 antibody against the integrin subunit $\alpha 4$, which, as already mentioned, is marketed only in US), vedolizumab (a humanized IgG1 monoclonal antibody blocking the enteric-specific $\alpha 4\beta 7$ integrin), and ustekinumab (a fully human IgG1 monoclonal antibody against the p40 subunit that is common in the IL-12 and IL-23 molecules) [10, 12–18].

The aim of the present systematic review is to analyze all available evidence from randomized controlled trials (RCTs) in literature regarding the efficacy for induction of remission or response of the aforementioned biological agents in CD patients who had already had a previous biologic treatment ("biological treatment-experienced patients"). To accomplish our aim, we performed a traditional meta-analysis to evaluate the effect of a second biological treatment versus placebo and a network meta-analysis to indirectly compare available drugs, since no head-to-head comparisons have been conducted.

2. Methods

2.1. Data Sources and Search. The study was conducted in accordance with the PRISMA statement [19]. A search of clinical trials in PubMed and Cochrane Library databases was performed using the following search strategy: "adalimumab OR infliximab OR certolizumab OR vedolizumab OR natalizumab OR ustekinumab AND crohn." The studies of interest were placebo-controlled, randomized studies; retrospective and observational studies were not included in any of the analyses. The search was not limited by language, but a large majority of the manuscripts were originally published in English.

2.2. Study Selection. Two investigators independently reviewed the titles of all identified citations to generate a list of potentially relevant articles for further review. The abstracts of these articles were reviewed to identify studies suitable for inclusion in our final analyses. For a manuscript to be eligible for our study, it had to satisfy the following eligibility criteria: (i) studies had to examine the effect of a single biological agent on induction of response or remission in CD; (ii) studies had to include in the analysis patients who had already received previously treatment with an anti-TNF agent; (iii) studies could not duplicate data already published; (iv) studies needed to be published as full manuscripts; (v) response or remission had to be defined by standardized quantitative scoring criteria (typically using the Crohn's Disease Activity Index (CDAI)); (vi) studies had to be placebo-controlled, randomized clinical trials with treatment and control arms. We did not include nonrandomized controlled trials given the concern for study heterogeneity.

2.3. Data Synthesis and Analysis. The odds ratio (OR) was used to measure treatment effects in all comparisons. Study-level ORs with 95% confidence intervals (CIs) were calculated in accordance with the intention-to-treat principle.

The meta-analysis was performed using the Mantel-Haenszel method calculating the fixed and random effect when indicated. Heterogeneity between studies was calculated by χ^2 test. Software MedCalc version 9.2 was used for statistical calculations.

For network meta-analysis, a frequentist approach was used with the graphical tools developed by Chaimani et al. for the STATA software [20]. In short, multivariate random-effects meta-analyses were fit to model the intervention effects across studies. Effect sizes for network meta-analysis were described with 95% credible intervals. The off-diagonal cells of the league tables calculated contain odds ratios and 95% confidence intervals from all pairwise comparisons in network meta-analyses. The contribution of direct evidence to the mixed estimates and the entire network was also calculated and plotted. Probabilities of each treatment being at a specific order and surface under the cumulative ranking area (SUCRA) values were estimated running 10,000 replications. SUCRA is used to provide a hierarchy of treatments for each outcome. The larger the SUCRA value was, the better the treatment was considered. STATA 13 MP software was used to conduct the network meta-analysis.

All p values are 2-tailed. For all tests (except for heterogeneity), a $p < 0.05$ indicates statistical significance.

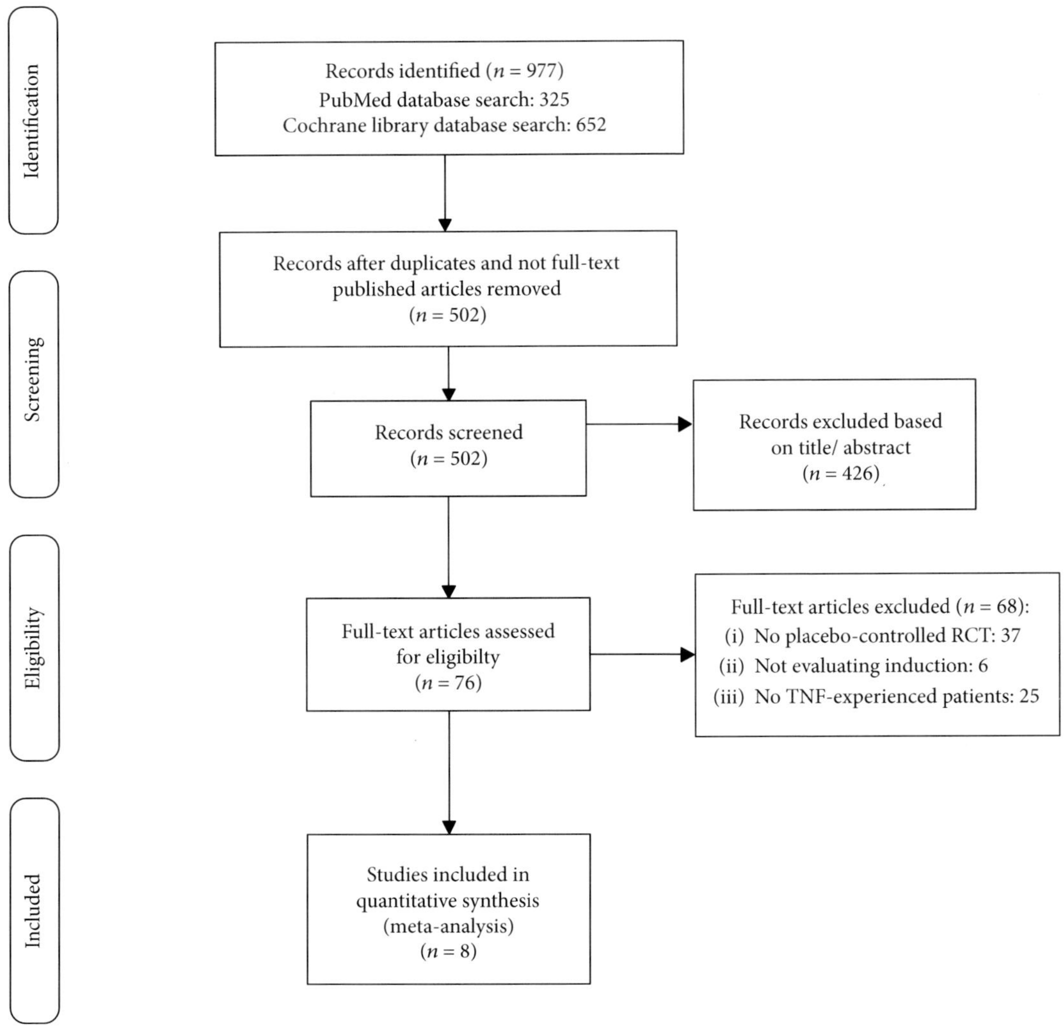

FIGURE 1: Summary of evidence search and selection for induction of response and remission in anti-TNF-experienced CD patients.

3. Results

3.1. Search Results. A flow diagram combining the search and selection process is presented in Figure 1. Initial literature search for clinical trials yielded a total of 977 citations, among which 325 from PubMed database and 652 from Cochrane library database. After exclusion of duplicates and nonfull-text published articles (i.e., conference proceedings and abstract of congress presentations), 502 studies were reviewed. Among those, 426 records were excluded after title and/or abstract evaluation, and the remaining 76 studies were evaluated in full-text. Sixty-eight studies were further excluded for the following reasons: not being placebo-controlled RCT ($n = 37$), not evaluating induction of remission ($n = 6$), and not including anti-TNF-experienced CD patients ($n = 25$). Finally, 8 studies [21–28] were included in the meta-analysis, with a total of 1281 treated and 733 placebo CD patients. Among those, 5 studies evaluated both remission and response, 2 only response and 1 only remission. In 4 studies, TNF-experienced patients represented the whole population analyzed, while in 4 studies, they represented a subgroup of patients. Characteristics of the 8 studies that fulfilled inclusion criteria are summarized in Table 1.

3.2. Direct Treatment Comparison (Treatment versus Placebo). Results of traditional meta-analysis showed that treatment with a second biologic drug in anti-TNF-experienced CD patients was superior to placebo in inducing remission (OR 2.2, 95% CI 1.7 to 3) and response (OR 1.9, 95% CI 1.5 to 2.5) (Figures 2a and 2b). Globally, 273/1159 (24%) of patients in the treatment group achieved remission comparing with 71/621 (11%) in the placebo group. In addition, clinical response was achieved by 519/1229 (42%) versus 192/706 (27%), respectively, ($p < 0.001$ for both; χ^2 test). Heterogeneity across studies was not significant ($p = 0.59$ and $p = 0.26$ for remission and response, resp.).

3.3. Indirect Treatment Comparison (Treatment versus Treatment). For the network meta-analysis, initially, the network diagrams were generated separately for the two outcomes of the included studies (i.e., remission and response after induction of secondary biological treatment) as shown

Table 1: Characteristics of the studies included in the meta-analysis.

Study (ref)	Drug	*N* drug/placebo	Inclusion	Outcome	Population characteristic	Time (wks)
Sandborn et al., PRECISE 1 [22]	Certolizumab	97/85	No primary nonresponders	Response	Subgroup	6
Sandborn et al., GAIN [23]	Adalimumab	159/166	No primary nonresponders	Remission/response	Whole	4
Sandborn et al. [24]	Ustekinumab	394/132	Primary/secondary nonresponse, adverse events	Remission/response (3 different doses)	Whole	8
Sandborn et al. [21]	Ustekinumab	25/27	Previous exposure	Response (2 different doses)	Subgroup	8
Sands, GEMINI 3 (25)	Vedolizumab	158/157	Primary/secondary nonresponse, adverse events	Remission/response	Whole	10
Sandborn et al. [26]	Vedolizumab	105/70	Primary/secondary nonresponse, adverse events	Remission/response	Subgroup	6
Sands et al. [27]	Natalizumab	52/27	Secondary nonresponders	Remission	Whole	10
Sandborn et al. [28]	Natalizumab	291/69	Not specified	Remission/response	Subgroup	10

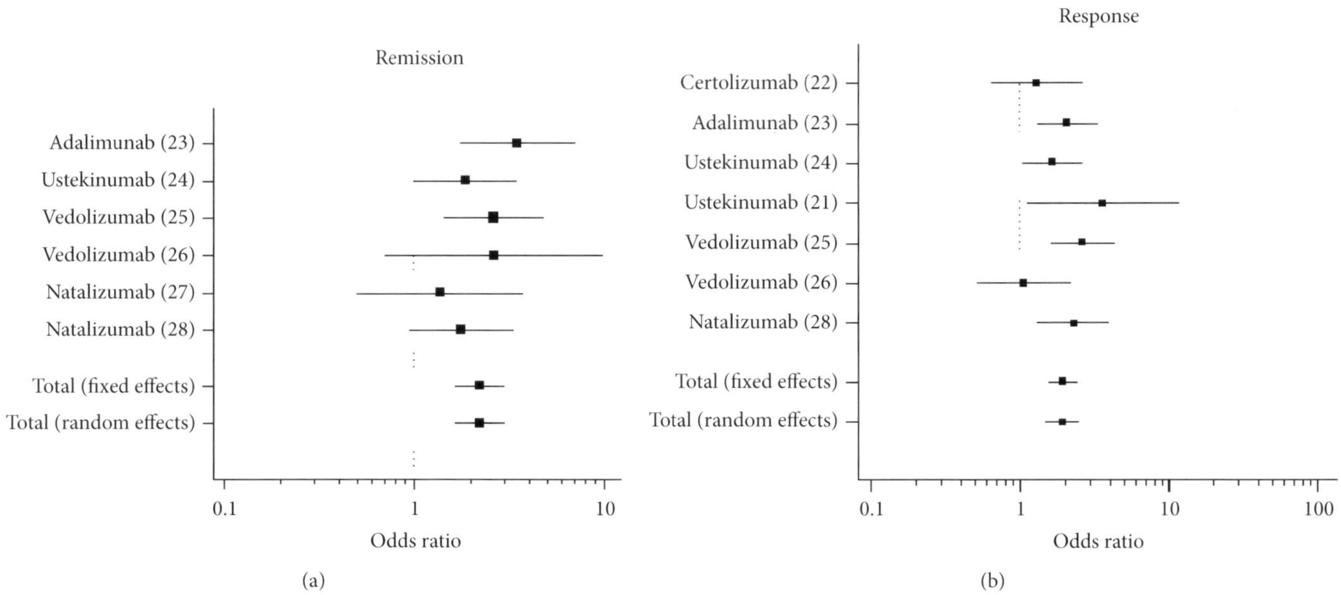

FIGURE 2: Traditional meta-analysis of published studies for induction of remission (a) and response (b) in anti-TNF-experienced CD patients. The name of the drug and the reference of the study is reported. Global comparison showed significant efficacy of treatment comparing with placebo.

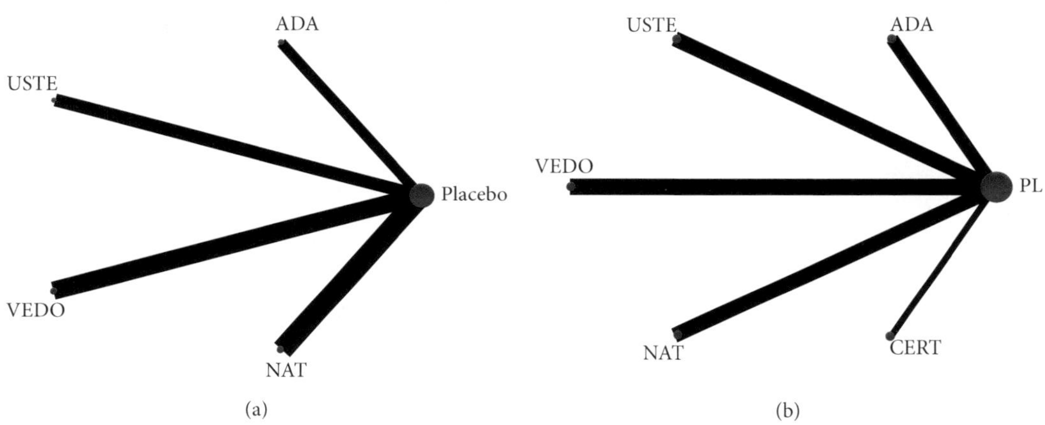

FIGURE 3: Network diagrams of published studies for induction of remission (a) and response (b) in anti-TNF-experienced CD patients. In brief, circles correspond to each intervention as a node while lines represent the direct comparisons. The size of each circle indicates the number of included participants for each corresponding treatment, and line thickness indicates the number of studies included in each comparison. Placebo as expected is represented by the biggest node. ADA = adalimumab; USTE = ustekinumab; VEDO = vedolizumab; NAT = natalizumab; CERT = certolizumab; PL = placebo.

in Figure 3. No direct comparisons were made between therapeutic regimens, so comparisons were performed in a pairwise manner as described above. Due to the criteria of our study design (only RCTs with two arms, the one being placebo administration), no inconsistency was observed in our model while calculated heterogeneity values were not significant.

Next, interval plots were calculated (relative efficacy is plotted as OR with 95% credible intervals). These plots demonstrate that no secondary biological agent was superior to others in a statistically significant level in inducing remission or response (Figure 4). Interestingly, our results indicate that the statistically significant superiority of biological agents in comparison to placebo persists in the network meta-analysis for remission but not for response.

Furthermore, so as to rank treatments, a SUCRA (i.e., the converted value reflecting the probability of a treatment being the best according to the ranking of each treatment) analysis was conducted and league tables were generated. Our calculations indicate that adalimumab showed relatively better efficacy in inducing remission than the other drugs followed up in second place by vedolizumab (Figure 5). Nevertheless, regarding the achievement of clinical response, the results were more ambivalent; natalizumab, ustekinumab, and adalimumab produced similar SUCRA values that were relatively better from vedolizumab and certolizumab (Figure 6).

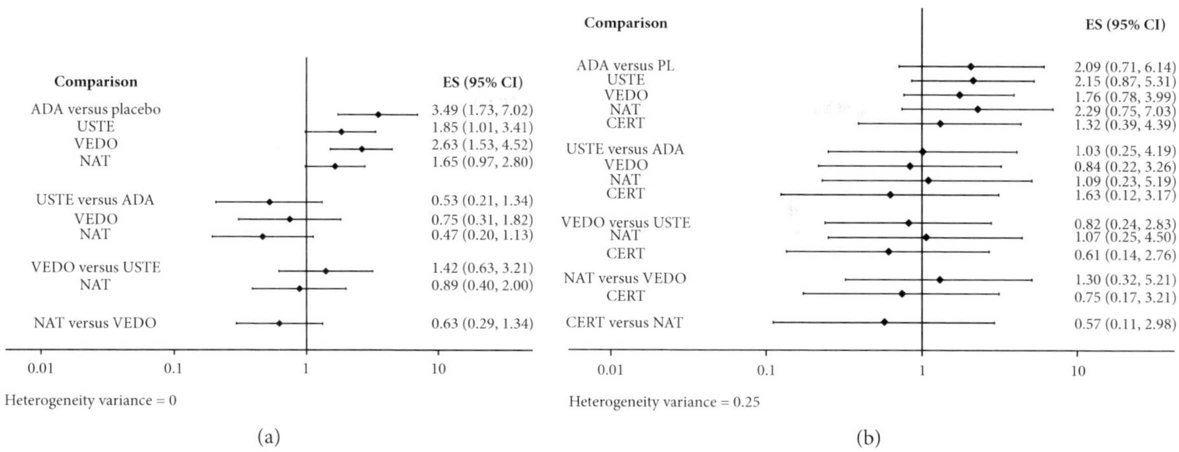

FIGURE 4: Network meta-analysis interval plot of published studies for induction of (a) remission and (b) response in anti-TNF-experienced CD patients. Odds ratios (ORs) with 95% confidence interval (CI) are reported. All the single drugs showed consistent efficacy comparing with placebo while no drug proved to be superior in a statistically significant level to all others in inducing remission. ADA = adalimumab; USTE = ustekinumab; VEDO = vedolizumab; NAT = natalizumab; CERT = certolizumab; PL = placebo.

SUCRA

Treatment	SUCRA	PrBest	Mean rank
PL	01.5	00.0	04.9
ADA	89.8	69.4	01.4
USTE	47.0	04.6	03.1
VEDO	74.0	24.5	02.0
NAT	37.7	01.5	03.5

(a)

OR > 1 means the treatment in top left is better

Adalimumab				
1.33 (0.55–3.23)	Vedolizumab			
1.88 (0.75–3.23)	1.42 (0.63–3.21)	Ustekinumab		
2.12 (0.88–5.0)	1.59 (0.74–3.45)	1.13 (0.5–2.5)	Natalizumab	
3.49 (1.73–7.02)	2.63 (1.53–4.52)	1.42 (1.01–3.41)	1.42 (0.97–2.80)	Placebo

(b)

FIGURE 5: Network meta-analysis and ranking of treatments for inducing remission in anti-TNF-experienced CD patients via (a) SUCRA analysis and (b) league table graph. Odds ratios (ORs) with 95% confidence interval (CI) are reported. ADA = adalimumab; USTE = ustekinumab; VEDO = vedolizumab; NAT = natalizumab; PL = placebo.

SUCRA response

Treatment	SUCRA	PrBest	Mean rank
PL	12.5	00.0	05.4
ADA	63.6	25.6	02.8
USTE	65.6	22.7	02.7
VEDO	54.2	10.9	03.3
NAT	68.0	32.6	02.6
CERT	36.1	08.1	04.2

(a)

OR > 1 means the treatment in top left is better

Natalizumab					
1.07 (0.25–4.5)	Ustekinumab				
1.09 (0.23–5.19)	1.03 (0.25–4.19)	Adalimumab			
1.30 (0.32–5.21)	1.22 (0.35–4.55)	1.16 (0.16–8.75)	Vedolizumab		
1.75 (0.34–9.1)	1.64 (0.37–7.14)	1.59 (0.32–8.33)	1.33 (0.31–5.88)	Certolizumab	
2.29 (0.75–7.03)	2.15 (0.87–5.31)	2.09 (0.71–6.14)	1.76 (0.78–3.99)	1.32 (0.39–4.39)	Placebo

(b)

FIGURE 6: Network meta-analysis and ranking of treatments for inducing response in anti-TNF-experienced CD patients via (a) SUCRA analysis and (b) league table graph. Odds ratios (ORs) with 95% confidence interval (CI) are reported. ADA = adalimumab; USTE = ustekinumab; VEDO = vedolizumab; NAT = natalizumab; PL = placebo.

4. Discussion

The utilization of anti-TNF monoclonal antibodies for the treatment of CD for the last 20 years has resulted in a substantial, anti-TNF-experienced population of patients. Included therein are patients that failed to respond, those who lost their initial response, and those who were forced to discontinue therapy due to toxicity concerns. Our present meta-analysis clearly demonstrates that there is an increasing number of choices for such anti-TNF failures, which include a second anti-TNF monoclonal antibody, the anti-integrins vedolizumab and natalizumab, and, lastly, the anti-IL-12/IL-23 antibody ustekinumab. According to our network meta-analysis, no single treatment appears to be superior in indirect comparison.

The efficacy of biologic treatment has been highlighted by different RCTs and recently summarized in a meta-analysis by Stidham et al. [29] that analyzed in a network meta-analysis 10 studies evaluating efficacy of anti-TNF agents in induction and maintenance of remission and response in CD patients, irrespectively of their prior exposure to anti-TNF therapy. They reported that biological agents exhibited consistently superiority versus placebo. On the other hand, no clear evidence of clinical superiority of one drug versus the others could be elicited. Another research group restricted their analysis to efficacy of biologic drugs in TNF naïve patients, finding 17 studies which evaluated 6 different biologic agents. The authors came to the conclusion that infliximab was found to surpass other agents in achieving remission in this group of patients [30]. To date, the only study specifically evaluating efficacy of biologic drugs in anti-TNF-experienced patients with CD is a recent meta-analysis by Gisbert et al. [7]. In this study, authors included not only RCTs but also case-controlled and retrospective studies. Their findings mainly focused on the cause of previous anti-TNF failure as the main factor determining response to a secondary biological agent. Thus, it was suggested that patients who had a primary nonresponse had a lower remission and response rate to a second anti-TNF, while patients with loss of response or intolerance to the first anti-TNF had higher rates of success. In accordance with that observation, the only two studies included in the present work who analyzed administration of a second anti-TNF (namely adalimumab [23] and certolizumab [22]) excluded patients with primary nonresponse. This is in line with the currently prevailing opinion that recommends utilization of a biological with a different mechanism of action (switch out of class) in such patients [8].

Our study included only RCTs and evaluated specifically anti-TNF-experienced CD patients. As shown by the traditional meta-analysis section, secondary biological treatment was significantly superior to placebo for both induction of remission and response. Since no head-to-head study directly comparing two biologic drugs is currently available, we indirectly compared secondary biologicals with one another by means of network meta-analysis. Our analysis based on a frequentist approach implies that in this patient population, no single drug clearly outcompetes the other candidates in achieving remission/response. Further studies, with a prospective design and with different biological-treatment arms (including novel agents), will answer the question of which medication best suits patients failing anti-TNF therapy. Moreover, prospective studies that will evaluate not only the effect of anti-TNF but also of anti-integrin and anti-IL12/23 administration in the future course of biologically naïve CD patients are warranted to elucidate optimal management of nonresponse or treatment-intolerant patients and open the way for highly effective personalized therapeutic interventions. Until such studies become available, the choice of drug needs to be empirically tailored to the characteristics of each case, as well as local availability and patient preference issues. Interestingly, analysis of the included studies clearly shows that a considerable proportion of these patients will not respond to a secondary biological intervention. Identification of clinical, genetic, and/or molecular characteristics that may predict a beneficial response to each drug is urgently needed for these "difficult-to-treat" patients.

We are aware that the present study has several limitations. First, in the included studies, TNF-experienced patients represented either the whole population, and this had been a specific consideration in the inclusion criteria (in four studies) or a part of the population included in which a subgroup analysis was performed (in four studies). This disparity could imply a degree of selection bias that has to be taken into account. Nevertheless, when analyzing separately these two categories of studies, only a trend was observed towards higher response rate in studies that included only anti-TNF-experienced patients versus studies that included anti-TNF naïve patients as well (OR: 2.4 (95% CI: 1.7–3.3) versus 1.9 (1.1–3.3) and 2.1 (1.6–2.7) versus 1.7 (1.1–2.8), for response and remission, respectively).

Second, the reason for discontinuation of the first anti-TNF or the precise timeframe and the duration of the first biological treatment was not always specified in the included trials. Considering that anti-TNF primary failure patients have been excluded from the adalimumab and certolizumab trials, a degree of heterogeneity is to be expected regarding the cause of discontinuation in the included studies. This in turn may have affected the response/remission rate across different studies. A case, for instance, could be made that patients with a primary nonresponse may represent a subgroup with a more "difficult to treat" disease. As a result, studies that exclude or enroll a low number of such patients may be more likely to have better results. This may partially explain the trend for better results observed for adalimumab in the network comparison. On the other hand, while this same subgroup of patients was excluded in the certolizumab trial as well, no similar improved efficacy was noted.

In view of the aforementioned known problems, we decided to include only RCTs and excluded case-controlled and retrospective studies in order to reduce heterogeneity. We also chose to examine as outcomes only the achievement of response and/or remission in these patients to a second-line biological treatment, as the definitions for these particular outcomes were comparable among different trials. Moreover, inclusion criteria regarding severity and characteristics of baseline disease were also found to be quite similar across the studies we analyzed. This approach resulted to the fact that heterogeneity among studies was shown to be not significant in our meta-analysis. Nonetheless, minor differences still exist, that is, in the evaluation time points (that ranged from four to ten weeks) and in drug administration protocols, that may confound our comparisons. Apart from that, the strict criteria we chose for inclusion in our review while helpful in limiting heterogeneity led to a relatively small number ($n = 8$) of studies with a total of 2014 anti-TNF-experienced patients (1281 receiving secondary biological treatment and 733 placebo) being selected, which may limit the strength of our analysis.

In conclusion, anti-TNF-experienced CD patients requiring second-line biological therapy constitute an important and constantly expanding clinical conundrum, as management strategies are not always clear. Our systematic review, including a well-executed traditional and network meta-analysis, demonstrates that in these cases, administration of second-line biological treatment results in significant efficacy regarding remission and response when compared to placebo but with no evidence of superiority for a specific therapeutic regimen. Although such findings are clearly encouraging, still an improved characterization and classification of CD patients is needed with the aid of relevant molecular biomarkers or clinical features in order to appropriately identify disease phenotypes with specific responses to selected therapeutic regimens. Our end goal should be a highly tailored therapy with improved efficacy and outcomes in all our patients, minimizing unnecessary drug exposure and adverse events.

Disclosure

Cristiano Pagnini and Spyros I. Siakavellas are joint first authors.

Authors' Contributions

Cristiano Pagnini and Giorgos Bamias conceived and designed the study. Cristiano Pagnini and Spyros I. Siakavellas conducted the literature search and performed the statistical analysis. Cristiano Pagnini and Spyros I. Siakavellas wrote the manuscript. Giorgos Bamias provided significant additional intellectual content for inclusion in the final form of the manuscript.

Acknowledgments

The authors wish to thank Lucia Cocomello and Arianna Sanna for their help in the literature search and study selection.

References

[1] C. Abraham and J. H. Cho, "Inflammatory bowel disease," *New England Journal of Medicine*, vol. 361, no. 21, pp. 2066–2078, 2009.

[2] D. C. Baumgart and W. J. Sandborn, "Crohn's disease," *The Lancet*, vol. 380, no. 9853, pp. 1590–1605, 2012.

[3] G. R. Lichtenstein, S. Yan, M. Bala, M. Blank, and B. E. Sands, "Infliximab maintenance treatment reduces hospitalizations, surgeries, and procedures in fistulizing Crohn's disease," *Gastroenterology*, vol. 128, no. 4, pp. 862–869, 2005.

[4] G. Van Assche, S. Vermeire, and P. Rutgeerts, "The potential for disease modification in Crohn's disease," *Nature Reviews Gastroenterology & Hepatology*, vol. 7, no. 2, pp. 79–85, 2010.

[5] S. Danese, G. Fiorino, C. Fernandes, and L. Peyrin-Biroulet, "Catching the therapeutic window of opportunity in early Crohn's disease," *Current Drug Targets*, vol. 15, no. 11, pp. 1056–1063, 2014.

[6] S. Hirschmann and M. F. Neurath, "Top-down approach to biological therapy of Crohn's disease," *Expert Opinion on Biological Therapy*, vol. 17, no. 3, pp. 285–293, 2017.

[7] J. P. Gisbert, A. C. Marín, A. G. McNicholl, and M. Chaparro, "Systematic review with meta-analysis: the efficacy of a second anti-TNF in patients with inflammatory bowel disease whose previous anti-TNF treatment has failed," *Alimentary Pharmacology & Therapeutics*, vol. 41, no. 7, pp. 613–623, 2015.

[8] S. Ben-Horin, U. Kopylov, and Y. Chowers, "Optimizing anti-TNF treatments in inflammatory bowel disease," *Autoimmunity Reviews*, vol. 13, no. 1, pp. 24–30, 2014.

[9] U. Wong and R. K. Cross, "Primary and secondary nonresponse to infliximab: mechanisms and countermeasures," *Expert Opinion on Drug Metabolism & Toxicology*, vol. 13, no. 10, pp. 1039–1046, 2017.

[10] C. Pagnini, K. O. Arseneau, and F. Cominelli, "Natalizumab in the treatment of Crohn's disease patients," *Expert Opinion on Biological Therapy*, vol. 17, no. 11, pp. 1433–1438, 2017.

[11] G. Fiorino, S. Rovida, C. Correale, A. Malesci, and S. Danese, "Emerging biologics in the treatment of inflammatory bowel disease: what is around the corner?," *Current Drug Targets*, vol. 11, no. 2, pp. 249–260, 2010.

[12] S. Danese, L. Vuitton, and L. Peyrin-Biroulet, "Biologic agents for IBD: practical insights," *Nature Reviews Gastroenterology & Hepatology*, vol. 12, no. 9, pp. 537–545, 2015.

[13] P. Deepak and W. J. Sandborn, "Ustekinumab and anti-interleukin-23 agents in Crohn's disease," *Gastroenterology Clinics of North America*, vol. 46, no. 3, pp. 603–626, 2017.

[14] T. Lobaton, S. Vermeire, G. Van Assche, and P. Rutgeerts, "Review article: anti-adhesion therapies for inflammatory bowel disease," *Alimentary Pharmacology & Therapeutics*, vol. 39, no. 6, pp. 579–594, 2014.

[15] A. Jauregui-Amezaga, M. Somers, H. De Schepper, and E. Macken, "Next generation of biologics for the treatment of Crohn's disease: an evidence-based review on ustekinumab," *Clinical and Experimental Gastroenterology*, vol. 10, pp. 293–301, 2017.

[16] P. G. Kotze, C. Ma, A. Almutairdi, and R. Panaccione, "Clinical utility of ustekinumab in Crohn's disease," *Journal of Inflammation Research*, vol. 11, pp. 35–47, 2018.

[17] M. Argollo, G. Fiorino, L. Peyrin-Biroulet, and S. Danese, "Vedolizumab for the treatment of Crohn's disease," *Expert Review of Clinical Immunology*, vol. 14, no. 3, pp. 179–189, 2018.

[18] M. Noman, M. Ferrante, R. Bisschops et al., "Vedolizumab induces long-term mucosal healing in patients with Crohn's

disease and ulcerative colitis," *Journal of Crohn's and Colitis*, vol. 11, no. 9, pp. 1085–1089, 2017.

[19] D. Moher, A. Liberati, J. Tetzlaff, D. G. Altman, and PRISMA Group, "Preferred reporting items for systematic reviews and meta-analyses: the PRISMA statement," *Annals of Internal Medicine*, vol. 151, no. 4, pp. 264–269, 2009.

[20] A. Chaimani, J. P. T. Higgins, D. Mavridis, P. Spyridonos, and G. Salanti, "Graphical tools for network meta-analysis in STATA," *PLoS One*, vol. 8, no. 10, article e76654, 2013.

[21] W. J. Sandborn, B. G. Feagan, R. N. Fedorak et al., "A randomized trial of ustekinumab, a human interleukin-12/23 monoclonal antibody, in patients with moderate-to-severe Crohn's disease," *Gastroenterology*, vol. 135, no. 4, pp. 1130–1141, 2008.

[22] W. J. Sandborn, B. G. Feagan, S. Stoinov et al., "Certolizumab pegol for the treatment of Crohn's disease," *The New England Journal of Medicine*, vol. 357, no. 3, pp. 228–238, 2007.

[23] W. J. Sandborn, P. Rutgeerts, R. Enns et al., "Adalimumab induction therapy for Crohn disease previously treated with infliximab: a randomized trial," *Annals of Internal Medicine*, vol. 146, no. 12, pp. 829–838, 2007.

[24] W. J. Sandborn, C. Gasink, L. L. Gao et al., "Ustekinumab induction and maintenance therapy in refractory Crohn's disease," *The New England Journal of Medicine*, vol. 367, no. 16, pp. 1519–1528, 2012.

[25] B. E. Sands, B. G. Feagan, P. Rutgeerts et al., "Effects of vedolizumab induction therapy for patients with Crohn's disease in whom tumor necrosis factor antagonist treatment failed," *Gastroenterology*, vol. 147, no. 3, pp. 618–627.e3, 2014.

[26] W. J. Sandborn, B. G. Feagan, P. Rutgeerts et al., "Vedolizumab as induction and maintenance therapy for Crohn's disease," *The New England Journal of Medicine*, vol. 369, no. 8, pp. 711–721, 2013.

[27] B. E. Sands, R. Kozarek, J. Spainhour et al., "Safety and tolerability of concurrent natalizumab treatment for patients with Crohn's disease not in remission while receiving infliximab," *Inflammatory Bowel Diseases*, vol. 13, no. 1, pp. 2–11, 2007.

[28] W. J. Sandborn, J. F. Colombel, R. Enns et al., "Natalizumab induction and maintenance therapy for Crohn's disease," *The New England Journal of Medicine*, vol. 353, no. 18, pp. 1912–1925, 2005.

[29] R. W. Stidham, T. C. H. Lee, P. D. R. Higgins et al., "Systematic review with network meta-analysis: the efficacy of anti-TNF agents for the treatment of Crohn's disease," *Alimentary Pharmacology & Therapeutics*, vol. 39, no. 12, pp. 1349–1362, 2014.

[30] S. Singh, S. K. Garg, D. S. Pardi, Z. Wang, M. Hassan Murad, and E. V. Loftus Jr., "Comparative efficacy of biologic therapy in biologic-naïve patients with Crohn disease: a systematic review and network meta-analysis," *Mayo Clinic Proceedings*, vol. 89, no. 12, pp. 1621–1635, 2014.

12

On-Demand Therapy with Proton Pump Inhibitors for Maintenance Treatment of Nonerosive Reflux Disease or Mild Erosive Esophagitis

Zubair Khan,[1] Yaseen Alastal,[1] Muhammad Ali Khan,[2] Mohammad Saud Khan,[1] Basmah Khalil,[1] Shreesh Shrestha,[2] Faisal Kamal,[2] Ali Nawras,[1] and Colin W. Howden[2]

[1]*Division of Gastroenterology and Hepatology, University of Toledo Medical Center, Toledo, OH, USA*
[2]*Division of Gastroenterology and Hepatology, The University of Tennessee Health Science Center, Memphis, TN, USA*

Correspondence should be addressed to Muhammad Ali Khan; mkhan24@uthsc.edu

Academic Editor: Paolo Gionchetti

Background. Proton pump inhibitors (PPIs) are widely used for the long-term management of gastroesophageal reflux disease (GERD). However, concerns about the cost and/or inconvenience of continuous maintenance PPI treatment have led to the evaluation of various alternative approaches. *Aim.* To assess the effectiveness of on-demand PPI therapy in the maintenance treatment of nonerosive reflux disease (NERD) or mild erosive esophagitis (EE). *Methods.* We searched MEDLINE, EMBASE, Web of Science, and Cochrane Library from inception until October 2, 2017, for randomized controlled trials (RCTs) comparing on-demand PPI versus placebo or daily PPI in the management of NERD or mild EE (Savary-Miller grade 1). Discontinuation of therapy during the trial was used as a surrogate for patient dissatisfaction and failure of symptomatic control. We calculated pooled odds ratios (OR) to evaluate the efficacy of on-demand PPI treatment. Separate analyses were conducted for studies comparing on-demand PPI with daily PPI and with placebo. Subgroup analysis was done based on NERD studies alone and on studies of both NERD and mild EE. These were analyzed using a random effects model. *Results.* We included 10 RCTs with 4574 patients. On-demand PPI was superior to daily PPI (pooled OR = 0.50; 95% confidence interval (CI) = 0.35, 0.72). On subgroup analysis in NERD patients only, pooled OR was 0.44 (0.29, 0.66). In studies including patients with NERD and mild EE, pooled OR was 0.76 (0.36, 1.60). For studies comparing on-demand PPI with placebo, pooled OR was 0.21 (0.15, 0.29); subgroup analyses of studies evaluating NERD only and studies conducted in NERD and mild EE showed similar results (pooled OR was 0.22 (0.13, 0.36) and 0.18 (0.11, 0.31), resp.). *Conclusions.* On-demand PPI treatment is effective for many patients with NERD or mild EE. Although not FDA-approved, it may be adequate for those patients whose symptoms are controlled to their satisfaction.

1. Introduction

Gastroesophageal reflux disease (GERD) is a common disorder of the upper gastrointestinal tract. The prevalence of reflux symptoms is steadily rising throughout the industrialized world [1]. An estimated 20–40% of Western adult populations report chronic heartburn or regurgitation symptoms [2]. Different manifestations of GERD include nonerosive reflux disease (NERD) and erosive esophagitis (EE). Complications of GERD, which are generally confined to EE patients, include ulceration, stricture, and Barrett's esophagus with attendant risk of esophageal adenocarcinoma [3]. NERD, the most frequent manifestation of GERD, is present in around 70% of patients and characterized by the presence of typical GERD symptoms associated with pathological acid reflux but the absence of demonstrable esophageal mucosal injury on endoscopy [4, 5]. Despite the absence of mucosal injury on endoscopy, many patients with NERD experience severe symptoms and impairment in quality of life that may be equivalent to, or greater than, seen in patients with EE [6, 7]. Acid-suppressive therapy with proton pump inhibitors (PPI) has proved to be the most effective treatment strategy for both NERD and EE [8–10]. PPIs have shown superiority over histamine H_2-receptor antagonists for controlling symptoms as well as for healing erosions and preventing relapse [8, 10]. However, up to 75% patients with NERD and up to 90% of patients with EE may experience symptomatic relapse within six months of stopping treatment [11, 12]. Therefore, many patients subsequently receive long-term treatment to maintain adequate symptom control and, for EE patients, healing of erosions. However, this may have led to unnecessary use of these drugs, among NERD patients especially, adding to overall costs [13]. In the United States, the total expenditure for PPI treatment may be over $11 billion annually [14]. Due to the costs of PPI treatment, there have been efforts to develop effective and cost-efficient alternative long-term maintenance strategies for some GERD patients [15, 16], including "on-demand" PPI therapy, with patients taking a daily dose of a PPI when symptoms recur and stopping treatment when symptoms resolve. This is in contrast to intermittent treatment, in which patients take a regular daily dose of a PPI upon symptom relapse and continue it for a prespecified duration (typically 1 or 2 weeks) regardless of symptom response.

To evaluate the effectiveness of on-demand PPI treatment in patients with NERD or mild EE, we conducted a systematic review of randomized controlled trials (RCTs) comparing it with regular daily PPI treatment or placebo.

2. Methods

2.1. Data Sources and Search Strategy. We carried out this systematic review and meta-analysis in accordance with the guidelines of preferred reporting items for systematic review and meta-analysis (PRISMA) [17]. The search strategies were developed in Ovid MEDLINE, and the same keywords and subject headings were applied to Ovid EMBASE, Cochrane, Scopus, and ISI Web of Science databases from inception through November 2, 2016. The search terms included "Esophagitis" OR "Gastroesophageal reflux" OR "GERD" OR "Nonerosive reflux disease" OR "NERD" OR "Erosive esophagitis" OR "EE" AND "Proton pump inhibitors" OR "PPIs" AND "on-demand" OR "on demand" OR "daily" AND "Placebo." A medical librarian with more than 20 years of experience performed this search.

2.2. Study Selection and Inclusion and Exclusion Criteria. Two authors (Z.K. and Y.A.) searched for original studies based on the previously defined search strategy. We searched for RCTs comparing on-demand PPI treatment with either placebo or daily PPI in the maintenance treatment of NERD and/or mild EE. NERD was defined as the presence of classic GERD symptoms in the absence of esophageal mucosal injury during upper endoscopy (Savary-Miller Grade 0 and LA class M). Mild EE was defined as having esophagitis with Savary-Miller Grade 1 or LA class A. The main outcome measure used to assess treatment efficacy was discontinuation of therapy during the trial. Continuation of therapy during a trial was used as a surrogate for patient satisfaction and control of GERD symptoms. Hence, the proportion of patients who discontinued therapy during a trial was taken as an indirect measure of failure of symptomatic control of GERD. Studies were excluded if they did not contain raw or usable data or were published only in abstract form. We also excluded duplicate publications, expert opinion, and letters. We also searched bibliographies of retrieved articles to enhance the yield of our search strategy. All articles were downloaded into Endnote 7.0, a bibliographic database manager, and any duplicate citations were identified and removed.

2.3. Data Extraction and Quality Assessment. Two reviewers (Z.K. and Y.A.) assessed the eligibility of selected studies and extracted data using customized data extraction forms. Any disagreement between reviewers was discussed with a third reviewer (M.A.K.), and agreement was reached by consensus. Extracted data included study design, the year and country of publication, inclusion and exclusion criteria, PPI regimen used for on-demand and continuous groups, classification of esophagitis, outcome studied (number of patients discontinuing on-demand treatment due to inadequate symptom control), follow-up duration, and patient demographics.

We used the Cochrane tool for assessing risk of bias for RCTs. Two reviewers (Z.K. and Y.A.) performed quality assessment with any disagreement to be discussed with a third reviewer (M.A.K.). We used the GRADE framework to interpret our findings [18].

2.4. Data Synthesis and Statistical Analysis. Our main outcome of interest was the effectiveness of on-demand PPI treatment versus placebo or daily PPI in the management of NERD and/or mild EE. The primary efficacy endpoint used was the premature discontinuation of treatment. We analyzed pooled data using a random effects model and calculated odds ratios (ORs) with their 95% confidence interval (CI). We conducted separate analyses for studies comparing on-demand PPI with daily PPI and with placebo. We performed additional subgroup analyses based on NERD studies alone and on studies including patients with either NERD or mild EE. Cochrane's Q test and I^2 statistics were used to assess heterogeneity among studies. A P value of <0.1 for the Cochrane Q test or an I^2 value of $>50\%$ signified the presence of heterogeneity.

We constructed funnel plots and used Egger's precision test to assess publication bias. Statistical analysis was performed using RevMan, version 5.3 for Windows (Cochrane Collaboration, the Nordic Cochrane Center, Copenhagen, Denmark, 2014).

3. Results

3.1. Search Strategy Yield and Identification of Studies. The search strategy identified 409 articles, of which 35 were removed as duplicates. Of the remaining 374 articles, 347 were removed after title and abstract review. The remaining 27 full-text articles were reviewed, of which 10 RCTs [19–28] with 4574 patients were included in the meta-analysis as shown in PRISMA flowchart (Supplementary Materials (available here)). Among the patients, 2797 received on-demand PPI, 843 received daily PPI and 934 received

Table 1: Characteristics of studies comparing on-demand PPI with daily PPI.

References	Country	Center (multi, single)	Study design	Inclusion criteria	Exclusion criteria	PPI regimen for continuous therapy	PPI regimen for on-demand therapy	Outcome studied	Follow-up period	Esophagitis class
[19]	UK (92 general practices, 28 hospitals)	Multicenter	Single-blind (investigator), randomized, parallel group study	NERD with resolution of heartburn after 2 to 4 weeks of esomeprazole 20	Patients with persistent heartburn and structural diseases	Lansoprazole 15 mg PO once daily	Esomeprazole 20 mg	Time to discontinuation due to unwillingness to continue	6 months	Not applicable
[20]	Single university hospital Japan	Single center	Prospective parallel randomized open-label study	Patients with modified LA class M after having 8-week treatment with PPIs	Patients with cancer, serious liver disease, kidney disease, heart disease, a hematological disorder, gastric ulcers, and/or duodenal ulcers	Omeprazole 20 mg	Omeprazole 20 mg	Symptom relief at 4, 8, 16, and 24 weeks in each study group with relief from symptoms as the primary endpoint	6 months	Modified LA class M
[21]	Austria, France, Germany, South Africa, and Spain (61 centers)	Multicenter	Open-label, randomized, parallel group	NERD who were heartburn-free after 4-week treatment with esomeprazole 20 mg daily	Reflux esophagitis	Esomeprazole 20 mg	Esomeprazole 20 mg	Discontinuation due to unsatisfactory treatment	6 months	Not applicable
[22]	58 active centers: 29 in Germany, 12 in France, 11 in Switzerland, and 6 in Hungary	Multicenter	Open-label, randomized, parallel group	NERD + mild esophagitis treated with pantoprazole 20 mg PO daily for 4 weeks	Patients with persistent symptoms and heartburn, erosive esophagitis	Pantoprazole 20 mg	Pantoprazole 20 mg	The symptoms (as assessed in the patient's diary) were considered controlled until the time of failure, which was defined as the first point at which one of the following events occurred: (1) GERD symptoms of at least moderate severity were present for 3 or more consecutive days despite medication (event time = the first of these 3 days); (2) use of >1 tablet of study medication on >3 consecutive days (event time = the first of these 3 days); or (3) premature withdrawal from the study due to lack of efficacy (event time = the date of withdrawal)	6 months	Savary-Miller grade 0 or 1

Table 2: Characteristics of studies comparing on-demand PPI with placebo.

References	Country	Center (multi, single)	Study design	Inclusion criteria	Exclusion criteria	PPI regimen for continuous therapy	PPI regimen for on-demand therapy	Primary outcome studied	Follow-up period	Esophagitis class
[23]	Sweden & Denmark (25 centers)	Multicenter	Double-blind, randomized, placebo controlled	NERD with resolution of heartburn after short-term treatment (4 to 8 weeks)	Erosive, ulcerative PUD	N/A	Omeprazole 20, omeprazole 10, placebo	Discontinuation of medicine due to unwillingness to continue	6 months	N/A
[24]	65 centers in Denmark, Finland, Norway, and Sweden	Multicenter	Randomized, double-blind, parallel group	Endoscopy-negative GERD treated with 4 weeks of omep 20 or Eso 20	Patients requiring concomitant drugs, NSAIDS, quinidine, etc. excluded	N/A	Esomeprazole 20 mg on demand, placebo on demand	Time to discontinuation of on-demand therapy due to unwillingness to continue	6 months	N/A
[25]	116 centers in the UK, the Republic of Ireland, and Canada	Multicenter	Randomized, double-blind, parallel-group study	Patients with NERD treated with Eso 40, 20, or Omep 20 for 4 weeks	Patients requiring concomitant drugs, NSAIDS, quinidine, etc. excluded	N/A	Esomeprazole 40 mg on demand, esomeprazole 20 mg on demand, placebo on demand	Time to study discontinuation due to unwillingness to continue for any reason	6 months	N/A
[26]	International (Greece, Italy, the Netherlands, Spain, France, Portugal, Sweden, Denmark, Ireland, Belgium, United Kingdom, Russia, Poland, and Lithuania)	Multicenter	Randomized, double-blind, placebo-controlled, withdrawal study	NERD treated with rabeprazole 10 mg PO daily for 4 weeks	Patients with erosive disease and no relief of heartburn in acute 4-week phase	N/A	Rabeprazole 10 mg on demand, placebo on demand	The proportion of patients discontinuing treatment in the on-demand phase because of inadequate heartburn control	6 months	N/A
[27]	Germany 36 centers	Multicenter	Randomized, double-blind, placebo-controlled, parallel-group comparison	Nonerosive GERD or reflux esophagitis grade 1 according to Savary–Miller classification underwent 4 weeks of pantoprazole 20 mg PO OD for 4 weeks	Patients symptomtic after acute phase or nonerosive GERD or reflux esophagitis grade 2 to 4 according to Savary–Miller classification	N/A	Pantoprazole 40 mg on demand, pantoprazole 20 mg on demand, placebo on demand	Discontinuation rate due to insufficient control of heartburn	6 months	Savary-Miller grade 0 or 1

Table 2: Continued.

References	Country	Center (multi, single)	Study design	Inclusion criteria	Exclusion criteria	PPI regimen for continuous therapy	PPI regimen for on-demand therapy	Primary outcome studied	Follow-up period	Esophagitis class
[28]	40 centers in Germany and five in Lithuania	Multicenter	Randomized, double-blind, placebo-controlled parallel-group comparison	Nonerosive GERD or reflux esophagitis grade 1 according to Savary–Miller classification underwent 4 weeks of pantoprazole 20 mg PO OD for 4 weeks	Patients symptomtic after acute phase or nonerosive GERD or reflux esophagitis grades 2 to 4 according to Savary–Miller classification	N/A	Pantoprazole 20 mg on demand, placebo on demand	The number of patients unwilling to continue the therapy and the corresponding reasons for it were analyzed using the Kaplan–Meier analysis	7 months	Savary-Miller grade 0 or 1

Table 3: Patient characteristics and demographics of included trials.

Study	*N*, on demand/cont	Mean age ± SD	Male (%)
Tsai et al. [19]	(1) Eso 20 mg on demand = 311	51 ± 13.8	46%
	(2) Lanso 15 mg continuous = 311	51 ± 13.8	41.8%
Nagahara et al. [20]	Omeprazole 20 mg continuous = 18 Omeprazole 20 mg on demand = 17	56.2 ± 12.8	21/35 = 60%
Bayerdörffer et al. [21]	(1) Eso 20 mg on demand = 301	48.2 ± 13.6	40.5%
	(2) Eso 20 mg continuous = 297	47.6 ± 15.1	43.8%
Janssen et al. [22]	Pantoprazole 20 mg on demand = 215	50.4 (SD 13.6)	46.5%
	Pantoprazole 20 mg continuous = 217	51.8 (SD 13.5)	47.5%
Lind et al. [23]	(1) Omeprazole 20 on demand = 139 (*n*)	52 (19–79) *R*	38.1%
	(2) Omeprazole 10 on demand = 142	51 (20–81) *R*	45.8%
	(3) Placebo = 143	48 (20–79) *R*	42.7%
Talley et al. [24]	(1) Eso 20 mg on demand = 170	49 (19–78) *R*	55%
	(2) Placebo on demand = 172	49 (21–79) *R*	57%
Talley et al. [25]	(1) Esomeprazole 40 mg on demand = 293	48	46.1%
	(2) Esomeprazole 20 mg on demand = 282	48.4	47.9%
	(3) Placebo on demand = 146	48.2	39.7%
Bytzer et al. [26]	(1) Rabeprazole 10 mg on demand = 279	47 (0.81 SE)	44%
	(2) Placebo on demand = 139	48 (1.23 SE)	41%
Scholten et al. [27]	Pantoprazole 40 mg on demand = 218	54 ± 14	47.3%
	Pantoprazole 20 mg on demand = 217	52 ± 14	52.5%
	Placebo on demand = 108	52 ± 14	53.7%
Kaspari et al. [28]	Pantoprazole 20 mg on demand = 213	50.7 ± 13.7 years	46%
	Placebo on demand = 226	51.0 ± 14.5 years	43.3%

placebo. Four RCTs [19–22] compared a daily PPI regimen with on-demand treatment. Three of these were confined to patients with NERD [19–21], while the fourth [22] also included patients with mild EE. Six trials compared on-demand treatment with placebo [23–28]; four only included patients with NERD [23–26], and two included both patients with NERD or mild EE [27, 28]. Tables 1–3 highlight the characteristics of included studies.

3.2. Meta-Analysis

3.2.1. On Demand versus Daily PPI. For studies comparing on-demand PPI therapy with daily PPI therapy, 5.8% of patients discontinued treatment in the on-demand group compared to 11.0% in the daily PPI group. The pooled OR with 95% confidence interval (CI) was 0.50 (0.35, 0.72), with no heterogeneity ($I^2 = 0\%$) (Figure 1). On subgroup analysis of the three RCTs that included only NERD patients, results were similar; 5.7% of patients in the on-demand PPI group and 12.1% of patients in the daily PPI group discontinued treatment prematurely (OR = 0.44; 95% CI = 0.29 to 0.66). However, on subgroup analysis of the study that included patients with either NERD or mild EE, there was no significant difference between treatments (OR = 0.76; 95% CI = 0.36 to 1.60). With on-demand treatment, 6.0% of patients discontinued treatment prematurely compared with 7.8% on daily PPI treatment.

3.2.2. On-Demand PPI Treatment versus Placebo. The proportions of patients prematurely discontinuing treatment were 11.6% with on-demand PPI therapy and 39.2% with placebo (pooled OR = 0.21; 95% CI = 0.15 to 0.29). There was significant heterogeneity among studies ($I^2 = 66\%$) (Figure 2). On subgroup analysis of studies conducted only in NERD patients, on-demand PPI treatment was superior to placebo; proportions of patients prematurely discontinuing treatment were 12.3% and 39.8%, respectively (OR = 0.22; 95% CI = 0.13 to 0.36). Among studies evaluating patients with either NERD or mild EE, proportions of patients discontinuing treatment prematurely were 10.2% and 38.0% (OR = 0.18; 95% CI = 0.11 to 0.31), respectively.

4. Discussion

We found that on-demand PPI therapy was superior to both placebo and daily PPI therapy as maintenance treatment for patients with NERD or mild EE. In general, more patients were willing to continue on-demand PPI treatment than either of the alternatives studied. Furthermore, adherence to treatment and patient satisfaction were higher with on-demand PPI treatment compared to continuous PPI treatment. On-demand treatment may help to improve overall patient satisfaction since patients may feel more in control of their treatment and can take a dose of PPI according to their perceived needs and symptoms [18]. However, the

Study or subgroup	On demand Events	On demand Total	Daily PPI Events	Daily PPI Total	Weight	Odds ratio M-H, random, 95% CI	Year
1.4.1 NERD only							
Tsai, 2004	19	311	41	311	41.1%	0.43 (0.24, 0.76)	2004
Nagahara, 2014	4	17	6	18	6.0%	0.62 (0.14, 2.73)	2014
Bayerdörffer, 2016	4	17	6	18	6.0%	0.42 (0.21, 0.82)	2016
Subtotal (95% CI)		629		626	76.3%	0.44 (0.29 0.66)	
Total events	36		76				
Heterogeneity: $Tau^2 = 0.00$; $Chi^2 = 0.23$, df = 2 ($P = 0.89$); $I^2 = 0\%$							
Test for overall effect: $Z = 3.89$ ($P < 0.0001$)							
1.4.2 NERD + mild esophagitis							
Janssen, 2005	13	215	17	217	23.7%	0.76 (0.36, 1.60)	2005
Subtotal (95% CI)		215		217	23.7%	0.76 (0.36, 1.60)	
Total events	13		17				
Heterogeneity: not applicable							
Test for overall effect: $Z = 0.73$ ($P = 0.47$)							
Total (955 CI)		844		843	100.0%	0.50 (0.35, 0.72)	
Total events	49		93				
Heterogeneity: $Tau^2 = 0.00$; Chi^2=1.82, df= 2 ($P = 0.61$); $I^2 = 0\%$							
Test for overall effect: $Z = 3.76$ ($P = 0.0002$)							
Test for subgroup differences: $Chi^2 = 1.59$, df = 1 ($P = 0.21$), $I^2 = 37.1\%$							

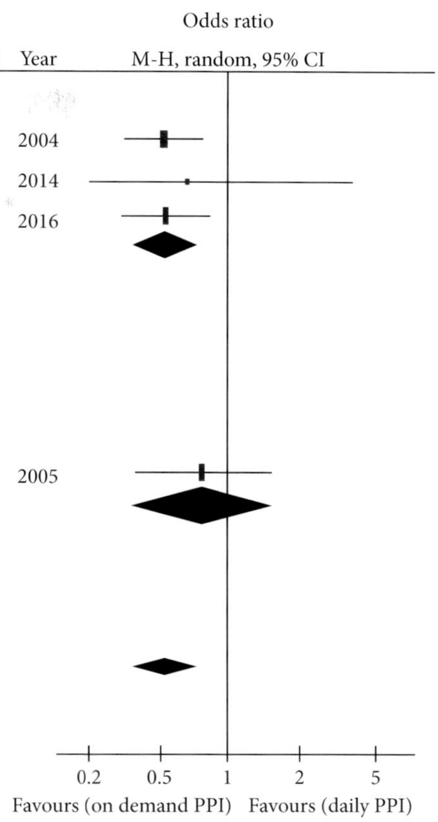

FIGURE 1: Forest plot comparing on-demand PPI with daily PPI.

usefulness of on-demand PPI treatment compared to daily PPI was less obvious when patients with mild EE were included in the analysis.

Our analysis is different from two previously conducted analyses. Jiang et al. [29] concluded that on-demand treatment with PPIs is superior to continuous or placebo therapy, but did not perform subgroup analysis of NERD and mild EE. A recently published Cochrane review showed that on-demand deprescribing may lead to an increase in gastrointestinal symptoms (e.g., dyspepsia and regurgitation) in patients with NERD or mild grades of EE (Los Angeles grades A and B or Savary-Miller grades 1 and 2) [30]. Besides having a broad definition for on-demand deprescribing, this review did not differentiate NERD from mild EE; Savary-Miller grading for most of the included patients was >1. In our analysis, the only included were patients with Savary-Miller grade 0 (NERD) or 1 (mild EE). We excluded studies that included EE patients with Savary-Miller grade higher than 1, since those would represent moderate and severe EE.

Since the risk of progression of NERD or mild EE to more advanced disease is low, symptom control is the main objective of management [31–33]. Many patients experience intermittent symptoms of short duration. These symptoms can be effectively managed with on-demand PPI treatment. This symptom-driven approach for the long-term management of NERD also simulates many patients' actual use of these medicines [16]. Many patients who are prescribed daily PPI treatment may actually consume them on an as needed basis. Up to 29% of patients who were prescribed continuous PPI treatment decreased the frequency of use without a recommendation from their providers, and only 21% of patients prescribed continuous PPI treatment fill their prescriptions in a manner to remain fully compliant with the recommended dosing schedule [34, 35]. The most commonly cited reasons for not continuing treatment are inconvenience and cost. However, studies [36–38] evaluating the on-demand strategy versus continuous PPI treatment for EE have shown that the on-demand strategy is inferior. On-demand PPI treatment is, therefore, not appropriate or adequate for patients with EE of Savary-Miller grade 2 or above.

As well as patient preference and satisfaction for on-demand PPI treatment, cost of long-term treatment is also important. The consistently demonstrated efficacy and the favorable safety profile of PPI treatment have led to its widespread use in GERD patients [13]. There has been a substantial increase in the cost of GERD management with medicines contributing to overall costs. This has led to increasing concern from health care authorities and third-party payers [36]. On-demand PPI treatment might reduce overall consumption by up to one third. Tsai et al. [19], who compared on-demand esomeprazole with daily lansoprazole in 622 patients for six months, found that patients in the esomeprazole on-demand group took treatment on approximately one-third of the days (0.3 times per day) whereas

Study or subgroup	On demand Events	On demand Total	Daily PPI Events	Daily PPI Total	Weight	Odds ratio M-H, random, 95% CI	Year
1.3.1 NERD only							
Lind, 1999	66	281	63	143	18.4%	0.39 (0.25, 0.60)	1999
Talley, 2001	24	170	87	172	16.2%	0.16 (0.09, 0.27)	2001
Talley, 2002	55	575	61	146	18.4%	0.15 (0.10, 0.23)	2002
Bytzer, 2004	16	279	28	139	13.4%	0.24 (0.13, 0.46)	2004
Subtotal (95% CI)		1305		600	66.4%	0.22 (0.13, 0.36)	
Total events	161		239				
Heterogeneity: $Tau^2 = 0.18$; $Chi^2 = 11.58$, df = 3 ($P = 0.009$); $I^2 = 74\%$							
Test for overall effect: $Z = 6.09$ ($P < 0.0001$)							
1.3.2 NERD + mild esophagitis							
Scholten, 2005	41	435	46	108	16.8%	0.14 (0.09, 0.23)	2005
Kaspari, 2005	25	213	81	226	16.8%	0.24 (0.14, 0.39)	2005
Subtotal (95% CI)		648		334	33.6%	0.18 (0.11, 0.31)	
Total events	66		127				
Heterogeneity: $Tau^2 = 0.08$; $Chi^2 = 2.21$, df = 1 ($P = 0.14$); $I^2 = 55\%$							
Test for overall effect: $Z = 6.36$ ($P < 0.00001$)							
Total (955 CI)		1953		934	100.0%	0.21 (0.15, 0.29)	
Total events	227		366				
Heterogeneity: $Tau^2 = 0.12$; $Chi^2 = 14.50$, df = 5 ($P = 0.01$); $I^2 = 66\%$							
Test for overall effect: $Z = 8.97$ ($P < 0.00001$)							
Test for subgroup differences: $Chi^2 = 0.23$, df = 1 ($P < 0.63$), $I^2 = 0\%$							

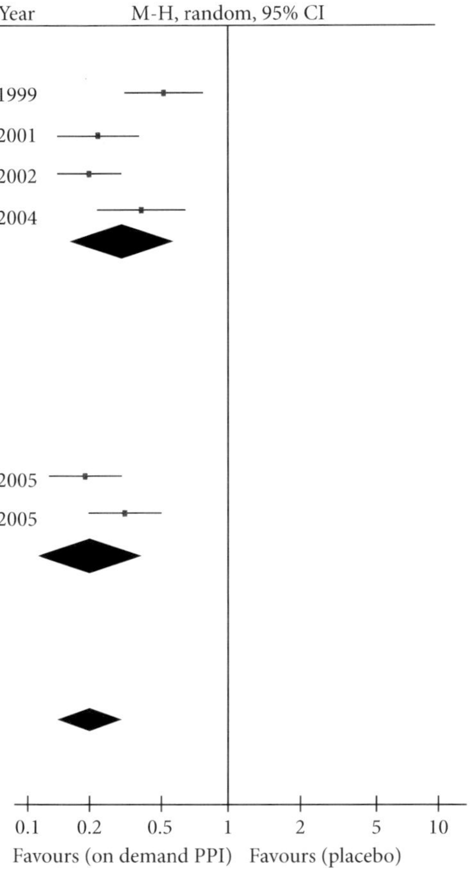

FIGURE 2: Forest plot comparing on-demand PPI with placebo.

those receiving lansoprazole daily took treatment on approximately 4 of every 5 days (0.8 times per day) despite being instructed to take them every day. Bayerdörffer et al. [21] found similar results with mean daily drug consumption of 0.41 tablets in the on-demand group and 0.91 tablets in the continuous daily group. Therefore, on-demand treatment may be a cost-effective strategy for the long-term management of patients with NERD or mild EE. It can be effective in controlling symptoms and is convenient for, and acceptable to, many patients. Those patients with NERD or mild EE who do not obtain adequate relief with on-demand PPI treatment can be considered for regular, daily PPI treatment in the lowest effective dose.

The studies included in our analysis defined NERD based on symptoms and endoscopic findings without physiological demonstration of abnormal gastroesophageal reflux (acidic or weekly acidic), which could be a limitation. Also, most of the studies used only Savary-Miller grading for classifying esophagitis. The studies that classified esophagitis using the LA classification were very limited and did not differentiate between LA grades A and B. We tried to be conservative while defining mild esophagitis and so confined our analysis to studies with either LA grades M or A and considered LA grade B to be indicative of moderate—rather than mild—esophagitis.

5. Conclusion

On-demand PPI treatment appears to be effective for the long-term management of many patients with NERD or mild EE. After the initial control of symptoms with a course of PPI treatment, on-demand PPI treatment can be appropriately considered for the long-term management of such patients.

Abbreviations

PPIs:	Proton pump inhibitors
GERD:	Gastroesophageal reflux disease
EE:	Erosive esophagitis
NERD:	Nonerosive reflux disease
PRISMA:	Preferred reporting items for systematic review and meta-analysis
RCT:	Randomized clinical trial
OR:	Odds ratio.

Disclosure

The abstract of this review was presented in the Digestive Disease Week 2017 held in Chicago.

Authors' Contributions

Zubair Khan helped in the study design, data collection, statistical analysis, manuscript drafting, and final approval of the manuscript. Yaseen Alastal helped in the study design, data collection, statistical analysis, manuscript drafting, critical revision, and final approval of the manuscript. Muhammad Ali Khan helped in the development of search strategies, data collection, manuscript drafting, and final approval of the manuscript. Mohammad Saud Khan helped in the study design, manuscript drafting, and final approval of the manuscript. Basmah Khalil, Shreesh Shrestha, and Faisal Kamal helped in the data collection, manuscript drafting, and final approval of the manuscript. Ali Nawras helped in the manuscript drafting, critical revision for intellectual content, and final approval of the manuscript. Colin W. Howden helped in the statistical analysis, manuscript drafting, critical revision for intellectual content, and final approval of the manuscript.

References

[1] H. B. El–serag, "Time trends of gastroesophageal reflux disease: a systematic review," *Clinical Gastroenterology and Hepatology*, vol. 5, no. 1, pp. 17–26, 2007.

[2] L. Frank, L. Kleinman, D. Ganoczy et al., "Upper gastrointestinal symptoms in North America: prevalence and relationship to healthcare utilization and quality of life," *Digestive Diseases and Sciences*, vol. 45, no. 4, pp. 809–818, 2000.

[3] F. Pace and G. B. Porro, "Gastroesophageal reflux disease: a typical spectrum disease (a new conceptual framework is not needed)," *The American Journal of Gastroenterology*, vol. 99, no. 5, pp. 946–949, 2004.

[4] N. Vakil, S. V. van Zanten, P. Kahrilas, J. Dent, R. Jones, and the Global Consensus Group, "The Montreal definition and classification of gastroesophageal reflux disease: a global evidence-based consensus," *American Journal of Gastroenterology*, vol. 101, no. 8, pp. 1900–1920, 2006.

[5] H. B. El-Serag, "Epidemiology of non-erosive reflux disease," *Digestion*, vol. 78, no. 1, Supplement 1, pp. 6–10, 2008.

[6] J. C. Y. Wu, C. M. Y. Cheung, V. W. S. Wong, and J. J. Y. Sung, "Distinct clinical characteristics between patients with nonerosive reflux disease and those with reflux esophagitis," *Clinical Gastroenterology and Hepatology*, vol. 5, no. 6, pp. 690–695, 2007.

[7] M. Kulig, A. Leodolter, M. Vieth et al., "Quality of life in relation to symptoms in patients with gastro-oesophageal reflux disease– an analysis based on the ProGERD initiative," *Alimentary Pharmacology & Therapeutics*, vol. 18, no. 8, pp. 767–776, 2003.

[8] P. Moayyedi and N. J. Talley, "Gastro-oesophageal reflux disease," *Lancet*, vol. 367, no. 9528, pp. 2086–2100, 2006.

[9] B. van Pinxteren, K. E. Sigterman, P. Bonis, J. Lau, and M. E. Numans, "Short-term treatment with proton pump inhibitors, H2-receptor antagonists and prokinetics for gastro-oesophageal reflux disease-like symptoms and endoscopy negative reflux disease," *Cochrane Database of Systematic Reviews*, no. 3, article CD002095, 2006.

[10] C. Donnellan, N. Sharma, C. Preston, and P. Moayyedi, "Medical treatments for the maintenance therapy of reflux oesophagitis and endoscopic negative reflux disease," *Cochrane Database of Systematic Reviews*, vol. 2, article CD003245, 2004.

[11] B. B. Dean, A. D. Gano Jr., K. Knight, J. J. Ofman, and R. Fass, "Effectiveness of proton pump inhibitors in nonerosive reflux disease," *Clinical Gastroenterology and Hepatology*, vol. 2, no. 8, pp. 656–664, 2004.

[12] Y. Kinoshita, K. Ashida, M. Hongo, and The Japan Rabeprazole Study Group for NERD, "Randomised clinical trial: a multicentre, double-blind, placebo-controlled study on the efficacy and safety of rabeprazole 5 mg or 10 mg once daily in patients with non-erosive reflux disease," *Alimentary Pharmacology and Therapeutics*, vol. 33, no. 2, pp. 213–224, 2011.

[13] J. J. Heidelbaugh, A. H. Kim, R. Chang, and P. C. Walker, "Overutilization of proton-pump inhibitors: what the clinician needs to know," *Therapeutic Advances in Gastroenterology*, vol. 5, no. 4, pp. 219–232, 2012.

[14] N. J. Shaheen, R. A. Hansen, D. R. Morgan et al., "The burden of gastrointestinal and liver diseases, 2006," *The American Journal of Gastroenterology*, vol. 101, no. 9, pp. 2128–2138, 2006.

[15] D. C. Metz, J. M. Inadomi, C. W. Howden, S. J. V. van Zanten, and P. Bytzer, "On-demand therapy for gastroesophageal reflux disease," *The American Journal of Gastroenterology*, vol. 102, no. 3, pp. 642–653, 2007.

[16] J. M. Inadomi, R. Jamal, G. H. Murata et al., "Step-down management of gastroesophageal reflux disease," *Gastroenterology*, vol. 121, no. 5, pp. 1095–1100, 2001.

[17] A. Liberati, D. G. Altman, J. Tetzlaff et al., "The PRISMA statement for reporting systematic reviews and meta-analyses of studies that evaluate healthcare interventions: explanation and elaboration," *BMJ*, vol. 339, no. jul21 1, article b2700, 2009.

[18] D. Atkins, D. Best, P. A. Briss et al., "Grading quality of evidence and strength of recommendations," *BMJ*, vol. 328, no. 7454, p. 1490, 2004.

[19] H. H. Tsai, R. Chapman, A. Shepherd et al., "Esomeprazole 20 mg on-demand is more acceptable to patients than continuous lansoprazole 15 mg in the long-term maintenance of endoscopy-negative gastro-oesophageal reflux patients: the COMMAND study," *Alimentary Pharmacology & Therapeutics*, vol. 20, no. 6, pp. 657–665, 2004.

[20] A. Nagahara, M. Hojo, D. Asaoka, H. Sasaki, and S. Watanabe, "A randomized prospective study comparing the efficacy of on-demand therapy versus continuous therapy for 6 months for long-term maintenance with omeprazole 20 mg in patients with gastroesophageal reflux disease in Japan," *Scandinavian Journal of Gastroenterology*, vol. 49, no. 4, pp. 409–417, 2014.

[21] E. Bayerdörffer, M.-A. Bigard, W. Weiss et al., "Randomized, multicenter study: on-demand versus continuous maintenance treatment with esomeprazole in patients with non-erosive gastroesophageal reflux disease," *BMC Gastroenterology*, vol. 16, no. 1, p. 48, 2016.

[22] W. Janssen, E. Meier, G. Gatz, and B. Pfaffenberger, "Effects of pantoprazole 20 mg in mildgastroesophageal reflux disease:

once-daily treatment in the acute phase, and comparison of on-demand versus continuous treatment in the long term," *Current Therapeutic Research, Clinical and Experimental*, vol. 66, no. 4, pp. 345–363, 2005.

[23] T. Lind, T. Havelund, L. Lundell et al., "On demand therapy with omeprazole for the long-term management of patients with heartburn without oesophagitis—a placebo-controlled randomized trial," *Alimentary Pharmacology & Therapeutics*, vol. 13, no. 7, pp. 907–914, 1999.

[24] N. J. Talley, K. Lauritsen, H. Tunturi-Hihnala et al., "Esomeprazole 20 mg maintains symptom control in endoscopy-negative gastro-oesophageal reflux disease: a controlled trial of 'on-demand' therapy for 6 months," *Alimentary Pharmacology & Therapeutics*, vol. 15, no. 3, pp. 347–354, 2001.

[25] N. J. Talley, T. L. Venables, J. R. B. Green et al., "Esomeprazole 40 mg and 20 mg is efficacious in the long-term management of patients with endoscopy-negative gastro-oesophageal reflux disease: a placebo-controlled trial of on-demand therapy for 6 months," *European Journal of Gastroenterology & Hepatology*, vol. 14, no. 8, pp. 857–863, 2002.

[26] P. Bytzer, A. Blum, D. de Herdt, D. Dubois, and the trial investigators, "Six-month trial of on-demand rabeprazole 10 mg maintains symptom relief in patients with non-erosive reflux disease," *Alimentary Pharmacology and Therapeutics*, vol. 20, no. 2, pp. 181–188, 2004.

[27] T. Scholten, C. P. M. Dekkers, K. Schütze, T. Körner, M. Bohuschke, and G. Gatz, "On-demand therapy with pantoprazole 20 mg as effective long-term management of reflux disease in patients with mild GERD: the ORION trial," *Digestion*, vol. 72, no. 2-3, pp. 76–85, 2005.

[28] S. Kaspari, L. Kupcinskas, H. Heinze, and P. Berghöfer, "Pantoprazole 20 mg on demand is effective in the long-term management of patients with mild gastro-oesophageal reflux disease," *European Journal of Gastroenterology & Hepatology*, vol. 17, no. 9, pp. 935–941, 2005.

[29] Y. X. Jiang, Y. Chen, X. Kong, Y. L. Tong, and S. C. Xu, "Maintenance treatment of mild gastroesophageal reflux disease with proton pump inhibitors taken on-demand: a meta-analysis," *Hepato-Gastroenterology*, vol. 60, no. 125, pp. 1077–1082, 2013.

[30] T. A. Boghossian, F. J. Rashid, W. Thompson et al., "Deprescribing versus continuation of chronic proton pump inhibitor use in adults," *Cochrane Database of Systematic Reviews*, vol. 3, article CD011969, 2017.

[31] N. Manabe, M. Yoshihara, A. Sasaki, S. Tanaka, K. Haruma, and K. Chayama, "Clinical characteristics and natural history of patients with low-grade reflux esophagitis," *Journal of Gastroenterology and Hepatology*, vol. 17, no. 9, pp. 949–954, 2002.

[32] J. Labenz, M. Nocon, T. Lind et al., "Prospective follow-up data from the ProGERD study suggest that GERD is not a categorial disease," *The American Journal of Gastroenterology*, vol. 101, no. 11, pp. 2457–2462, 2006.

[33] M. Fullard, J. Y. Kang, P. Neild, A. Poullis, and J. D. Maxwell, "Systematic review: does gastro-oesophageal reflux disease progress?," *Alimentary Pharmacology & Therapeutics*, vol. 24, no. 1, pp. 33–45, 2006.

[34] A. P. Hungin, G. Rubin, and H. O'Flanagan, "Factors influencing compliance in long-term proton pump inhibitor therapy in general practice," *The British Journal of General Practice*, vol. 49, no. 443, pp. 463-464, 1999.

[35] A. P. Hungin, G. P. Rubin, and H. O'Flanagan, "Long-term prescribing of proton pump inhibitors in general practice," *The British Journal of General Practice*, vol. 49, no. 443, pp. 451–453, 1999.

[36] F. Johnsson, B. Moum, M. Vilien, O. Grove, M. Simren, and M. Thoring, "On-demand treatment in patients with oesophagitis and reflux symptoms: comparison of lansoprazole and omeprazole," *Scandinavian Journal of Gastroenterology*, vol. 37, no. 6, pp. 642–647, 2009.

[37] S. Sjostedt, R. Befrits, A. Sylvan et al., "Daily treatment with esomeprazole is superior to that taken on-demand for maintenance of healed erosive oesophagitis," *Alimentary Pharmacology & Therapeutics*, vol. 22, no. 3, pp. 183–191, 2005.

[38] F. Pace, M. Tonini, S. Pallotta, P. Molteni, and G. B. Porro, "Systematic review: maintenance treatment of gastro-oesophageal reflux disease with proton pump inhibitors taken 'on-demand'," *Alimentary Pharmacology & Therapeutics*, vol. 26, no. 2, pp. 195–204, 2007.

13

Comparison of the Long-Term Outcomes of Endoscopic Papillary Large Balloon Dilation Alone versus Endoscopic Sphincterotomy for Removal of Bile Duct Stones

Tao Li, Jun Wen, Like Bie, and Biao Gong

Digestive Endoscopy Center, Department of Gastroenterology, Ruijin Hospital, Affiliated to Shanghai Jiao Tong University School of Medicine, Shanghai, China

Correspondence should be addressed to Biao Gong; gbercp616@163.com

Academic Editor: Tatsuya Toyokawa

Background and Aims. Endoscopic papillary large balloon dilation (EPLBD) alone is an alternative to endoscopic sphincterotomy (EST) for treatment of common bile duct (CBD) stones. However, limited data exists regarding comparison of the long-term outcomes for these techniques. In this study, we compared the long-term outcomes after EST with those after EPLBD alone for removal of CBD stones. *Methods.* The records of patients with EST or EPLBD alone referred for CBD stones retrieval between June 2008 and July 2015 were retrospectively reviewed. Complete stone clearance, ERCP-related adverse events, and late biliary complications during long-term follow-up were analyzed. *Results.* Basic patient characteristics were similar between the groups that underwent EST ($n = 60$) and EPLBD alone ($n = 161$). EPLBD compared with EST resulted in similar outcomes in terms of complete stone clearance (99.4% versus 100%, $P = 0.54$) and ERCP-related adverse events (6.8% versus 6.7%, $P = 1.00$). The mean duration of the follow-up was 74.5 months and 71.6 months who underwent EST and EPLBD alone, respectively ($P = 0.42$). Late biliary complications were occurred frequently in the EST group than in the EPLBD alone group (11 [18.6%] versus 16 [10.2%]), although the difference did not reach statistical significance ($P = 0.11$). Multivariate analysis showed that mechanical lithotripsy ([OR], 2.815; 95% CI, 1.148–6.902; $P = 0.024$) was significantly associated with late biliary complications. *Conclusion.* As an alternative to EST, EPLBD has similar efficacy and safety for managing CBD stones. During long-term follow-up, patients who underwent EPLBD alone may have fewer late biliary complications compared with those after EST. In addition, mechanical lithotripsy may be an independent risk factor for late biliary complications.

1. Introduction

Endoscopic sphincterotomy (EST) is a well-established standard method for extraction of common bile duct (CBD) stones. However, adverse events such as bleeding, perforation, pancreatitis, and cholangitis occur in 5% to 10% of patients who underwent EST [1–3]. Furthermore, EST causes a permanent reduction in biliary sphincter function and results in additional late biliary complications [4]. To remedy this disadvantage, the technique of endoscopic papillary large balloon dilatation (EPLBD) using a balloon larger than 12 mm was introduced for removal of large CBD stones [5, 6]. Since then, several studies have reported that EPLBD with or without EST produced satisfactory results with large CBD stone clearance without an increased risk of severely adverse events [7–11]. In addition, some authors also showed that the short-term therapeutic outcomes and complications related to EPLBD for treatment of large bile duct stones are comparable to those after EST [12]. However, up to now, there is no consensus yet on the long-term efficacy and safety of EPLBD alone compared with those after EST for treatment of CBD stones. Therefore, in this study, we aimed to compare the long-term outcomes between EPLBD alone and EST for the management of CBD stones. In addition, risk factors associated with late biliary complications were also analyzed.

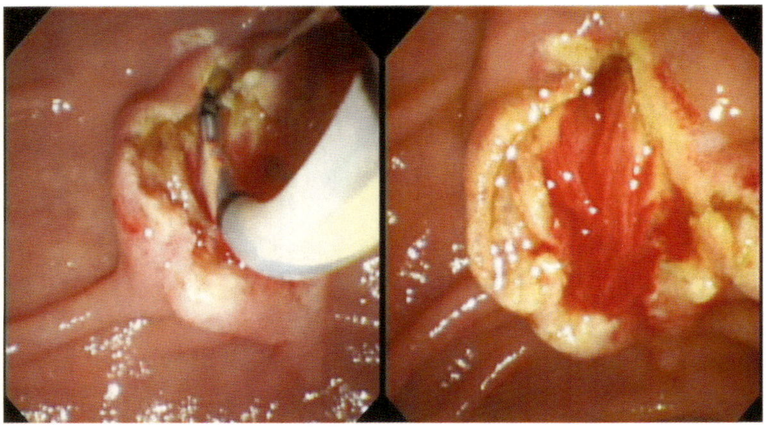

FIGURE 1: Complete endoscopic sphincterotomy was performed.

2. Materials and Methods

2.1. Patients. The study was conducted based on data recorded in a prospectively maintained registry of patients who underwent EPLBD alone or EST referred for bile duct stone retrieval between June 2008 and July 2015 in our center. Patients were retrospectively selected based on the following inclusion criteria: [1] age over 18 years, [2] a large or multiple CBD stones (≥10 mm or ≥3 stones), [3] CBD stones visualized during endoscopic retrograde cholangiopancreatography (ERCP). However, patients were excluded if they met the following criteria: [1] concomitant intrahepatic stones or pancreaticobiliary malignancies, [2] distal CBD with stricture, [3], coagulation disorders (such as international normalized ratio [INR] > 1.5 and platelet count < 50,000/mL). Patients' clinical information, including demographic characteristics, present and past medical history, laboratory and imaging results, ERCP procedures, and related adverse events were collected and analyzed. Analysis of these data was approved by the institutional review board.

2.2. Endoscopic Procedures. After communicating with the patients, written informed consent for the endoscopic procedure was signed from all patients. ERCP was performed using a side-viewing endoscope (TJF-240, JF-260V; Olympus Co. Ltd., Tokyo, Japan) by two experienced endoscopists (Biao Gong and Like Bie). When selective cannulation was achieved, a diagnostic cholangiogram was performed to assess the size and number of bile duct stones, the diameter of CBD. Either EST or EPLBD alone was chosen at discretion of the endoscopists to enlarge the bile duct opening of the duodenum. The choice of methods depended on the preference of the endoscopist in most cases. In addition, we preferred EPLBD to EST in the following cases: (1) the presence of periampullary diverticulum and (2) patients with surgically altered anatomy. But when the distal bile duct was not sufficiently dilated for some patients, excessive balloon dilation beyond the diameter of the distal bile duct may increase the risk of perforation; therefore, we selected the EST. For patients in the EST group, a complete sphincterotomy was performed with a pull-type sphincterotome and the sphincter was divided up to the transverse duodenal fold. A complete sphincterotomy was defined by the free passage of a fully bowed sphincterotome and the presence of spontaneous bile drainage (Figure 1). For patients in the EPLBD alone group, a large-size balloon dilator ≥ 12 mm (CRE wire-guided dilator, Boston Scientific, MA, USA) was passed over a prepositioned guidewire, positioning the deflated balloon across the main duodenal papilla. The size of the balloon was chosen according to the size of the bile duct, the papillary orifice, and the largest CBD stone, but it did not exceed the diameter of the distal CBD. The balloon was then gradually filled with diluted contrast medium and remained inflated until the waist of the balloon had disappeared on fluoroscopy. Subsequently, the fully expanded balloon was maintained in position for 60 seconds. EPLBD alone was defined as dilation of major duodenal papilla and distal CBD endoscopically using a balloon dilation catheter of diameter from 12 to 20 mm to facilitate the removal of difficult bile duct stones without any EST (Figure 2). Besides, the maximum diameter of the balloon used was no more than 15 mm in our center. The stones were retrieved from the bile duct with a basket or a retrieval balloon. Mechanical lithotripsy (ML, Lithotriptoren; MTW Endoskopie, Germany) was used to crush the stones if needed. After complete stone removal, an occlusion cholangiogram was obtained in the end of the procedure. Prophylactic antibiotics were not routinely administered before ERCP.

2.3. Evaluation of Clinical and Endoscopic Data. Complete stone clearance was defined as the absence of filling defects on occlusion cholangiogram. Overall success rate was defined as the rate of complete CBD stone retrieval irrespective of the use of ML or number of ERCP sessions. Adverse events after ERCP were sorted and graded according to the consensus guidelines [13, 14].

2.4. Measurements during Follow-Up. All the patients were followed up periodically after complete stone clearance. During the follow-up, a blood sample for liver function tests were scheduled at every 6 months and the abdominal ultrasonography was checked at least once yearly after removal of CBD stones. If the patient was unable to visit outpatient clinic, the

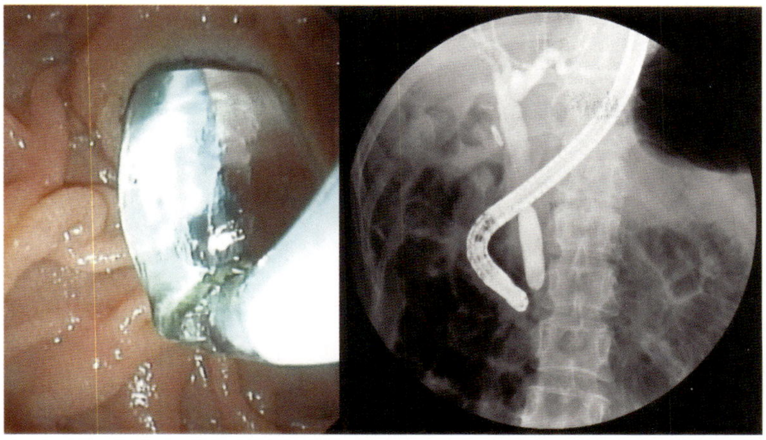

FIGURE 2: Endoscopic papillary large balloon dilation alone was performed.

TABLE 1: Baseline characteristics of the study patients who underwent EPLBD and EST.

	EST ($n = 60$)	EPLBD ($n = 161$)	P value
Age, mean(SD), years	67.0 (14.6)	70.1 (14.6)	0.17
Sex, male/female	32/28	76/85	0.45
Diameter of CBD (mm), mean (SD)	14.9 (3.3)	14.9 (2.8)	0.85
Number of CBDS, mean (SD)	1.2 (0.6)	1.3 (1.2)	0.58
Maximum stone size (mm), mean (SD)	12.1 (2.8)	12.7 (3.6)	0.2
Periampullary diverticulum, n (%)	14 (23.3%)	85 (52.8%)	0.01
Status of gallbladder			
Previous cholecystectomy, n (%)	29 (48.3%)	67 (41.6%)	0.45
Cholecystectomy after ERCP, n (%)	7 (11.7%)	14 (8.7%)	0.61
Gallbladder with stones in situ, n (%)	7 (11.7%)	35 (21.7%)	0.12
Gallbladder without stones in situ, n (%)	17 (28.3%)	45 (28.1%)	>0.99

The values are shown in mean ± standard deviation (SD). EPLBD: endoscopic papillary large balloon dilation; EST: endoscopic sphincterotomy; CBD: common bile duct; ERCP: endoscopic retrograde cholangiopancreatography; CBDS: common bile duct stone.

patients' primary follow-up information was contacted by telephone. If clinical symptoms are indicative of biliary complications, such as stone recurrence and cholangitis, additional workups, such as imaging modalities (computed tomography (CT) or magnetic resonance cholangiopancreatography (MRCP)) and/or ERCP, were performed to confirm them. Late biliary complications occurring at least 30 days after complete stone removal were classified by symptoms, laboratory data, and imaging findings. Stone recurrence was defined as a newly detected CBD stone by cholangiography after the determination of complete stone removal. Cholangitis was diagnosed when patients had at least three of the following: pain, fever, jaundice, and elevation of hepatobiliary enzyme levels.

2.5. Statistical Analysis. Baseline patient characteristics and basic outcome variables are presented as means and standard deviations (SD) for continuous variables or a frequency and a percentage for categorical variables. Statistical analysis was performed by using the chi-squared test or the Fisher exact test for noncontinuous variables and the Student t-test for continuous variables. The distributions of the occurrence of late biliary complications over time were estimated by the Kaplan-Meier product moment method, and the log-rank test was used to assess differences between the groups. To evaluate the risk factors for late biliary complications, potential risk factors were initially assessed by univariate analysis. The predictive risk factors with a P value < 0.2 in univariate analysis were then included in a multivariate logistic regression analysis. P values of <0.05 was considered to be statistically significant. Data analyses were performed using the IBM SPSS Statistics for Windows (version 20.0; IBM Corp, Armonk, New York, USA).

3. Results

3.1. Patient Demographics. Database analysis identified 221 patients referred for CBD stone retrieval during the study period; 60 patients were enrolled in the EST group, and 161 patients were enrolled in the EPLBD alone group. Patients' characteristics are summarized in Table 1. There were no between-group differences in patient demographic details, number and size of CBD stones, and CBD diameter. However, the presence of the periampullary diverticulum was slightly different in the two groups. 29 (48.3%) patients from the EST group and 67 (41.6%) patients from

Table 2: Comparison of procedural details between the EPLBD group and the EST group.

	EST ($n = 60$)	EPLBD ($n = 161$)	P value
Complete stone removal, n (%)	60 (100%)	160 (99.4%)	0.54
In first session	59 (98.3%)	158 (98.8%)	0.81
In second session	1 (1.7%)	2 (1.2%)	
Number of mechanical lithotripsy, n (%)	17 (28.3%)	29 (18.0%)	0.1
Method of stone removal, n (%)			
Retrieval basket	26 (43.3%)	75 (46.9%)	0.65
Balloon catheter	9 (15%)	19 (11.9)	0.51
Retrieval basket and balloon catheter	22 (36.7%)	61 (38.1%)	0.88
Mechanical lithotripsy basket	3 (5.0%)	5 (3.1%)	0.69
Hospital days, mean (SD)	7.4 (2.5)	7.8 (3.3)	0.49

Table 3: Comparison of the adverse events between the EST and EPLBD groups.

	EST ($n = 60$)	EPLBD ($n = 161$)	P value
Pancreatitis	2 (3.3%)	8 (5.0%)	0.73
Mild	2	7	
Moderate	0	1	
Severe	0	0	
Hemorrhage	0	0	—
Cholangitis	2 (3.3%)	3 (1.9%)	0.62
Perforation	0	0	—
Overall adverse events	4 (6.7%)	11 (6.8%)	1.00

the EPLBD alone group had undergone a previous cholecystectomy ($P = 0.45$). Cholecystectomy was performed within 1 month after EST in 7 patients (of 14 with gallbladder in situ with stones) and in 14 patients (of 49 with gallbladder in situ with stones) after EPLBD alone. No significant difference was observed in the gallbladder status between the two groups.

3.2. Immediate Treatment Outcome. The overall complete stone clearance rate was 100% (60/60) in the EST group and 99.4% (160/161) in the EPLBD alone group ($P = 0.54$) (Table 2). The causes of failure in one patient were larger stone impaction and difficulty in removing it, and the patient underwent surgery in the end. A total of 98.3% of patients in the EST group and 98.8% of patients in the EPLBD alone group had stones cleared in the first session ($P = 0.81$), respectively. The use of ML was more frequently in the EST group than in the EPLBD alone group (17 [28.3%] versus 29 [18%]), although the difference did not reach statistical significance ($P = 0.10$). In addition, there is no difference in the mean length of hospital stay between the EST and EPLBD alone groups (7.4 versus 7.8, $P = 0.49$).

3.3. ERCP-Related Adverse Events. ERCP-related adverse events occurred in 6.7% of patients in the EST group and 6.8% of patients in the EPLBD alone group, respectively. The details are shown in Table 3. The incidence of post-ERCP pancreatitis (3.3% versus 5.0%, $P = 0.73$) and cholangitis (3.3% versus 1.9%, $P = 0.62$) were not significantly different between the EST and EPLBD alone groups. All of these patients improved with conservative management. Severe complications, including perforation, bleeding, and severe pancreatitis did not develop in any patients. None of the patients died after ERCP procedures.

3.4. Outcomes of the Long-Term Follow-Up. Follow-up data was collected every year after complete stone clearance, and final updates were done in October 2017. Five patients were lost during the follow-up period. Six patients died during the follow-up period. The causes of death were not related to biliary complications. No significant difference was observed between the EST and EPLBD alone groups in the mean duration of follow-up from the end of complete stone clearance to the last observation or death (74.5 ± 20.2 versus 71.6 ± 24.5 months, respectively, $P = 0.42$) (Table 4). The incidence of late biliary complications occurred frequently in the EST group than in the EPLBD alone group (11 [18.6%] versus 16 [10.2%]), although the difference did not reach statistical significance ($P = 0.11$). Kaplan-Meier analysis also revealed no difference of the incidence of late biliary complications between the EST and EPLBD groups (log-rank test, $P = 0.223$) (Figure 3). Stone recurrence were observed in 16 and 8 patients for the EPLBD alone and EST groups (10.2% versus 13.6%, $P = 0.47$), respectively. All recurrent stones were successfully extracted by ERCP procedure again. In addition, a significantly higher incidence of cholangitis without stone recurrence was observed in the EST group than in the EPLBD alone group (3 [5.1%] versus 0 [0%]; $P = 0.02$). These patients were treated with antibiotics, and their symptoms resolved in a few days.

3.5. Risk Factors for Late Biliary Complications. To examine predictive risk factors for late biliary complications, potential risk factors of patient characteristics and ERCP procedures were compared between the late biliary complication group ($n = 26$) and without late biliary complication group ($n = 190$). ML was identified as a risk factor for late biliary complication based on univariate analysis. The multivariate

TABLE 4: Comparison of the late biliary complications during follow-up between the EST and EPLBD groups.

	EST ($n = 59$)	EPLBD ($n = 157$)	P value
Duration of follow-up (months), mean (SD)	74.5 (20.2)	71.6 (24.5)	0.42
Recurrent bile duct stones, n (%)	8 (13.6%)	16 (10.2%)	0.47
Cholangitis without stone recurrence, n (%)	3 (5.1%)	0	0.02
Total biliary complications, n (%)	11 (18.6%)	16 (10.2%)	0.11

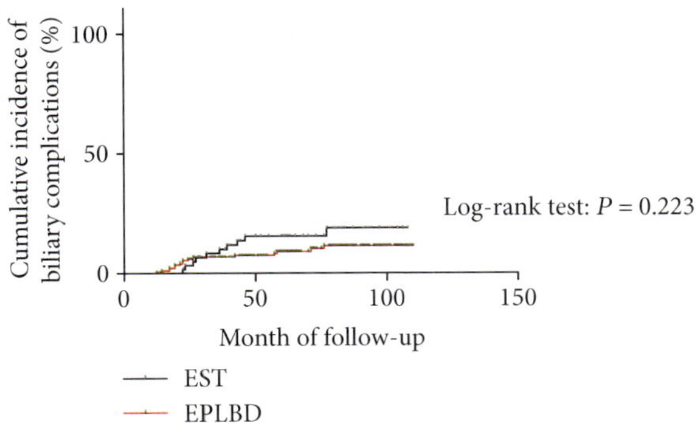

FIGURE 3: Cumulative incidence of late biliary complications. The red line indicates the EPLBD group, and the black line corresponds to the EST group. Kaplan-Meier estimates of the proportion of patients with late biliary complications in the endoscopic sphincterotomy (EST) ($n = 59$) and endoscopic papillary large balloon dilation alone (EPLBD) ($n = 157$) groups ($P = 0.223$ by log-rank test).

analysis also showed that ML ([OR], 2.815; 95% CI, 1.148–6.902; $P = 0.024$) was significantly associated with late biliary complications (Table 5).

4. Discussion

EST is the most commonly used method as a standard technique for the treatment of CBD stones [13]. However, EST has many early complications including hemorrhage, cholangitis, and perforation and late complications associated with dysfunction of the sphincter [15, 16]. To overcome this disadvantage, EPLBD with or without a preceding EST was introduced for removal of larger bile duct stones [5, 6]. In addition, EPLBD is especially suitable for patients with an unfavorable anatomy for EST, such as for patients who have underwent Roux-en-Y or Billroth II gastrectomy [17–19].

Periampullary diverticulum is known to be associated with an increased frequency of pancreatobiliary diseases, because the ampullary area in patients with periampullary diverticula is composed of thin mucosa without sphincter muscle. Besides, the periampullary diverticulum tends to distort the anatomy of the duodenum and the sphincter. So this altered state makes EST more difficult and dangerous for these patients [2, 20]. So in our present study, we preferred EPLBD alone in patients with periampullary diverticulum.

In our study, both EST and EPLBD alone for management of bile duct stones resulted in similar outcomes with respect to complete stone clearance (100% versus 99.4%), which is similar to previous results regarding overall stone clearance [12, 21, 22]. In addition, ML might be used more often in the EST group compared to the EPLBD group for removal of large or multiple stones in our study (17 [28.3%] versus 29 [18%]). Our results were consistent with previous studies [21, 23, 24], because the widened ampullary orifice made by EPLBD alone facilitates easier extraction of relatively large bile duct stones and may reduce the need for ML compared to EST.

Major adverse events typically related to both EST and EPLBD are pancreatitis, bleeding, and perforation. In the current study, ERCP-related adverse events were similar between the two groups (6.7% versus 6.8%, $P = 1.00$). With respect to the post-ERCP pancreatitis, many concerns have been raised about pancreatitis after balloon dilation with increasing balloon size. However, in this study, the risk of post-ERCP pancreatitis was not increased with EPLBD compared to EST (5.0% versus 3.3%). Recently, some studies also reported that the increase in balloon size does not affect the development of pancreatitis after EPLBD for bile duct stone removal [9, 25]. Based on these results, post-ERCP pancreatitis associated with EPLBD may occur at a lower incidence rate and with a similar incidence compared to EST. Furthermore, although severe complications did not develop in our study, it should be mentioned that EPLBD may cause very serious bleeding and perforation [26, 27]. The most likely explanation would be that large-diameter balloon dilation would tear the ducts and result in bleeding and perforation.

Several studies have investigated the long-term outcomes of EST. The incidence of biliary complications such as stone recurrence and cholangitis was reported in 9.2% to 17.7% of the patients which is similar to ours [28–31]. Park et al. [8] in a retrospective study of EPLBD alone for the treatment of large CBD stones reported that the incidence of biliary complications such as stone recurrence and cholangitis was 16.8% during a mean follow-up period of 1398 days. However, up to now, few studies have investigated comparison of the long-term outcomes of EPLBD alone versus EST for removal of bile duct stones. In our present study, the median duration of the follow-up from the end of the complete stone clearance to the last observation or death was 74.5 months and 71.6 months who underwent EST and EPLBD alone, respectively ($P = 0.42$), which we believe was sufficient to determine the incidence of late biliary complications. In the current study, the incidence of stone recurrence in the EPLBD alone group (10.2%) was not significantly different from the EST group (13.6%) which is similar to previous studies [4, 8, 32–34]. As far as we know, several studies have

Table 5: Univariate and multivariate analyses for risk factors of the late biliary complications.

	Late complication $n = 26$	Without late complication $n = 190$	P value
Age (y)	67.0 (16.4)	69.6 (14.5)	0.398
Sex, male/female	12/14	94/96	0.836
Diameter of CBD (mm), mean (SD)	15.7 (3.2)	14.8 (2.9)	0.140
Number of CBDS, mean (SD)	1.3 (0.7)	1.3 (1.1)	0.997
Maximum stone size (mm), mean (SD)	12.2 (2.6)	12.6 (3.5)	0.570
Periampullary diverticulum, n (%)	14 (53.8%)	91 (47.9%)	0.677
Mechanical lithotripsy, n (%)	11 (42.3%)	34 (17.9)	0.008
Previous cholecystectomy, n (%)	15 (57.7%)	100 (52.6%)	0.679
Gallbladder with stones in situ, n (%)	7 (26.9%)	34 (17.9%)	0.288
Gallbladder without stones in situ, n (%)	4 (15.4%)	56 (29.6%)	0.164
	Odds ratio	95% Confidence interval	P value
Mechanical lithotripsy	2.815	1.148–6.902	0.024

demonstrated a severe permanent impairment of sphincter of Oddi function after EST; subsequent duodenobiliary reflux and bacterial contamination after EST can cause late biliary complications such as cholangitis and stone formation [4, 35]. However, EPLBD used large-diameter balloon (≥12 mm); extensive dilation of the sphincter may lead to the tearing of the sphincter muscles, and the degree of papillary damage would be more serious in EPLBD compared to EPBD. Recently, a prospective randomized study revealed that EPLBD alone resulted in persistent and comparable loss of sphincter of Oddi function [36]. Therefore, it appears that EPLBD alone could permanently disrupt sphincter function and cause long-term adverse events in the same manner as EST. However, further study is needed to provide related data that demonstrate it. In addition, a higher incidence of cholangitis without stone recurrence was observed in the EST group than in the EPLBD alone group. We thought it might be related to sphincterotomy stenosis. Because dilatation of the bile duct was detected by MRCP for these patients, dilated CBD may promote bile stasis and bacterial contamination, which play essential roles in a mechanism of cholangitis.

In the present study, multivariate analysis showed that ML was the key factor accounting for the increased incidence of late biliary complications which is in line with the previous study [37]. When CBD stones were not removed, ML was required, which raises the possibility that residual stone fragments, undetectable by cholangiography, might have acted as nidi for stone formation. So we recommend that a regular follow-up be improved for these high-risk patients.

Some limitations of our study must be highlighted: the retrospective design which was conducted at a single center could have resulted in a selection bias; future randomized controlled trials and multicenter study are expected in order to provide the optimal endoscopic therapy for these patients.

In conclusion, as an alternative to EST, EPLBD alone has similar efficacy and safety for treatment of CBD stones. During long-term follow-up, patients who underwent EPLBD alone may have fewer late biliary complications compared with those after EST. In addition, ML may be an independent risk factor for late biliary complications.

Abbreviations

EPLBD: Endoscopic papillary large balloon dilation
EST: Endoscopic sphincterotomy
CBD: Common bile duct
CT: Computed tomography
MRCP: Magnetic resonance cholangiopancreatography
ERCP: Endoscopic retrograde cholangiopancreatography
ML: Mechanical lithotripsy.

Authors' Contributions

Biao Gong designed the research; Like Bie performed the research; Jun Wen worked on clinical data acquisition; and Tao Li performed data analysis and wrote the manuscript, and Biao Gong supervised it. All authors approved the final version of the text.

Acknowledgments

The authors thank all the staffs from the Digestive Endoscopy Center, Ruijin Hospital Affiliated to Shanghai Jiao Tong University School of Medicine for their help in this study.

References

[1] S. Sherman, T. A. Ruffolo, R. H. Hawes, and G. A. Lehman, "Complications of endoscopic sphincterotomy. A prospective series with emphasis on the increased risk associated with

sphincter of Oddi dysfunction and nondilated bile ducts," *Gastroenterology*, vol. 101, no. 4, pp. 1068–1075, 1991.

[2] J. W. C. Leung, F. K. L. Chan, J. J. Y. Sung, and S. C. S. Chung, "Endoscopic sphincterotomy-induced hemorrhage: a study of risk factors and the role of epinephrine injection," *Gastrointestinal Endoscopy*, vol. 42, no. 6, pp. 550–554, 1995.

[3] J. Boender, G. A. J. J. Nix, M. A. J. de Ridder et al., "Endoscopic papillotomy for common bile duct stones: factors influencing the complication rate," *Endoscopy*, vol. 26, no. 02, pp. 209–216, 1994.

[4] I. Yasuda, N. Fujita, H. Maguchi et al., "Long-term outcomes after endoscopic sphincterotomy versus endoscopic papillary balloon dilation for bile duct stones," *Gastrointestinal Endoscopy*, vol. 72, no. 6, pp. 1185–1191, 2010.

[5] G. Ersoz, O. Tekesin, A. O. Ozutemiz, and F. Gunsar, "Biliary sphincterotomy plus dilation with a large balloon for bile duct stones that are difficult to extract," *Gastrointestinal Endoscopy*, vol. 57, no. 2, pp. 156–159, 2003.

[6] S. Jeong, S. H. Ki, D. H. Lee et al., "Endoscopic large-balloon sphincteroplasty without preceding sphincterotomy for the removal of large bile duct stones: a preliminary study," *Gastrointestinal Endoscopy*, vol. 70, no. 5, pp. 915–922, 2009.

[7] D. Karsenti, E. Coron, G. Vanbiervliet et al., "Complete endoscopic sphincterotomy with vs. without large-balloon dilation for the removal of large bile duct stones: randomized multicenter study," *Endoscopy*, vol. 49, no. 10, pp. 968–976, 2017.

[8] J. S. Park, S. Jeong, B. W. Bang, A. R. Kang, and D. H. Lee, "Endoscopic papillary large balloon dilatation without sphincterotomy for the treatment of large common bile duct stone: long-term outcomes at a single center," *Digestive Diseases and Sciences*, vol. 61, no. 10, pp. 3045–3053, 2016.

[9] J. S. Park, T. N. Kim, and K. H. Kim, "Endoscopic papillary large balloon dilation for treatment of large bile duct stones does not increase the risk of post-procedure pancreatitis," *Digestive Diseases and Sciences*, vol. 59, no. 12, pp. 3092–3098, 2014.

[10] A. Y. B. Teoh, F. K. Y. Cheung, B. Hu et al., "Randomized trial of endoscopic sphincterotomy with balloon dilation versus endoscopic sphincterotomy alone for removal of bile duct stones," *Gastroenterology*, vol. 144, no. 2, pp. 341–345.e1, 2013.

[11] H. G. Yoon, J. H. Moon, H. J. Choi et al., "Endoscopic papillary large balloon dilation for the management of recurrent difficult bile duct stones after previous endoscopic sphincterotomy," *Digestive Endoscopy*, vol. 26, no. 2, pp. 259–263, 2014.

[12] M. J. Oh and T. N. Kim, "Prospective comparative study of endoscopic papillary large balloon dilation and endoscopic sphincterotomy for removal of large bile duct stones in patients above 45 years of age," *Scandinavian Journal of Gastroenterology*, vol. 47, no. 8-9, pp. 1071–1077, 2012.

[13] P. B. Cotton, G. Lehman, J. Vennes et al., "Endoscopic sphincterotomy complications and their management: an attempt at consensus," *Gastrointestinal Endoscopy*, vol. 37, no. 3, pp. 383–393, 1991.

[14] P. B. Cotton, G. M. Eisen, L. Aabakken et al., "A lexicon for endoscopic adverse events: report of an ASGE workshop," *Gastrointestinal Endoscopy*, vol. 71, no. 3, pp. 446–454, 2010.

[15] S. G. Sheth and D. A. Howell, "What are really the true late complications of endoscopic biliary sphincterotomy?," *The American Journal of Gastroenterology*, vol. 97, no. 11, pp. 2699–2701, 2002.

[16] M. L. Freeman, D. B. Nelson, S. Sherman et al., "Complications of endoscopic biliary sphincterotomy," *The New England Journal of Medicine*, vol. 335, no. 13, pp. 909–919, 1996.

[17] C. W. Choi, J. S. Choi, D. H. Kang et al., "Endoscopic papillary large balloon dilation in Billroth II gastrectomy patients with bile duct stones," *Journal of Gastroenterology and Hepatology*, vol. 27, no. 2, pp. 256–260, 2012.

[18] T. Itoi, K. Ishii, A. Sofuni et al., "Large balloon dilatation following endoscopic sphincterotomy using a balloon enteroscope for the bile duct stone extractions in patients with Roux-en-Y anastomosis," *Digestive and Liver Disease*, vol. 43, no. 3, pp. 237–241, 2011.

[19] K. H. Kim and T. N. Kim, "Endoscopic papillary large balloon dilation for the retrieval of bile duct stones after prior Billroth II gastrectomy," *Saudi Journal of Gastroenterology*, vol. 20, no. 2, pp. 128–133, 2014.

[20] K. H. Kim and T. N. Kim, "Endoscopic papillary large balloon dilation in patients with periampullary diverticula," *World Journal of Gastroenterology*, vol. 19, no. 41, pp. 7168–7176, 2013.

[21] Y. Feng, H. Zhu, X. Chen et al., "Comparison of endoscopic papillary large balloon dilation and endoscopic sphincterotomy for retrieval of choledocholithiasis: a meta-analysis of randomized controlled trials," *Journal of Gastroenterology*, vol. 47, no. 6, pp. 655–663, 2012.

[22] K. Tsuchida, M. Iwasaki, M. Tsubouchi et al., "Comparison of the usefulness of endoscopic papillary large-balloon dilation with endoscopic sphincterotomy for large and multiple common bile duct stones," *BMC Gastroenterology*, vol. 15, no. 1, p. 59, 2015.

[23] T. H. Kim, H. J. Oh, J. Y. Lee, and Y. W. Sohn, "Can a small endoscopic sphincterotomy plus a large-balloon dilation reduce the use of mechanical lithotripsy in patients with large bile duct stones?," *Surgical Endoscopy*, vol. 25, no. 10, pp. 3330–3337, 2011.

[24] T. Itoi, F. Itokawa, A. Sofuni et al., "Endoscopic sphincterotomy combined with large balloon dilation can reduce the procedure time and fluoroscopy time for removal of large bile duct stones," *The American Journal of Gastroenterology*, vol. 104, no. 3, pp. 560–565, 2009.

[25] Y. H. Youn, H. C. Lim, J. H. Jahng et al., "The increase in balloon size to over 15 mm does not affect the development of pancreatitis after endoscopic papillary large balloon dilatation for bile duct stone removal," *Digestive Diseases and Sciences*, vol. 56, no. 5, pp. 1572–1577, 2011.

[26] T. H. Lee, S. H. Park, C. K. Lee, I. K. Chung, S. J. Kim, and C. H. Kang, "Life-threatening hemorrhage following large-balloon endoscopic papillary dilation successfully treated with angiographic embolization," *Endoscopy*, vol. 41, no. S 02, pp. E241–E242, 2009.

[27] P. Katsinelos, G. Chatzimavroudis, I. Pilpilidis et al., "Benign retropneumoperitoneum developed after endoscopic sphincterotomy and large balloon dilation of biliary sphincter for removal of large biliary stones: a case report," *Cases Journal*, vol. 1, no. 1, p. 279, 2008.

[28] M. Sugiyama and Y. Atomi, "Risk factors predictive of late complications after endoscopic sphincterotomy for bile duct stones: long-term (more than 10 years) follow-up study," *The American Journal of Gastroenterology*, vol. 97, no. 11, pp. 2763–2767, 2002.

[29] G. Costamagna, A. Tringali, S. K. Shah, M. Mutignani, G. Zuccala, and V. Perri, "Long-term follow-up of patients

after endoscopic sphincterotomy for choledocholithiasis, and risk factors for recurrence," *Endoscopy*, vol. 34, no. 4, pp. 273–279, 2002.

[30] M. Tanaka, S. Takahata, H. Konomi et al., "Long-term consequence of endoscopic sphincterotomy for bile duct stones," *Gastrointestinal Endoscopy*, vol. 48, no. 5, pp. 465–469, 1998.

[31] J. J. G. H. M. Bergman, S. van der Mey, E. A. J. Rauws et al., "Long-term follow-up after endoscopic sphincterotomy for bile duct stones in patients younger than 60 years of age," *Gastrointestinal Endoscopy*, vol. 44, no. 6, pp. 643–649, 1996.

[32] H. H. Chan, K. H. Lai, C. K. Lin et al., "Endoscopic papillary large balloon dilation alone without sphincterotomy for the treatment of large common bile duct stones," *BMC Gastroenterology*, vol. 11, no. 1, p. 69, 2011.

[33] H. Kogure, T. Tsujino, H. Isayama et al., "Short- and long-term outcomes of endoscopic papillary large balloon dilation with or without sphincterotomy for removal of large bile duct stones," *Scandinavian Journal of Gastroenterology*, vol. 49, no. 1, pp. 121–128, 2014.

[34] K. Y. Kim, J. Han, H. G. Kim et al., "Late complications and stone recurrence rates after bile duct stone removal by endoscopic sphincterotomy and large balloon dilation are similar to those after endoscopic sphincterotomy alone," *Clinical Endoscopy*, vol. 46, no. 6, pp. 637–642, 2013.

[35] I. Yasuda, E. Tomita, M. Enya, T. Kato, and H. Moriwaki, "Can endoscopic papillary balloon dilation really preserve sphincter of Oddi function?," *Gut*, vol. 49, no. 5, pp. 686–691, 2001.

[36] Y. K. Cheon, T. Y. Lee, S. N. Kim, and C. S. Shim, "Impact of endoscopic papillary large-balloon dilation on sphincter of Oddi function: a prospective randomized study," *Gastrointestinal Endoscopy*, vol. 85, no. 4, pp. 782–790.e1, 2017.

[37] Y. Lu, J. C. Wu, L. Liu, L. K. Bie, and B. Gong, "Short-term and long-term outcomes after endoscopic sphincterotomy versus endoscopic papillary balloon dilation for bile duct stones," *European Journal of Gastroenterology & Hepatology*, vol. 26, no. 12, pp. 1367–1373, 2014.

14

Safety of Propofol versus Nonpropofol-Based Sedation in Children Undergoing Gastrointestinal Endoscopy

Neeraj Narula,[1] Sameer Masood,[2] Samira Shojaee,[3] Brandon McGuinness,[1] Saama Sabeti,[2] and Arianne Buchan[4]

[1]*Department of Medicine (Division of Gastroenterology) and Farncombe Family Digestive Health Research Institute, McMaster University, Hamilton, ON, Canada*
[2]*Harvard TH Chan School of Public Health, Boston, MA, USA*
[3]*Department of Medicine (Division of Pulmonary and Critical Care Medicine), Virginia Commonwealth University, Richmond, VA, USA*
[4]*Department of Medicine, The Ottawa Hospital, Ottawa, ON, Canada*

Correspondence should be addressed to Neeraj Narula; neeraj.narula@medportal.ca

Academic Editor: Tatsuya Toyokawa

Background. The majority of children who undergo gastrointestinal (GI) endoscopy require anesthesia or procedural sedation for comfort, cooperation, and procedure efficiency. The safety profile of propofol is not well established in children but has been studied in the literature. *Objective.* The aim of this study is to evaluate and compare the safety of propofol-only sedation for GI endoscopy procedures to other anesthetic regimes in the pediatric population. *Methods.* A search was conducted in the MEDLINE, Embase, and Cochrane Library databases. Randomized clinical trials and prospective cohorts were included in the study. *Results.* No significant difference was noted in total complications between the two cohorts with a pooled OR of 1.31 (95% CI: 0.57–3.04, $chi^2 = 0.053$, $I^2 = 54.31\%$). The pooled rate of complications in the studies was 23.4% for those receiving propofol only and 18.2% for those receiving other anesthetic regimens. Sensitivity analysis was performed removing a study with a very different control comparison compared to the rest of the studies included. Once excluded, there was minimal heterogeneity in the remaining studies and a significant difference in overall complications was detected, with more complications seen in the propofol-only group compared to the other anesthetic groups (OR 1.87, 95% CI 1.09–3.20). *Conclusion.* Significantly higher incidence of cardiorespiratory complications was noted in the propofol-only versus other anesthetic regimens in pediatric patients undergoing GI endoscopy in this meta-analysis. However, the overall quality of the evidence is very low. *How to Apply This Knowledge for Routine Clinical Practice.* Clinicians providing sedation to a pediatric population for GI endoscopy should consider there may be increased risks when using a propofol-only regimen, but further study is needed.

1. Introduction

Gastrointestinal (GI) endoscopic procedures are performed for diagnostic and therapeutic purposes in pediatric gastrointestinal diseases. Most children however do not tolerate these procedures without sedation or general anesthesia [1]. Proper sedation is particularly important for successful procedure completion, as well as preventing unpleasant experiences, which could complicate performing future procedures in children who will be frequently requiring them [2].

The goals of sedation are to ensure patient safety, provide analgesia and amnesia, control behavior during the procedure, enable successful completion of the procedure, and return the patient to pretreatment level of consciousness as fast as possible [3]. The most commonly used medication combinations for pediatric sedation include ketamine, propofol, midazolam, fentanyl, and pethidine [4]. Each of these drugs, however, can cause respiratory depression [5, 6].

The adverse respiratory profile of most sedatives creates the need for a sedative drug that can be used safely and efficiently with limited adverse effects during sedation in pediatric patients undergoing upper endoscopic procedures. Propofol (2,6-diisopropylphenol), an intravenously administered anesthetic released for use in 1989, has become popular as an agent for induction and maintenance of anesthesia [7]. The main advantages of propofol are rapid induction of anesthesia and smooth maintenance of sedation with good preservation of cardiovascular parameters [8–11].

Recovery from propofol is also remarkably rapid, occurring within 6 to 8 minutes and with fewer complications such as agitation, nausea, or vomiting, in the postprocedure period, which facilitates early discharge [12]. This favorable efficacy of propofol has made it a popular anesthetic agent for GI endoscopy. However, most experience with propofol relates to its use in adults [12, 13]. The safety of propofol in the pediatric age group has been documented during surgical, ophthalmologic, urologic, radiologic, and dental procedures [14–16]. However, data regarding its use for pediatric GI endoscopic procedures are limited and remain a matter of debate. In this meta-analysis, we present a review and meta-analysis of the existing literature evaluating the safety of a propofol-only sedation regimen compared to other sedation regimens during endoscopic procedures in the pediatric population.

2. Method Section

A search of Medline and Embase was performed using OVID for article retrieval and removal of duplicates. Using the same search terms, this search was also carried out in the Cochrane database of randomized controlled trials. Duplicates were removed manually by the reviewer for the Cochrane registry results. The following search terms were used:

(1) Titles or abstracts containing endoscopy or esophagoscopy or aesophagoscopy or colonoscopy or sigmoidoscopy or endoscopic or enteroscopy or esophagogastroduodenoscopy or aesophagogastroduodenoscopy or gastroscopy or digestive system or gastrointestinal

(2) Titles or abstracts containing propofol or diprivan or propoven

(3) Titles containing anesthesia or anaesthesia or anesthetic or anaesthetic or sedat*

(4) 1 and 2 or 3

(5) Filters for age 0–18 and publication year > 1980 which were applied appropriate to the respective database. For the Cochrane database, a childhood hedge which was applied:

Titles or abstracts containing child* or children or teen* or preteen* or pre-teen* or baby or babies or adolescent or youth or juvenile or toddler or pubescent or prepubescent or infant or newborn or pediatric or paediatric

To assess the sensitivity of the age filter, the childhood hedge was compared to the filter within Medline with no difference noted. The anesthesia term was restricted to a title search, due to a significant number of nonrelevant trials, returning with an abstract and title search. This search strategy was trialed against a list of previously identified trials, with none being excluded.

Titles and abstracts were screened independently by two investigators (Saama Sabeti, Brandon McGuinness). Inclusion criteria for progression to full-text review included the following: prospective cohort studies, randomized controlled trials (RCTs), pediatric population (<18 years old), GI endoscopy under sedation, and at least one propofol-only sedation arm. We decided to include studies where the control arm may have received propofol as well, but in addition to other anesthetic drugs, as the propofol dose used in this circumstance is often less than that used when relying on propofol only. Exclusion criteria included adult population, non-English, no propofol-only arm, no sedation comparisons, general anesthesia comparison, non-GI endoscopy procedure, not assessing outcomes of interest, and study designs other than prospective cohort studies or RCTs. The primary outcome of interest was total cardiac and respiratory complications. We also looked at secondary outcomes of cardiac and respiratory complications individually.

Once included studies had been determined, using a standardized data extraction form, two independent reviewers recorded data from the full text. For conference abstracts or articles where the full text was not available, data was collected from the abstract. The quality of the evidence was assessed for each included study. The Cochrane Risk of Bias Tool was used for randomized controlled trials, and the Newcastle-Ottawa scale was used for prospective cohort studies.

3. Statistical Analysis

Meta-analysis of aggregate patient data was conducted by combining the odds ratios of individual studies into a pooled odds ratio using a random effects model. Intention-to-treat data was extracted from all studies. We tested for heterogeneity using the chi-squared test and the I^2 test. The I^2 test describes the percentage of variability in effect estimates that is due to heterogeneity rather than chance, wherein an I^2 test greater than 50% suggests significant heterogeneity. A random effects model was used given the variation among study designs, as this provides a more conservative estimate than a fixed effects model. Metaregression was performed to analyze for an association between the quality of the study and the outcome of interest. This was specified a priori as a possible source of heterogeneity within our result pool, as prospective trials would be at a higher risk of confounding by indication. Another source of heterogeneity which was specified a priori was differences between studies in the sedation regimen used in the control group. For the assessment of publication bias, we performed funnel plots and calculated Egger's regression intercept for studies that report therapeutic response; a one-tailed p value < 0.05 was considered statistically significant. Analyses were performed with Comprehensive Meta-Analysis statistical software (version 2.2; Biostat, Englewood, NJ).

4. Results

In total, the search resulted in 625 titles and abstracts to be screened. The search process is summarized in a Prisma flow diagram (Figure 1). Forty studies progressed to a full-text review. After the full-text review, there were 2 studies excluded for being published in a non-English language, 21 studies excluded for involving an adult population, 5 studies excluded for not including a propofol-only arm, 1 study excluded for not having an intervention group, 1 study excluded for having a general anesthesia comparator as opposed to conscious sedation, and 2 studies excluded for an incorrect study design. The final list of 7 studies [17–23] selected to undergo data extraction included 3 RCTs for which full text was available and 4 prospective studies, 2 of which had full text available but 2 of which were only available in abstract form (full text exists but is not available online [17]; conference abstract only [23]).

Raw data is summarized in Table 1. This was subsequently condensed into combined cardiovascular and respiratory complications (Table 2). Adverse cardiovascular outcomes were defined as hypotension or bradycardia. Adverse respiratory outcomes were defined as apneic episodes, depressed respiratory rate, or hypoxia. A combined total cardiorespiratory adverse event outcome was assigned for each study. One study [22] included only data measured as the median integrated pulmonary index (IPI), a combined measure of both cardiac and respiratory parameters. This however was not directly correlated with harm in the study, and no harm data was reported. Therefore, for the purpose of analysis, it was excluded. The median IPI however was lower (1 Q1:1 Q3:7) than that for the propofol + midazolam (7 Q1:6 Q3:8) or propofol + midazolam + fentanyl group (7 Q1:6 Q3:8). These results are consistent with the subsequent analysis. All remaining studies included data regarding respiratory complications. Four of the included studies reported the number of cardiovascular complications. Nausea and emesis as well as recovery time were not included in the final analysis as it was only reported in one and three studies, respectively.

4.1. Total Cardiovascular and Respiratory Complications. Six studies reported total complications from endoscopy and included 273 subjects who received propofol only and 319 subjects received other anesthetic regimens. There was no significant difference in total complications between the two cohorts, as the pooled OR for total complications among the six studies was 1.31 (95% CI: 0.57–3.04, Cochrane's Q statistic p value = 0.053, $I^2 = 54.31\%$) (Figure 2). The pooled rate of complications in the studies is 23.4% for those receiving propofol only and 18.2% for those receiving other anesthetic regimens.

4.2. Respiratory Complications. Six studies reported respiratory complications from endoscopy and included 273 subjects who received propofol only and 319 subjects received other anesthetic regimens. There was no significant difference in respiratory complications between the two cohorts, with a pooled OR for respiratory complications among the six studies of 1.18 (95% CI: 0.46–3.08, Cochrane's Q statistic p value = 0.07, $I^2 = 52\%$) (Figure 3). The pooled rate of respiratory complications in the studies is 11.0% for those receiving propofol only and 10.7% for those receiving other anesthetic regimens.

4.3. Cardiovascular Complications. Four studies reported cardiovascular complications from endoscopy and included 140 subjects who received propofol only and 140 subjects received other anesthetic regimens. There was no significant difference in cardiovascular complications between the two cohorts, with a pooled OR for cardiovascular complications among the four studies of 1.70 (95% CI: 0.90–3.20, Cochrane's Q statistic p value = 0.44, $I^2 = 0\%$) (Figure 4). The pooled rate of cardiovascular complications in the studies is 24.3% for those receiving propofol only and 17.1% for those receiving other anesthetic regimens.

4.4. Sensitivity Analysis and Publication Bias. Sensitivity analyses were performed using the one-study removed technique (Figure 5). A significant difference in overall complications was detected once the Prunty et al. study was removed, with less complications seen in the other anesthetic regimens compared to propofol only (OR 1.87, 95% CI 1.09–3.20). The study by Prunty et al. used a four-drug combination in the control arm, including propofol, and it is possible that they observed an excess of respiratory complications due to this. Inclusion of this study in the overall meta-analysis led to more complication events occurring in the control arm and as a result led to no significant difference in total complications between those receiving propofol only and other anesthetic regimens in the overall meta-analysis. We felt this study was inherently different from the remaining studies included in the meta-analysis given the excessive number of drugs used on the control arm. Once this study was excluded, there was minimal heterogeneity between the remaining studies detected (Cochrane's Q statistic p value = 0.63, $I^2 = 0\%$). Metaregression was performed to adjust for study type (RCT compared to cohort studies). No significant difference was seen between RCTs and cohort studies ($p = 0.87$) (Figure 6). We conducted a subgroup analysis of cardiovascular versus respiratory complications to determine if one subgroup had a more significant effect seen in total complications (excluding the study by Prunty et al. given its contribution to increasing heterogeneity). We did not detect any significant difference between cardiovascular and respiratory complications ($p = 0.08$) (Figure 7).

Figure 8 is a funnel plot for studies that report on total complications. Symmetrical distribution of the studies on the plot suggests no publication bias. Egger's test similarly showed no publication bias (p value = 0.46) but may have limited ability to detect publication bias given the small number of studies included.

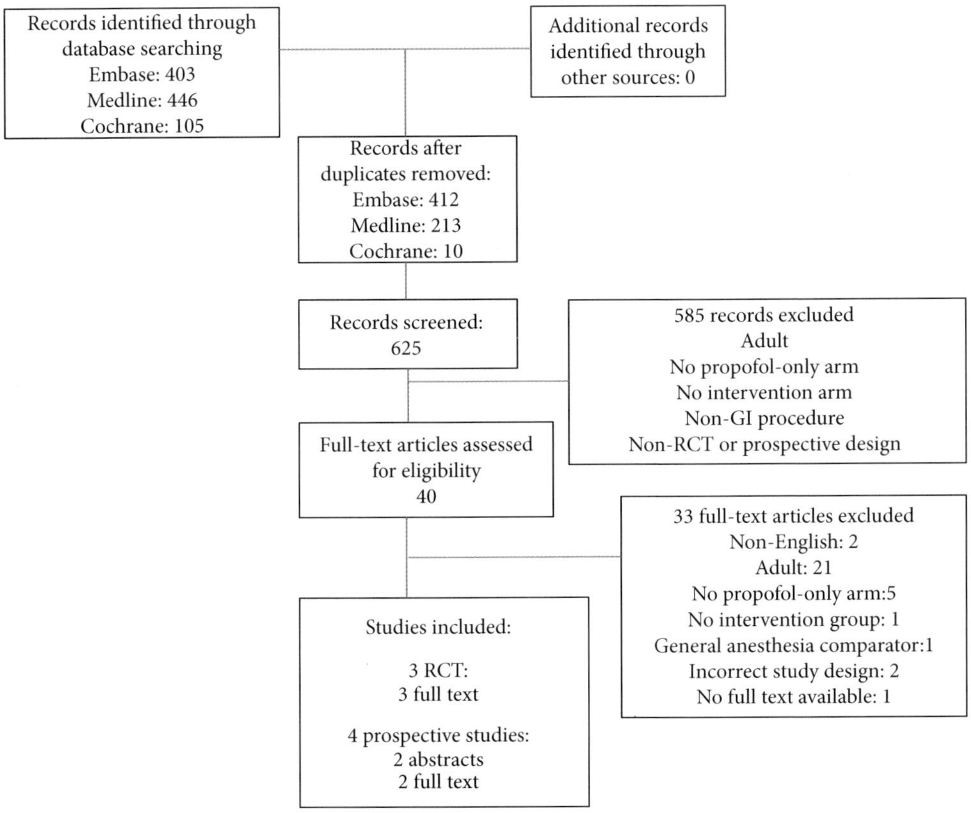

Figure 1: Prisma flow diagram. Retrieved studies and process of screening. Total included studies included 3 randomized controlled trials and 4 prospective cohort studies. All exclusion criteria were determined a priori.

Bias assessment for each study is provided in supplementary materials (available here). The overall quality of the included studies is summarized in Table 3 and Supplementary Figure S1. Randomized controlled trials frequently did not specify the method of allocation or blinding. Within the observational trials, none demonstrated good comparability between the trial arms. Therefore, there was a high risk of confounding by indication within the included studies. According to the GRADE system for assessing quality, evidence from randomized controlled trials begins with a "high" rating. We downgraded the rating because of the risk of bias in the studies, given that patients and clinicians were not blinded, as well as impreciseness of the treatment effect and inconsistency in results. The overall GRADE rating applied to the randomized controlled trials was "low." Evidence from observational evidence begins with a "low" rating. We downgraded the rating to "very low" due to the risk of bias in some of the observational studies, mainly due to inclusion of abstracts where the risk of bias was largely unclear, as well as imprecision of the treatment effect due to a small size. Details are available in Table 3.

5. Discussion

Our results show that there was a statistically significant difference in combined cardiorespiratory complications between propofol-only and other sedation regimens in pediatric patients undergoing GI endoscopy, when excluding the study by Prunty et al. which we felt used an inappropriate control group for the purposes of our safety analysis. There was no difference in the subgroup analysis when complications were divided into cardiovascular and respiratory.

Our study focused on the safety of propofol compared to other sedation regimens in pediatric patients, specifically in relation to respiratory or cardiovascular complications. To our knowledge, there has not been a previous meta-analysis addressing this topic. A previous systematic review examined 10 studies (6 RCTs, 4 non-RCTs) looking at procedural sedation for GI endoscopy in children [24]. This systematic review concluded that propofol-based sedation was a safe option with low rates of major respiratory complications with the use of propofol and did not find a significant difference in adverse events compared to other sedative regimens [24]. However, since this study did not perform a meta-analysis and its conclusions were based on a review of heterogeneous studies, the overall safety was difficult to quantify.

Previous studies in the adult population have shown that propofol is an effective and safe agent to use for sedation in GI endoscopy procedures [25]. Most studies in children have centered around effectiveness, including which physician specialty is best suited to administer the sedation [26]. The efficacy of propofol as a sedative agent for endoscopy is well established, largely in part due to its rapid onset, short-acting nature, low cost, and decades of experience using it in adults. However, safety data on propofol in children undergoing endoscopy is lacking and concern has been raised due to its potential to induce respiratory depression

Table 1: Detail summarizing the 3 randomized controlled trials and 4 prospective studies included in the meta-analysis.

Study	Age	Procedure	Treatment arms	N	Dose	Adverse events (n) Bradycardia	Hypotension	Desaturation	Respiratory depression	Total airway
Singh et al., 1996 [17] Prospective cohort (abstract) $N = 100$	4–15	Endoscopy, colonoscopy	Propofol	50	3–3.5 mg/kg				2 (apnea)	
			Propofol + diazemul or pentazocine	50	Propofol 2.5–3 mg/kg, diazemul 2.5 mg, pentazocine 5 mg				2 (apnea)	
Barbi et al., 2003* [18] RCT (full text) $N = 122$	0.5–17	Upper GI	Propofol	60	n/a		27	8		
			Propofol + ketamine	62	n/a		17	9		
Paspatis et al., 2006** [19] RCT (full text) $N = 54$	3–17	Upper GI	Propofol	28	0.5 mg/kg repeat doses	4	1	6		
			Propofol + midazolam premed (PO)	26	Propofol: 0.5 mg/kg repeat doses (max 20 mg)	4	0	4		
Hammer et al., 2009 [20] Prospective cohort (full text) $N = 24$	3–10	EGD	Propofol	12	Avg: 2.8–4 mcg/ml	0	2		4	
			Propofol + dexmedetomidine	12	Dex: bolus (10 min) 1 mcg/kg; maintenance: 0.5 mcg/kg/hr; propofol: avg 2.8–4 mcg/ml	3	0		1	
Hasanin and Sira 2014 [21] RCT (full text) $N = 80$	1–14	Upper and lower endoscopy	Propofol	40	Bolus: 2 mg/kg; maintenance: 100 mcg/kg/min	0	0	6	0	
			Dexmedetomidine	40	Bolus: 2.5 mcg/kg; maintenance: 2 mg/kg/hr	0	0	0	0	
Garah et al., 2015 [22] Prospective cohort (full text) $N = 109$	1–18	Upper endoscopy, colonoscopy, both	Propofol	5						IPI 1 (IQR 6)
			Propofol + midazolam	89						IPI 7 (IQR 2)
			Propofol + midazolam fentanyl	15						IPI 7 (IQR 2)
Prunty et al., 2015 [23] Prospective cohort (abstract) $N = 212$	n/a	EGD	Propofol	83				3	0	33
			Propofol + glycopyrrolate + fentanyl + midazolam	129				15	2	17

EGD: esophagogastroduodenoscopy. *Definition of hypotension: mean arterial pressure (MAP) decrease of >20 mm hg; definition of desaturation: SpO2 < 92%. **Definition of bradycardia: 20% decrease in heart rate; definition of hypotension: MAP decrease > 10 mm hg; definition of desaturation: hypoxemia < 92% for 10 seconds.

TABLE 2: Condensed data set. Data was collapsed into the following categories from the raw data, Table 1, using the following criteria; cardiovascular depression included hypotension or bradycardia; respiratory depression included hypoxia, decreased respiratory rate, or apnea.

Study	Group	Cardiovascular depression (n)	Respiratory depression (n)
Singh et al., 1996	Propofol ($n = 50$)		2
	Propofol + diazemul or pentazocine ($n = 50$)		2
Barbi et al., 2003	Propofol ($n = 60$)	27	8
	Propofol + ketamine ($n = 62$)	17	9
Paspatis et al., 2006	Propofol ($n = 28$)	5	6
	Propofol + midazolam ($n = 26$)	4	4
Hammer et al., 2009	Propofol ($n = 12$)	2	4
	Propofol + dexmedetomidine ($n = 12$)	3	1
Hasanin and Sira, 2014	Propofol ($n = 40$)	0	6
	Dexmedetomidine ($n = 40$)	0	0
Prunty et al., 2015	Propofol ($n = 83$)		3
	Propofol + glycopyrrolate + fentanyl + midazolam ($n = 129$)		17

Study name	Odds ratio	Lower limit	Upper limit	Z Value	p Value
	Statistics for each study				
Hasanin and Sira, 2014	15.261	0.830	280.719	1.834	0.067
Paspatis et al., 2006	1.456	0.472	4.491	0.654	0.513
Barbi et al., 2003	1.944	0.946	3.996	1.809	0.070
Hammer et al., 2009	2.000	0.384	10.409	0.824	0.410
Prunty et al., 2015	0.247	0.070	0.871	−2.174	0.030
Singh et al., 1996	1.000	0.135	7.392	0.000	1.000
	1.314	0.569	3.036	0.640	0.522

Odds ratio and 95% CI

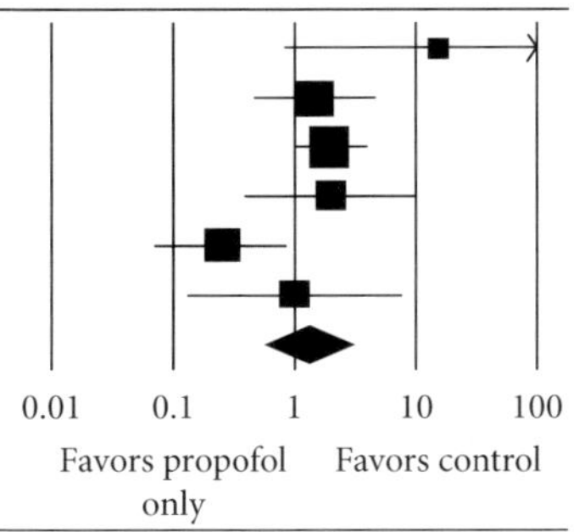

FIGURE 2: Comparison of total complications in children receiving propofol only versus other anesthetic regimens.

Study name	Odds ratio	Lower limit	Upper limit	Z Value	p Value
	Statistics for each study				
Hasanin and Sira, 2014	15.261	0.830	280.719	1.834	0.067
Paspatis et al., 2006	1.500	0.371	6.061	0.569	0.569
Barbi et al., 2003	0.918	0.344	2.445	−0.172	0.864
Hammer et al., 2009	5.500	0.513	59.014	1.408	0.159
Prunty et al., 2015	0.247	0.070	0.871	−2.174	0.030
Singh et al., 1996	1.000	0.135	7.392	0.000	1.000
	1.184	0.455	3.079	0.346	0.729

Odds ratio and 95% CI

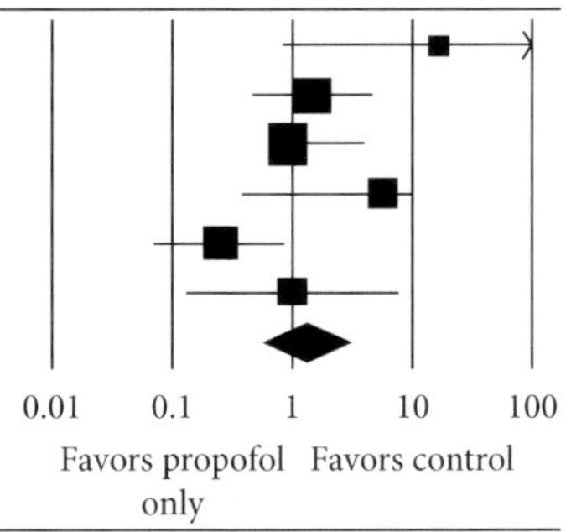

FIGURE 3: Comparison of respiratory complications in children receiving propofol versus under anesthetic regimens.

and cardiovascular instability [26]. A survey of pediatric gastroenterologists found that there is a wide variation in practice with respect to sedation for GI endoscopy in pediatric patients, and this included experience with propofol [27].

There have been several meta-analyses designed to answer this question in the adult population. Most recently, in 2017, Wadhwa et al. published a meta-analysis that compared propofol to other anesthetics for GI endoscopy in the

Study name	Statistics for each study: Odds ratio	Lower limit	Upper limit	*Z* Value	*p* Value
Paspatis et al., 2006	1.196	0.284	5.041	0.243	0.808
Barbi et al., 2003	2.166	1.018	4.608	2.006	0.045
Hammer et al., 2009	0.600	0.081	4.447	−0.500	0.617
	1.697	0.900	3.199	1.634	0.102

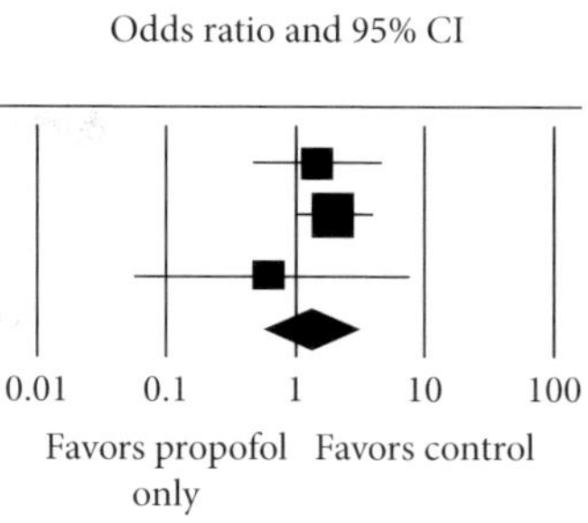

FIGURE 4: Comparison of cardiac complications in children receiving propofol versus under anesthetic regimens.

Study name	Statistics for each study: Odds ratio	Lower limit	Upper limit	*Z* Value	*p* Value
Hasanin and Sira, 2014	1.115	0.502	2.478	0.268	0.789
Paspatis et al., 2006	1.322	0.439	3.981	0.496	0.620
Barbi et al., 2003	1.192	0.393	3.611	0.310	0.757
Hammer et al., 2009	1.237	0.459	3.338	0.421	0.674
Prunty et al., 2015	1.867	1.090	3.198	2.272	0.023
Singh et al., 1996	1.382	0.527	3.625	0.658	0.511
	1.314	0.569	3.036	0.640	0.522

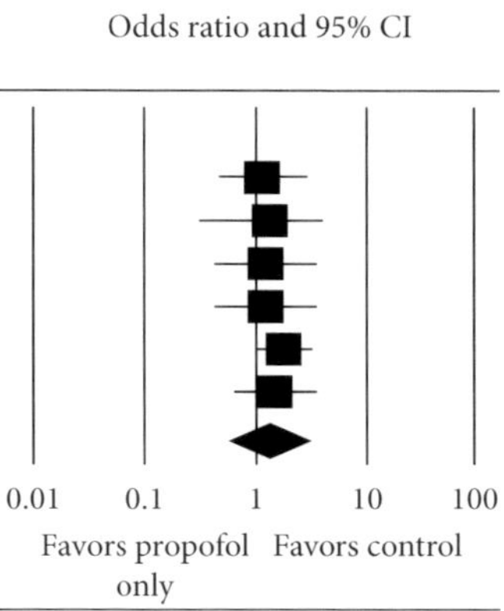

FIGURE 5: Sensitivity analysis with one study removed.

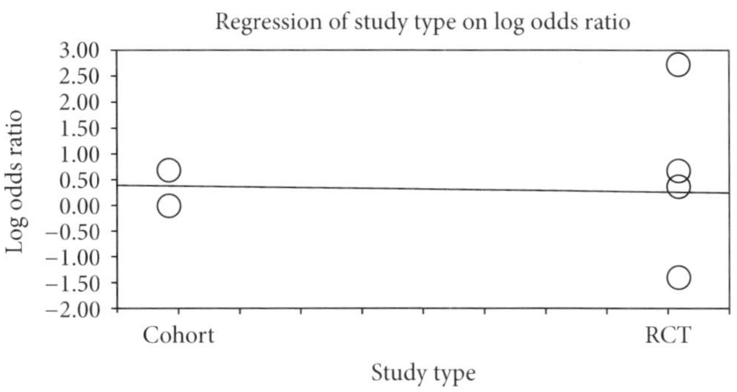

FIGURE 6: Plot of metaregression.

adult population [25]. The authors concluded that based on a meta-analysis of 27 original studies, there was no significant difference in cardiopulmonary adverse events between these two groups [25]. Notably, our meta-analysis showed that results differed in a pediatric population.

Our study has several strengths. It is the first meta-analysis done specifically on the pediatric population which attempts to answer an important question. We strictly included prospective studies, which minimized bias seen in previous observational studies. The focus of the analysis on overall cardiorespiratory complications is an important distinction from other complications due to their direct relationship to mortality. Furthermore, the meta-analysis also provided insights into the current state of evidence, including the need for standardized reporting of adverse outcomes during procedural sedation and the lack of publication bias being a significant factor in the study findings. Stratifying our studies based on the study design did not change our overall findings, which adds credibility and consistency to our overall findings as study design bias did not affect the results.

Several limitations were identified in this meta-analysis. First, very few studies exist that address the study question. Only a total of 6 studies were included and generated a pooled sample size of only 592 patients. The individual studies all had small sample sizes, the largest of which was Prunty et al. which included 212 patients [23]. As compared to a recent meta-analysis done in the adult population which included 27 studies totaling 2518 patients [25], we believe that the lack of studies and small sample size were in part due to the generally lower number of research studies done in pediatric populations which was the focus of our question.

Second, the quality of the studies identified in this meta-analysis was assessed using the GRADE criteria. We concluded that the quality of the RCTs and the prospective studies included ranked very low. The main reasons for the poor quality included unclear randomization protocols, lack of blinding, and lack of concealment of allocation.

Group by Cardiac or resp	Study name	Statistics for each study				
		Odds ratio	Lower limit	Upper limit	Z Value	p Value
c	Paspatis et al.,2006	1.196	0.284	5.041	0.243	0.808
c	Barbi et al., 2003	2.166	1.018	4.608	2.006	0.045
c	Hammer et al., 2009	0.600	0.081	4.447	-0.500	0.617
c		1.645	0.825	3.279	1.414	0.157
r	Hasanin and Sira, 2014	15.261	0.830	280.719	1.834	0.067
r	Paspatis et al., 2006	1.500	0.371	6.061	0.569	0.569
r	Barbi et al., 2003	0.918	0.344	2.445	-0.172	0.864
r	Hammer et al.,2009	5.500	0.513	59.014	1.408	0.159
r		1.000	0.135	7.392	0.000	1.000
r		1.461	0.710	3.008	1.029	0.303
r		1.555	0.944	2.560	1.734	0.083
Overall						

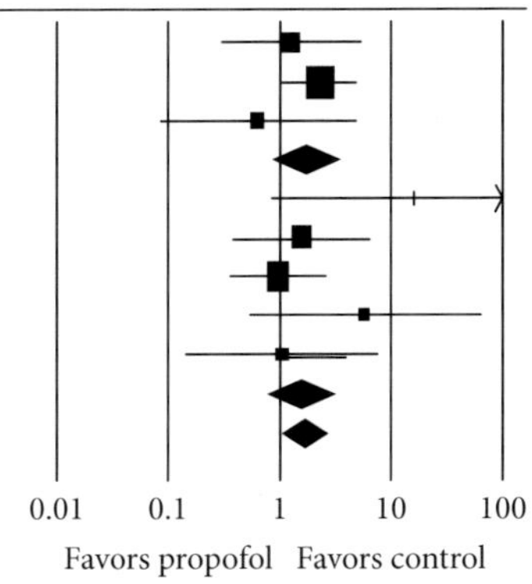

Figure 7: Subgroup analysis.

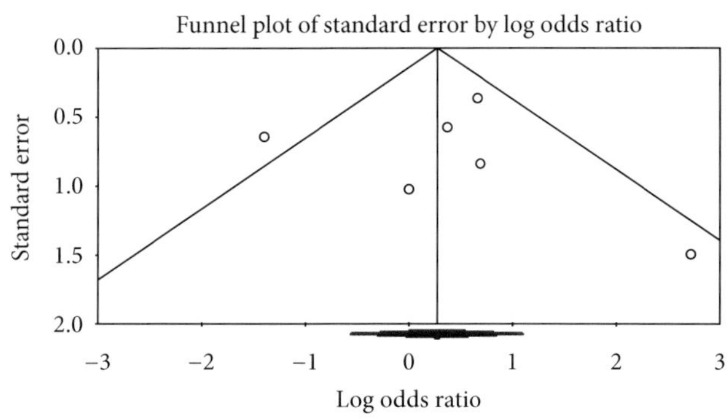

Figure 8: Funnel plot for publication bias.

Third, the other major weakness of this meta-analysis was heterogeneity. To address this issue, we performed the "one-study" removed analysis (removed Prunty et al.) and found that it significantly reduced the heterogeneity. A priori, we had a concern that the variation in comparison arm sedation regimens between studies was a large source for heterogeneity. Prunty et al. included four different sedative agents (propofol + glycopyrrolate + fentanyl + midazolam) in the comparison arm [23]. It is possible that combining multiple sedatives may in fact increase the risk of adverse events through an additive or synergistic mechanism. This also makes the study different from the rest, as the other comparison arms consist of only one or two sedative agents. Therefore, we opted to present results of the "one-study" removed analysis excluding Prunty et al. With this study excluded, there was a statistically significant increase in combined cardiovascular and respiratory adverse events using propofol only. It is important to note however that while I^2 became 0% with this change, there are still differences between the studies and wide confidence intervals. We may not have the power to detect differences within studies. For example, we were interested in cardiovascular complications including hypotension. Only 4 studies [18–21] included hypotension as an adverse effect, and even between these studies, the outcome measure was defined differently. Barbi et al. defined hypotension as a drop in systolic blood pressure (SBP) over 20 mmHg [18], whereas Paspatis et al. defined it as a drop in SBP over 10 mmHg [19]. Given the inconsistencies in outcomes between the studies, the different outcome measures reported were grouped to create broader categories consisting of respiratory complications, cardiovascular complications, and combined to report total complications. Similarly, procedural details differed between studies; one notable example was by the type of endoscopy. The majority of studies included upper GI endoscopy, but one included lower GI endoscopy as well [21]. These results were not presented separately; therefore, we could not perform metaregression based on the procedure type. As well, patient details including the reason for undergoing endoscopy and comorbid conditions were not clearly reported and may have influenced complication rates. Finally, the sedation regimen varied within the comparison arm between studies. Of the 5 studies included in the "one-study" removed analysis, 4 studies contained a propofol + additional sedative comparison arm consisting of propofol + dexmedetomidine [20], midazolam + propofol [19], ketamine + propofol [18], and diazemul or pentazocine + propofol [17]. Only one study did not contain propofol in the comparison arm, instead of using dexmedetomidine as the comparator [21]. It is therefore important to interpret our results in the context of these studies. We are unable to draw a conclusion regarding an ideal sedative regime; however, there may be an increase in total cardiorespiratory complications when using propofol only.

6. Conclusion

Our meta-analysis found a significant difference in combined cardiorespiratory adverse events when propofol-only sedation was used for pediatric patients undergoing endoscopy compared to other sedation regimens. The odds of combined adverse events was higher in pediatric patients who received propofol only for sedation during GI endoscopy (OR 1.87, 95% CI 1.09–3.20). This is not in keeping with prior studies

Table 3: Overall quality assessment, on basis of the Grading of Recommendations Assessment, Development, and Evaluation (GRADE) criteria.

Study	Starting level of evidence	Reasons for decreasing the level of evidence					Reasons to increase level of evidence (strong association, plausible confounding, and bias adjustment)	Final level of evidence
		Risk of bias	Inconsistency	Indirectness	Imprecision	Publication bias		
Randomized trials—3	High	↓	↓	↔	↓	↔	↔	Very Low
Observational trials—4	Low	↓	↔	↔	↓	↔	↔	Very low

or with a recent meta-analysis done in the adult population. This meta-analysis was designed to specifically examine cardiorespiratory adverse events. It did not address the efficacy of propofol compared to other sedation regimens. We would recommend that the findings from this meta-analysis be taken in conjunction with data on efficacy in order to best guide clinical practice.

There were multiple limitations encountered in this study, including very low-quality evidence; therefore, we believe further higher quality evidence is needed. We recommend a well-designed, large study focusing on well-defined safety outcome measures to convincingly answer our study question. A large multicenter prospective cohort study where patients undergoing different sedation regimens were observed and recorded would be the most feasible and practical way to definitively answer this question. Until then, health care providers providing sedation to children should consider the possibility of increased risk in total complications and weigh this against possible benefits in using propofol only.

References

[1] J. L. Koh, D. D. Black, I. K. Leatherman, R. D. Harrison, and M. L. Schmitz, "Experience with an anesthesiologist interventional model for endoscopy in a pediatric hospital," *Journal of Pediatric Gastroenterology and Nutrition*, vol. 33, no. 3, pp. 314–318, 2001.

[2] R. L. Claar, L. S. Walker, and J. A. Barnard, "Children's knowledge, anticipatory anxiety, procedural distress, and recall of esophagogastroduodenoscopy," *Journal of Pediatric Gastroenterology and Nutrition*, vol. 34, no. 1, pp. 68–72, 2002.

[3] S. Amornyotin, P. Aanpreung, U. Prakarnrattana, W. Chalayonnavin, S. Chatchawankitkul, and W. Srikureja, "Experience of intravenous sedation for pediatric gastrointestinal endoscopy in a large tertiary referral center in a developing country," *Pediatric Anesthesia*, vol. 19, no. 8, pp. 784–791, 2009.

[4] Scottish Intercollegiate Guidelines Network, "SIGN guideline 58: safe sedation of children undergoing diagnostic and therapeutic procedures," *Pediatric Anesthesia*, vol. 18, no. 1, pp. 11-12, 2008.

[5] P. L. Bailey, N. L. Pace, M. A. Ashburn, J. W. B. Moll, K. A. East, and T. H. Stanley, "Frequent hypoxemia and apnea after sedation with midazolam and fentanyl," *Anesthesiology*, vol. 73, no. 5, pp. 826–830, 1990.

[6] ASA Task Force on Sedation and Analgesia by Non-Anesthesiologists, "Practice guidelines for sedation and analgesia by non-anesthesiologists," *Anesthesiology*, vol. 96, pp. 1004–1017, 2002.

[7] H. M. Bryson, B. R. Fulton, and D. Faulds, "Propofol: an update of its use in anaesthesia and conscious sedation," *Drugs*, vol. 50, no. 3, pp. 513–559, 1995.

[8] M. D. Reed, T. S. Yamashita, C. M. Marx, C. M. Myers, and J. L. Blumer, "A pharmacokinetically based propofol dosing strategy for sedation of the critically ill, mechanically ventilated pediatric patient," *Critical Care Medicine*, vol. 24, no. 9, pp. 1473–1481, 1996.

[9] S. J. Hunter and C. A. B. McLaren, "Propofol for inpatient dental anaesthesia. A comparison of propofol as sole anaesthetic agent with thiopentone and halothane for inpatient dental anaesthesia," *Anesthesia*, vol. 43, no. s1, pp. 81–84, 1988.

[10] R. S. Hannallah, J. T. Britton, P. G. Schafer, R. I. Patel, and J. M. Norden, "Propofol anaesthesia in paediatric ambulatory patients: a comparison with thiopentone and halothane," *Canadian Journal of Anesthesia*, vol. 41, no. 1, pp. 12–18, 1994.

[11] S. Barst, A. Markowitz, Y. Yossefy, A. Abramson, P. Lebowitz, and R. Bienkowski, "Propofol reduces the incidence of vomiting after tonsillectomy in children," *Pediatric Anesthesia*, vol. 5, no. 4, pp. 249–252, 1995.

[12] J. L. Apfelbaum, T. H. Grasela, C. C. Hug Jr. et al., "The initial clinical experience of 1819 physicians in maintaining anesthesia with propofol: characteristics associated with prolonged time to awakening," *Anesthesia and Analgesia*, vol. 77, Supplement 4, pp. 510–514, 1993.

[13] A. Dubois, E. Balatoni, J. P. Peeters, and M. Baudoux, "Use of propofol for sedation, and general anesthesia—what is best?," *Gastrointestinal Endoscopy*, vol. 41, pp. 173–175, 1995.

[14] A. Levatt, N. Colombo, E. M. Arosio et al., "Propofol anaesthesia in spontaneously breathing paediatric patients during magnetic resonance imaging," *Acta Anaesthesiologica Scandinavica*, vol. 40, no. 5, pp. 561–565, 1996.

[15] W. J. Moore and S. Underwood, "Propofol as sole agent for paediatric day-case dental surgery," *Anesthesia*, vol. 49, no. 9, pp. 811–813, 1994.

[16] R. H. McDowall, C. S. Scher, and S. M. Barst, "Total intravenous anesthesia for children undergoing brief diagnostic or therapeutic procedures," *Journal of Clinical Anesthesia*, vol. 7, no. 4, pp. 273–280, 1995.

[17] R. K. A. Singh, H. K. Galhotra, and A. S. Raj Kumar, "Propofol induction and maintenance of sedation for outpatient paediatric endoscopy," *Journal of Anaesthesiology Clinical Pharmacology*, vol. 12, no. 2, pp. 97–101, 1996.

[18] E. Barbi, F. Marchetti, T. Gerarduzzi et al., "Pretreatment with intravenous ketamine reduces propofol injection pain," *Paediatric Anaesthesia*, vol. 13, no. 9, pp. 764–768, 2003.

[19] G. A. Paspatis, I. Charoniti, M. Manolaraki et al., "Synergistic sedation with oral midazolam as a premedication and intravenous propofol versus intravenous propofol alone in upper gastrointestinal endoscopies in children," *Journal of Pediatric Gastroenterology and Nutrition*, vol. 43, no. 2, pp. 195–199, 2006.

[20] G. B. Hammer, W. J. Sam, M. I. Chen, B. Golianu, and D. R. Drover, "Determination of the pharmacodynamic interaction of propofol and dexmedetomidine during esophagogastroduodenoscopy in children," *Pediatric Anesthesia*, vol. 19, no. 2, pp. 138–144, 2009.

[21] A. S. Hasanin and A. M. Sira, "Dexmedetomidine versus propofol for sedation during gastrointestinal endoscopy in pediatric patients," *Egyptian Journal of Anaesthesia*, vol. 30, no. 1, pp. 21–26, 2014.

[22] J. Garah, O. E. Adiv, I. Rosen, and R. Shaoul, "The value of integrated pulmonary index (IPI) monitoring during endoscopies in children," *Journal of Clinical Monitoring and Computing*, vol. 29, no. 6, pp. 773–778, 2015.

[23] M. Prunty, P. Wankum, E. Birisci, J. Anderson, and A. Dalabih, "375: decreased airway complications with glycopyrrolate prophylaxis for endoscopy: a prospective trial," *Critical Care Medicine*, vol. 43, no. 12, p. 95, 2015.

[24] E. J. A. H. Van Beek and P. L. J. M. Leroy, "Safe and effective procedural sedation for gastrointestinal endoscopy in children," *Journal of Pediatric Gastroenterology and Nutrition*, vol. 54, no. 2, pp. 171–185, 2012.

[25] V. Wadhwa, D. Issa, S. Garg, R. Lopez, M. R. Sanaka, and J. J. Vargo, "Similar risk of cardiopulmonary adverse events between propofol and traditional anesthesia for gastrointestinal endoscopy: a systematic review and meta-analysis," *Clinical Gastroenterology and Hepatology*, vol. 15, no. 2, pp. 194–206, 2017.

[26] M. E. Fredette and J. R. Lightdale, "Endoscopic sedation in pediatric practice," *Gastrointestinal Endoscopy Clinics of North America*, vol. 18, no. 4, pp. 739–751, 2008.

[27] J. R. Lightdale, L. B. Mahoney, S. M. Schwarz, and C. A. Liacouras, "Methods of sedation in pediatric endoscopy: a survey of NASPGHAN members," *Journal of Pediatric Gastroenterology and Nutrition*, vol. 45, no. 4, pp. 500–502, 2007.

15

Development and Validation of the Coeliac Disease Food Attitudes and Behaviours Scale

Rose-Marie Satherley,[1] **Ruth Howard**,[2] **and Suzanne Higgs**[2]

[1]*School of Populations Sciences and Health Services Research, Guy's Campus, King's College London, 5th Floor Addison House, London SE1 1UL, UK*
[2]*School of Psychology, University of Birmingham, 52 Pritchatts Road, Edgbaston, Birmingham B15 2SB, UK*

Correspondence should be addressed to Rose-Marie Satherley; rose-marie.satherley@kcl.ac.uk

Academic Editor: Luca Elli

Objectives. Previous studies on coeliac disease suggest that attitudes towards the gluten-free diet may contribute to the development of disordered eating. This study describes the development and validation of the Coeliac Disease Food Attitudes and Behaviours scale (CD-FAB) to measure these behaviours in coeliac disease. *Research Methods and Procedures.* Focus groups were used to develop 33 potential questionnaire items. These items were reviewed by service users and then distributed online to 157 adults with coeliac disease. Items were removed based on ceiling/floor effects, high interitem correlations (>0.7) and factor analysis. 11 items were retained. Exploratory factor analysis was then conducted. The psychometric properties of the final version of the CD-FAB were assessed via using an online platform. *Results.* The CD-FAB had 11 items distributed across one factor assessing attitudes and behaviours towards food. These factors explained 44.1% of the variance in responding. The CD-FAB and its subscales had high internal consistency (Cronbach's alpha > 0.7) and psychometric validation indicated good convergent and discriminant validity. High scores on the CD-FAB are associated with psychological distress and an impaired quality of life. *Conclusions.* The CD-FAB is a reliable and valid measure of food attitudes and behaviours in coeliac disease. As a new disease-specific instrument, it may be a useful tool for evaluating food concerns in individuals with coeliac disease in a clinical setting and for further exploring the development of disordered eating patterns in coeliac disease. Further research is required to assess the full potential of the CD-FAB.

1. Introduction

Coeliac disease (CD) is managed by a strict, life-long gluten-free diet (GFD), which leads to improvement in the majority of CD-related symptoms [1]. However, following the GFD may harm some individuals' relationship with food, increasing the risk of disordered eating [2]. Disordered eating describes a spectrum of eating behaviours, ranging from clinical eating disorders, including anorexia and bulimia nervosa [3], to skipping meals and restricting certain foods [4].

A two-pathway model of disordered eating has been used to understand disordered eating attitudes and behaviours in CD [2]. The first pathway describes those who experience distress around weight change associated with diagnosis that triggers disordered eating attitudes and behaviours. The second pathway describes a hypervigilance around food that triggers disordered eating attitudes and behaviours. Case studies of comorbid CD and disordered eating, although limited by small sample sizes, are concordant with systematic studies suggesting that 22–29% of individuals with CD score above clinical cut-offs for disordered eating [5–7]. However, evidence for clinically diagnosed eating disorders is mixed. Evidence from Sweden and the UK had demonstrated an increased risk of anorexia nervosa in CD [8, 9], whereas Babio et al. [10] found no greater risk for eating disorder in individuals with CD when compared to healthy controls.

Following the GFD requires vigilance around food and knowledge of food preparation and so current disordered eating measures may incorrectly classify behaviours essential for the management of CD as disordered. The binge eating scale (BES) [11] and the Eating Attitudes Test (EAT-26) [12] have been used to identify disordered eating CD [6]. However, some individuals with CD who score below the clinical cut-off on these measures describe apparent disordered eating attitudes and behaviours, with a cognitive focus on fears about cross-contamination and food safety [13]. Although control around food is essential for those following a GFD, these beliefs about food may result in disordered eating attitudes and behaviours [13]. To better understand how these beliefs develop from adaptive coping mechanisms to disordered attitudes and behaviours, they must be measureable in CD.

This article reports the development of a CD Food Attitudes and Behaviours Scale (CD-FAB) to identify disordered eating attitudes and behaviours resulting from beliefs around cross-contamination and food safety, including the psychometric properties comprising subscale structure, reliability and validity, and psychosocial correlates.

2. Methods

A mixed methods approach using three studies was used to develop the CD-FAB (Figure 1).

3. Study 1: Item Generation

Online focus groups, moderated by the first author, were used to generate CD-FAB items. Individuals with a self-reported, biopsy-confirmed diagnosis of CD (18–69 years) were recruited from online forums. Individuals reporting CD diagnosis via blood test, physician report, or self-report, without intestinal biopsy, were excluded from the analyses. Interested individuals emailed the first author to complete a screening questionnaire and to confirm focus group attendance. Verbal consent, over the phone, and online consent was provided before attending the focus group. Participants experiencing other dietary-controlled conditions (e.g., cystic fibrosis and diabetes mellitus) or food allergies were excluded.

Eight open-ended questions were designed to answer the key questions of the study: (1) the construct of food attitudes in CD and (2) the everyday interactions with food in CD. The five stages in the two-pathway model of disordered eating in gastrointestinal disease (diagnosis of CD, adaptation to diagnosis, illness beliefs, dietary management, and eating patterns) were used to frame questions [2]. Closure of the focus group was based on data saturation, by repeatedly comparing data across participants, which occurred when no new information was obtained from the focus group.

3.1. Data Analysis. Thematic analysis identified key themes related to food attitudes, concerns, and eating behaviours [14]. The first author (experienced in qualitative analysis and under the supervision of experienced academics) read through the transcripts noting initial thoughts; transcripts were reread allowing data immersion. Subsequently, the coding phase began. Codes identified characteristics related to food attitudes, concerns, and eating behaviours; similar codes were grouped, creating themes. Emerging themes were used to develop items for the CD-FAB. Each item was transformed into a 7-point Likert scale (strongly agree to strongly disagree). Questions were phrased so that higher scores indicated greater food concerns; four items were reverse scored to minimise response bias. Individuals from the focus group rated the 33 pilot items on clarity, adequacy, and relevance to the focus group discussion. Three service users with CD, recruited via email from the Birmingham Coeliac UK committee who did not take part in the focus groups, commented on the clarity, adequacy, and relevance of the questions. These questions were rated on a 5-point scale (1: strongly agree to 5: strongly disagree); those items that consistently scored low were removed.

4. Results of Item Generation

Twelve individuals took part in the focus group (10 females, mean age = 29.1 years, SD = 8.16; mean time since diagnosis = 6.2 years, SD = 4.69). Three had a CD diagnosis for over 10 years (see Table 1).

4.1. Thematic Analysis. Four themes were identified: *handling of food*, *trust*, *risk-taking*, and *food safety*. *Handling of food* refers to feelings around gluten-containing products, including preparing gluten-containing food for others, having gluten in the home, and touching gluten-containing foods. Some participants said that they would prepare gluten-containing foods for others and had no concerns being around gluten, as long as they did not consume gluten. Other participants described a fear around food that was attributed to their need to be vigilant about food content; gluten was not allowed in the home and feelings of anxiety increased when they were in close proximity to gluten. "*I get concerned in supermarkets when the gluten-free bread is next to the normal bread. I know they're all wrapped up but it scares me*" *(Ashley).*

The second theme, *trust*, described the need for control during food preparation, especially where others were involved. Concerns stemmed from the belief that others may not be vigilant around cross-contamination. To reduce concerns around eating food prepared by others, trust in the individual preparing food was needed. "*I don't let him prepare my food. I like to be in control of my food, I can't trust others to do it*" *Charlie).* Clem described the impact of trust on the ability to eat outside the home "*Going out for a meal I always have to double check. If they (the restaurant) sound unsure I won't go. I need to trust them*" *(Clem).*

Risk-taking reflects the ability to consume foods in new environments. Twelve participants indicated that an element of risk was necessary to live a normal life. A lack of risk-taking led to isolation from events involving food. "*I have to take small risks if I want to have a normal life!*" *(Jamie).*

Food safety describes the eating strategies employed to manage food concerns. Although most participants were willing to try new gluten-free foods, some viewed food as the enemy. These individuals experienced anxiety around food and felt safer not eating. A limited range of food was

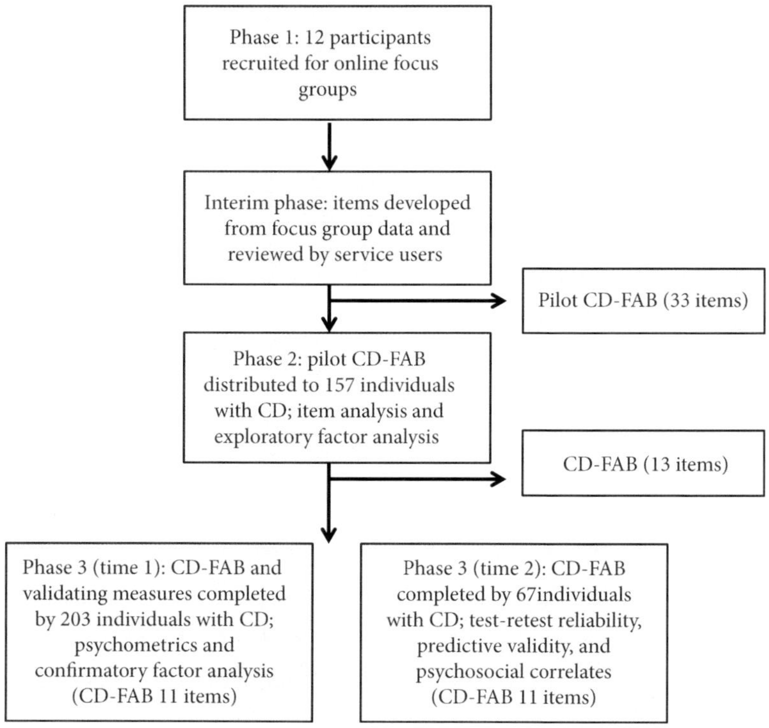

FIGURE 1: Flow chart of the CD-FAB development and validation process.

TABLE 1: Participant characteristics for focus groups (study 1: item generation).

Pseudonym	Gender	Age (years)	Years since diagnosis
Alex	Male	36	1
Ari	Female	23	4
Ashley	Female	19	2
Charlie	Female	26	3
Clem	Female	47	2
Eddie	Female	28	3
Frances	Female	24	13
Jamie	Female	31	12
Sam	Female	29	4
Sean	Female	27	7
Tyler	Male	20	9
Wren	Female	39	14

consumed, or long periods of food restriction to promote safety and prevent gastrointestinal symptoms were reported. *"I cope with my fear of getting glutened by not eating." (Ashley).* These attitudes were related to the participant's ability to recall their symptoms and adverse food experiences prior to diagnosis. *"I don't go to restaurants. They remind me of being ill. I didn't like that, so I don't eat much" (Alex).*

4.2. Item Development. The identified themes were used to generate 33 items for the CD-FAB. After the review, 13 items were reworded and 3 items were removed to create the 30 items in the pilot CD-FAB to be used in study two.

5. Study 2: Item Analysis and Exploratory Factor Analysis

Study two identified items for the final scale. The pilot CD-FAB was distributed to a new sample of people with CD recruited from our research database (November–December 2015). This database consists of 157 adults (18–69 years) with self-reported biopsy confirmed diagnosis of CD, recruited from online forums, who had previously volunteered to take part in research. As in study 1, individuals reporting CD diagnosis via blood test, physician report, or self-report, without intestinal biopsy, were excluded from the analyses. All 157 individuals were approached and directed to an online questionnaire, which included demographic information (age and years with diagnosis) and the pilot CD-FAB.

5.1. Data Analysis. Only items that contributed to the questionnaire's explanatory power were retained (see Table 2 for removal criteria) [15]. One theoretically relevant item was retained due to its salience during the focus group, *"I am afraid to touch gluten-containing foods,"* despite the removal criteria.

Principle component analysis with orthogonal rotation was used to identify loading patterns within the CD-FAB. The scree plot and factor eigenvalues > 1 identified the most appropriate factor solution.

6. Results of Item Analysis and Exploratory Factor Analysis

One hundred and two individuals (96 females) completed the pilot stage (mean age = 8.6 years; SD = 16.73; 9.6 years with

TABLE 2: Removal criteria for CD-FAB items.

Spread of responses across options	High endorsement of a single item suggests poor discriminatory power. Items were considered for removal if >80% or <20% were an agree-type statement or a disagree-type statement	16 removed
Internal consistency	Items with a corrected item-domain total correlation < 0.3 or in a domain with a poor Cronbach's alpha < 0.7 were considered for removal	1 removed
Timing of administration of questionnaire	Needs to be applicable to people from the point of coeliac disease diagnosis onwards, so all individuals with coeliac disease can complete the scale	2 reworded
Clarity and relevance of items	Difficult to understand items were reworded or considered for removal	13 reworded
Items deemed theoretically important	These items were retained despite meeting the above criteria because they were deemed theoretically important	1 retained

TABLE 3: Factor loadings for CD-FAB items.

	Item number	Factor loading
Cronbach's alpha for scale		
I am afraid to eat outside my home	2	0.78
I am comfortable eating gluten-free food from other people's kitchens*	11	0.77
I am afraid to touch gluten-containing foods	3	0.75
I get concerned being near others when they are eating gluten	1	0.73
My concerns about cross-contamination prevent me from going to social events involving food	8	0.71
I get worried when eating with strangers	5	0.70
I enjoy going out for meals as much as I did before my diagnosis*	10	0.69
Being contaminated by gluten in the past has not stopped me from enjoying restaurants*	12	0.69
I will only eat food that I have prepared myself	7	0.65
If I ask questions, I can normally find gluten-free food to eat*	13	0.64
I will happily prepare gluten for others	9	0.58
I find it hard to eat gluten-free foods that look like the gluten-containing foods that have made me ill in the past	6	0.45
I have a lack of variety in my diet	4	0.35

* represents items that are reverse scored. Numerical values represent factor loadings.

CD diagnosis; SD = 18.24; response rate = 65%). Twelve were excluded, as they did not report a biopsy-confirmed diagnosis of CD.

6.1. Content and Internal Reliability. The CD-FAB was reduced from 30 to 13 items based on the criteria described in Table 1. The Cronbach's alpha for the overall scale was acceptable (0.89).

6.2. Exploratory Factor Analysis. The Kaiser-Meyer-Olkin and Bartlett's test of sphericity assumptions were met. A three-factor solution was extracted. Given the high intercorrelations among the three factors, a stricter eigenvalue of 2 was used, producing a one-factor solution explaining 44.1% of the variance (Table 3).

7. Study 3: Confirmatory Factor Analysis, Psychometrics, and Psychosocial Correlates

Study three assessed the feasibility, reliability, and psychometric properties of the CD-FAB and validated the underlying factor structure. The psychosocial correlates of the CD-FAB were also explored (see Table 4 for CD-FAB).

Recruitment posters in food outlets across the University of Birmingham, UK, directed interested individuals to an online survey (January–March 2016). Individuals were asked not to complete the questionnaire if they had completed study one. All participants who completed the questionnaire (time 1) were invited to complete the CD-FAB and items assessing predictive validity four weeks later (time 2). Online questionnaires to assess the psychosocial correlates were distributed at time 2 with the CD-FAB. Two hundred individuals with self-reported, biopsy-confirmed CD were targeted, as this is a sufficient sample size for confirmatory factor analysis (CFA) [16]. The inclusion/exclusion criteria were as described in study one.

7.1. Data Analysis. Floor and ceiling effects determined feasibility of the CD-FAB score; these were considered when more than 15% of respondents achieved the lowest/highest possible score.

TABLE 4: The Coeliac Disease Food Attitudes and Behaviours scale (CD-FAB). Instructions: this questionnaire is designed to explore food attitudes and beliefs in coeliac disease. Some questions may not apply to you; this is because we are trying to assess a range of beliefs about coeliac disease and managing the gluten-free diet. Please fill out the form below as accurately, honestly, and completely as possible. There are no right or wrong answers. All of your responses are confidential. Please tick the box that best describes your response to the question.

	Strongly agree (7)	Agree (6)	Somewhat agree (5)	Neither agree nor disagree (4)	Somewhat disagree (3)	Disagree (2)	Strongly disagree (1)
Because of my coeliac disease...							
I get concerned being near others when they are eating gluten							
I am afraid to eat outside my home							
I am afraid to touch gluten-containing foods							
I get worried when eating with strangers							
I find it hard to eat gluten-free foods that look like the gluten-containing foods that have made me ill in the past							
I will only eat food that I have prepared myself							
My concerns about cross-contamination prevent me from going to social events involving food							
Despite having coeliac disease...							
I enjoy going out for meals as much as I did before my diagnosis*							
I am comfortable eating gluten-free food from other people's kitchens*							
Being contaminated by gluten in the past has not stopped me from enjoying restaurants*							
If I ask questions, I can normally find gluten-free food to eat*							

Reverse items with * and add all scores to make total score.

CFA was used to confirm the one factor model found in study two, based on the goodness fit and assessed using several indices: the comparative fit index (CFI; >0.95 indicates acceptable fit), Tucker-Lewis index (TLI; >0.95 indicates acceptable fit), and root mean square errors of approximation (RMSEA; <0.08 indicates acceptable fit) [17]. Modification indices determined changes made to improve model fit. CD-FAB scores were calculated by summing the responses on each item. CD-FAB scores ranged between 13 and 91, with higher scores indicating greater CD-related food concerns and compensatory behaviours.

Correlation coefficients were used to assess test-retest reliability of the CD-FAB scores; for 50 participants, a correlation coefficient > 0.7 is indicative of strong reliability [18].

Psychosocial correlates were explored by applying a tertiary split to CD-FAB scores, dividing individuals into high, medium, and low scorers based on the 33rd and 66th percentiles. Analysis of variance was used to compare psychosocial outcomes across the three groups, and *t*-tests were used to compare the means across the low and high scorers on the CD-FAB.

7.2. Measures

7.2.1. Food Neophobia Scale (FNS) [19]. Convergent validity was assessed using the FNS, as this has previously been used to assess food anxieties in CD[6]. The FNS measures willingness to try new food, with lower scores indicating a greater willingness to try new foods. The scale consists of 10 items and is the standard measure of food nephobia [19]. Correlations were sought to determine the degree to which the CD-FAB score reflected a fear of trying new foods. We anticipated a moderately positive relationship between total CD-FAB score and FNS scores, as individuals with high CD-FAB scores may also be fearful of trying new foods.

7.2.2. Depression, Anxiety, Stress Scale 21 (DASS-21) [20]. The *Anxiety* subscale from the DASS-21 was used to assess convergent validity. This subscale measures behavioural feelings of anxiety over the last four weeks with higher scores indicating greater anxiety. The DASS-21 has strong psychometric properties; with higher scores indicating greater anxiety [21]. To demonstrate convergent validity, total scores on the CD-FAB should correlate with scores on the *Anxiety* subscale. At time 2, all subscales of the DASS-21 were distributed to explore the relationship between CD-FAB scores, depression, anxiety, and stress.

7.2.3. CD Quality of Life Scale (CD-QoL) [22]. The *Treatment* subscale was used to assess discriminative validity. This subscale assesses satisfaction with one's treatment (the GFD). No relationship between these scores was anticipated. At time 2, all subscales of the CD-QoL were distributed to explore the relationship between CD-FAB scores and quality of life.

7.2.4. Behavioural Item. Known groups discriminant validity was assessed using the behavioural item, *"Do you consider yourself to be anxious around food?"* This item was rated yes/no. A further behavioural item "*How many times have you eaten outside the home over the last month?*" was assessed at time 2, to assess predictive validity. We anticipated that individuals scoring high on the total CD-FAB score at time 1 would eat outside the home less than those with lower CD-FAB scores at time 2.

7.2.5. Gluten-Free Management. Gluten-free dietary management was rated on a 5-point Likert scale, in response to the question *"In general, how strictly do you maintain a gluten-free diet?" ranging from '1) All of the time'; 2) 'Most of the time'; 3) 'Some of the time'; 4) 'Now and then'; 5) 'Not at all'* [23].

8. Results of Confirmatory Factor Analysis and Psychometrics

8.1. Participants at Time 1. 203 (35 males, 2 "other") participants took part in the validation stage with a mean age of 30.9 years (SD = 11.4) and 6.2 years with CD diagnosis (SD = 8.4). Nineteen participants were excluded as they reported a self-diagnosis and not a biopsy-proven diagnosis of CD. This sample was older than the participants recruited for study two (t (1, 285) = −4.21, $p < 0.001$). No difference was found in years since the diagnosis across the two samples (t (1, 286) = −1.81, $p = 0.072$). 56.1% of participants with CD reported following their GFD "*all of the time.*" Of the remainder, 1% were completely nonadherent, and 42.9% were partially adherent to the GFD.

8.2. Participants at Time 2. 112 of those recruited at time 1 consented to be contacted at time 2; of these, 67 completed the second questionnaire (54 females; mean age = 32.8, SD = 16.51; mean years with diagnosis = 7.5, SD = 11.42; response rate = 60%).

When comparing participant contact details to those recruited in study one, there was a 3% overlap across the samples. These individuals were removed from the analysis.

8.2.1. Reliability and Feasibility. Floor and ceiling effects ranged between 0.5 and 1%. The CD-FAB total score showed good internal consistency (Cronbach's alpha = 0.89).

8.2.2. Confirmatory Factor Analysis. All items loaded onto the total CD-FAB score (Figure 2). Figure 2 shows the structural equation model containing the standardised path estimates between the items and factors for the final model. Items 4 (*I have a lack of variety in my diet*) and 9 (*I will happily prepare gluten for others*) were removed from the model due to low factor loadings and improved model fit after removal. Despite item 6 (*I find it hard to eat gluten-free foods that look like the gluten-containing-foods that have made me ill in the past*) having a low factor loading (0.56), this item was retained, as removal did not improve model fit. Model fit could be improved by covarying the errors on items 1 and 3, 1 and 5, 7 and 8, and 10 and 12. The resulting model fit was acceptable (TLI = 0.95; CFI = 0.93; RMSEA = 0.08). The resulting CD-FAB contained 11 items with total scores ranging from 11 to 77 (Cronbach's alpha for 11-item CD-FAB remained at 0.89). These calculations were used in subsequent analyses.

8.3. Convergent Validity. Total CD-FAB positively correlated with the FNS ($r = .274, p < 0.001$) and the *Anxiety* subscale of the DASS-21 ($r = 0.188$, $p = 0.016$). Correlation coefficients were <0.7, indicating a weak relationship.

8.4. Discriminant Validity. Beliefs about the effectiveness of the GFD were not related to CD-FAB scores ($r = -0.002$, $p = 0.98$), indicating good discriminant validity.

8.5. Known Groups Validity. 37.2% of participants considered themselves to feel anxious around food. These individuals had significantly higher CD-FAB scores ($m = 48.2$, SD = 6.3) than those who were not anxious around food ($m = 40.6$, SD = 7.5, $p < 0.001$)

8.5.1. Predictive Validity. CD-FAB scores taken at time 1 were associated with responses to the item "*How many times have you eaten outside the home over the last month?*" taken at time 2 ($r = -0.37$, $p = 0.048$),

8.5.2. Test-Retest Reliability. Test-retest correlation coefficients between the total CD-FAB scores at time 1 and time 2 were strong ($r = 0.92$, $p < 0.001$).

8.5.3. Psychosocial Correlates. The top third of CD-FAB scores were associated with increased psychological distress and a more impaired quality of life when compared to low scores ($p < 0.01$). No significant differences were found between medium and high scorers (Table 5).

Low CD-FAB scorers were in the "normal" ranges for DASS-21, whereas the medium and high scorers were within the "mild" and "moderate" ranges [20]. No differences were found across age and BMI for CD-FAB scores.

9. General Discussion

The recent research has highlighted the association between disordered eating and CD [5–9]. Qualitative studies suggest that existing measures of disordered eating do not identify all atypical eating patterns reported in CD [13]. Beliefs around cross-contamination and food safety have been implicated in the development of disordered eating attitudes and behaviours in CD [13], but there are no tools to measure these factors. We developed and validated a self-report food attitudes and behaviours measure for adults with CD.

The CD-FAB set out to measure the four themes identified in focus groups, which explored underlying food attitudes, concerns, and eating behaviour themes (i.e., *handling of food, trust, risk-taking, and food safety*). One factor emerged but items targeting each of the themes were retained within this factor. This factor explained 44.1% of the variance in scores. High scores described greater concerns around food alongside avoidance and changes in the diet to cope with these concerns.

The CD-FAB has a high Cronbach's alpha (0.89), indicating strong psychometric properties and good predictive

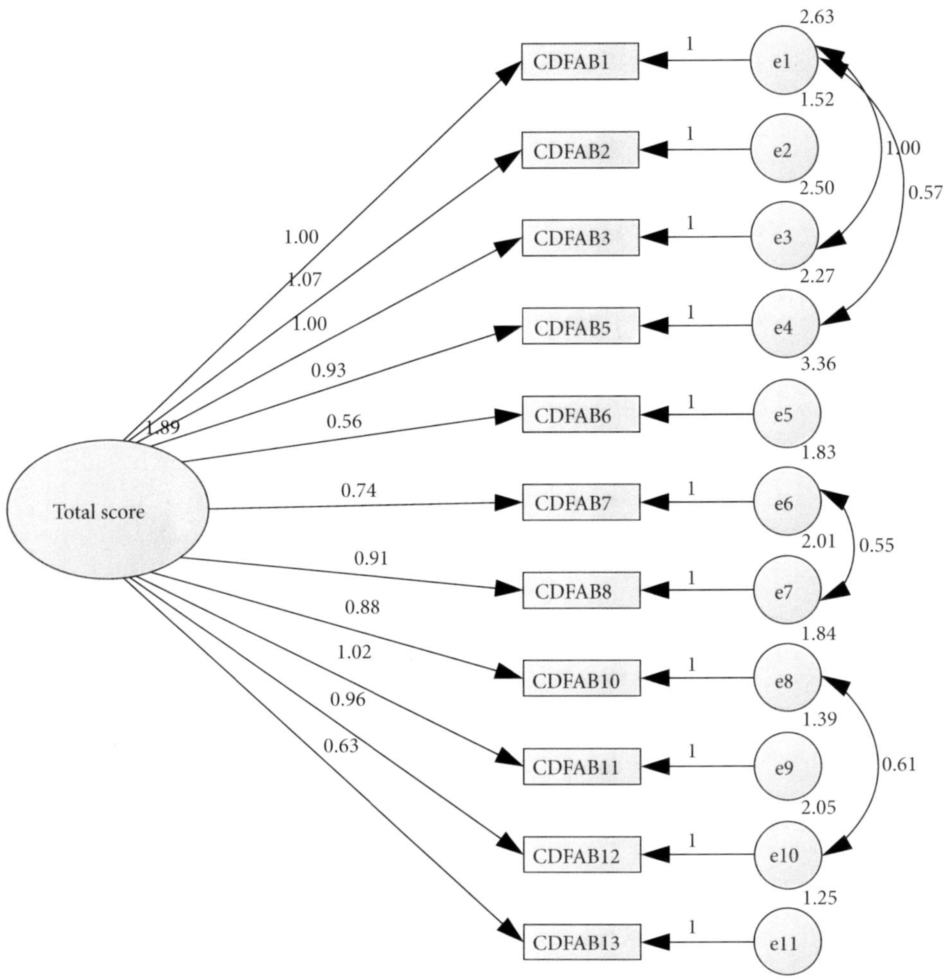

Figure 2: Confirmatory factor analysis with standardised item loadings onto the one CD-FAB factor. The numbers shown on the diagram from right to left are (1) covariance of the errors, (2) error terms (E), and (3) path coefficients of indicators.

validity. Test-retest reliability over 4 weeks was excellent. This may indicate that CD food attitudes and behaviours are a stable trait, supporting previous literature highlighting this issue [24]. Additionally, the CD-FAB has good discriminant validity, showing no correlation with the CD-QoL *Treatment* subscale. The direction and magnitude of the correlations between the CD-FAB and the FNS and *Anxiety* subscale of the DASS-21 were weak, indicating limited convergent validity. However, the use of the DASS-21 to assess trait anxiety may be problematic if the CD-FAB assessed situational concerns, future research should explore the use of a state measure of anxiety alongside the CD-FAB to further explore convergent validity claims of the CD-FAB. Individuals with high CD-FAB scores felt more socially limited and concerned about their CD and its health consequences compared to low scorers, suggesting high scores on the CD-FAB indicate impaired psychosocial well-being.

A strength of this study lies in the use of participant involvement to create the CD-FAB. This information alongside a priori themes, including a framework developed by Satherley, Howard, and Higgs [2], was used to make these items relevant to participant experiences. Constructs identified by respondents related to social settings, gastrointestinal symptoms, and eating behaviours are measured for the first time by the CD-FAB. Pertinent examples of this are that eating at social events is less enjoyable after a CD diagnosis as the GFD can lead to feelings of embarrassment, isolation, and a fear of gastrointestinal symptoms, [24] for some, this fear of symptoms and anxiety around food may lead to disordered eating attitudes and behaviours [13].

Despite the strengths of the current study, future research needs to examine long-term changes in CD-FAB scores, particularly during the first year of diagnosis, to explore typical and atypical adaptation to CD and the GFD. The high dropout rate between time 1 and time 2 completion of the CD-FAB is a further limitation of this study. Given this high dropout, future investigations should consider recruiting a larger subject population for follow-up analyses. Furthermore, participants in the developmental stages of the CD-FAB were predominantly female, which reflects the higher prevalence of both eating concerns and CD in females [25, 26]. However, further validation of the CD-FAB should reflect a better balance between males and females. Additionally, despite the exclusion of participants who did not report a biopsy confirmation of their CD

Table 5: Demographic and psychosocial outcomes using the tertiary split on the CD-FAB. Data are presented as means.

	Low scorers	Medium scorers	High scorers	F statistic
Demographic outcomes				
Age (years)	32.3	29.0	29.0	1.75
BMI	22.6	22.7	21.9	0.29
Psychosocial outcomes				
Depression	8.6	13.5^{a}	13.5^{b}	3.81^{*}
Anxiety	6.6	10.1^{a}	11.6^{b}	4.34^{*}
Stress	11.6	16.9^{a}	15.8^{b}	4.13^{*}
Total DASS-21	26.7	40.5^{a}	40.9^{b}	5.3^{*}
FNS	27.4	31.3	33.9^{b}	10.7^{**}
Total quality of life	71.1	57.9^{aa}	53.6^{bb}	16.03^{**}
Limitations	31.4	24.4^{aa}	21.9^{bb}	17.32^{**}
Health	17.1	13.6^{aa}	12.4^{bb}	10.92^{**}
Treatment	5.5	5.5	5.5	0.032
Dysphoria	17.1	14.6^{a}	14.2^{bb}	7.12^{**}

$^{*}p = 0.05$; $^{**}p < 0.001$ for ANOVA across all three groups; $^{a}p = 0.05$; $^{aa}p < 0.001$ for t-test across low and medium scorers; $^{b}p = 0.05$; $^{bb}p < 0.001$ for t-test across low and high CD-FAB scorers.

diagnosis throughout the procedures, self-report is not sufficient to ensure CD diagnosis. Given the confusion among CD diagnosis and symptomatic overlap with non-coeliac gluten sensitivity and irritable bowel syndrome, it is possible that individuals without a biopsy-confirmed diagnosis of CD could have been included in these studies. Given this limitation, further validation is needed in a sample of biopsy-confirmed individuals with CD recruited from clinical settings.

Measurement of symptom severity needs to be conducted alongside further assessment of the CD-FAB to control for impact of symptom severity on associated behaviours, affect, and cognition. In addition, a more thorough assessment of GFD adherence and an exploration of eating disorder history would aid in further understanding scores on the CD-FAB. Finally, expert review was not used to assess content validity, but the involvement of service users with CD in generating the items and providing feedback on the overall CD-FAB provides evidence for content validity.

These limitations do not detract from the clinical utility of the CD-FAB. The instrument may be used as an outcome measure in clinical research, enabling a greater understanding of CD-related eating patterns that are not currently captured by current tools. There is a need to establish clinical cut-off points; further guidance regarding the interpretation of CD-FAB scores (e.g., referral to dietician, clinical psychologist, or specialist eating disorder service) can be given following the identification of population norms and health implications.

The CD-FAB is a brief, self-report questionnaire that shows good reliability and validity in measuring disordered eating attitudes and behaviours in CD. The measure may be a useful tool to help understand eating attitudes and behaviours in adults with CD.

Abbreviations

BES:	Binge eating scale
CD:	Coeliac disease
CD-FAB:	Coeliac Disease Food Attitudes and Behaviours scale
CD-QoL:	Coeliac disease quality of life scale
CFI:	Comparative fit index
DASS-21:	Depression anxiety stress scale
EAT-26:	Eating attitudes test
FNS:	Food Neophobia Scale
GFD:	Gluten-free diet
RMSEA:	Root mean square of errors approximation
TLI:	Tucker-Lewis index.

Ethical Approval

The Psychology Research Ethics Committee, University of Birmingham, UK, granted ethical approval (ERN_15-0370A). All work was conducted in accordance with the Declaration of Helsinki (1964), with individuals' understanding and consent.

Authors' Contributions

Rose-Marie Satherley collected and analysed data and wrote the initial draft. Suzanne Higgs and Ruth Howard reviewed analyses, advised on interpretation, and contributed to the final version of this article. Rose-Marie Satherley is the guarantor of this paper. All authors approved the final version of the manuscript.

References

[1] NICE, "Coeliac Disease: Recognition and assessment of disease," March 2016, http://www.nice.org.uk/nicemedia/pdf/cg061niceguideline.pdf.

[2] R. Satherley, R. Howard, and S. Higgs, "Disordered eating in gastrointestinal disorders," *Appetite*, vol. 84, pp. 240–250, 2014.

[3] American Psychiatric Association, *Diagnostic and Statistical Manual of Mental Disorders: DSM-5*, American Psychiatric Publishing, WA, USA, 5 edition, 2013.

[4] C. Grilo, *Eating and Weight Disorders*, Psychology Press, New York, NY, USA, 2006.

[5] D. Arigo, A. M. Anskis, and J. M. Smyth, "Psychiatric comorbidities in women with celiac disease," *Chronic Illness*, vol. 8, pp. 45–55, 2012.

[6] D. A. Leffler, M. Dennis, J. B. Edwards-George, and C. P. Kelly, "The interaction between eating disorders and celiac disease: an exploration of 10 cases," *European Journal of Gastroenterology & Hepatology*, vol. 19, no. 3, pp. 251–255, 2007.

[7] R. Satherley, R. Howard, and S. Higgs, "The prevalence and predictors of disordered eating in women with coeliac disease," *Appetite*, vol. 107, pp. 260–267, 2016.

[8] A. Karwautz, G. Wagner, G. Berger, U. Sinnreich, V. Grylli, and W. D. Huber, "Eating pathology in adolescents with celiac disease," *Psychosomatics*, vol. 49, no. 5, pp. 399–406, 2008.

[9] C. J. Wotton, A. James, and M. J. Goldacre, "Coexistence of eating disorders and autoimmune diseases: record linkage cohort study, UK," *International Journal of Eating Disorders*, vol. 49, no. 7, pp. 663–672, 2016.

[10] K. Marild, K. Stordal, C. M. Bulik et al., "Celiac disease and anorexia nervosa: a nationwide study," *Pediatrics*, vol. 139, no. 5, article e20164367, 2017.

[11] N. Babio, M. Alcazar, G. Castillejo et al., "Risk of eating disorders in patients with celiac disease," *Journal of Pediatric Gastroenterology and Nutrition*, vol. 66, no. 1, pp. 53–57, 2018.

[12] J. Gormally, S. Black, S. Daston, and D. Rardin, "The assessment of binge eating severity among obese persons," *Addictive Behaviors*, vol. 7, no. 1, pp. 47–55, 1982.

[13] D. M. Garner, M. P. Olmsted, Y. Bohr, and P. E. Garfinkel, "The eating attitudes test: psychometric features and clinical correlates," *Psychological Medicine*, vol. 12, no. 4, pp. 871–878, 1982.

[14] R. Satherley, R. Howard, and S. Higgs, "Disordered eating patterns in coeliac disease: a framework analysis," *Journal of Human Nutrition and Dietetics*, vol. 30, no. 6, pp. 724–736, 2017.

[15] V. Braun and V. Clarke, "Using thematic analysis in psychology," *Qualitative Research in Psychology*, vol. 3, no. 2, pp. 77–101, 2006.

[16] J. P. Stevens, *Applied Multivariate Statistics for the Social Sciences*, Erlbaum, Hillsdale, NJ, USA, 2nd edition, 1992.

[17] P. Kline, *An Easy Guide to Factor Analysis*, Routledge, London, 1994.

[18] L. T. Hu and P. M. Bentler, "Cutoff criteria for fit indexes in covariance structure analysis: conventional criteria versus new alternatives," *Structural Equation Modelling*, vol. 6, no. 1, pp. 1–55, 1999.

[19] J. M. Bland and D. G. Altman, "Statistical methods for assessing agreement between two methods of clinical measurement," *The Lancet*, vol. 327, no. 8476, pp. 307–310, 1986.

[20] P. Pliner and K. Hobden, "Development of a scale to measure the trait of food neophobia in humans," *Appetite*, vol. 19, no. 2, pp. 105–120, 1992.

[21] S. H. Lovibond and P. F. Lovibond, *Manual for the Depression Anxiety Stress Scales*, Psychology Foundation, Sydney, 2nd edition, 1995.

[22] T. A. Brown, B. F. Chorpita, W. Korotitsch, and D. H. Barlow, "Psychometric properties of the Depression Anxiety Stress Scales (DASS) in clinical samples," *Behaviour Research and Therapy*, vol. 35, no. 1, pp. 79–89, 1997.

[23] S. D. Dorn, L. Hernandez, M. T. Minaya et al., "The development and validation of a new coeliac disease quality of life survey (CD-QOL)," *Alimentary Pharmacology and Therapeutics*, vol. 31, no. 6, pp. 666–675, 2010.

[24] S. Ford, R. Howard, and J. Oyebode, "Psychosocial aspects of coeliac disease: a cross-sectional survey of a UK population," *British Journal of Health Psychology*, vol. 17, no. 4, pp. 743–757, 2012.

[25] A. Sverker, G. Hensing, and C. Hallert, "'Controlled by food' – lived experiences of coeliac disease," *Journal of Human Nutrition and Dietetics*, vol. 18, no. 3, pp. 171–180, 2005.

[26] P. Sing, A. Arora, T. A. Strand et al., "Global prevalence of celiac disease: systematic review and meta-analysis," *Clinical Gastroenterology and Hepatology*, vol. 16, no. 6, pp. 823–836.e2, 2018.

16

Cellular Stress Responses and Gut Microbiota in Inflammatory Bowel Disease

Siyan "Stewart" Cao

Department of Medicine, University of California, San Francisco, San Francisco, CA 94143, USA

Correspondence should be addressed to Siyan "Stewart" Cao; siyan.cao@ucsf.edu

Academic Editor: Paul Enck

Progresses in the past two decades have greatly expanded our understanding of inflammatory bowel disease (IBD), an incurable disease with multifaceted and challenging clinical manifestations. The pathogenesis of IBD involves multiple processes on the cellular level, which include the stress response signaling such as endoplasmic reticulum (ER) stress, oxidative stress, and hypoxia. Under physiological conditions, the stress responses play key roles in cell survival, mucosal barrier integrity, and immunomodulation. However, they can also cause energy depletion, trigger cell death and tissue injury, promote inflammatory response, and drive the progression of clinical disease. In recent years, gut microflora has emerged as an essential pathogenic factor and therapeutic target for IBD. Altered compositional and metabolic profiles of gut microbiota, termed dysbiosis, are associated with IBD. Recent studies, although limited, have shed light on how ER stress, oxidative stress, and hypoxic stress interact with gut microorganisms, a potential source of stress in the microenvironment of gastrointestinal tract. Our knowledge of cellular stress responses in intestinal homeostasis as well as their cross-talks with gut microbiome will further our understanding of the pathogenesis of inflammatory bowel disease and probably open avenues for new therapies.

1. Introduction

Inflammatory bowel disease (IBD) affects more than 3.1 million people in the United States and 2.5 million in Europe and is increasing in incidence worldwide especially in regions such as Eastern and South Asia [1, 2]. IBD including Crohn's disease (CD) and ulcerative colitis (UC) are characterized by chronic intestinal inflammation as well as extraintestinal manifestations, which are likely triggered by a combination of genetic predispositions and environmental factors such as diet, infection, and medication use [3]. The complex pathophysiology of IBD involves multiple cell populations in the gastrointestinal tract and numerous signaling pathways from energy homeostasis to innate immune response. Cellular stress signaling, including endoplasmic reticulum (ER) stress, oxidative stress, and hypoxic stress, has been implicated in multiple human pathologies such as metabolic disease, neurodegenerative disease, cardiovascular disease, cancer, and autoimmune disease. Recent evidence suggests that stress signaling plays a key role in mucosal homeostasis in the gut. As an integral component of the gastrointestinal environment, the gut microbiome has been shown to promote intestinal health as a physiological stressor. Meanwhile, through complex interactions with the stress pathways in the host cells, these microorganisms may contribute to the pathogenesis of IBD by inducing cell death and differentiation, epithelial barrier breakdown, and inflammatory response. Recently, targeting cellular stress signaling and the gut microbiota have been proposed as new therapies for UC and CD. The understanding of both sides and the bridge between the two will likely spur the progresses in this arena.

2. Cellular Stress Signaling in Gastrointestinal Tract

2.1. ER Stress. Approximately one-third of all proteins synthesized in the cell travel across the ER where they are folded into their proper three-dimensional structures with post-translational modifications including disulfide bond formation, glycosylation, hydroxylation, and lipidation. Protein folding in the ER is subject to numerous insults such as increased mRNA translation, elevated demand of protein secretion, genetic mutations of client proteins, deficiency of ER chaperones or foldases, ER redox or calcium perturbations, bacterial and viral infection, ATP depletion, nutrient deficiency, and pharmacological and toxicological insults. The accumulation of unfolded or misfolded proteins in the ER lumen activates the unfolded protein response (UPR), which is signaled through three ER transmembrane proteins: inositol-requiring enzyme 1α (IRE1α), dsRNA-activated protein kinase-related ER protein kinase (PERK), and activating transcription factor 6α (ATF6α). All three transmembrane sensors are maintained in an inactive state through interaction between their ER luminal domains and the protein chaperone immunoglobulin heavy chain-binding protein (BiP). A recent study showed that the ER luminal cochaperone ERdj4/DNAJB9 is required for the complex formation between BiP and the luminal domain of IRE1a, thereby maintaining IRE1a in a monomeric, inactive state in the absence of ER stress [4]. Upon ER stress, accumulated unfolded/misfolded proteins in the ER lumen bind and sequester BiP, thereby triggering dissociation of BiP from IRE1α, PERK, and ATF6α [5–7]. All three branches of the UPR have been involved in intestinal mucosal homeostasis and the pathogenesis of IBD.

The most evolutionarily conserved ER stress transducer is IRE1α, which contains both endoribonuclease and kinase domains within its cytosolic region. During ER stress, IRE1α activates via dimerization and auto-transphosphorylation, which then leads to removal of a 26-nucleotide intron from the mRNA encoding an active and stable transcription factor XBP1s. The activity of XBP1s has been linked to cellular proteostasis by inducing the expression of various genes involved in ER protein translocation, protein folding and modification, quality-control mechanisms, biogenesis of the ER and Golgi compartments, and ER-associated protein degradation (ERAD) [5, 6]. In addition to the cleavage of *Xbp1* mRNA, IRE1α regulates the UPR, cell death and differentiation, and inflammation via regulated IRE1a-dependent decay (RIDD) of various mRNAs and miRNAs, which was recently shown to orchestrate the survival of conventional dendritic cell in the gut [8]. Furthermore, IRE1α also cross-talks with a number of other stress-related signaling pathways including autophagy, nuclear factor-κB (NF-κB), mitogen-activated protein (MAP) kinases, and the c-Jun N-terminal kinase (JNK) pathways [6].

The IRE1α-XBP1 pathway has been well known to play an essential role in immunity and inflammation. XBP1 is required for the differentiation of plasma cells, dendritic cells, $CD8^+$ T cells, and eosinophils, as well as the production of several cytokines in macrophages [9, 10]. XBP1 is one of the first UPR effectors to associate with IBD. Findings from both animal and human studies suggested an essential role of XBP1-mediated adaptive UPR signaling in the intestinal homeostasis. Loss of *Xbp1* in murine intestinal epithelial cells (IECs) hyperactivates IRE1α, which results in a NF-κB and JNK-dependent inflammatory response. A recent study showed that the selective autophagy receptor optineurin may interact with and target IRE1α for degradation, thereby containing IRE1a aggregation and hyperactivation in IECs [11]. XBP1 deficiency leads to Paneth cell death, spontaneous small bowel inflammation, and susceptibility to bacterial infection [12]. Interestingly, ablation of *Xbp1* in Paneth cells alone (using *Defa6*-Cre) is sufficient to produce similar phenotype of spontaneous ileitis as observed in the previous model [13]. In addition to Paneth cells, the goblet cells in the large bowel were also affected by *Xbp1* deletion as shown by impaired mucin secretion. These animals were more susceptible to dextran sodium sulfate- (DSS-) induced colitis, which is probably caused by multiple mechanisms including the absence of XBP1-mediated adaptive UPR, proapoptotic effectors such as CCAAT-enhancer-binding protein homologous protein (CHOP), cellular inflammatory response in the settings of IRE1α activation, and its downstream signaling [14]. In colonic mucosal tissues from mice and humans, *Xbp1* was targeted by a colitis-induced miRNA, miR665, which was shown to promote apoptosis and DSS-induced colitis in mice [15]. A recent study suggested that loss of *Xbp1* in the IECs leads to increased expression of natural killer group 2 member D ligand (NKG2DL) mouse UL16-binding protein-like transcript 1 via CHOP, which likely contributes to the recruitment of NKG2D-expressing group 1 innate lymphoid cells and mucosal inflammation [16]. In addition, a human deep-sequencing study identified hypomorphic, rare variants of *XBP1* that associate with both CD and UC [12]. Despite that hyperactivation of IRE1α seems to contribute to mucosal inflammation, the deletion of *Ire1α* in murine IECs resulted in the loss of colonic goblet cells, impaired barrier function, and subsequent spontaneous colitis and rectal bleeding. There was a decreased *Xbp1* mRNA splicing, as expected, and an increased CHOP in the colonocytes of the mutant animals [14]. Although the IRE1α and XBP1 deficiencies in IECs cause mucosal inflammation from different mechanisms, it seems that both models involve proapoptotic UPR signaling such as CHOP. It would be interesting to test whether the ablation of *Chop* in IECs rescues the phenotypes (see more discussions below). It is also worthwhile to notice that *Xbp1* deletion produced more dramatic abnormalities in the small intestine, while the loss of IRE1α generated phenotype mainly in the large bowel. It is unclear whether this is due to the differential roles of IRE1α versus XBP1 in different IECs (Paneth cells versus goblet cells) or it is related to the microflora in specific animal facilities [17–19].

PERK is an ER transmembrane protein with a serine/threonine kinase domain on its cytosolic side. The activated PERK directly phosphorylates the eukaryotic mRNA translation initiation factor eIF2α, which dampens global protein synthesis and therefore relieving protein folding overload in the ER [5, 20, 21]. Meanwhile, the phosphorylated eIF2α undergoes selective translation of some mRNAs including that of activating transcription factor 4 (ATF4), which induces various genes involved in ER protein translocation and folding, antioxidative response, autophagy, and amino acid metabolism. ATF4 also engages apoptotic and inflammatory pathways through the transactivation of *Chop* and *Bcl-2* family members, as well as *Mcp1*, *Il6*, and *Tnfα* [5, 22]. The role of eIF2α phosphorylation in murine IECs was studied using mice with IEC-specific expression of nonphosphorylatable eIF2α [23]. Electron microscopy of Paneth cells in the mutant mice revealed a decreased number of secretory granules, a fragmented ER, and damaged mitochondria, which resembled the morphology of the Paneth cells deficient of autophagy mediator ATG16L1 or ATG5 [24]. The mutant mice exhibited a diminished secretion of lysozyme and cryptdins in their small bowel, which were likely responsible for the increased susceptibility to Salmonella infection. Interestingly, the ER-associated translation of *Lysozyme* and *Cryptdin* mRNAs was specifically impaired, which is associated with reduced expression of ER protein translocation machinery in the absence of eIF2a phosphorylation [5, 23]. A recent study showed that lysozyme is transported via secretory autophagy in Paneth cells, a process requiring bacteria-induced PERK-eIF2α activation [25]. In addition, eIF2α phosphorylation is linked to mucosal homeostasis in the large bowel. The unaffected mucosal tissue of UC patients exhibited decreased eIF2α phosphorylation, which may indicate a defective integrated stress response in colonic epithelial cells [26]. Most data so far support a protective role of eIF2α phosphorylation in IECs for intestinal homeostasis. In contrast, the overexpression of transcription factor *Chop* exacerbated DSS-induced colitis, which seems due to impaired epithelial cell proliferation rather than increased apoptosis [27]. Consistently, a recent study showed that the absence of CHOP alleviates bile duct ligation-induced loss of stemness in intestinal stem cells, although the underlying mechanism is unclear [28]. Besides ER stress, eIF2α phosphorylation serves as the regulatory hub of the so-called integrated stress response, which can also be initiated by three other serine/threonine eIF2α kinases in response to distinct stimuli including viral infection (via the double-stranded RNA-activated protein kinase, a.k.a. PKR), amino acid deprivation (via the general control nonderepressible 2, a.k.a. GCN2), and heme deficiency (via the heme-regulated eIF2α kinase, a.k.a. HRI) [6, 29]. PKR has been implicated in a broad spectrum of infectious and inflammatory processes in addition to its well-known antiviral response [30–33]. PKR is activated in murine colonic epithelial cells during DSS-induced colitis. The deletion of *Pkr* exacerbated epithelial cell death and colonic inflammation, which are likely due to reduced ER chaperones and other prosurvival pathways such as Akt/PKB and the signal transducer and activator of transcription 3 [34, 35]. A recent study linked GCN2 to intestinal inflammation. The genetic ablation of *Gcn2* in either IECs or CD11c$^+$ antigen-presenting cells leads to Th17 cell activation and intestinal inflammation, which are likely due to impaired autophagy, elevated reactive oxygen species, and subsequent inflammasome activation [36].

Unlike IRE1α and PERK, ATF6α contains a basic leucine zipper transcription factor domain within its cytosolic region. Upon dissociation of BiP during ER stress, ATF6α translocates to the Golgi apparatus, where it is cleaved by endopeptidases S1P and S2P. The released ATF6α p50 fragment then travels to the nucleus and induces genes that are involved in protein folding and ERAD [7]. The *Atf6a*$^{-/-}$ mice reconstituted with wild-type bone marrow cells are more vulnerable to DSS-induced colitis, likely due to diminished expression of ER chaperones including BiP and P58^{IPK} and increased proapoptotic UPR signaling including CHOP in the colonocytes [37].

2.2. Oxidative Stress. Oxygen metabolism produces reactive oxygen species (ROS) including superoxide, hydroxyl radicals, hydrogen peroxide, hypochlorous acid, and lipid hydroperoxides [38]. The electron transport chain in mitochondria generates a large proportion of ROS [39, 40]. Other sources of endogenous ROS in mammals include the ER, peroxisomes, nucleus as well as the cytosol, and extracellular matrix. Under physiological conditions, the cell is protected from ROS by its antioxidant capacity. However, an excessive ROS production or insufficient antioxidative response can cause lipid and protein modifications, DNA damage, altered membrane permeability, inflammatory response, and cell death, all of which can contribute to the pathogenesis of IBD [41–44]

Multiple cell types in the gastrointestinal tract can be both perpetrators and victims of oxidative stress. Induced by inflammatory cytokines, the IECs produce superoxide and nitric oxide that can damage cytoskeleton proteins and alter tight junctions, subsequently leading to barrier disruption and exacerbation of mucosal inflammation [45, 46]. Upon activation, neutrophils and macrophages in the intestine generate more ROS, which forms a vicious circle of mucosal injury and inflammation [47, 48]. Furthermore, oxidative stress can be initiated by environmental factors, such as luminal antigens, cigarette smoking, alcohol, drugs, xenobiotics, radiation, and chemotherapy, all of which contribute to IBD [3, 49]. Tobacco smoking is one of best known environmental risk factors for CD, whereas it is considered as an alleviating factor of UC. How smoking affects CD risks is not fully understood. Several mechanisms have been proposed. First of all, the gas and tar of cigarette smoke contain a large amount of ROS. Second, cigarette smoke can affect the ROS production in the cell. For example, metal ions from tobacco smoke promote the generation of highly reactive hydroxyl radical from hydrogen peroxide [50]. The activity of inducible nitric oxide synthase is elevated in the small intestine after nicotine administration, although the underlying mechanism remains unclear. Third, tobacco smoke can impair the antioxidative response via multiple mechanisms including the inactivation of superoxide dismutase [51–53]. In recent years, the genetic variations of several antioxidant enzyme genes have been associated with IBD. Some examples include the genes encoding superoxide dismutase 2, glutathione S-transferase, NAD(P)H:quinone oxidoreductase 1, paraoxonase 1, and nuclear factor- (erythroid-derived 2) like 2 [54–61]. Interestingly, the loss of peroxiredoxin 6, an important antioxidative protein, partially protected mice against both acute and chronic DSS-induced colitis, likely by promoting a compensatory elevation of other antioxidative enzymes in the gastrointestinal tract [62]. However, it is unclear whether peroxiredoxin 6 has similar function in different cell populations (e.g. IECs versus immune cells) during intestinal inflammation. This data suggests that the network of antioxidative mechanisms in the gut may be more complex than we previously appreciated.

2.3. Hypoxia. The association between mucosal hypoxia and intestinal inflammation has been demonstrated by hypoxic staining of mucosal tissues in animal models of colitis as well as elevated hypoxia-induced transcription factors in inflamed intestinal samples from individuals with IBD [63–68]. There is also an interesting finding that travelling to altitude > 2000 meters or taking flights increased the risk of IBD exacerbations within 4 weeks of travel, suggesting the role of hypoxia in the course of IBD [69]. Under normal conditions, there is a steep oxygen gradient from the intestinal lumen towards the submucosa in mammalian gastrointestinal tract [68, 70]. Intestinal mucosa becomes more hypoxic during inflammation due to increased oxygen consumption by infiltrated immune cells as well as decreased oxygen supply due to local microvascular occlusion and thrombosis [71, 72]. Mammalian cells have developed evolutionarily conserved mechanisms, including the prolyl hydroxylase domain protein- (PHD-) hypoxia-inducible factors (HIFs) pathway and NF-κB, to code with hypoxic stress [73].

The degree of hypoxia in the GI tract was measured with different measures. The level of intestinal hypoxia under normal conditions, termed physiologic hypoxia, is indispensable for intestinal homeostasis [74]. Low-grade hypoxia promotes intestinal barrier function by inducing the expression of genes such as trefoil factor 3, mucin-3, multidrug resistance protein 1, CD39, CD73, and creatine kinases in IECs [75–78]. In addition to signal transduction via HIFs, PHD3 has been shown to stabilize the tight junction protein occludin in IECs by preventing its interaction with the E3 ligase Itch in a hydroxylase-independent manner [79]. Using a zebrafish model, intestinal *hif1ab* was shown to bind to a hypoxia-inducible response element of mammalian anterior gradient 2 (AGR2) that encodes an ER protein disulfide-isomerase [80]. *AGR2* is associated with IBD and required for the differentiation and maturation of intestinal goblet cells in mice [81–84]. Furthermore, physiological level hypoxia in IECs is important for the constitutive expression of β defensin, an antimicrobial peptide, and netrin-1 that impedes neutrophil infiltration into intestinal mucosa [85, 86]. In contrast, severe hypoxia can elicit an inflammatory response in the gut by targeting multiple cell types. IECs produce higher level of inflammatory cytokines such as TNFα and even enter apoptosis when the local oxygen drops below the physiological level [87, 88]. Mucosal immune cells are also affected by hypoxia during inflammation. Similar to IECs, pathologic hypoxia induces expression of proinflammatory cytokines in macrophages and dendritic cells [89–91]. Importantly, hypoxic macrophages were shown to downregulate autophagy in IECs, a protective signaling against mucosal inflammation. Upon hypoxia, HIF-1 induces Wnt1 expression in macrophages, which suppressed autophagy in cocultured epithelial cells via the activation of β-catenin and mTOR [92]. Knockout of the gene encoding PHD1, an inhibitor of the HIF signaling, drives macrophages towards an anti-inflammatory M2 phenotype and attenuates IL-1b production in dendritic cells in response to lipopolysaccharide [93]. In addition, dendritic cell-specific deletion of *Hif1α* in mice worsened DSS-induced colitis. This is likely due to impaired activation of Foxp3+ regulatory T cells in the settings of decreased thymic stromal lymphopoietin receptor and IL-10 in *Hif1a*$^{-/-}$ dendritic cells [94]. Interestingly, hypoxia-challenged neutrophils may actually survive longer, thereby delaying the resolution of inflammation [95, 96]. Hypoxia also elicits the expression of β2 integrin that promotes leukocyte adhesion and extravasation [97]. Upon severe hypoxia, endothelial cells release proinflammatory cytokines, prostaglandins, platelet-activating factor, and P-selectin, all of which contribute to neutrophil recruitment and mucosal inflammation [98, 99].

3. Cellular Stress Responses Interact with Microbiome in Gastrointestinal Tract

A role of the gut microbiota in the pathogenesis of IBD has long been studied. In particular, both UC and DC are associated with dysbiosis, defined as a decrease in gut bacterial diversity due to a shift from commensal to potentially pathogenic species [100–102]. For example, the Firmicutes phylum usually decreases in the fecal samples of patients with CD compared to healthy individuals, while the Proteobacteria phylum including *Escherichia coli* is often increased in proportional abundance in patients with UC or CD [101, 103–109]. Studies of pediatric cohorts have revealed substantial differences in gut bacterial populations between diseased and healthy children [110–112]. Importantly, dysbiosis has also been observed in the stool and mucosal samples from newly diagnosed, treatment-naive children with CD [113], suggesting that dysbiotic alternations might precede the onset of clinical disease. The gut microbiota also includes viruses and fungi, whose roles in IBD have been increasingly appreciated. Bacteriophages are the predominant species of the gut virome as shown by metagenomic analyses of viral particles from human stool samples [114, 115]. Altered bacteriophage composition has been associated with IBD. In particular, expansion of *Caudovirales* bacteriophages was observed in patients with CD [116, 117]. A recent study suggests that some phages have immunomodulatory functions on human peripheral mononuclear cells by downregulating CD14, TLR4 while upregulating IL-10, IL-1R antagonist, and suppressor of cytokine signaling 3 [118]. However, whether bacteriophages in the gut have similar properties is unclear. There are very limited data about the role of eukaryotic viruses in IBD [119]. Similarly, changes in fungal composition in the gut have been reported in both fecal and mucosa samples. Animal studies suggest that fungi may affect intestinal homeostasis by regulating host metabolism, mucosal immune response, and other microorganisms in the gut [120], although a causal relationship between specific fungal species and IBD remains undetermined.

3.1. ER Stress and Gut Microbiota. The interactions between bacteria and the ER in mammalian cells have long been recognized and investigated (Figure 1). As a biosynthetic factory of the cell, the ER is a nutrient-rich environment presumably free of antimicrobial or hydrolytic enzymes, making it a safe haven for the survival and proliferation of many intracellular bacteria. There are few studies so far that directly examined how gut commensals interact with the ER. However, several gastrointestinal pathogens have been shown to induce ER stress and the UPR both *in vitro* and *in vivo*. For example, *Helicobacter pylori* can elicit ER stress in gastric epithelial

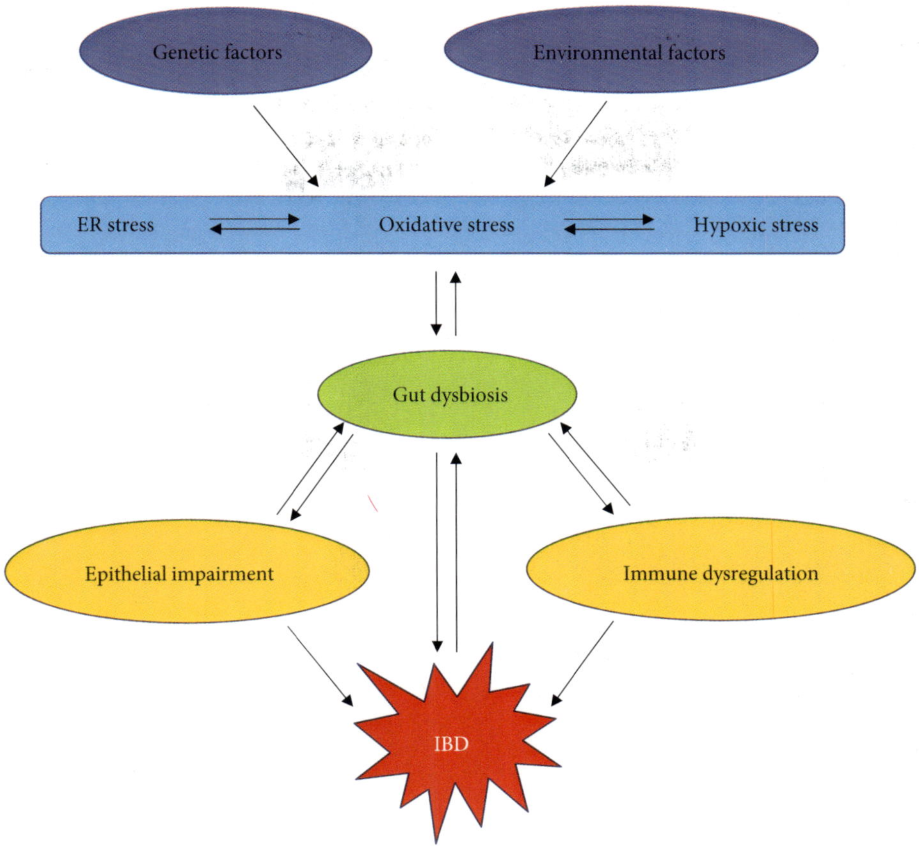

FIGURE 1: Cellular stress signaling interacts with the gut microbiome in the pathogenesis of IBD.

cells with its vacuolating cytotoxin VacA, which activates the PERK-eIF2α-CHOP pathway and causes mitochondrial damage and subsequent apoptosis [120]. ER stress induction is not restricted to ER-dwelling microorganisms. Secreted toxins enable extracellular bacteria to disrupt ER homeostasis without entering the cell. *Listeria monocytogenes* can activate all three branches of the UPR and downstream apoptotic signaling via secretion of cytolysin listeriolysin O (LLO), likely by disturbing ER calcium homeostasis through its pore-forming activity [121, 122]. Other bacteria produce and deliver proteins with enzymatic activities specifically targeting the UPR pathway. Shiga-toxigenic *Escherichia coli* secretes subtilase cytotoxin that cleaves the ER chaperone BiP, triggering the UPR activation and subsequent cell cycle arrest via translation attenuation and degradation of cyclin D1 [123–125]. Several gastrointestinal pathogens are known to exploit ER stress and the UPR for its survival and/or replication. ER stress may play a key role in the mucosal inflammatory response to microorganisms and their secreted molecules. For example, cholera toxin and Shiga toxin undergo retro-translocation to the ER, where they fold appropriately before arriving at their final destinations in the IECs. In the ER lumen, the A subunits of cholera toxin (CTA) and Shiga toxin (Stx1A) activate NF-κB through direct binding to IRE1α and subsequent activation of RIDD [126]. The UPR activation by pathogens and their molecules also involves the pattern recognition receptors including Toll-like receptors (TLRs) and nucleotide-binding oligomerization domain- (NOD-) like receptors (NLRs). In murine and human macrophages, ligands of TLR2/4 specifically activate the IRE1α-XBP1 pathway that requires recruitment of TNF receptor-associated factor 6 (TRAF6) to the TLR and subsequent ROS production by NADPH oxidase NOX2. The spliced XBP1 then induces the expression of *Tnfα* and *Il6* by binding to their promoter regions [127]. IRE1α is known to activate the JNK-dependent inflammatory signaling through the recruitment of TRAF2 [128]. A recent study showed that the interaction between TRAF2 and NOD1/NOD2 is indispensable in this process [129]. This is of particular interest because some genetic variants of both *NOD2* and *XBP1* have been implicated in Crohn's disease [10]. So far, most studies have focused on the interactions between pathogenic bacteria and the ER. There is lack of data on how commensal bacteria affect the ER function and homeostasis.

Viral invasion and replication can active the UPR in host cells. At least 36 eukaryotic viruses have been shown to trigger ER stress and induce downstream pathways including inflammatory and immune responses [130]. However, little is known about how gut virome affects the ER homeostasis in any cell type in the gastrointestinal tract. For the last decade, the findings that helminth infection may improve IBD have drawn our attention to the role of parasites in intestinal health [131, 132]. A recent study showed that infection of *Schistosoma japonicum* mitigated DSS-induced colitis in mice. Alleviated ER stress in the colonic tissues was shown to be partly responsible for the improved inflammation and mucosal cell apoptosis in infected mice, although the underlying mechanisms are unclear [133].

3.2. Oxidative Stress and Gut Microbiota. Oxidative stress in the gastrointestinal tract plays a multifactorial role in the pathogenesis of IBD. Previous studies have associated elevated ROS with dysbiosis in the gut. Given the radial oxygen gradient in the intestinal tract, bacteria residing on the colonic mucosa have higher oxygen tolerance and catalase expression relative to their luminal or stool-associated counterparts [134]. As inflammation usually drives an oxidative state, it might favor the outgrowth of aerotolerant phyla such as Actinobacteria and Proteobacteria in the gut, one example is the murine pathogen *Citrobacter rodentium* [135]. Furthermore, intestinal inflammation has been shown to upregulate the production of small molecules that function as terminal electron acceptors for facultative anaerobes such as Enterobacteriaceae [136, 137], thus contributing to dysbiosis in the intestine.

During intestinal inflammation, the gut microbiota can contribute to ROS production directly and/or indirectly through the mucosal cells [43] (Figure 1). One example is *H. pylori* that generates ROS both by itself and by inducing neutrophils to produce ROS [138]. Some bacteria in the gut can enhance the production of nitric oxide and nitrous oxide by activating macrophages in the settings of inflammation-induced DNA damage [139, 140]. Importantly, the host DNA repair mechanisms can be altered by bacterial modulation. Some strains of enteropathogenic *E. coli* have been shown to interfere with the DNA mismatch repair by secreted toxins, leading to apoptotic cell death and carcinogenesis [141, 142].

3.3. Hypoxic Stress and Gut Microbiota. The gut microbiota influence intestinal health in a number of ways, one of which is the production of short-chain fatty acids (SCFA) including butyrate, propionate, and acetate [143]. In addition to being absorbed into the circulation, SCFAs serve as energy sources of colonocytes and are important for intestinal barrier function. Butyrate augments regulatory T cell function by activating G-protein coupled receptors and leads to epigenetic modification through the inhibition of histone deacetylases [97]. In addition, metabolism of butyrate has recently been shown to boost the oxygen consumption and to stabilize HIFs in murine IECs. Consistently, the level of hypoxia is lower with decreased expression of HIFs in germ-free mice [143]. Depletion of butyrate-producing Clostridia using antibiotics facilitated the expansion of *Salmonella* in the more aerobic (or less hypoxic) mucosal microenvironment [144]. These data indicate that the gut microbiota composition dramatically impacts intestinal oxygenation versus hypoxia status, which orchestrates the composition of aerobes versus anaerobes and gut dysbiosis. A recent study linked the peroxisome proliferator-activated receptor-γ (PPARγ) to the bioavailability of oxygen in the microbial composition and intestinal homeostasis. Butyrate in the colon activates the nuclear receptor PPARγ, which drives the β-oxidation of butyrate in the colonocytes. This process is highly oxygen-consuming and thereby generates a hypoxic environment that limits the expansion of facultative anaerobic bacteria including the Enterobacteriaceae [145]. The ileal mucosa of patients with CD is predominantly colonized by adherent-invasive *Escherichia coli* (AIEC) [146], which requires the interaction between type 1 pili on AIEC and CEACAM6 receptors on the IECs [147]. Another study revealed potentially methylated dinucleotide CpGs within the hypoxia-responsive elements (HREs) of CEACAM6 promoter and the inverse correlation between the methylation and CEACAM6 expression in the IECs [148]. This data highlight a role of HRE methylation and HIF-1 in the regulation of AIEC colonization and ileal mucosal inflammation. Furthermore, hypoxia is a known regulator of autophagy and NLR signaling, two key innate immune mechanisms associated with IBD. A recent study showed that hypoxia suppresses NF-κB and NLRP3 signaling via hypoxia-induced autophagy in IECs, thereby relieving colitis in mice [149]. This data suggests that hypoxia is an important regulator of the microbial-epithelial interaction and innate immunity in the gut (Figure 1).

Importantly, the luminal oxygen level diminishes significantly from the small intestine to large intestine, together with other factors such as antimicrobial peptides and pH, creating distinct habitats for commensal bacteria. Fast-growing facultative anaerobes that effectively utilize simple carbohydrates while tolerating oxidative stress, bile acids, and antimicrobial peptides dominate in the small intestine [150]. For example, certain *Clostridium* spp. and some members of the phylum Proteobacteria are enriched in ileostomy samples from humans [151]. In contrast, the cecum and colon cultivate a more diverse community of bacteria. Fermentative polysaccharide-degrading anaerobes, notably the Bacteroidaceae and Clostridia, flourish in the large bowel thanks to its more hypoxic environment, slower transit time, a lack of simple carbon sources, and lower levels of antimicrobials [152]. The longitudinal gradient of oxygenation plays an important role in the intestinal homeostasis, either dependent or independent of the microbiota. It remains unclear whether the hypoxia gradient along the GI tract contributes to the longitudinal distribution of disease in UC versus CD.

4. Discussions

The complex pathophysiology of IBD is linked to the tremendous complexity of interactions between the host cells and microorganisms in the gastrointestinal tract. Gut microflora is a key component of the mammalian digestive system and has been shown to play a critical role in intestinal health in humans. Although the causative relationship between dysbiosis and the pathogenesis of IBD has not yet been established, data from both animal and human studies suggest that the altered composition and metabolic profiles are not merely a byproduct of intestinal inflammation. It is evident that gut microbiome can influence intestinal homeostasis by interacting with multiple types of cells in the gut through numerous signaling pathways. During evolution, cellular stress responses have developed as important players in the cross-talks with gut microorganisms, an essential component of environmental stress one faces on a daily basis. Both *in vitro* and *in vivo* studies have shown how gut microorganisms and their molecules activate cellular stress pathways, which can produce distinct effects on cell fate and tissue homeostasis. Recent studies found that the ER stress/UPR, antioxidative stress response, and hypoxic stress response may contribute to IBD via multiple mechanisms such as changes in cellular metabolism, altered differentiation and survival of cells, epithelial barrier impairment, proinflammatory response, and fibrosis and wound healing. The picture is further complicated by the fact that ER stress, oxidative stress, and hypoxia interact extensively during intestinal inflammation [10, 153, 154]. Future studies should focus on the network of cellular stress responses in the interaction with gut microbiome using tools such as systems biology.

There is evidence from animal studies that deletion of a single gene associated with the stress signaling (e.g., *Xbp1*) or transfer of colitogenic bacteria to wild-type mice is sufficient to cause inflammation [11, 155, 156]. However, such examples are sparse in humans and the vast majority of IBD cases are probably multifactorial involving both host genetics and environmental factors. It is possible that an altered stress response from either genetic or epigenetic defects can initiate clinical disease of IBD, when the individuals encounter certain microorganisms/molecules in the gut that target these pathways and/or their compensatory pathways directly or indirectly. One example of this susceptibility gene-microbial interaction in mice is that a combination of impaired autophagy (from a mutated *Atg16L1*) and colonization of murine norovirus results in Paneth cell dysfunction, resembling the abnormalities seen in some patients with Crohn's ileitis [157]. Microbiome GWAS (mGWAS) has shed light on how host genetics may interact with gut microbiota in IBD pathogenesis by combining human genome sequencing and 16s rRNA or metagenome sequencing of microbiome [158]. Using these tools, the human lactase gene *LCT* was associated with the abundance of *Bifidobacterium* in a small mGWAS and validated in subsequent cohorts [159]. Future mGWAS with larger sample sizes are likely to achieve higher statistical power [154]. Longitudinal studies that start tracking genetically susceptible individuals before the onset of clinical disease may shed light on the causality between certain microorganism populations and IBD. Following this strategy, a recently published study showed an alternation of intestinal virome that occurred before the development of type-1 diabetes-associated serum auto-antibodies in genetically susceptible children [160].

Bacteria are by far the most studied microorganisms in the gut. Some gastrointestinal pathogens are known to disturb ER function and modulate the UPR either by physically invading the ER lumen or via their secreted molecules. However, how specific gut commensal populations influence host's stress signaling remains elusive. It is likely that the interactions between the host and the commensal microorganisms follow rules different from those between the host and pathogens. Given the findings that certain bacterial species can trigger intestinal inflammation upon transfer to wild-type mice, it would be worthwhile to explore how these microorganisms affect cellular stress responses in the gastrointestinal tract. In addition, some bacterial metabolites can affect mucosal homeostasis via interactions with IECs and immune cells. Future studies should explore how these molecules cross-talk with the stress signaling pathways in these cells. While many mutations in the stress pathways alone do not cause clinical disease in mice, these models provide unique opportunities to study the interactions between susceptibility genes and specific populations of the microbiome in intestinal inflammation. While many human viruses have been shown to compromise ER function during their invasion and/or replication, the relevance of gut virome to ER stress or other stress pathways is unknown. Similarly, the potential interactions between the stress pathways and fungal species in the gut remain to be determined. The exploration into these puzzles will not only further our understanding of IBD but also spur the efforts in developing novel therapies for this disease.

Acknowledgments

The author thanks Dr. Randal Kaufman at Sanford Burnham Prebys Medical Discovery Institute, Dr. Nicholas Davidson at Washington University in St. Louis, and Dr. Averil Ma at the University of California, San Francisco, for discussions.

References

[1] J. M. Dahlhamer, E. P. Zammitti, B. W. Ward, A. G. Wheaton, and J. B. Croft, "Prevalence of inflammatory bowel disease among adults aged ≥18 years — United States, 2015," *MMWR. Morbidity and Mortality Weekly Report*, vol. 65, no. 42, pp. 1166–1169, 2016.

[2] G. G. Kaplan, "The global burden of IBD: from 2015 to 2025," *Nature Reviews Gastroenterology & Hepatology*, vol. 12, no. 12, pp. 720–727, 2015.

[3] A. N. Ananthakrishnan, C. N. Bernstein, D. Iliopoulos et al., "Environmental triggers in IBD: a review of progress and evidence," *Nature Reviews Gastroenterology & Hepatology*, vol. 15, no. 1, pp. 39–49, 2017.

[4] N. Amin-Wetzel, R. A. Saunders, M. J. Kamphuis et al., "A J-protein co-chaperone recruits BiP to monomerize IRE1 and repress the unfolded protein response," *Cell*, vol. 171, no. 7, pp. 1625–1637.e13, 2017.

[5] J. Han and R. J. Kaufman, "Physiological/pathological ramifications of transcription factors in the unfolded protein response," *Genes & Development*, vol. 31, no. 14, pp. 1417–1438, 2017.

[6] C. Hetz and F. R. Papa, "The unfolded protein response and cell fate control," *Molecular Cell*, vol. 69, no. 2, pp. 169–181, 2018.

[7] S. S. Cao and R. J. Kaufman, "Unfolded protein response," *Current Biology*, vol. 22, no. 16, pp. R622–R626, 2012.

[8] S. J. Tavernier, F. Osorio, L. Vandersarren et al., "Regulated IRE1-dependent mRNA decay sets the threshold for dendritic cell survival," *Nature Cell Biology*, vol. 19, no. 6, pp. 698–710, 2017.

[9] M. Wang and R. J. Kaufman, "Protein misfolding in the endoplasmic reticulum as a conduit to human disease," *Nature*, vol. 529, no. 7586, pp. 326–335, 2016.

[10] J. Grootjans, A. Kaser, R. J. Kaufman, and R. S. Blumberg, "The unfolded protein response in immunity and inflammation," *Nature Reviews Immunology*, vol. 16, no. 8, pp. 469–484, 2016.

[11] M. Tschurtschenthaler, T. E. Adolph, J. W. Ashcroft et al., "Defective ATG16L1-mediated removal of IRE1α drives Crohn's disease–like ileitis," *The Journal of Experimental Medicine*, vol. 214, no. 2, pp. 401–422, 2017.

[12] A. Kaser, A.-H. Lee, A. Franke et al., "XBP1 links ER stress to intestinal inflammation and confers genetic risk for human inflammatory bowel disease," *Cell*, vol. 134, no. 5, pp. 743–756, 2008.

[13] T. E. Adolph, M. F. Tomczak, L. Niederreiter et al., "Paneth cells as a site of origin for intestinal inflammation," *Nature*, vol. 503, no. 7475, pp. 272–276, 2013.

[14] H.-S. Zhang, Y. Chen, L. Fan et al., "The endoplasmic reticulum stress sensor IRE1α in intestinal epithelial cells is essential for protecting against colitis," *Journal of Biological Chemistry*, vol. 290, no. 24, pp. 15327–15336, 2015.

[15] M. Li, S. Zhang, Y. Qiu et al., "Upregulation of miR-665 promotes apoptosis and colitis in inflammatory bowel disease by repressing the endoplasmic reticulum stress components XBP1 and ORMDL3," *Cell Death & Disease*, vol. 8, no. 3, article e2699, 2017.

[16] S. Hosomi, J. Grootjans, M. Tschurtschenthaler et al., "Intestinal epithelial cell endoplasmic reticulum stress promotes MULT1 up-regulation and NKG2D-mediated inflammation," *Journal of Experimental Medicine*, vol. 214, no. 10, pp. 2985–2997, 2017.

[17] S. S. Cao, "Endoplasmic reticulum stress and unfolded protein response in inflammatory bowel disease," *Inflammatory Bowel Diseases*, vol. 21, no. 3, pp. 636–644, 2015.

[18] S. S. Cao, "Epithelial ER stress in Crohn's disease and ulcerative colitis," *Inflammatory Bowel Diseases*, vol. 22, no. 4, pp. 984–993, 2016.

[19] S. S. Cao, K. L. Luo, and L. Shi, "Endoplasmic reticulum stress interacts with inflammation in human diseases," *Journal of Cellular Physiology*, vol. 231, no. 2, pp. 288–294, 2016.

[20] R. J. Kaufman, M. V. Davies, V. K. Pathak, and J. W. Hershey, "The phosphorylation state of eucaryotic initiation factor 2 alters translational efficiency of specific mRNAs," *Molecular and Cellular Biology*, vol. 9, no. 3, pp. 946–958, 1989.

[21] P. Murtha-Riel, M. V. Davies, B. J. Scherer, S. Y. Choi, J. W. Hershey, and R. J. Kaufman, "Expression of a phosphorylation-resistant eukaryotic initiation factor 2 alpha-subunit mitigates heat shock inhibition of protein synthesis," *Journal of Biological Chemistry*, vol. 268, no. 17, pp. 12946–12951, 1993.

[22] J. Han, S. H. Back, J. Hur et al., "ER-stress-induced transcriptional regulation increases protein synthesis leading to cell death," *Nature Cell Biology*, vol. 15, no. 5, pp. 481–490, 2013.

[23] S. S. Cao, M. Wang, J. C. Harrington, B.-M. Chuang, L. Eckmann, and R. J. Kaufman, "Phosphorylation of eIF2α is dispensable for differentiation but required at a posttranscriptional level for paneth cell function and intestinal homeostasis in mice," *Inflammatory Bowel Diseases*, vol. 20, no. 4, pp. 712–722, 2014.

[24] K. Cadwell, J. Y. Liu, S. L. Brown et al., "A key role for autophagy and the autophagy gene *Atg16l1* in mouse and human intestinal Paneth cells," *Nature*, vol. 456, no. 7219, pp. 259–263, 2008.

[25] S. Bel, M. Pendse, Y. Wang et al., "Paneth cells secrete lysozyme via secretory autophagy during bacterial infection of the intestine," *Science*, vol. 357, no. 6355, pp. 1047–1052, 2017.

[26] X. Tréton, E. Pédruzzi, D. Cazals-Hatem et al., "Altered endoplasmic reticulum stress affects translation in inactive colon tissue from patients with ulcerative colitis," *Gastroenterology*, vol. 141, no. 3, pp. 1024–1035, 2011.

[27] N. Waldschmitt, E. Berger, E. Rath et al., "C/EBP homologous protein inhibits tissue repair in response to gut injury and is inversely regulated with chronic inflammation," *Mucosal Immunology*, vol. 7, no. 6, pp. 1452–1466, 2014.

[28] R. Liu, X. Li, Z. Huang et al., "CHOP-induced loss of intestinal epithelial stemness contributes to bile duct ligation-induced cholestatic liver injury," *Hepatology (Baltimore, Md.)*, vol. 67, no. 4, pp. 1441–1457, 2017.

[29] S. Taniuchi, M. Miyake, K. Tsugawa, M. Oyadomari, and S. Oyadomari, "Integrated stress response of vertebrates is regulated by four eIF2α kinases," *Scientific Reports*, vol. 6, no. 1, article 32886, 2016.

[30] A. Dalet, E. Gatti, and P. Pierre, "Integration of PKR-dependent translation inhibition with innate immunity is required for a coordinated anti-viral response," *FEBS Letters*, vol. 589, no. 14, pp. 1539–1545, 2015.

[31] A. Dhar, "The role of PKR as a potential target for treating cardiovascular diseases," *Current Cardiology Reviews*, vol. 13, no. 1, pp. 28–31, 2017.

[32] C. M. Hull and P. C. Bevilacqua, "Discriminating self and non-self by RNA: roles for RNA structure, misfolding, and modification in regulating the innate immune sensor PKR," *Accounts of Chemical Research*, vol. 49, no. 6, pp. 1242–1249, 2016.

[33] N. Sud, A. C. Rutledge, K. Pan, and Q. Su, "Activation of the dsRNA-activated protein kinase PKR in mitochondrial dysfunction and inflammatory stress in metabolic syndrome," *Current Pharmaceutical Design*, vol. 22, no. 18, pp. 2697–2703, 2016.

[34] S. S. Cao, B. Song, and R. J. Kaufman, "PKR protects colonic epithelium against colitis through the unfolded protein response and prosurvival signaling," *Inflammatory Bowel Diseases*, vol. 18, no. 9, pp. 1735–1742, 2012.

[35] S. S. Cao and R. J. Kaufman, "PKR in DSS-induced colitis: a matter of genetic background and maternal microflora?," *Inflammatory Bowel Diseases*, vol. 19, no. 3, pp. E49–E50, 2013.

[36] R. Ravindran, J. Loebbermann, H. I. Nakaya et al., "The amino acid sensor GCN2 controls gut inflammation by inhibiting inflammasome activation," *Nature*, vol. 531, no. 7595, pp. 523–527, 2016.

[37] S. S. Cao, E. M. Zimmermann, B.-. M. Chuang et al., "The unfolded protein response and chemical chaperones reduce protein misfolding and colitis in mice," *Gastroenterology*, vol. 144, no. 5, pp. 989–1000.e6, 2013.

[38] K. Bedard and K.-H. Krause, "The NOX family of ROS-generating NADPH oxidases: physiology and pathophysiology," *Physiological Reviews*, vol. 87, no. 1, pp. 245–313, 2007.

[39] E. A. Novak and K. P. Mollen, "Mitochondrial dysfunction in inflammatory bowel disease," *Frontiers in Cell and Development Biology*, vol. 3, 2015.

[40] R. O. Poyton, P. R. Castello, K. A. Ball, D. K. Woo, and N. Pan, "Mitochondria and hypoxic signaling: a new view," *Annals of the New York Academy of Sciences*, vol. 1177, no. 1, pp. 48–56, 2009.

[41] L. A. Ridnour, J. S. Isenberg, M. G. Espey, D. D. Thomas, D. D. Roberts, and D. A. Wink, "Nitric oxide regulates angiogenesis through a functional switch involving thrombospondin-1," *Proceedings of the National Academy of Sciences of the United States of America*, vol. 102, no. 37, pp. 13147–13152, 2005.

[42] M. Valko, D. Leibfritz, J. Moncol, M. T. D. Cronin, M. Mazur, and J. Telser, "Free radicals and antioxidants in normal physiological functions and human disease," *The International Journal of Biochemistry & Cell Biology*, vol. 39, no. 1, pp. 44–84, 2007.

[43] T. Tian, Z. Wang, and J. Zhang, "Pathomechanisms of oxidative stress in inflammatory bowel disease and potential antioxidant therapies," *Oxidative Medicine and Cellular Longevity*, vol. 2017, Article ID 4535194, 18 pages, 2017.

[44] C. Pereira, R. Coelho, D. Grácio et al., "DNA damage and oxidative DNA damage in inflammatory bowel disease," *Journal of Crohn's & Colitis*, vol. 10, no. 11, pp. 1316–1323, 2016.

[45] A. Banan, S. Choudhary, Y. Zhang, J. Z. Fields, and A. Keshavarzian, "Ethanol-induced barrier dysfunction and Its prevention by growth factors in human intestinal monolayers: evidence for oxidative and cytoskeletal mechanisms," *The Journal of Pharmacology and Experimental Therapeutics*, vol. 291, no. 3, pp. 1075–1085, 1999.

[46] R. Rao, R. D. Baker, and S. S. Baker, "Inhibition of oxidant-induced barrier disruption and protein tyrosine phosphorylation in Caco-2 cell monolayers by epidermal growth factor," *Biochemical Pharmacology*, vol. 57, no. 6, pp. 685–695, 1999.

[47] C. G. Knutson, A. Mangerich, Y. Zeng et al., "Chemical and cytokine features of innate immunity characterize serum and tissue profiles in inflammatory bowel disease," *Proceedings of the National Academy of Sciences of the United States of America*, vol. 110, no. 26, pp. E2332–E2341, 2013.

[48] P. Pacher, J. S. Beckman, and L. Liaudet, "Nitric oxide and peroxynitrite in health and disease," *Physiological Reviews*, vol. 87, no. 1, pp. 315–424, 2007.

[49] S. Danese, M. Sans, and C. Fiocchi, "Inflammatory bowel disease: the role of environmental factors," *Autoimmunity Reviews*, vol. 3, no. 5, pp. 394–400, 2004.

[50] H. Wang, M. Yu, M. Ochani et al., "Nicotinic acetylcholine receptor $\alpha 7$ subunit is an essential regulator of inflammation," *Nature*, vol. 421, no. 6921, pp. 384–388, 2003.

[51] R. Eliakim, F. Karmeli, P. Cohen, S. N. Heyman, and D. Rachmilewitz, "Dual effect of chronic nicotine administration: augmentation of jejunitis and amelioration of colitis induced by iodoacetamide in rats," *International Journal of Colorectal Disease*, vol. 16, no. 1, pp. 14–21, 2001.

[52] X. Guo, J. K. S. Ko, Q.-B. Mei, and C. H. Cho, "Aggravating effect of cigarette smoke exposure on experimental colitis is associated with leukotriene B_4 and reactive oxygen metabolites," *Digestion*, vol. 63, no. 3, pp. 180–187, 2001.

[53] X. Guo, W. P. Wang, J. K. S. Ko, and C. H. Cho, "Involvement of neutrophils and free radicals in the potentiating effects of passive cigarette smoking on inflammatory bowel disease in rats," *Gastroenterology*, vol. 117, no. 4, pp. 884–892, 1999.

[54] R. D. Mittal, P. K. Manchanda, H. K. Bid, and U. C. Ghoshal, "Analysis of polymorphisms of tumor necrosis factor-α and polymorphic xenobiotic metabolizing enzymes in inflammatory bowel disease: study from northern India," *Journal of Gastroenterology and Hepatology*, vol. 22, no. 6, pp. 920–924, 2007.

[55] T. Kosaka, J. Yoshino, K. Inui et al., "Involvement of NAD(P)H:quinone oxidoreductase 1 and superoxide dismutase polymorphisms in ulcerative colitis," *DNA and Cell Biology*, vol. 28, no. 12, pp. 625–631, 2009.

[56] A. Karban, C. Hartman, R. Eliakim et al., "Paraoxonase (PON)1 192R allele carriage is associated with reduced risk of inflammatory bowel disease," *Digestive Diseases and Sciences*, vol. 52, no. 10, pp. 2707–2715, 2007.

[57] T. Arisawa, T. Tahara, T. Shibata et al., "Nrf2 gene promoter polymorphism is associated with ulcerative colitis in a Japanese population," *Hepato-Gastroenterology*, vol. 55, no. 82-83, pp. 394–397, 2008.

[58] A. Karban, N. Krivoy, H. Elkin et al., "Non-Jewish Israeli IBD patients have significantly higher glutathione S-transferase *GSTT1*-null frequency," *Digestive Diseases and Sciences*, vol. 56, no. 7, pp. 2081–2087, 2011.

[59] N. Senhaji, Y. Kassogue, M. Fahimi, N. Serbati, W. Badre, and S. Nadifi, "Genetic polymorphisms of multidrug resistance gene-1 (*MDR1/ABCB1*) and glutathione S-transferase gene and the risk of inflammatory bowel disease among Moroccan patients," *Mediators of Inflammation*, vol. 2015, 8 pages, 2015.

[60] A. Varzari, I. V. Deyneko, E. Tudor, and S. Turcan, "Polymorphisms of glutathione S-transferase and methylenetetrahydrofolate reductase genes in Moldavian patients with ulcerative colitis: genotype-phenotype correlation," *Meta Gene*, vol. 7, pp. 76–82, 2016.

[61] J. Mrowicki, M. Mrowicka, I. Majsterek, M. Mik, A. Dziki, and Ł. Dziki, "Evaluation of effect CAT -262C/T, SOD + 35A/C, GPx1 Pro197Leu polymorphisms in patients with IBD in the Polish population," *Polish Journal of Surgery*, vol. 88, no. 6, pp. 321–327, 2016.

[62] H. Melhem, M. R. Spalinger, J. Cosin-Roger et al., "Prdx6 deficiency ameliorates DSS colitis: relevance of compensatory antioxidant mechanisms," *Journal of Crohn's & Colitis*, vol. 11, no. 7, pp. 871–884, 2017.

[63] J. Karhausen, G. T. Furuta, J. E. Tomaszewski, R. S. Johnson, S. P. Colgan, and V. H. Haase, "Epithelial hypoxia-inducible factor-1 is protective in murine experimental colitis," *Journal of Clinical Investigation*, vol. 114, no. 8, pp. 1098–1106, 2004.

[64] A. Giatromanolaki, E. Sivridis, E. Maltezos et al., "Hypoxia inducible factor 1α and 2α overexpression in inflammatory bowel disease," *Journal of Clinical Pathology*, vol. 56, no. 3, pp. 209–213, 2003.

[65] C. Xu and W. Dong, "Role of hypoxia-inducible factor-1α in pathogenesis and disease evaluation of ulcerative colitis," *Experimental and Therapeutic Medicine*, vol. 11, no. 4, pp. 1330–1334, 2016.

[66] P. Hindryckx, A. Waeytens, D. Laukens et al., "Absence of placental growth factor blocks dextran sodium sulfate-induced colonic mucosal angiogenesis, increases mucosal hypoxia and aggravates acute colonic injury," *Laboratory Investigation*, vol. 90, no. 4, pp. 566–576, 2010.

[67] S. Schreiber, S. Nikolaus, and J. Hampe, "Activation of nuclear factor κB in inflammatory bowel disease," *Gut*, vol. 42, no. 4, pp. 477–484, 1998.

[68] E. Brown and C. T. Taylor, "Hypoxia-sensitive pathways in intestinal inflammation," *The Journal of Physiology*, 2017.

[69] S. R. Vavricka, G. Rogler, S. Maetzler et al., "High altitude journeys and flights are associated with an increased risk of flares in inflammatory bowel disease patients," *Journal of Crohn's & Colitis*, vol. 8, no. 3, pp. 191–199, 2014.

[70] E. M. Fisher, M. Khan, R. Salisbury, and P. Kuppusamy, "Noninvasive monitoring of small intestinal oxygen in a rat model of chronic mesenteric ischemia," *Cell Biochemistry and Biophysics*, vol. 67, no. 2, pp. 451–459, 2013.

[71] O. A. Hatoum, H. Miura, and D. G. Binion, "The vascular contribution in the pathogenesis of inflammatory bowel disease," *American Journal of Physiology-Heart and Circulatory Physiology*, vol. 285, no. 5, pp. H1791–H1796, 2003.

[72] E. L. Campbell, W. J. Bruyninckx, C. J. Kelly et al., "Transmigrating neutrophils shape the mucosal microenvironment through localized oxygen depletion to influence resolution of inflammation," *Immunity*, vol. 40, no. 1, pp. 66–77, 2014.

[73] S. Van Welden, A. C. Selfridge, and P. Hindryckx, "Intestinal hypoxia and hypoxia-induced signalling as therapeutic targets for IBD," *Nature Reviews Gastroenterology & Hepatology*, vol. 14, pp. 596–611, 2017.

[74] S. P. Colgan, A. L. Dzus, and C. A. Parkos, "Epithelial exposure to hypoxia modulates neutrophil transepithelial migration," *Journal of Experimental Medicine*, vol. 184, no. 3, pp. 1003–1015, 1996.

[75] K. Synnestvedt, G. T. Furuta, K. M. Comerford et al., "Ecto-5′-nucleotidase (CD73) regulation by hypoxia-inducible factor-1 mediates permeability changes in intestinal epithelia," *Journal of Clinical Investigation*, vol. 110, no. 7, pp. 993–1002, 2002.

[76] G. T. Furuta, J. R. Turner, C. T. Taylor et al., "Hypoxia-inducible factor 1–dependent induction of intestinal trefoil factor protects barrier function during hypoxia," *The Journal of Experimental Medicine*, vol. 193, no. 9, pp. 1027–1034, 2001.

[77] N. A. Louis, K. E. Hamilton, G. Canny, L. L. Shekels, S. B. Ho, and S. P. Colgan, "Selective induction of mucin-3 by hypoxia in intestinal epithelia," *Journal of Cellular Biochemistry*, vol. 99, no. 6, pp. 1616–1627, 2006.

[78] K. M. Comerford, T. J. Wallace, J. Karhausen, N. A. Louis, M. C. Montalto, and S. P. Colgan, "Hypoxia-inducible factor-1-dependent regulation of the multidrug resistance (MDR1) gene," *Cancer Research*, vol. 62, no. 12, pp. 3387–3394, 2002.

[79] Y. Chen, H.-S. Zhang, G.-H. Fong et al., "PHD3 stabilizes the tight junction protein occludin and protects intestinal epithelial barrier function," *Journal of Biological Chemistry*, vol. 290, no. 33, pp. 20580–20589, 2015.

[80] Y.-R. Lai, Y.-F. Lu, H.-W. Lien, C. J. Huang, and S. P. L. Hwang, "Foxa2 and Hif1ab regulate maturation of intestinal goblet cells by modulating agr2 expression in zebrafish embryos," *Biochemical Journal*, vol. 473, no. 14, pp. 2205–2218, 2016.

[81] W. Zheng, P. Rosenstiel, K. Huse et al., "Evaluation of *AGR2* and *AGR3* as candidate genes for inflammatory bowel *disease*," *Genes & Immunity*, vol. 7, no. 1, pp. 11–18, 2006.

[82] Y.-C. Chen, Y.-F. Lu, I.-C. Li, and S. P. L. Hwang, "Zebrafish Agr2 is required for terminal differentiation of intestinal goblet cells," *PLoS One*, vol. 7, no. 4, article e34408, 2012.

[83] F. Zhao, R. Edwards, D. Dizon et al., "Disruption of Paneth and goblet cell homeostasis and increased endoplasmic reticulum stress in *Agr2−/−* mice," *Developmental Biology*, vol. 338, no. 2, pp. 270–279, 2010.

[84] T. Pelaseyed, J. H. Bergström, J. K. Gustafsson et al., "The mucus and mucins of the goblet cells and enterocytes provide the first defense line of the gastrointestinal tract and interact with the immune system," *Immunological Reviews*, vol. 260, no. 1, pp. 8–20, 2014.

[85] C. J. Kelly, L. E. Glover, E. L. Campbell et al., "Fundamental role for HIF-1α in constitutive expression of human β defensin-1," *Mucosal Immunology*, vol. 6, no. 6, pp. 1110–1118, 2013.

[86] P. Rosenberger, J. M. Schwab, V. Mirakaj et al., "Hypoxia-inducible factor–dependent induction of netrin-1 dampens inflammation caused by hypoxia," *Nature Immunology*, vol. 10, no. 2, pp. 195–202, 2009.

[87] C. T. Taylor, A. L. Dzus, and S. P. Colgan, "Autocrine regulation of epithelial permeability by hypoxia: role for polarized release of tumor necrosis factor α," *Gastroenterology*, vol. 114, no. 4, pp. 657–668, 1998.

[88] C. T. Taylor, N. Fueki, A. Agah, R. M. Hershberg, and S. P. Colgan, "Critical role of cAMP response element binding protein expression in hypoxia-elicited induction of epithelial tumor necrosis factor-α," *Journal of Biological Chemistry*, vol. 274, no. 27, pp. 19447–19454, 1999.

[89] J. K. Yun, T. S. McCormick, C. Villabona, R. R. Judware, M. B. Espinosa, and E. G. Lapetina, "Inflammatory mediators are perpetuated in macrophages resistant to apoptosis induced by hypoxia," *Proceedings of the National Academy of Sciences of the United States of America*, vol. 94, no. 25, pp. 13903–13908, 1997.

[90] T. Köhler, B. Reizis, R. S. Johnson, H. Weighardt, and I. Förster, "Influence of hypoxia-inducible factor 1α on dendritic cell differentiation and migration," *European Journal of Immunology*, vol. 42, no. 5, pp. 1226–1236, 2012.

[91] F. Blengio, F. Raggi, D. Pierobon et al., "The hypoxic environment reprograms the cytokine/chemokine expression profile of human mature dendritic cells," *Immunobiology*, vol. 218, no. 1, pp. 76–89, 2013.

[92] D. Ortiz-Masiá, J. Cosín-Roger, S. Calatayud et al., "Hypoxic macrophages impair autophagy in epithelial cells through Wnt1: relevance in IBD," *Mucosal Immunology*, vol. 7, no. 4, pp. 929–938, 2014.

[93] M. Sun, C. He, W. Wu et al., "Hypoxia inducible factor-1α-induced interleukin-33 expression in intestinal epithelia contributes to mucosal homeostasis in inflammatory bowel disease," *Clinical & Experimental Immunology*, vol. 187, no. 3, pp. 428–440, 2017.

[94] K. Flück, G. Breves, J. Fandrey, and S. Winning, "Hypoxia-inducible factor 1 in dendritic cells is crucial for the activation of protective regulatory T cells in murine colitis," *Mucosal Immunology*, vol. 9, no. 2, pp. 379–390, 2016.

[95] S. Hannah, K. Mecklenburgh, I. Rahman et al., "Hypoxia prolongs neutrophil survival in vitro," *FEBS Letters*, vol. 372, no. 2-3, pp. 233–237, 1995.

[96] K. I. Mecklenburgh, S. R. Walmsley, A. S. Cowburn et al., "Involvement of a ferroprotein sensor in hypoxia-mediated

inhibition of neutrophil apoptosis," *Blood*, vol. 100, no. 8, pp. 3008–3016, 2002.

[97] L. Kong, J. Wang, W. Han, and Z. Cao, "Modeling heterogeneity in direct infectious disease transmission in a compartmental model," *International Journal of Environmental Research and Public Health*, vol. 13, no. 3, pp. 3–253, 2016.

[98] C. Michiels, T. Arnould, I. Knott, M. Dieu, and J. Remacle, "Stimulation of prostaglandin synthesis by human endothelial cells exposed to hypoxia," *American Journal of Physiology-Cell Physiology*, vol. 264, no. 4, pp. C866–C874, 1993.

[99] C. Michiels, T. Arnould, and J. Remacle, "Endothelial cell responses to hypoxia: initiation of a cascade of cellular interactions," *Biochimica et Biophysica Acta (BBA) - Molecular Cell Research*, vol. 1497, no. 1, pp. 1–10, 2000.

[100] S. J. Ott, M. Musfeldt, D. F. Wenderoth et al., "Reduction in diversity of the colonic mucosa associated bacterial microflora in patients with active inflammatory bowel disease," *Gut*, vol. 53, no. 5, pp. 685–693, 2004.

[101] C. Manichanh, L. Rigottier-Gois, E. Bonnaud et al., "Reduced diversity of faecal microbiota in Crohn's disease revealed by a metagenomic approach," *Gut*, vol. 55, no. 2, pp. 205–211, 2006.

[102] J. Ni, G. D. Wu, L. Albenberg, and V. T. Tomov, "Gut microbiota and IBD: causation or correlation?," *Nature Reviews Gastroenterology & Hepatology*, vol. 14, no. 10, pp. 573–584, 2017.

[103] H. Sokol, B. Pigneur, L. Watterlot et al., "*Faecalibacterium prausnitzii* is an anti-inflammatory commensal bacterium identified by gut microbiota analysis of Crohn disease patients," *Proceedings of the National Academy of Sciences of the United States of America*, vol. 105, no. 43, pp. 16731–16736, 2008.

[104] A. W. Walker, J. D. Sanderson, C. Churcher et al., "High-throughput clone library analysis of the mucosa-associated microbiota reveals dysbiosis and differences between inflamed and non-inflamed regions of the intestine in inflammatory bowel disease," *BMC Microbiology*, vol. 11, no. 1, p. 7, 2011.

[105] U. Gophna, K. Sommerfeld, S. Gophna, W. F. Doolittle, and S. J. O. Veldhuyzen van Zanten, "Differences between tissue-associated intestinal microfloras of patients with Crohn's disease and ulcerative colitis," *Journal of Clinical Microbiology*, vol. 44, no. 11, pp. 4136–4141, 2006.

[106] D. N. Frank, A. L. St. Amand, R. A. Feldman, E. C. Boedeker, N. Harpaz, and N. R. Pace, "Molecular-phylogenetic characterization of microbial community imbalances in human inflammatory bowel diseases," *Proceedings of the National Academy of Sciences of the United States of America*, vol. 104, no. 34, pp. 13780–13785, 2007.

[107] M. Martinez-Medina, X. Aldeguer, F. Gonzalez-Huix, D. Acero, and J. L. Garcia-Gil, "Abnormal microbiota composition in the ileocolonic mucosa of Crohn's disease patients as revealed by polymerase chain reaction-denaturing gradient gel electrophoresis," *Inflammatory Bowel Diseases*, vol. 12, no. 12, pp. 1136–1145, 2006.

[108] A. Rehman, P. Rausch, J. Wang et al., "Geographical patterns of the standing and active human gut microbiome in health and IBD," *Gut*, vol. 65, no. 2, pp. 238–248, 2016.

[109] M. Baumgart, B. Dogan, M. Rishniw et al., "Culture independent analysis of ileal mucosa reveals a selective increase in invasive *Escherichia coli* of novel phylogeny relative to depletion of Clostridiales in Crohn's disease involving the ileum," *The ISME Journal*, vol. 1, no. 5, pp. 403–418, 2007.

[110] A. Assa, J. Butcher, J. Li et al., "Mucosa-associated ileal microbiota in new-onset pediatric Crohn's disease," *Inflammatory Bowel Diseases*, vol. 22, no. 7, pp. 1533–1539, 2016.

[111] R. Kellermayer, S. A. V. Mir, D. Nagy-Szakal et al., "Microbiota separation and C-reactive protein elevation in treatment-naïve pediatric granulomatous Crohn disease," *Journal of Pediatric Gastroenterology and Nutrition*, vol. 55, no. 3, pp. 243–250, 2012.

[112] R. Shah, J. L. Cope, D. Nagy-Szakal et al., "Composition and function of the pediatric colonic mucosal microbiome in untreated patients with ulcerative colitis," *Gut Microbes*, vol. 7, no. 5, pp. 384–396, 2016.

[113] D. Gevers, S. Kugathasan, L. A. Denson et al., "The treatment-naive microbiome in new-onset Crohn's disease," *Cell Host & Microbe*, vol. 15, no. 3, pp. 382–392, 2014.

[114] A. Reyes, M. Haynes, N. Hanson et al., "Viruses in the faecal microbiota of monozygotic twins and their mothers," *Nature*, vol. 466, no. 7304, pp. 334–338, 2010.

[115] S. Minot, R. Sinha, J. Chen et al., "The human gut virome: inter-individual variation and dynamic response to diet," *Genome Research*, vol. 21, no. 10, pp. 1616–1625, 2011.

[116] J. Wagner, J. Maksimovic, G. Farries et al., "Bacteriophages in gut samples from pediatric Crohn's disease patients: metagenomic analysis using 454 pyrosequencing," *Inflammatory Bowel Diseases*, vol. 19, no. 8, pp. 1598–1608, 2013.

[117] J. M. Norman, S. A. Handley, M. T. Baldridge et al., "Disease-specific alterations in the enteric virome in inflammatory bowel disease," *Cell*, vol. 160, no. 3, pp. 447–460, 2015.

[118] J. D. Van Belleghem, F. Clement, M. Merabishvili, R. Lavigne, and M. Vaneechoutte, "Pro- and anti-inflammatory responses of peripheral blood mononuclear cells induced by *Staphylococcus aureus* and *Pseudomonas aeruginosa* phages," *Scientific Reports*, vol. 7, no. 1, p. 8004, 2017.

[119] W. S. Magin, H. J. Van Kruiningen, and J.-F. Colombel, "Immunohistochemical search for viral and bacterial antigens in Crohn's disease," *Journal of Crohn's & Colitis*, vol. 7, no. 2, pp. 161–166, 2013.

[120] Y. Akazawa, H. Isomoto, K. Matsushima et al., "Endoplasmic reticulum stress contributes to *Helicobacter pylori* VacA-induced apoptosis," *PLoS One*, vol. 8, no. 12, article e82322, 2013.

[121] N. O. Gekara, L. Groebe, N. Viegas, and S. Weiss, "*Listeria monocytogenes* desensitizes immune cells to subsequent Ca^{2+} signaling via listeriolysin O-induced depletion of intracellular Ca^{2+} stores," *Infection and Immunity*, vol. 76, no. 2, pp. 857–862, 2008.

[122] H. Pillich, M. Loose, K.-P. Zimmer, and T. Chakraborty, "Activation of the unfolded protein response by *listeria monocytogenes*," *Cellular Microbiology*, vol. 14, no. 6, pp. 949–964, 2012.

[123] A. W. Paton, T. Beddoe, C. M. Thorpe et al., "AB_5 subtilase cytotoxin inactivates the endoplasmic reticulum chaperone BiP," *Nature*, vol. 443, no. 7111, pp. 548–552, 2006.

[124] J. J. Wolfson, K. L. May, C. M. Thorpe, D. M. Jandhyala, J. C. Paton, and A. W. Paton, "Subtilase cytotoxin activates PERK, IRE1 and ATF6 endoplasmic reticulum stress-signalling pathways," *Cellular Microbiology*, vol. 10, no. 9, pp. 1775–1786, 2008.

[125] N. Morinaga, K. Yahiro, G. Matsuura, J. Moss, and M. Noda, "Subtilase cytotoxin, produced by Shiga-toxigenic *Escherichia coli*, transiently inhibits protein synthesis of Vero cells via degradation of BiP and induces cell cycle arrest at G1 by downregulation of cyclin D1," *Cellular Microbiology*, vol. 10, no. 4, pp. 921–929, 2008.

[126] J. A. Cho, A.-H. Lee, B. Platzer et al., "The unfolded protein response element IRE1α senses bacterial proteins invading the ER to activate RIG-I and innate immune signaling," *Cell Host & Microbe*, vol. 13, no. 5, pp. 558–569, 2013.

[127] F. Martinon, X. Chen, A.-H. Lee, and L. H. Glimcher, "TLR activation of the transcription factor XBP1 regulates innate immune responses in macrophages," *Nature Immunology*, vol. 11, no. 5, pp. 411–418, 2010.

[128] F. Urano, X. Wang, A. Bertolotti et al., "Coupling of stress in the ER to activation of JNK protein kinases by transmembrane protein kinase IRE1," *Science*, vol. 287, no. 5453, pp. 664–666, 2000.

[129] A. M. Keestra-Gounder, M. X. Byndloss, N. Seyffert et al., "NOD1 and NOD2 signalling links ER stress with inflammation," *Nature*, vol. 532, no. 7599, pp. 394–397, 2016.

[130] S. Li, L. Kong, and X. Yu, "The expanding roles of endoplasmic reticulum stress in virus replication and pathogenesis," *Critical Reviews in Microbiology*, vol. 41, no. 2, pp. 150–164, 2015.

[131] M. Heylen, N. E. Ruyssers, E. M. Gielis et al., "Of worms, mice and man: an overview of experimental and clinical helminth-based therapy for inflammatory bowel disease," *Pharmacology & Therapeutics*, vol. 143, no. 2, pp. 153–167, 2014.

[132] A. S. Cheifetz, R. Gianotti, R. Luber, and P. R. Gibson, "Complementary and alternative medicines used by patients with inflammatory bowel diseases," *Gastroenterology*, vol. 152, no. 2, pp. 415–429.e15, 2017.

[133] Y. Liu, Q. Ye, Y.-L. Liu, J. Kang, Y. Chen, and W. G. Dong, "Schistosoma japonicum attenuates dextran sodium sulfate-induced colitis in mice via reduction of endoplasmic reticulum stress," *World Journal of Gastroenterology*, vol. 23, no. 31, pp. 5700–5712, 2017.

[134] L. Albenberg, T. V. Esipova, C. P. Judge et al., "Correlation between intraluminal oxygen gradient and radial partitioning of intestinal microbiota," *Gastroenterology*, vol. 147, no. 5, pp. 1055–1063.e8, 2014.

[135] C. A. Lopez, B. M. Miller, F. Rivera-Chavez et al., "Virulence factors enhance Citrobacter rodentium expansion through aerobic respiration," *Science*, vol. 353, no. 6305, pp. 1249–1253, 2016.

[136] S. E. Winter, C. A. Lopez, and A. J. Bäumler, "The dynamics of gut-associated microbial communities during inflammation," *EMBO Reports*, vol. 14, no. 4, pp. 319–327, 2013.

[137] J. D. Lewis, E. Z. Chen, R. N. Baldassano et al., "Inflammation, antibiotics, and diet as environmental stressors of the gut microbiome in pediatric Crohn's disease," *Cell Host & Microbe*, vol. 22, no. 2, p. 247, 2017.

[138] O. Handa, Y. Naito, and T. Yoshikawa, "*Helicobacter pylori*: a ROS-inducing bacterial species in the stomach," *Inflammation Research*, vol. 59, no. 12, pp. 997–1003, 2010.

[139] T. Irrazábal, A. Belcheva, S. E. Girardin, A. Martin, and D. J. Philpott, "The multifaceted role of the intestinal microbiota in colon cancer," *Molecular Cell*, vol. 54, no. 2, pp. 309–320, 2014.

[140] J. O. Lundberg, E. Weitzberg, J. A. Cole, and N. Benjamin, "Nitrate, bacteria and human health," *Nature Reviews Microbiology*, vol. 2, no. 7, pp. 593–602, 2004.

[141] O. D. K. Maddocks, A. J. Short, M. S. Donnenberg, S. Bader, and D. J. Harrison, "Attaching and effacing Escherichia coli downregulate DNA mismatch repair protein in vitro and are associated with colorectal adenocarcinomas in humans," *PLoS One*, vol. 4, no. 5, article e5517, 2009.

[142] O. D. K. Maddocks, K. M. Scanlon, and M. S. Donnenberg, "An *Escherichia coli* effector protein promotes host mutation via depletion of DNA mismatch repair proteins," *mBio*, vol. 4, no. 3, pp. e00152–e00113, 2013.

[143] C. J. Kelly, L. Zheng, E. L. Campbell et al., "Crosstalk between microbiota-derived short-chain fatty acids and intestinal epithelial HIF augments tissue barrier function," *Cell Host & Microbe*, vol. 17, no. 5, pp. 662–671, 2015.

[144] F. Rivera-Chávez, L. F. Zhang, F. Faber et al., "Depletion of butyrate-producing clostridia from the gut microbiota drives an aerobic luminal expansion of Salmonella," *Cell Host & Microbe*, vol. 19, no. 4, pp. 443–454, 2016.

[145] M. X. Byndloss, E. E. Olsan, F. Rivera-Chávez et al., "Microbiota-activated PPAR-γ signaling inhibits dysbiotic Enterobacteriaceae expansion," *Science*, vol. 357, no. 6351, pp. 570–575, 2017.

[146] H. M. Martin, B. J. Campbell, C. A. Hart et al., "Enhanced *Escherichia coli* adherence and invasion in Crohn's disease and colon cancer," *Gastroenterology*, vol. 127, no. 1, pp. 80–93, 2004.

[147] F. A. Carvalho, N. Barnich, A. Sivignon et al., "Crohn's disease adherent-invasive *Escherichia coli* colonize and induce strong gut inflammation in transgenic mice expressing human CEACAM," *The Journal of Experimental Medicine*, vol. 206, no. 10, pp. 2179–2189, 2009.

[148] J. Denizot, A. Desrichard, A. Agus et al., "Diet-induced hypoxia responsive element demethylation increases CEACAM6 expression, favouring Crohn's disease-associated *Escherichia coli* colonisation," *Gut*, vol. 64, no. 3, pp. 428–437, 2015.

[149] J. Cosin-Roger, S. Simmen, H. Melhem et al., "Hypoxia ameliorates intestinal inflammation through NLRP3/mTOR downregulation and autophagy activation," *Nature Communications*, vol. 8, no. 1, p. 98, 2017.

[150] K. B. M. S. Islam, S. Fukiya, M. Hagio et al., "Bile acid is a host factor that regulates the composition of the cecal microbiota in rats," *Gastroenterology*, vol. 141, no. 5, pp. 1773–1781, 2011.

[151] E. G. Zoetendal, J. Raes, B. van den Bogert et al., "The human small intestinal microbiota is driven by rapid uptake and conversion of simple carbohydrates," *The ISME Journal*, vol. 6, no. 7, pp. 1415–1426, 2012.

[152] G. P. Donaldson, S. M. Lee, and S. K. Mazmanian, "Gut biogeography of the bacterial microbiota," *Nature Reviews Microbiology*, vol. 14, no. 1, pp. 20–32, 2016.

[153] S. S. Cao and R. J. Kaufman, "Endoplasmic reticulum stress and oxidative stress in cell fate decision and human disease," *Antioxidants & Redox Signaling*, vol. 21, no. 3, pp. 396–413, 2014.

[154] W. C. Chong, M. D. Shastri, and R. Eri, "Endoplasmic reticulum stress and oxidative stress: a vicious nexus implicated in bowel disease pathophysiology," *International Journal of Molecular Sciences*, vol. 18, no. 4, 2017.

[155] W. S. Garrett, G. M. Lord, S. Punit et al., "Communicable ulcerative colitis induced by T-bet deficiency in the innate immune system," *Cell*, vol. 131, no. 1, pp. 33–45, 2007.

[156] N. W. Palm, M. R. de Zoete, T. W. Cullen et al., "Immunoglobulin A coating identifies colitogenic bacteria in inflammatory bowel disease," *Cell*, vol. 158, no. 5, pp. 1000–1010, 2014.

[157] K. Cadwell, K. K. Patel, N. S. Maloney et al., "Virus-plus-susceptibility gene interaction determines Crohn's disease gene Atg16L1 phenotypes in intestine," *Cell*, vol. 141, no. 7, pp. 1135–1145, 2010.

[158] A. B. Hall, A. C. Tolonen, and R. J. Xavier, "Human genetic variation and the gut microbiome in disease," *Nature Reviews Genetics*, vol. 18, no. 11, pp. 690–699, 2017.

[159] R. Blekhman, J. K. Goodrich, K. Huang et al., "Host genetic variation impacts microbiome composition across human body sites," *Genome Biology*, vol. 16, no. 1, p. 191, 2015.

[160] G. Zhao, T. Vatanen, L. Droit et al., "Intestinal virome changes precede autoimmunity in type I diabetes-susceptible children," *Proceedings of the National Academy of Sciences of the United States of America*, vol. 114, no. 30, pp. E6166–E6175, 2017.

17

Diagnostic Potential of Systemic Eosinophil-Associated Cytokines and Growth Factors in IBD

Katarzyna Neubauer,[1] Malgorzata Matusiewicz,[2] Iwona Bednarz-Misa,[2] Sabina Gorska,[3] Andrzej Gamian,[2,3] and Malgorzata Krzystek-Korpacka[2]

[1]*Department of Gastroenterology and Hepatology, Wroclaw Medical University, 50-556 Wroclaw, Poland*
[2]*Department of Medical Biochemistry, Wroclaw Medical University, 50-368 Wroclaw, Poland*
[3]*Laboratory of Medical Microbiology, Ludwik Hirszfeld Institute of Immunology and Experimental Therapy, Polish Academy of Sciences, 53-114 Wroclaw, Poland*

Correspondence should be addressed to Katarzyna Neubauer; kasianeu@gmail.com

Academic Editor: Amosy M'Koma

Despite the acknowledged contribution of eosinophils to the disease pathogenesis, available data on cytokines closely related to the peripheral eosinophils in inflammatory bowel disease (IBD) are scattered. We assessed the concentrations of eosinophil-associated cytokines and growth factors in the group of 277 individuals (101 patients with Crohn's disease (CD), 77 with ulcerative colitis (UC), 16 with irritable bowel syndrome (IBS), and 83 healthy controls) and referred to IBD activity and the levels of hsCRP. As compared to IBS patients or healthy controls, patients with CD had significantly higher levels of IL5, IL8, IL12(p70), GM-CSF, and TNFα and patients with UC, the levels of eotaxin, IL4, IL5, IL8, IL12(p70), IL13, GM-CSF, and TNFα were also higher. As compared to CD patients, patients with UC had significantly higher levels of eotaxin, IL4, IL5, IL8, and IL1. In turn, the concentrations of hsCRP were significantly higher in CD than UC. Except for IL13, all cytokines and hsCRP positively correlated with CDAI. In UC, a positive correlation with MDAI was observed for hsCRP, GM-CSF, IL12(p70), and IFNγ and a negative one for IL8. The concentrations of hsCRP, GM-CSF, IFNγ, IL12(p70), and RANTES were higher in UC patients with active than inactive disease whereas those of IL8 and TNFα were significantly lower. Eotaxin, determined individually or in a panel with IFNγ and hsCRP, showed fair accuracy in differentiating CD from UC. If confirmed on a larger representation of IBS patients, IL8 might support differential diagnosis of organic and functional conditions of the bowel. GM-CSF, in turn, demonstrated to be an excellent indicator of bowel inflammation and may be taken into consideration as a noninvasive marker of mucosal healing. In summary, eosinophil-associated cytokines are elevated in IBD, more pronouncedly in UC, and may support the differential diagnosis of IBD and aid in monitoring of mucosal healing.

1. Introduction

Crohn's disease (CD) and ulcerative colitis (UC) are two main types of inflammatory bowel disease (IBD), a group of chronic inflammatory conditions of the bowel. IBD incidence is increasing worldwide, both in pediatric and adult populations [1, 2]. The disease is characterized by the wide spectrum of intestinal and extraintestinal complications. Pathogenesis of IBD is multifactorial and still not fully elucidated. Nevertheless, the consensus is that the crucial role is played by an impaired immune response to the gut microbiota, evoked by environmental triggers and/or genetic factors [3, 4]. The adaptive immunity seems to play the first fiddle in the pathogenesis of IBD [4]. However, the inflamed mucosa is infiltrated also by cytokine-rich innate immune cells [5] and their unceasing activation contributes to local and systemic inflammations [6].

IBD diagnostics and differential diagnostics pose a challenge for clinicians. IBD symptoms are nonspecific and overlapping. Establishing diagnosis requires a performance of series of laboratory, endoscopic, radiologic, and histologic tests. Those tests are expensive, often invasive, related to some risk, and poorly acceptable by patients. Biochemical markers currently used in clinical practice are insufficient and not recommended to serve as therapeutic targets [7]. Therefore, as a key part of the precision medicine strategy, the alternative, noninvasive biomarkers of IBD are intensively searched for [8, 9].

Eosinophils are acidophilic multifunctional granulocytes involved in inflammation and immunity that remain outside the mainstream research on IBD. However, they are a rich source of cytotoxic proteins, pro- and anti-inflammatory cytokines, chemokines, and growth factors and are likely to contribute to both inflammatory and regenerative phases of the disease. Accordingly, peripheral eosinophils of IBD patients are primed and preactivated. They display increased responsiveness, adhesiveness, migration, and degranulation [10, 11] and are characterized by upregulated secretion of their mediators, for example, eosinophilic cationic protein [12] or eotaxin [13, 14]. Peripheral eosinophilia is associated with less favorable outcome, that is, higher incidence of primary sclerosing cholangitis or need for surgical intervention [15]. Interestingly, prevalence of peripheral eosinophilia significantly differs between CD and UC. It has been reported to occur more often in UC patients, both in pediatric [16] and adult [15] populations. Locally, increased number and activation of eosinophils have been repeatedly observed in areas of active inflammation. Functionally, as evidenced in animal models of colitis, eosinophils seem to exert proinflammatory and promotility effects in IBD, thus contributing to diarrhea, tissue inflammation, and destruction, as well as fibrosis and formation of strictures. Additionally, they have been suggested to contribute to tissue repair and remodeling (reviewed in [17–19]). However, knowledge concerning eosinophils and quiescent bowel remains inconsistent.

Despite the acknowledged contribution of eosinophils to the disease pathogenesis, available data on cytokines closely related to the development and activity of peripheral eosinophils in IBD patients are either scattered or nonexistent. Herein, we assessed cytokines and growth factors crucial for eosinophil proliferation and differentiation (GM-CSF, IL5, and IL4), for their release from bone marrow (IL5), for their survival (IL5, IL13, GM-CSF, and IL4) and priming in circulation (IL5, GM-CSF, IL4, and TNFα), and for extravasation (IL4, IFNγ, TNFα, IL8, and eotaxin) and homing into the gut (eotaxin, RANTES, IL5, IL8, IL13, GM-CSF, and TNFα) as well as responsible for inducing production and secretion of their mediators (TNFα, IFNγ, IL-5, GM-CSF, and eotaxin) (reviewed in [10, 17, 20]). We also evaluated IL12 as a key inductor of eosinophil apoptosis and as a mediator of antieosinophil actions of glucocorticosteroids [10]. This paper focuses on the potential of eosinophil-associated cytokines and growth factors as biomarkers in IBD, in reference to high-sensitive C-reactive protein, an inflammatory marker commonly used in IBD clinics [8].

2. Materials and Methods

2.1. Study Population. Study population consisted of 277 individuals: 101 patients with Crohn's disease, 77 with ulcerative colitis, 16 with irritable bowel syndrome (IBS), and 83 healthy controls. IBD and IBS patients were recruited from the Department of Gastroenterology and Hepatology of Wroclaw Medical University, Poland. Individuals with indeterminate colitis or the coexistence of other severe systemic diseases, malignancies, liver diseases, or pregnancies were not included. The clinical activity of the disease was assessed using the Crohn's Disease Activity Index (CDAI) for CD and the Mayo Disease Activity Index (MDAI) for UC. Severity of bowel inflammation in UC patients was assessed using a Mayo endoscopic score. IBD patients were treated with 5′-aminosalicylate (5′-ASA) derivatives. Healthy controls were recruited from among students of our university and hospital staff or from among outpatients of Research, Science, and Educational Center of Dementia Diseases, Scinawa, Poland, diagnosed with mild cognitive disorders (no significant medical history) or from blood donors from the Regional Center for Blood Donation and Therapeutics in Wroclaw, Poland. Female to male ratio in study groups was as follows: 50/51 in CD, 34/43 in UC, 12/4 in IBS, and 38/45 in controls, $p = 0.147$. Age distribution was as follows (medians with 95% CI): 31 yrs (30–36.9) in CD, 40 yrs (33.8–45) in UC, 53 yrs (25–57) in IBS, and 35 yrs (18–87) in controls ($p = 0.104$).

2.2. Ethical Considerations. The study protocol was accepted by the Medical Ethics Committee of Wroclaw Medical University (KB-575/2011). The study was conducted in accordance with the Helsinki Declaration of 1975, as revised in 1983, and an informed consent was obtained from all patients.

2.3. Analytical Methods. Blood was drawn by venipuncture, following an overnight fast, allowed to clot for 30 minutes, and centrifuged (15 minutes, 720 ×g). Resulting sera were collected, aliquoted, and kept frozen at −80° until examination. We applied a flow cytometry-based method utilizing magnetic microspheres conjugated with monoclonal antibodies (Luminex xMAP® Technology) to measure the concentrations of eotaxin, GM-CSF, IFNγ, IL4, IL5, IL8, IL12(p70), IL13, RANTES, and TNFα. Analytes were measured in duplicate using Bio-Plex Pro™ human cytokine, chemokine, and growth factor magnetic bead-based assays according to the instructions provided by the manufacturer but with a lower serum dilution factor and the Bio-Plex 200 platform with HRF (Bio-Rad, USA). Standard curves were drawn using 5-PL logistic regression, and the data were analyzed using Bio-Plex Manager 6.0 software. Data on high-sensitive C-reactive protein (hsCRP), measured using an enhanced immunoturbidimetric method with the CRPex-HS CRP test (Good Biotech Corp., Taichung, Taiwan), were retrieved from our earlier study on this population (available exclusively for IBD patients).

2.4. Statistical Analysis. Normality of data distribution was tested using the χ^2 test and homogeneity of variances using Levene's test. Data were log-transformed if necessary and presented as geometric means or medians accompanied by 95% confidence interval. Multigroup comparisons were conducted using one-way ANOVA or the Kruskal-Wallis H test. Two-group comparisons were conducted using t-test for independent samples (with Welch correction if appropriate) or the Mann–Whitney U test. Correlation analysis with the disease activity scores was conducted using the Spearman test. Frequency analysis was conducted using the χ^2 test or Fisher's exact test. Receiver operating characteristic (ROC) curve analysis was conducted to evaluate the strength of observed associations and the suitability of analytes as disease markers. A backward stepwise method of logistic regression, followed by the Hosmer and Lemeshow goodness-of-fit test and ROC analysis, was used to assess the discriminative power of combined marker evaluation. Model building was preceded by the analysis of linearity, collinearity, and interactions of candidate variables. To validate the final model, we applied the V-fold cross-validation. Z statistics was used to evaluate the significance of difference between area under ROC curves (AUCs; measure of test accuracy) obtained for training and validation sets. All calculated probabilities were two-tailed, and p values ≤ 0.05 were considered statistically significant. The statistical analysis was conducted using MedCalc statistical software version 15.8 (MedCalc Software bvba, Ostend, Belgium; https://www.medcalc.org; 2015) and Medical Bundle ver. 3.0., an add-in to Statistica 12 PL (StatSoft Polska Sp. z o.o. 2016; http://www.statsoft.pl).

3. Results

3.1. Eosinophil-Associated Cytokines in Bowel Diseases. Patients with UC had significantly higher levels of eotaxin, IL4, IL5, IL8, and IL13 than patients with CD or IBS and healthy controls. They also had higher levels of TNFα, GM-CSF, and IL12(p70) than IBS patients and healthy controls but not CD patients. The levels of RANTES and IFNγ were higher in UC patients but only in comparison to healthy controls (Figure 1).

Patients with CD had significantly higher levels of IL5, IL8, IL12(p70), GM-CSF, and TNFα than IBS patients and healthy controls and higher levels of IL13, IFNγ, and RANTES as compared to healthy controls (Figure 1).

Patients with IBS had significantly higher levels of IL12(p70) and IFNγ than healthy controls but lower levels of IL8 (Figure 1).

The concentrations of hsCRP in IBD patients were higher in CD than UC: 30.7 mg/l (25.9–55.8) and 6.1 mg/l (3.2–17.8), $p < 0.0001$, respectively.

3.2. Cytokine Relation to IBD Activity. From among evaluated cytokines, IL12(p70) was the sole cytokine that differed significantly between CD patients with active and inactive disease: 72.7 pg/ml (63–84) and 74.2 pg/ml (29–78), $p = 0.034$, respectively.

In UC, active disease was associated with more pronouncedly elevated levels of GM-CSF (47 pg/ml (39–57) versus 23.3 pg/ml (15–36), $p < 0.001$), IFNγ (95 pg/ml (83–154) versus 65 pg/ml (57–81), $p = 0.001$), IL12(p70) (81.8 pg/ml (66–102) versus 42.4 pg/ml (27–66), $p = 0.003$), and RANTES (10.1 ng/ml (9–13) versus 8.1 ng/ml (6–10), $p = 0.053$) than inactive disease. However, active UC was accompanied by lower levels of IL8 (70 pg/ml (58–85) versus 103 pg/ml (82–130), $p = 0.021$) and TNFα (38.5 pg/ml (32–46) versus 55.5 pg/ml (46–67), $p = 0.007$).

Except for IL13, all evaluated cytokines and growth factors weakly to moderately correlated with CDAI. In turn, only IL13 and GM-CSF displayed a positive association with MDAI (Table 1).

Of the examined cytokines, GM-CSF, IL12(p70), and IFNγ positively correlated with the degree of endoscopic inflammation in UC patients (Table 1). IL8 displayed a negative correlation due to high cytokine levels in patients without inflammation. When the analysis was restricted to patients with inflamed mucosa, the association tended to be positive ($p = 0.107$).

The levels of hsCRP were significantly higher in active than inactive CD: 38.6 mg/l (27–65) and 1.74 mg/l (0.7–21), $p = 0.002$, respectively. They were also higher in active than inactive UC: 18 mg/l (5.5–22.6) and 1.75 mg/l (0.3–3.8), $p < 0.001$, respectively. There was a positive correlation between hsCRP and the indices of clinical activity of CD and UC as well as endoscopic inflammation in UC (Table 1).

3.3. Eosinophil-Associated Cytokines as Differential Markers in IBD. Symptomatology of UC and CD may sometimes overlap, rendering both IBD types difficult to distinguish. Moreover, there is still a group of patients with unclassified IBD, in whom the definitive distinction between UC and CD is not possible despite of all recommended tests [21]. Of the evaluated eosinophil-associated cytokines, eotaxin (149.3 pg/ml (124.8–178.7) versus 103.4 pg/ml (91.6–116.7), $p < 0.001$), IFNγ (127.6 pg/ml (100.4–162.3) versus 94.2 pg/ml (78.2–113.4), $p = 0.046$), and IL13 (22.1 pg/ml (18.1–27.1) versus 16.9 pg/ml (14–6.19.7), $p = 0.035$) were more pronouncedly elevated in active UC than CD. In turn, hsCRP was significantly higher in active CD than UC (26.6 mg/l (17.2–41.2) versus 8.9 mg/l (4.3–18.4), $p = 0.011$). We applied ROC analysis to evaluate the suitability of these cytokines and hsCRP as individual differential markers (Figure 2(a)). As depicted in Table 2, eotaxin displayed superior accuracy as a marker of active UC, followed by hsCRP as a marker of active CD.

In order to discern the independent predictors of the disease type and evaluate the power of their combined assessment, we applied logistic regression. All cytokines, the levels of which significantly differed between active UC and CD, were selected as potential explanatory variables, and active CD was coded as 0 while active UC coded as 1. Data on CRP levels were unavailable for a few patients; thus, the analysis was limited to 115 patients with active IBD (45 with UC and 70 with CD). First, a univariate regression analysis was conducted for each variable and all variables were found to significantly affect the dependent variable. Next, candidate variables were tested for linearity, collinearity, and interactions. The model was built with eotaxin, IL13, IFNγ, and hsCRP (ratio of analyzed variables to cases was 29), and a backward stepwise method was used. Eotaxin ($b = 3.3$, $p = 0.002$; OR = 27 (4–210); constant = −9, $p < 0.001$), hsCRP ($b = -0.54$, $p = 0.020$; OR = 0.58 (0.37–0.92)), and IFNγ ($b = 1.1$, $p = 0.069$; OR = 2.95 (1–9.5)) contributed to model's predictive power and were retained in

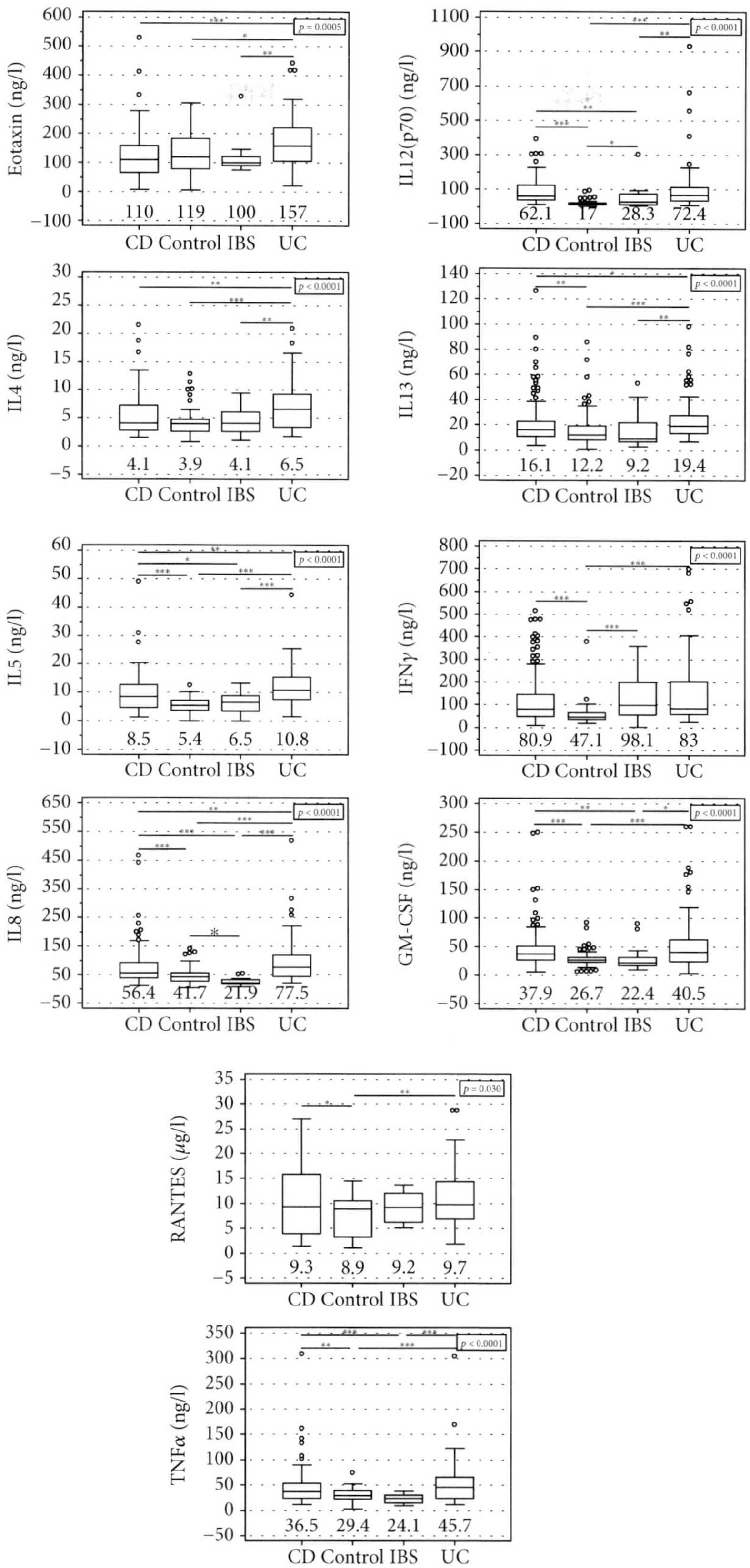

FIGURE 1: Systemic eosinophil-associated cytokines in patients with inflammatory bowel disease or irritable bowel syndrome and healthy controls. Data presented as medians (bar within box) with interquartile range (box) and 91% CI (whiskers) and analyzed with Kruskal-Wallis *H* test. Open circles mark outlying observations. Horizontal bars with asterisks indicate statistically significant between-group differences: $^{*}p < 0.05$, $^{**}p < 0.01$, and $^{***}p < 0.001$. CD: Crohn's disease; CONTROL: controls; IBS: irritable bowel syndrome; UC: ulcerative colitis.

Table 1: Correlation between eosinophil-associated cytokines, chemokines, and growth factors and disease activity.

Cytokine	Clinical activity CD (CDAI)	Clinical activity UC (Mayo)	Endoscopic activity in UC
Eotaxin	0.28, $p = 0.009$	ns	ns
GM-CSF	0.30, $p = 0.005$	0.33, $p = 0.003$	0.56, $p < 0.0001$
IL4	0.35, $p = 0.001$	ns	ns
IL5	0.38, $p < 0.001$	ns	ns
IL8	0.38, $p < 0.001$	ns	−0.38, $p = 0.005$
IL12(p70)	0.35, $p < 0.001$	0.511, $p < 0.0001$	0.49, $p < 0.001$
IL13	ns	ns	ns
IFNγ	0.25, $p = 0.019$	0.45, $p < 0.0001$	0.55, $p < 0.0001$
RANTES	0.24, $p = 0.028$	ns	ns
TNFα	0.22, $p = 0.037$	ns	ns
hsCRP	0.40, $p < 0.001$	0.66, $p < 0.0001$	0.46, $p < 0.001$

ns: not significant.

the final model whereas IL13 was not included. The overall fit of the three-parameter model was $\chi^2 = 25.8$, $p < 0.0001$, and the results of the Hosmer and Lemeshow test were $\chi^2 = 5.3$, $p = 0.731$ indicating a good logistic regression model fit. The model predictive power was fair (Table 2) and allowed for a correct classification of 72.2% of cases; however, the model's pseudo R-squared was rather low: Nagelkerke $R^2 = 0.273$. The accuracy of a validated model (V-fold cross-validation) was comparable (Table 2). Lack of significant difference in accuracy between training and validation sets suggests that the predictive power of the model was not overestimated.

3.4. Eosinophil-Associated Cytokines as Negative Markers of Mucosal Healing (MH) in UC. Data on endoscopic findings were available for UC patients, among whom 16 had no signs of active bowel inflammation (coded as 1 for the purpose of ROC analysis and logistic regression) and 37 had an ongoing inflammation (coded as 0). Of patients with active inflammation, 10 were assigned Mayo endoscopic score 1, 15 score 2, and 12 score 3.

GM-CSF, IFNγ, and IL12(p70) as well as hsCRP were significantly correlated with Mayo endoscopic subscore (Table 1). Individually, the accuracy of GM-CSF as the marker of mucosal healing was superior to those of other cytokines and hsCRP (Figure 2(b), Table 3).

Logistic regression (backward stepwise methods) was applied to discern the independent predictors of mucosal healing and to evaluate the power of potential multimarker assays. GM-CSF, IFNγ, IL12(p70), and hsCRP were tested as potential explanatory variables. However, they were found to be interrelated; GM-CSF was positively correlated with hsCRP ($r = 0.56$, $p < 0.00001$), IL12(p70) ($r = 0.404$, $p = 0.003$), and IFNγ ($r = 0.035$, $p = 0.011$). Also, hsCRP was correlated with IFNγ ($r = 0.36$, $p = 0.014$). As such, we attempted to build three separate models: one exclusively with GM-CSF, second containing IFNγ and IL12(p70) combined together, and third with hsCRP and IL12(p70) combined together. However, testing for linearity and collinearity excluded two latter combinations of variables. At the end, only a model with GM-CSF was built. Regression coefficient for GM-CSF was $b = -7.7$, $p < 0.001$; OR was 0.0005 (0–0.0335); constant = 10.33, $p < 0.001$. The overall model fit was $\chi^2 = 30.5$, $p < 0.00001$, and the results of the Hosmer and Lemeshow test were $\chi^2 = 6.8$, $p = 0.658$ indicating a good logistic regression model fit. The model predictive power was excellent (Table 3) and allowed for a correct classification of 87% of cases. The model's pseudo R-squared was high as well: Nagelkerke $R^2 = 0.619$. The accuracy of the V-fold cross-validated model was comparable proving the model predictive power not to be overestimated (Table 3).

3.5. Eosinophil-Associated Cytokines as Markers Differentiating between IBD and IBS. Functional bowel disorders like IBS display a similar set of symptoms to IBD making their differential diagnosis difficult. Herein, we evaluated the eosinophil-associated cytokines as potential differential markers.

As depicted in Figure 1, IL5, IL8, IL12(p70), TNFα, and GM-CSF were significantly higher in both CD and UC than in IBS. Of these, IL8 had the highest AUC and Youden index. At optimal cut-off values, IL5 and TNFα displayed superior specificity, IL12(p70) and GM-CSF displayed superior sensitivity, and the sensitivity and specificity of IL8 was equally high (Figure 2(c), Table 4).

Logistic regression was applied to discern the independent indicators of active IBD (coded as 1 and IBS coded as 0). Candidate variables (IL5, IL8, IL12(p70), GM-CSF, and TNFα) were tested for linearity, collinearity, and interactions. IL5, IL8, and TNFα occurred to be interrelated with the following correlation coefficients: $r = 0.74$ for IL5 and IL8, $r = 0.6$ for IL5 and TNFα, and $r = 0.62$ for IL8 and TNFα. As such, three separate models were tested: each model included GM-CSF and IL12(p70) and either IL5, IL8, or TNFα. Of these, the model with IL8 (IL8, GM-CSF, and IL12(p70)) displayed the best fit. However, following the analysis of variable contribution to the model's predictive power, exclusively IL8 was retained. Regression coefficient for IL8 was $b = 4.49$, $p < 0.0001$; OR was 89.4 (11.8–679); constant = −13.9, $p < 0.0001$. The overall model fit was $\chi^2 = 43.3$, $p < 0.00001$, and the results of the Hosmer and Lemeshow test were $\chi^2 = 5.3$, $p = 0.727$ indicating a good logistic regression model fit. The model predictive power was excellent (Table 4) and allowed for a correct classification of 93% of cases. The model's pseudo R-squared (Nagelkerke R^2) was 0.502. AUC obtained after V-fold cross-validation was slightly lower, but there was no significant difference compare to AUC of a training set proving the model predictive power not to be overestimated (Table 4).

4. Discussion

Eosinophils are gaining an increasing attention as the cells of unique properties among leukocytes, which can damage or repair surrounding tissue and modulate the activity of immune cells [22]. Accordingly, the infiltration of lamina propria by eosinophils has been shown to be an early histological marker of UC [23] and a predictor of clinical relapse [24] as well as poor response of UC patients to medical therapy [25]. Recently, local eosinophilia has been reported to be

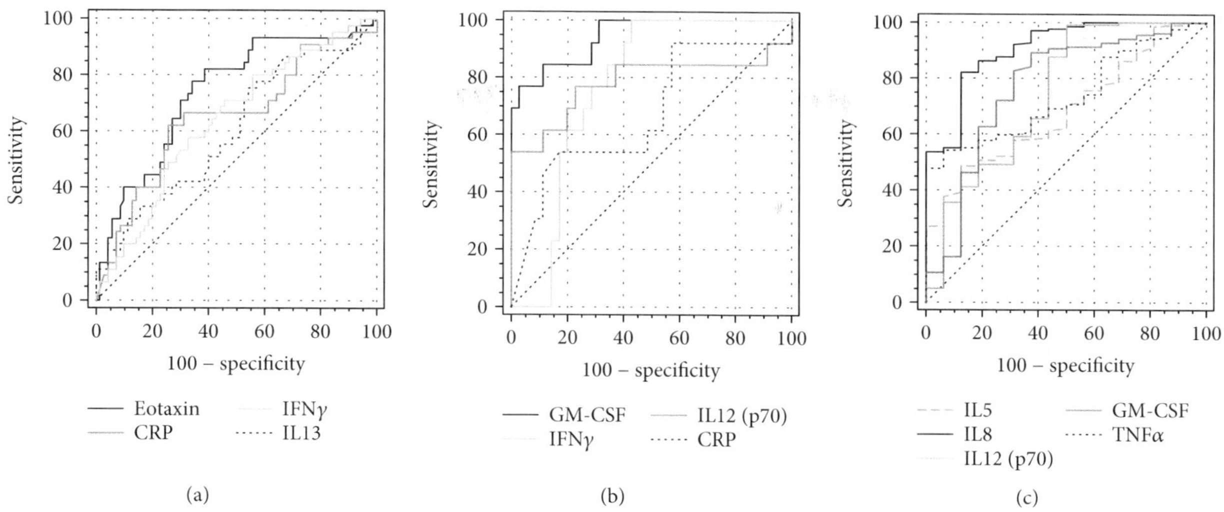

FIGURE 2: Eosinophil-associated cytokines as biomarkers in IBD-receiver operating characteristic (ROC) curves. (a) Eosinophil-associated cytokines as markers differentiating active UC and CD; (b) eosinophil-associated cytokines as mucosal healing markers; (c) eosinophil-associated cytokines as markers differentiating active IBD and IBS.

TABLE 2: Diagnostic power of eosinophil-associated cytokines as markers differentiating active UC from CD.

(a)

Marker	AUC (95% CI), $p_{AUC=0.5}$	Cut-off	Sens.&Spec.	*J* index
Eotaxin	0.708 (0.62–0.78), $p < 0.0001$	>138 pg/ml	71 and 68%	0.391
IL13	0.604 (0.52–0.69), $p = 0.032$	>20.8 pg/ml	51 and 69%	0.203
IFNγ	0.594 (0.51–0.68), $p = 0.054$	>64.5 pg/ml	76 and 44%	0.199
hsCRP*	0.657 (0.57–0.74), $p = 0.003$	≥19.9 mg/l	74 and 60%	0.347

(b)

Panel	AUC (95% CI)		Difference
	Learning set	Validation set	*z* statistics, *p*
Eotaxin, hsCRP, IFNγ	0.78 (0.7–0.87)	0.73 (0.63–0.82)	0. 818, $p = 0.414$

*hsCRP was tested as an indicator of CD. AUC: area under ROC curve; Sens.&Spec.: sensitivity and specificity; *J* index: Youden index.

TABLE 3: Diagnostic power of eosinophil-associated cytokines as negative markers of mucosal healing in UC.

(a)

Marker	AUC (95% CI), $p_{AUC=0.5}$	Cut-off	Sens.&Spec.	*J* index
GM-CSF	0.907 (0.80–0.97), $p < 0.001$	≤16.7 pg/ml	69 and 97%	0.661
IFNγ	0.782 (0.65–0.88), $p < 0.001$	≤83.2 pg/ml	100 and 60%	0.595
IL12(p70)	0.709 (0.57–0.83), $p = 0.033$	≤21.6 pg/ml	50 and 100%	0.500
hsCRP	0.673 (0.52–0.80), $p < 0.001$	≤0.5 mg/l	54 and 83%	0.367

(b)

Panel	AUC (95% CI), $p_{AUC=0.5}$		Difference
	Learning set	Validation set	*z* statistics, *p*
GM-CSF	0.907 (0.80–0.97)	0.884 (0.78–0.99)	0.335, $p = 0.738$

AUC: area under ROC curve; Sens.&Spec.: sensitivity and specificity; *J* index: Youden index.

Table 4: Diagnostic power of eosinophil-associated cytokines as markers differentiating active IBD from IBS.

(a)

Marker	AUC (95% CI), $p_{AUC=0.5}$	Cut-off	Sens.&Spec.	J index
IL5	0.69 (0.61–0.76), $p = 0.003$	>9.68 pg/ml	48.6 and 87.5%	0.361
IL8	0.91 (0.85–0.95), $p < 0.0001$	>36.8 pg/ml	82.1 and 87.5%	0.696
IL12(p70)	0.75 (0.67–0.81), $p = 0.002$	>22.6 pg/ml	99.3 and 50%	0.493
TNFα	0.74 (0.66–0.81), $p < 0.0001$	>34 pg/ml	54.3 and 93.8%	0.480
GM-CSF	0.77 (0.7–0.84), $p < 0.001$	>24 pg/ml	89.3 and 62.5%	0.518

(b)

Panel	AUC (95% CI), $p_{AUC=0.5}$		Difference
	Learning set	Validation set	z statistics, p
IL8	0.91 (0.85–0.95), $p < 0.0001$	0.87 (0.76–0.98), $p < 0.0001$	0.503, $p = 0.615$

AUC: area under ROC curve; Sens.&Spec.: sensitivity and specificity; J index: Youden index.

related to the stricturing phenotype of CD [26]. Peripheral eosinophilia has been observed in IBD as well and linked to poor prognosis [15]. Peripheral eosinophils isolated from IBD patients have been characterized as primed, displaying increased responsiveness, adhesiveness, migration, and degranulation [10, 11]. Still, little is known on cytokines involved in managing growth, distribution, and priming of eosinophils as well as in aiding their homing into the gut. Except for eotaxin, which has become a novel therapeutic target in UC [27], eosinophil-associated cytokines, such as GM-CSF, IL3, IL5, and IL13, have not been comprehensively analyzed in the context of IBD. Available data are scanty, mostly derived from the analysis of small cohorts, and obtained exclusively from multiplexed analyses intended for screening purposes, in which cytokines less abounded in sera frequently balance at the verge of lower detection limits of the tests, making their evaluation problematic [28–30]. Herein, the dilution of our samples was adjusted to enable credible analysis of these analytes. It allowed us to show that compared to healthy individuals, IBD patients had significantly higher concentrations of all evaluated eosinophil-associated cytokines and growth factors, although the elevation of eotaxin and IL4 was observed exclusively in UC patients.

Differential diagnosis of UC and CD might be challenging [21]. In this respect, it is easy to perform and noninvasive cytokine assays would be welcomed to assist clinicians in the diagnostic process. In line with higher prevalence of local [31] and peripheral eosinophilia [16] in UC than CD, we found several of eosinophil-associated cytokines to be more pronouncedly elevated in UC. We evaluated suitability of eotaxin, IL13, IFNγ, and hsCRP as differential markers assessed individually as well as a multicytokine panel. Individually, eotaxin performance was fair and superior to other markers. Eotaxin is a critical chemoattractant specific for eosinophils, and an elevation of its circulating concentrations in IBD has already been reported by several groups [13, 14, 28, 29, 32]. However, previous comparative analyses of eotaxin in CD and UC have been conducted exclusively in small cohorts and yielded contradictory results [13, 14, 28, 32]. The addition of IFNγ and hsCRP improved the discriminative power of the assay as compared to sole determination of eotaxin but not markedly. Of note, Iboshi et al. [33] found the expression of IFNγ to be more accentuated in UC than in CD.

Chronic bowel inflammation is a hallmark of IBD. The assessment of its severity is imperative for the determination of the disease activity and establishment of a therapeutic approach. It became particularly crucial in view of the recent change of priorities in IBD therapy from control of symptoms to the restriction of inflammation [1]. Mucosal healing (MH), currently assessed exclusively by endoscopy, is related to more favorable clinical outcomes and has lately become one of the therapeutic endpoints in clinical trials. However, clinical trials have shown a poor correlation between clinical symptoms and endoscopy. It is estimated that almost half of CD patients with clinical remission are still presenting with endoscopic features of active disease whereas almost 40% of patients with inactive disease in endoscopy are displaying clinical symptoms of the disease [34]. Since clinical indices are not sufficient, biomarkers, which could be applied in MH evaluation, as well as in monitoring the disease course, predicting its relapse, and recognizing flare, are intensively sought after [34–36]. Herein, hsCRP, GM-CSF, IFNγ, and IL12(p70) were significantly and positively correlated with the degree of bowel inflammation, expressed as Mayo endoscopic subscore. Of these, GM-CSF has emerged as a superior MH marker in UC. GM-CSF displayed high accuracy, falling within the range typical for biomarkers applied in clinical practice (85–95%). Importantly, GM-CSF accuracy remained high following its validation. Taking into account the invasiveness and a risk for complications associated with endoscopy, serum-based MH markers such as GM-CSF might help to assist in the selection of patients and limit the need for invasive examinations. GM-CSF has been the only cytokine other than eotaxin significantly elevated in sera of UC patients in Coburn et al.'s study [29]. GM-CSF controls proliferation and differentiation if eosinophils in the bone marrow provide survival signals and induce the release of their granule proteins. GM-CSF is also responsible for eosinophil priming in circulation and acts as their chemoattractant [20, 37]. However, as reviewed by Han et al. [38], data available on GM-CSF functionality in the bowel are equivocal. A beneficial role has been attributed to this growth factor in the small intestine, where it might contribute to maintaining intestinal barrier function, likely through stimulating proliferation of intestinal epithelial cells (IECs). Accordingly, no difference in GM-CSF expression has been noted between inflamed and noninflamed IECs. On the other hand, colonic mucosa has been shown to overexpress GM-CSF when inflamed or cancerous and the growth factor had no effect on colonic cell proliferation. Despite unresolved issue of GM-CSF function in IBD, growth factor-based therapies have been attempted and yielded promising results. In animal models of colitis, GM-CSF application has resulted in an improvement of clinical symptoms and histological findings as well as in accelerated ulcer healing. In human CD, a therapy with recombinant GM-CSF has lessened the disease severity (reviewed in [38]). In the light of these findings, our observation on GM-CSF increase in IBD patients might represent a protective mechanism. However, healing capabilities of GM-CSF might be counteracted by concomitant elevation in the levels of GM-CSF autoantibodies. Their presence in IBD patients and the association with a more aggressive disease phenotype have been previously reported and implied in functional GM-CSF deficiency caused by antibody interference with GM-CSF binding to its receptor [39, 40].

It is estimated that the endoscopy in about half of adult and 70% of pediatric patients presenting with symptoms indicative of IBD yields negative results. These patients are subsequently diagnosed with functional bowel disorders, for example, IBS, the condition which share many clinical symptoms with IBD. In this respect, a reliable but less invasive differential tool is needed [41]. From among eosinophil-associated cytokines analyzed by us, IL5, IL8, IL12(p70), TNFα, and GM-CSF were significantly higher in both CD and UC than in IBS. Of these, IL8 had superior accuracy in differentiating IBS and IBD and allowed for a correct classification of 93% of patients. IL8 is a cytokine which is the most loosely associated with eosinophils. Although secreted by these leukocytes and acting as their chemoattractant [20], IL8 is primarily responsible for neutrophil trafficking. Correspondingly, another neutrophil-associated protein, namely, calprotectin, has been claimed as having adequate sensitivity and specificity to assist in differentiating IBD from IBS. Even though IL8 herein displayed an excellent accuracy, validated using V-fold cross-validation technique, our results should be interpreted with care and treated as indicative only because of the small number of patients with IBS included in our cohort.

5. Conclusions

Our results obtained on a large cohort of patients showed that the concentrations of circulating eosinophil-associated cytokines are elevated in IBD and that this elevation is more accentuated in UC. Evaluated as prospective differential markers, eotaxin, individually and in a panel with IFNγ and hsCRP, showed fair accuracy in differentiating CD from UC. IL8, if confirmed on a larger representation of IBS patients, might, in turn, support differential diagnosis of organic (IBD) and functional (IBS) conditions of the bowel. GM-CSF demonstrated to be an excellent indicator of bowel inflammation and may be taken into consideration as a noninvasive marker of mucosal healing.

Ethical Approval

The study protocol was approved by the Medical Ethics Committee of Wroclaw Medical University (KB-575/2011).

Acknowledgments

This work was supported by National Science Centre (DEC-2011/01/D/NZ5/02835).

References

[1] P. Papay, A. Ignjatovic, K. Karmiris et al., "Optimising monitoring in the management of Crohn's disease: a physician's perspective," *Journal of Crohn's and Colitis*, vol. 7, no. 8, pp. 653–669, 2013.

[2] N. A. Molodecky, I. S. Soon, D. M. Rabi et al., "Increasing incidence and prevalence of the inflammatory bowel diseases with time, based on systematic review," *Gastroenterology*, vol. 142, no. 1, pp. 46–54.e42, 2012.

[3] K.-A. G. Buela, S. Omenetti, and T. T. Pizarro, "Cross-talk between type 3 innate lymphoid cells and the gut microbiota in inflammatory bowel disease," *Current Opinion in Gastroenterology*, vol. 31, no. 6, pp. 449–455, 2015.

[4] I. Loddo and C. Romano, "Inflammatory bowel disease: genetics, epigenetics, and pathogenesis," *Frontiers in Immunology*, vol. 6, p. 551, 2015.

[5] C. B. Larmonier, K. W. Shehab, F. K. Ghishan, and P. R. Kiela, "T lymphocyte dynamics in inflammatory bowel diseases: role of the microbiome," *BioMed Research International*, vol. 2015, Article ID 504638, 9 pages, 2015.

[6] A. Tommasini, A. Pirrone, G. Palla et al., "The universe of immune deficiencies in Crohn's disease: a new viewpoint for an old disease?," *Scandinavian Journal of Gastroenterology*, vol. 45, no. 10, pp. 1141–1149, 2010.

[7] L. Peyrin-Biroulet, W. Sandborn, B. E. Sands et al., "Selecting therapeutic targets in inflammatory bowel disease (STRIDE): determining therapeutic goals for treat-to-target," *The American Journal of Gastroenterology*, vol. 110, no. 9, pp. 1324–1338, 2015.

[8] S. Vermeire, G. van Assche, and P. Rutgeerts, "Laboratory markers in IBD: useful, magic, or unnecessary toys?," *Gut*, vol. 55, no. 3, pp. 426–431, 2006.

[9] R. K. Boyapati, R. Kalla, J. Satsangi, and G. T. Ho, "Biomarkers in search of precision medicine in IBD," *The American Journal of Gastroenterology*, vol. 111, no. 12, pp. 1682–1690, 2016.

[10] M. Lampinen, M. Carlson, L. D. Hakansson, and P. Venge, "Cytokine-regulated accumulation of eosinophils in inflammatory disease," *Allergy*, vol. 59, no. 8, pp. 793–805, 2004.

[11] L. C. Coppi, S. M. Thomazzi, M. L. S. Ayrizono et al., "Comparative study of eosinophil chemotaxis, adhesion, and degranulation in vitro in ulcerative colitis and Crohn's disease," *Inflammatory Bowel Diseases*, vol. 13, no. 2, pp. 211–218, 2007.

[12] A. Wędrychowicz, P. Tomasik, S. Pieczarkowski, K. Kowalska-Duplaga, Z. Grzenda-Adamek, and K. Fyderek, "Clinical value of serum eosinophilic cationic protein assessment in children with inflammatory bowel disease," *Archives of Medical Science*, vol. 6, no. 6, pp. 1142–1146, 2014.

[13] W. Chen, B. Paulus, D. Shu, I. Wilson, and V. Chadwick, "Increased serum levels of eotaxin in patients with inflammatory bowel disease," *Scandinavian Journal of Gastroenterology*, vol. 36, no. 5, pp. 515–520, 2001.

[14] A. Mir, M. Minguez, J. Tatay et al., "Elevated serum eotaxin levels in patients with inflammatory bowel disease," *The American Journal of Gastroenterology*, vol. 97, no. 6, pp. 1452–1457, 2002.

[15] A. Barrie, M. E. Mourabet, K. Weyant et al., "Recurrent blood eosinophilia in ulcerative colitis is associated with severe disease and primary sclerosing cholangitis," *Digestive Diseases and Sciences*, vol. 58, no. 1, pp. 222–228, 2013.

[16] G. Sadi, Q. Yang, B. Dufault, C. Stefanovici, J. Stoffman, and W. el-Matary, "Prevalence of peripheral eosinophilia at diagnosis in children with inflammatory bowel disease," *Journal of Pediatric Gastroenterology and Nutrition*, vol. 62, no. 4, pp. 573–576, 2016.

[17] S. Al-Haddad and R. H. Riddell, "The role of eosinophils in inflammatory bowel disease," *Gut*, vol. 54, no. 12, pp. 1674-1675, 2005.

[18] J. Wedemeyer and K. Vosskuhl, "Role of gastrointestinal eosinophils in inflammatory bowel disease and intestinal tumours," *Best Practice & Research. Clinical Gastroenterology*, vol. 22, no. 3, pp. 537–549, 2008.

[19] S. P. Hogan, A. Waddell, and P. C. Fulkerson, "Eosinophils in infection and intestinal immunity," *Current Opinion in Gastroenterology*, vol. 29, no. 1, pp. 7–14, 2013.

[20] F. Davoine and P. Lacy, "Eosinophil cytokines, chemokines, and growth factors: emerging roles in immunity," *Frontiers in Immunology*, vol. 5, p. 570, 2014.

[21] G. E. Tontini, M. Vecchi, L. Pastorelli, M. F. Neurath, and H. Neumann, "Differential diagnosis in inflammatory bowel disease colitis: state of the art and future perspectives," *World Journal of Gastroenterology*, vol. 21, no. 1, pp. 21–46, 2015.

[22] C. Bandeira-Melo and P. F. Weller, "Mechanisms of eosinophil cytokine release," *Memórias do Instituto Oswaldo Cruz*, vol. 100, Supplement 1, pp. 73–81, 2005.

[23] J. A. Bass, C. A. Friesen, A. D. Deacy et al., "Investigation of potential early histologic markers of pediatric inflammatory bowel disease," *BMC Gastroenterology*, vol. 15, no. 1, p. 129, 2015.

[24] S. Park, T. Abdi, M. Gentry, and L. Laine, "Histological disease activity as a predictor of clinical relapse among patients with ulcerative colitis: systematic review and meta-analysis," *The American Journal of Gastroenterology*, vol. 111, no. 12, pp. 1692–1701, 2016.

[25] P. Zezos, K. Patsiaoura, A. Nakos et al., "Severe eosinophilic infiltration in colonic biopsies predicts patients with ulcerative colitis not responding to medical therapy," *Colorectal Disease*, vol. 16, no. 12, pp. O420–O430, 2014.

[26] J. C. Masterson, K. E. Capocelli, L. Hosford et al., "Eosinophils and IL-33 perpetuate chronic inflammation and fibrosis in a pediatric population with stricturing Crohn's ileitis," *Inflammatory Bowel Diseases*, vol. 21, no. 10, pp. 2429–2440, 2015.

[27] V. Yadav, F. Varum, R. Bravo, E. Furrer, D. Bojic, and A. W. Basit, "Inflammatory bowel disease: exploring gut pathophysiology for novel therapeutic targets," *Translational Research*, vol. 176, pp. 38–68, 2016.

[28] O. Y. Korolkova, J. N. Myers, S. T. Pellom, L. Wang, and A. E. M'koma, "Characterization of serum cytokine profile in predominantly colonic inflammatory bowel disease to delineate ulcerative and Crohn's colitides," *Clinical Medicine Insights: Gastroenterology*, vol. 8, 2015.

[29] L. A. Coburn, S. N. Horst, R. Chaturvedi et al., "High-throughput multi-analyte Luminex profiling implicates eotaxin-1 in ulcerative colitis," *PLoS One*, vol. 8, no. 12, article e82300, 2013.

[30] G. Kleiner, V. Zanin, L. Monasta et al., "Pediatric patients with inflammatory bowel disease exhibit increased serum levels of proinflammatory cytokines and chemokines, but decreased circulating levels of macrophage inhibitory protein-1β, interleukin-2 and interleukin-17," *Experimental and Therapeutic Medicine*, vol. 9, no. 6, pp. 2047–2052, 2015.

[31] C. Flores, C. F. Francesconi, and L. Meurer, "Quantitative assessment of CD30^{+} lymphocytes and eosinophils for the histopathological differential diagnosis of inflammatory bowel disease," *Journal of Crohn's & Colitis*, vol. 9, no. 9, pp. 763–768, 2015.

[32] T. Adar, S. Shteingart, A. Ben-Ya'acov et al., "The importance of intestinal eotaxin-1 in inflammatory bowel disease: new insights and possible therapeutic implications," *Digestive Diseases and Sciences*, vol. 61, no. 7, pp. 1915–1924, 2016.

[33] Y. Iboshi, K. Nakamura, E. Ihara et al., "Multigene analysis unveils distinctive expression profiles of helper T-cell-related genes in the intestinal mucosa that discriminate between ulcerative colitis and Crohn's disease," *Inflammatory Bowel Diseases*, vol. 20, no. 6, pp. 967–977, 2014.

[34] J. Florholmen, "Mucosal healing in the era of biologic agents in treatment of inflammatory bowel disease," *Scandinavian Journal of Gastroenterology*, vol. 50, no. 1, pp. 43–52, 2015.

[35] M. F. Neurath and S. P. L. Travis, "Mucosal healing in inflammatory bowel diseases: a systematic review," *Gut*, vol. 61, no. 11, pp. 1619–1635, 2012.

[36] K. Pazdrak, T. W. Young, C. Straub, S. Stafford, and A. Kurosky, "Priming of eosinophils by GM-CSF is mediated by protein kinase CβII-phosphorylated L-plastin," *Journal of Immunology*, vol. 186, no. 11, pp. 6485–6496, 2011.

[37] L. Egea, Y. Hirata, and M. F. Kagnoff, "GM-CSF: a role in immune and inflammatory reactions in the intestine," *Expert Review of Gastroenterology & Hepatology*, vol. 4, no. 6, pp. 723–731, 2010.

[38] X. Han, K. Uchida, I. Jurickova et al., "Granulocyte-macrophage colony-stimulating factor autoantibodies in murine ileitis and progressive ileal Crohn's disease," *Gastroenterology*, vol. 136, no. 4, pp. 1261–1271.e3, 2009.

[39] G. Gathungu, M. O. Kim, J. P. Ferguson et al., "Granulocyte-macrophage colony-stimulating factor autoantibodies: a marker of aggressive Crohn's disease," *Inflammatory Bowel Diseases*, vol. 19, no. 8, pp. 1671–1680, 2013.

[40] F. S. Lehmann, E. Burri, and C. Beglinger, "The role and utility of faecal markers in inflammatory bowel disease," *Therapeutic Advances in Gastroenterology*, vol. 8, no. 1, pp. 23–36, 2014.

[41] R. Sherwood and N. Walsham, "Fecal calprotectin in inflammatory bowel disease," *Clinical and Experimental Gastroenterology*, vol. 9, pp. 21–29, 2016.

18

The EndoBarrier: Duodenal-Jejunal Bypass Liner for Diabetes and Weight Loss

Aruchuna Ruban, Hutan Ashrafian, and Julian P. Teare

Department of Surgery and Cancer, Imperial College, London, UK

Correspondence should be addressed to Aruchuna Ruban; aruchuna@doctors.org.uk

Academic Editor: Ramesh P Arasaradnam

The rapid rise of obesity and type 2 diabetes poses a global threat to healthcare and is a major cause of mortality and morbidity. Bariatric surgery has revolutionised the treatment of both these conditions but is invasive and associated with an increased risk of complications. The EndoBarrier is a device placed endoscopically in the duodenum, which is designed to mimic the effects of gastric bypass surgery with the aim of inducing weight loss and improving glycaemic control. This review outlines the current clinical evidence of the device, its efficacy, potential mechanisms of action, and utility in clinical practice.

1. Introduction

Obesity has reached epidemic proportions with the WHO estimating that approximately 2.3 billion adults worldwide are overweight and more than 700 million are obese [1]. Obesity is associated with the development of other comorbidities, in particular diabetes, which currently affects 422 million adults worldwide [2]. The current favoured treatment for patients with type 2 diabetes (T2DM) who are obese is referral for bariatric surgery. In the 2nd Diabetes Surgery Summit in 2015, several national diabetes societies such as the American Diabetes Association (ADA) and Diabetes UK have recommended the use of bariatric surgery in obese type 2 diabetics reporting diabetes remission rates of between 30–60% following surgery [3]. However, with a greater demand being placed on bariatric surgery, there is a drive to develop nonsurgical alternatives to combat the ever-rising obesity and diabetes epidemic.

One potential alternative is the EndoBarrier, an endoluminal duodenal-jejunal bypass liner (DJBL) developed by GI Dynamics (GID) Inc., Lexington, MA. In this state-of-the-art review, we present the current clinical trial data available on the EndoBarrier and explore its potential mode of action, safety profile, and potential applications in the management of obesity and T2DM.

2. The Device

The EndoBarrier is a single-use endoscopic implant, which consists of the liner, delivery system, and retrieval system. The actual liner portion is an impermeable fluoropolymer that spans 60 cm into the small intestine (Figure 1). Located at the proximal end of the liner are anchors with barbs made of nitinol allowing the device to affix and be secured to the duodenal bulb, proximal to the ampulla of Vater but distal to the pylorus. These anchors also have drawstrings attached to them to facilitate subsequent removal of the device at the end of treatment. Once deployed in the duodenum, the device can remain for a maximum treatment period of 12 months. The liner is open at both ends promoting the passage of chyme from the stomach bypassing the duodenum and into the jejunum. Concurrently, pancreatic juices and bile will enter the duodenum from the ampulla of Vater running along the outside of the sleeve avoiding contact with gastric contents until these exit the sleeve in the jejunum (Figure 2). The desired effect is for the sleeve to mimic the

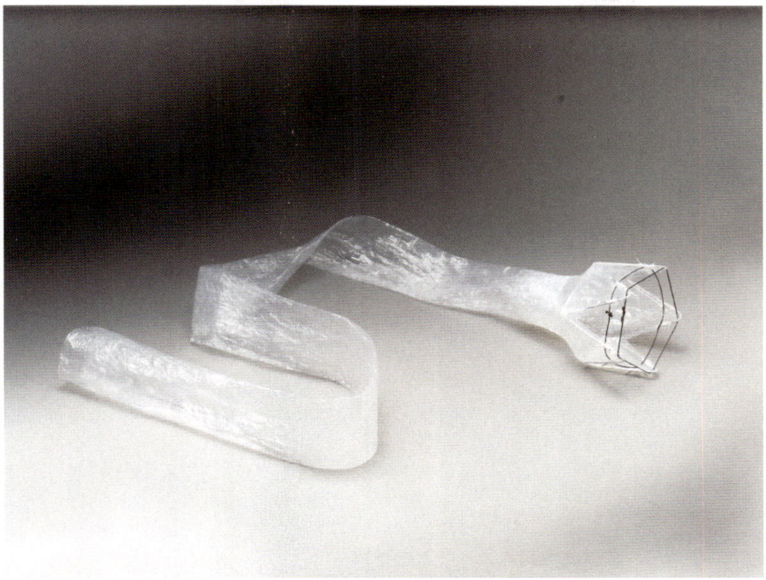

Figure 1: The EndoBarrier device.

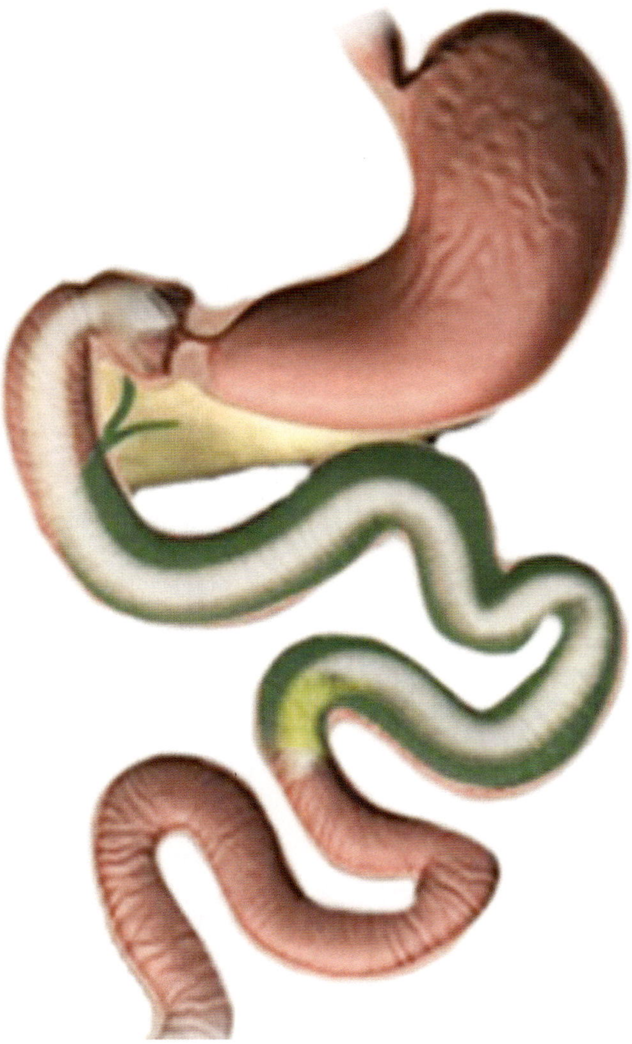

Figure 2: Bile flowing around the outside of the sleeve coming into contact with nutrients distally in the jejunum.

Table 1: Advantages and disadvantages of the EndoBarrier procedure.

Advantages	Disadvantages
Can be performed without the need for a general anaesthetic under conscious sedation	Two operators required for both implant and explant.
Easy to perform	Fluoroscopy is essential, and this involves a small dose of radiation to the patient.
Patient can be discharged at home the same day	Patients must take protein pump inhibitors for the duration of treatment with the device.
Easily reversible	Patients must commence a liquid diet prior to EndoBarrier placement and for a short duration afterwards.

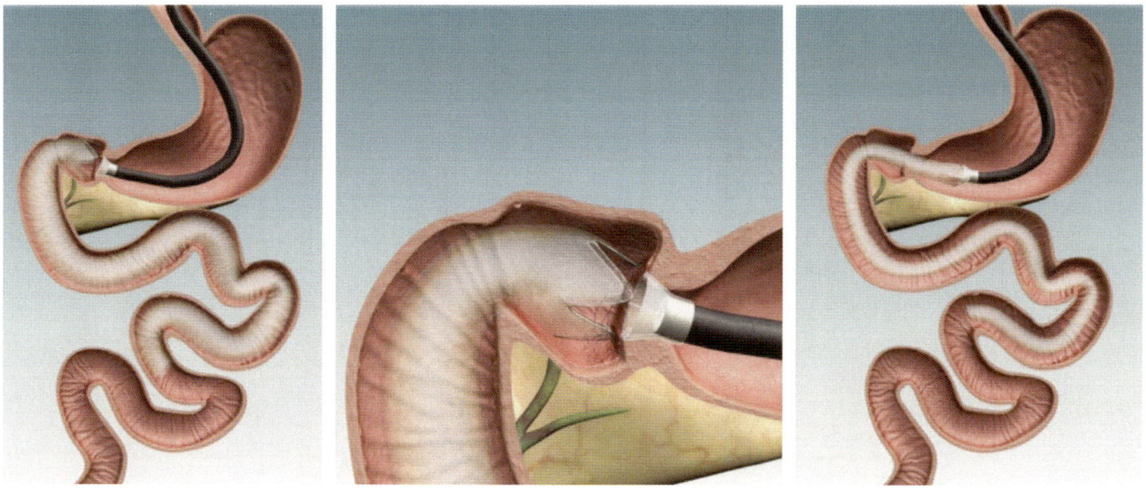

Figure 3: Duodenal sleeve implantation.

duodenal-jejunal exclusion portion of gastric bypass surgery, thus recreating the beneficial effects seen in postsurgery on glucose homeostasis and energy metabolism, but without enduring permanent alterations to the intestinal anatomy and avoiding the risks associated with undergoing invasive surgery.

2.1. Procedural Overview. All patients undergoing EndoBarrier implantation will adhere to strict dietary advice, which involves following a liquid diet of nutritional drink supplements for at least 1 week prior to their implant date and for 1-2 weeks of postprocedure. The purpose of following this regime is to facilitate clear views during endoscopy for implantation of the device and to minimise the risk of a food bolus obstruction of the liner in the first few weeks of postprocedure.

Both general and conscious sedation can be used for this procedure, which also requires fluoroscopic imaging for guidance in the insertion or removal of the liner. A thorough endoscopic examination of the upper GI tract is conducted prior to device placement to ensure suitability and to detect any potential anatomical variants such as a short duodenal bulb or peptic ulcer disease, which may preclude the device from being inserted. GID, the manufacturer of the device, advocates prescribing a proton pump inhibitor (e.g., omeprazole 40 mg twice daily) three days prior to insertion and to continue this whilst the device is in situ up until two weeks after the device is removed to minimise the risk of potential bleeding from the implant. Furthermore, to reduce the potential for infection, GID also suggests administering a single dose of broad-spectrum antibiotic (e.g., 2 g ceftriaxone) 1-2 hours prior to implantation.

The advantages and disadvantages of the EndoBarrier implant and explant procedure are summarised in Table 1.

2.2. Implantation. Implantation takes on average 45 minutes to perform. The patient is placed in left lateral decubitus position, and a surveillance gastroscopy is performed after which the endoscope is placed in the first part of the duodenum. A guidewire is advanced as distally as possible into the duodenum through the working channel of the gastroscope and the gastroscope is removed. The EndoBarrier delivery system (coaxial catheter system with capsule containing the EndoBarrier sleeve) is advanced over the guidewire until the capsule sits comfortably in the pylorus. This is aided by a dotted line marked on the capsule, which allows the correct positioning of the device in the pylorus, so the distal end sits in the duodenal bulb ready to deploy the sleeve. The guidewire is then removed. The delivery system has 5 steps, which are followed in order to release the device from its protective capsule into the ideal position, which should be 5–10 mm from the pylorus with the proximal barbs anchored in the duodenal bulb and the sleeve running distal to this (Figure 3). Peristalsis will ensure the sleeve unravels across its 60 cm length into the duodenum. A water-soluble contrast such as gastrografin is then used to confirm the positioning of the device and to prove it is patent. The patient is usually discharged at home the same day following recovery from the anaesthetic.

2.3. Explantation. Explantation takes on average 30 minutes to perform. The patient is placed in left lateral decubitus position, and a surveillance gastroscopy is performed. The endoscope is then removed, and a protective hood is placed at the end of the endoscope. This circular hood is made out of a durable plastic polymer and is designed to hold within it the sharp anchors located at the proximal end of the liner. The endoscope is reintroduced into the duodenum, and the anchors of the device are identified. Each of the anchors has drawstrings attached to them. A specially designed grasper with a hook at the end contained in a protective plastic sheath is then passed down to the therapeutic channel of the scope until it arrives distal to the protective hood at the end of the endoscope. The retrieval hook is then advanced forward beyond its sheath and positioned around one of the drawstrings before being retracted, pulling the drawstring with it, thus collapsing down the device. Once the anchor is fully collapsed, the retrieval device is locked in position, and the endoscope with hood is advanced forward ensuring that all the collapsed anchors are captured within the hood, which can be confirmed by fluoroscopy. Under fluoroscopic guidance, the endoscope retrieval system and liner are removed together, making sure they can travel safely through the upper GI anatomy. Finally, the explant site is examined for signs of bleeding. The patient is usually discharged at home the same day following recovery from the anaesthetic.

3. Clinical Trial Data

To date, there have been five randomised controlled trials (RCTs) examining the efficacy of the EndoBarrier (Table 2). The largest of which was a multicentered trial performed in the Netherlands, in which 73 patients were randomised to receive either DJBL treatment in combination with dietary intervention or dietary intervention alone (the control group) [4].

A total of 35 patients successfully had the EndoBarrier implanted for a 6-month period. BMI at baseline was 35 kg/m^2 and 37 kg/m^2 in the device arm and control arm, respectively, and reduced to 31 kg/m^2 and 35 kg/m^2, respectively, over the 6-month period. HBA1c at baseline was 8.3% in both groups and reduced to 7.0% and 7.9% in the device and control arm, respectively. There was only one early device removal due to blockage of the DJBL with food. Patients were also followed up postremoval of the device after 6 months where BMI and HBA1c were measured. BMI was 32 kg/m^2 in the device group and 36 kg/m^2 in the control group, respectively, showing a slight increase following the device removal in the treatment arm. HBA1c was 7.3% and 8.0% at the end of the follow-up period in both groups, showing a mean reduction of 1% and 0.3% in both groups, respectively.

In another study of 41 patients, 26 had the device implanted compared to a control group on a low-calorie diet and had a mean excess weight loss of 19% for the device versus 6.9% in the control group [5]. Furthermore, out of 8 patients in the device arm with T2DM at baseline, improvements were seen in glucose levels and HBA1c in all but one of them.

Our research group at Imperial College conducted the first postmarketing clinical trial of the EndoBarrier in the UK consisting of 45 patients recruited from three centers (St. Mary's Hospital London, Southampton, and University Hospital Manchester) [9]. In this study, participants were aged 18–65 years with T2DM, with a BMI greater than 30 kg/m^2 and received the implant for a duration of one year. Mean HBA1c and BMI at baseline were 69 mmol (8.5%) and 39.9 kg/m^2, respectively. Of the 45 patients, 31 (69%) completed the 12-month study period. Average implantation time was 27 minutes, and fluoroscopic time was 7 min (SD 5.7). There were no procedure-related complications during implant or explant. There were 14 early withdrawals before the 12-month implant period, and two of these participants had device-related adverse events requiring premature explant for melaena and device migration resulting in abdominal pain, respectively. The other reasons for withdrawal included the development of other medical complications precluding EndoBarrier implantation and patient choice for early removal.

At 1 year at the time of explant, the average reduction in HBA1c was 0.8%. A mean reduction in BMI of 4.9 kg/m^2 was observed with a mean weight loss of 15 kg. These positive changes appeared to be maintained at the 6-month follow-up period with small but insignificant changes in these parameters after explantation.

A recent systematic review and meta-analysis assessing the effect of the EndoBarrier on glycaemic control in obese patients with T2DM yielded similar results [10]. This included 388 patients from the 5 RCTs listed above and additional 9 observational studies with an average device implantation time of 8.4 ± 4 months. HBA1c decreased by 1.3% at the time of explantation. The effect of the EndoBarrier on weight loss was also investigated, which included 10 studies with a total of 352 patients. Average weight loss was 11.3 kg at time of explantation corresponding to a BMI reduction of 4.1 kg/m^2. The average device implantation in this cohort of patients was 9.2 ± 3.1 months.

4. Potential Mechanisms of Action

There is currently a poor understanding of mechanisms underpinning how the device elicits its effects on weight loss and glycaemia. As the EndoBarrier is designed to mimic the bypass portion of the RYGB surgery, one might postulate that it works by similar mechanisms. One potential theory of how RYGB surgery works is the so-called BRAVE effects (bile flow changes, restriction of stomach size, anatomical gastrointestinal rearrangement, vagal manipulation, and enteric hormonal modulation) [11]. These changes are believed to take place within minutes of the RYGB surgery being performed and are considered as triggering gears that activate a multitude of subsequent downstream mechanisms (hindgut, foregut, and midgut theories), which might account for why glycaemic improvements are observed independent of any

Table 2: Summary of RCTs on the EndoBarrier.

Study	Number of patients	BMI	Implant duration (weeks)	Weight loss	Change in HBA1c	Stent removal rate
Gersin et al. [6]	47; 21 in treatment arm	46 kg/m^2	12	−8.2 kg ± 1.3 kg in treatment arm versus 2 kg ± 1.1 kg in sham arm	Not an endpoint	38%
Koehestanie et al. [4]	73; 34 in treatment arm	35 kg/m^2 device; 37 kg/m^2 in control	26	10.6 kg device; 5.3 kg in control	−1.3% versus 0.4% in control	3%
Rodriguez-Grunert et al. [7]	18; 12 in treatment arm	39 kg/m^2	24	−10.2 kg ± 1.3 kg in device arm versus 7.1 ± 4.3 kg in sham arm	−2.4 ± 0.7% versus −0.8 ± 0.4% in control	25%
Schouten et al. [5]	41; 30 in treatment arm	49 kg/m^2	12	19% in device; 6.9% in control	−1.1% versus 0.4% in control	15%
Tarnoff et al. [8]	35; 29 in treatment arm	42 kg/m^2 in device; 40 kg/m^2 in control	12	−10.3 kg ± 3.2 kg versus 2.6 kg ± 3.5 kg in the control group	Not an endpoint	20%

weight loss occurring. The EndoBarrier was designed to be an "endoscopic bypass" so that it has been envisaged to activate some of the same mechanisms as bariatric operations (historically based on foregut exclusion or the "foregut theory" where a putative anti-incretin is no longer released after surgical/interventional foregut exclusion). We consider some of the likely mechanisms including

(i) enteric hormonal modulation and the incretin theory,

(ii) alterations in the gut microbiota,

(iii) bile flow changes.

As very little data currently exists in the literature on how the EndoBarrier influences these above mechanisms, most of the evidence described below will be drawn from our experience post-RYGB surgery.

4.1. Incretin Theory. It is now widely accepted that altering the gastrointestinal anatomy following RYGB alters the flow of nutrients leading to important changes in gut-derived hormones by foregut exclusion and modified hindgut signals. This in turn positively influences the metabolic changes seen following surgery including improvement in glycaemic control and weight loss. Fundamental to this is the paradigm of the "incretin effect," which is the concept that insulin secretion is also directly influenced by hormonal cues resultant from food intake and energy expenditure [12]. In fact, it is estimated that the incretin effect accounts for as much as 50–70% of insulin secretion in response to an oral glucose load [13]. However, this incretin response is thought to be significantly impaired in patients who are obese or have T2DM [14]. Two key incretin hormones are glucagon-like peptide-1 (GLP-1) and glucagon-dependent insulinotropic polypeptide (GIP), which are both released following a meal from intestinal enteroendocrine cells known as L- and K-cells, respectively.

Following RYGB, undigested nutrients bypass the proximal intestine rapidly reaching the distal small bowel leading to an increase in GLP-1 levels by nutrient stimulation of L-cells [15]. GLP-1 stimulates insulin secretion from the pancreas, increases insulin sensitivity, and inhibits glucagon, thus reducing gluconeogenesis and hepatic glucose output. GLP-1 is also an anorexigenic hormone that acts centrally to increase satiety and reduce appetite [16]. It is a combination of these responses from increased levels of GLP-1, which is thought to play a pivotal role in the metabolic changes seen after RYGB.

GIP is primarily secreted in the proximal intestine, as this is where the majority K-cells are located and have various physiological effects including both postprandial secretion of insulin and glucagon release during hypoglycaemia or a euglycaemic state [17]. Following RYGB, the role of GIP is more unclear as there are conflicting reports of GIP levels with some studies showing an increase whilst others show decreased levels or no change at all [15, 18, 19]. Nevertheless, it is hypothesised that the blunting in levels of GIP observed in some studies following RYGB contributes to the antidiabetogenic effects of this type of surgery.

Various studies have investigated the changes in gut hormones following EndoBarrier implantation including a study by de Jonge et al. of 17 obese patients with T2DM who received the device for 6 months [20]. Fasting and postprandial levels of glucose, glucagon, and insulin were recorded as well as postprandial levels of GLP-1 and GIP. The authors found a reduction in both fasting and postprandial levels of glucose following EndoBarrier implantation, which coincided with a reduction in glucagon levels, although insulin levels were unchanged. Postprandial levels of GLP-1 increased significantly and conversely; GIP levels were found to decrease at 6 months. These findings are similar to the changes in gut hormones post-RYGB previously described.

In contrast to these findings, a small study by Koehestanie et al., in which fasting GIP, GLP-1, and ghrelin levels were measured at baseline, 1 week and 4 weeks in 12 obese diabetic patients, found no significant changes in GIP. Moreover, levels of GLP-1 appeared to decrease 1-week postimplant followed by an elevation back to baseline levels in the following 3 weeks [21]. There was no correlation identified between gut hormone changes and reductions in body weight and BMI.

Rohde et al. compared the effect of the EndoBarrier on postprandial physiology in 10 obese patients with normal glucose tolerance (NGT) and 9 age-, body weight-, and BMI-matched patients with T2DM. Parameters investigated included insulin, glucose, glucagon, gut hormone secretion, gall bladder emptying, and appetite and food intake using liquid mixed meal test and a subsequent ad libitum meal test at baseline, 1 week and 26 weeks following EndoBarrier implantation [22]. Basal plasma concentrations of GLP-1, GIP, and PYY were similar in the two groups before EndoBarrier implantation, and the device did not appear to affect basal concentrations significantly in any of the groups. Small but significant increases were observed in postprandial levels of GLP-1 and PYY levels at weeks 1 and 26 in the patient group with T2DM but not in those with NGT, and overall, the EndoBarrier did not appear to have any impact on levels of insulin, glucose, or glucagon following implantation.

Levels of ghrelin appear to increase following the EndoBarrier device in clinical trials, which contradict findings post-RYGB where a reduction in ghrelin levels is often seen [21, 23]. A potential explantation for this is that ghrelin is predominantly released from P1/D1 cells in the upper stomach and fundus, a part of the GI tract which is unaffected by the EndoBarrier implant unlike in RYGB. The rise in ghrelin could be a physiological response to dieting or in response to weight loss induced by the EndoBarrier. Clearly, larger numbers are required in order to draw any firm conclusion on the effects of EndoBarrier on the gut hormones.

4.2. Bile Flow Modulation. Bile acids (BAs) are believed to play an integral role in regulating satiety as well as influencing lipid, cholesterol, and glucose metabolism through complex interactions, which include stimulating the secretion of incretin hormones, GLP-1 and PYY, and disruption of the gut microbiota [24]. RYGB surgery appears to impact BA homeostasis by altering the enterohepatic circulation leading to increased levels of plasma BAs postsurgery compared with at baseline [25]. Potentially, this is another mechanism to explain the higher levels of incretin hormones seen in postbariatric surgery.

Fibroblast growth factor-19 (FGF-19) is a potent stimulator of BA synthesis, and in a small study of 30 obese patients with T2DM, levels were found to be markedly increased following EndoBarrier implantation for 10 months in these individuals [26]. This might provide a partial mechanism on how the device elicits its effects on improvements in glycaemic control.

Free BAs also interact closely with the microbiota found in the small intestine, so increased concentrations of these BAs may not only influence the overall number of bacteria in this region but also their composition.

4.3. Gut Microbiota. The gut microbiome has been implicated in numerous disease processes, and obesity is no different. Manipulation of the host gut microbiome using faecal transplantation has been shown to alter host phenotype as evidenced by improvements in insulin resistance observed in obese individuals following transplantation with lean microbiota [27]. Obese individuals have significant differences in their gut microbiota compared with lean individuals. Two particular groups of bacteria, which have found to be both beneficial and dominant in the gut, are the Bacteroidetes and the Firmicutes. A reduction in the proportion of Bacteroidetes has been observed in obese individuals when compared with lean individuals, and these species of bacteria appear to increase postbariatric surgery [28, 29]. Increased levels of Actinobacteria have also been found in observational studies of the gut microbiome of obese individuals compared with their lean twin [30].

Following RYGB, the gut microbiota alters with an increase in bacterial richness as a consequence of the changes in pH levels in the proximal small bowel, alteration in gastric motility and nutrient flow [31].

Numerous studies have shown an increase in certain bacterial species, which include Gammaproteobacteria following RYGB [32, 33]. Further explorations into the changes in gut microbiome following surgery are required, and this might in turn uncover new therapeutic strategies for the treatment of obesity and diabetes. To date, there have been no studies looking at the impact of the EndoBarrier on the gut microbiota, but one might hypothesize that similar microbial changes may be seen as in post-RYGB surgery.

4.4. Gastric Emptying. The EndoBarrier's effect on gastric emptying was investigated in a small study of 25 patients [34]. A delay in gastric emptying at 16-week post-EndoBarrier implant was found when compared to baseline, but this did not appear to correlate with any clinical outcomes such as weight loss or glycaemic control.

5. Safety Profile

By far, the most commonly reported side effect of the device is GI upset, including abdominal pain and nausea. These symptoms usually resolve as the patient acclimatises to having the device in situ, but a minority of patients (2%) are unable to tolerate these symptoms leading to early device removal. The other complications include GI bleeding (1.5%) and device migration (1.4%). Rarer complications such as cholestasis and pancreatitis can also occur.

Betzel et al. published safety data on 185 patients from 2011 to 2014 who received the EndoBarrier for one year [35]. In 31% of cases, devices were removed prematurely and predominantly from abdominal discomfort and nausea, with more serious adverse events reported as gastrointestinal bleeding, device migration, obstruction, and the development of liver abscesses.

Liver abscesses pose the most serious complication associated with the EndoBarrier with most cases reported late during the course of treatment, that is, towards the time of explanation at 9–12 months. The German DJBL registry reported 1 case in 66 patients who had received the EndoBarrier for one year having previously reported 4 cases in a 235 patient registry [36]. Three were documented at explantation with the other one occurring following early removal for device dislocation. All were managed with antibiotics and/or drained with no permanent sequelae.

The ENDO Trial was a multicenter, double-blinded, and randomised trial in the US to evaluate the safety and efficacy of the EndoBarrier on glycaemic control. Unfortunately, in March 2015, the Food and Drug Administration (FDA) halted the trial due to the development of 7 liver abscesses (3.5%), which was much higher than anticipated. The cause for these liver abscesses is unclear, but the theory is that the EndoBarrier creates a nidus of infection, which may spread to the liver bed.

Postmarket surveillance data from GID reports an incidence of 1%, which is also supported by the data from a worldwide registry established in 2017 by the Association of British Clinical Diabetologists [37]. From 492 EndoBarrier patients, there were 6 reported cases of liver abscesses. Early removal of device because of GI bleeding was 4%. Device migration was 3% with liner obstruction rare only accounting for 0.3% of cases.

6. Future Developments

Currently, the EndoBarrier is licensed for 1 year after which point it should be removed. A certain issue which arises is that the vast majority of patients may then lose the beneficial effects on glycaemic control and weight loss, which the device may have been exerting whilst in situ resulting in worsening of their diabetes and an increase in their BMI. An Australian study found that in 30 patients who were followed up for 6-month period immediate postremoval of the EndoBarrier, 72% gained weight with only 5 patients maintaining their weight loss and 4 patients losing further weight [38]. In the same study, 51 patients were followed up for a period of >6 months following explant with 69% regaining their weight and only 5 patients maintaining their weight and with 7 patients losing further weight. The study did not comment on how these particular patients managed to maintain their weight loss or indeed lose further weight.

To prevent this regression, occurring future therapeutic strategies may entail reimplantation of the device or developing a prototype that can remain in situ for longer than 1 year. GID has previously reported data demonstrating the feasibility and safety of reimplantation of the EndoBarrier in 5 patients who initially completed 12 months of EndoBarrier treatment but then proceeded to have the device reimplanted after 4 months for another 12 months. HbA1c fell from a baseline of 9.1% to 6.7% after the 1st explantation and from 7.8% upon 2nd implantation to 7.1% at explant with no reported complications [39]. Clearly, the numbers in this study are very small, but reimplantation of the EndoBarrier might be another treatment option to maintain the effect of the device.

A second-generation EndoBarrier device with a 1 mm increase in barb length was trialed in 80 patients in Chile. The subjects initially consented to the implant for one year but were then given the opportunity to keep the device in for up to 3 years if tolerated [40]. The percentage excess weight losses in the complete population at 52 weeks (71 patients), 104 weeks (40 patients), and 156 weeks (11 patients) were 44 ± 16, 40 ± 22, and 39 ± 20, respectively ($p < 0.001$). There were 17 T2DM subjects enrolled in the study with baseline HbA1c of 7.1 ± 1.6%, which significantly decreased to 6 ± 0.9 and 5.7 ± 0.7% after 12 and 24 months, respectively. Two diabetic subjects managed to complete 36 months of follow-up, and both maintained an HbA1c below 6%.

An ideal situation is the creation of a device which could remain in situ for longer thus providing a more permanent solution for these patients, but for this to happen, one must consider how to combat the unwanted side effects associated with having a duodenal sleeve implanted long term.

7. Conclusion

The EndoBarrier appears to be a promising device for the management of obese patients with type 2 diabetes, which is designed to mimic the clinical and physiological effects of bariatric surgery. It can induce moderate weight loss and improvements in glycaemic control in patients with an acceptable safety profile. However, currently, there is a paucity of data available with the majority of trials published containing small numbers of patients or from an unrandomised setting.

Its current position in the treatment algorithm for obesity and diabetes is unclear, and larger randomised controlled trials are required to help to try to answer this question. At present, we see the device's utility in the following situations:

(i) In obese patients with poorly controlled T2DM who decline or are unfit for surgery

(ii) An adjunct to surgery to induce weight loss in the superobese prior to bariatric surgery

(iii) To facilitate glycaemic improvement in patients requiring elective surgery but whose poor diabetes control precludes this surgical procedure from being performed

The EndoBarrier in its current form is unlikely to replace bariatric surgery but may act as a complementary intervention within the arsenal of antidiabetes/antiobesity therapies. Future work in this field should focus on developing the device so that it offers longer treatment duration whilst also improving its safety profile and tolerability. Such a minimally invasive device may then carry the potential to address some of the broader needs of the global diabesity population.

References

[1] WHO, "Obesity and overweight factsheet," 2018, http://www.who.int/news-room/fact-sheets/detail/obesity-and-overweight.

[2] WHO, "*Global Report on Diabetes*," 2016, http://www.who.int/diabetes/global-report/en/.

[3] R. V. Cohen, S. Shikora, T. Petry, P. P. Caravatto, and C. W. le Roux, "The diabetes surgery summit II guidelines: a disease-based clinical recommendation," *Obesity Surgery*, vol. 26, no. 8, pp. 1989–1991, 2016.

[4] P. Koehestanie, C. de Jonge, F. J. Berends, I. M. Janssen, N. D. Bouvy, and J. W. M. Greve, "The effect of the endoscopic duodenal-jejunal bypass liner on obesity and type 2 diabetes mellitus, a multicenter randomized controlled trial," *Annals of Surgery*, vol. 260, no. 6, pp. 984–992, 2014.

[5] R. Schouten, C. S. Rijs, N. D. Bouvy et al., "A multicenter, randomized efficacy study of the EndoBarrier gastrointestinal liner for presurgical weight loss prior to bariatric surgery," *Annals of Surgery*, vol. 251, no. 2, pp. 236–243, 2010.

[6] K. S. Gersin, R. I. Rothstein, R. J. Rosenthal et al., "Open-label, sham-controlled trial of an endoscopic duodenojejunal bypass liner for preoperative weight loss in bariatric surgery candidates," *Gastrointestinal Endoscopy*, vol. 71, no. 6, pp. 976–982, 2010.

[7] L. Rodriguez-Grunert, M. P. Galvao Neto, M. Alamo, A. C. Ramos, P. B. Baez, and M. Tarnoff, "First human experience with endoscopically delivered and retrieved duodenal-jejunal bypass sleeve," *Surgery for Obesity and Related Diseases*, vol. 4, no. 1, pp. 55–59, 2008.

[8] M. Tarnoff, L. Rodriguez, A. Escalona et al., "Open label, prospective, randomized controlled trial of an endoscopic duodenal-jejunal bypass sleeve versus low calorie diet for pre-operative weight loss in bariatric surgery," *Surgical Endoscopy*, vol. 23, no. 3, pp. 650–656, 2009.

[9] N. Patel, A. Mohanaruban, H. Ashrafian et al., "EndoBarrier®: a safe and effective novel treatment for obesity and type 2 diabetes?," *Obesity Surgery*, vol. 28, no. 7, pp. 1980–1989, 2018.

[10] P. Jirapinyo, A. V. Haas, and C. C. Thompson, "Effect of the duodenal-jejunal bypass liner on glycemic control in patients with type 2 diabetes with obesity: a meta-analysis with secondary analysis on weight loss and hormonal changes," *Diabetes Care*, vol. 41, no. 5, pp. 1106–1115, 2018.

[11] H. Ashrafian, T. Athanasiou, J. V. Li et al., "Diabetes resolution and hyperinsulinaemia after metabolic Roux-en-Y gastric bypass," *Obesity Reviews*, vol. 12, no. 5, pp. e257–e272, 2011.

[12] B. Jones, S. R. Bloom, T. Buenaventura, A. Tomas, and G. A. Rutter, "Control of insulin secretion by GLP-1," *Peptides*, vol. 100, pp. 75–84, 2018.

[13] W. Kim and J. M. Egan, "The role of incretins in glucose homeostasis and diabetes treatment," *Pharmacological Reviews*, vol. 60, no. 4, pp. 470–512, 2008.

[14] J. J. Holst, F. K. Knop, T. Vilsboll, T. Krarup, and S. Madsbad, "Loss of incretin effect is a specific, important, and early characteristic of type 2 diabetes," *Diabetes Care*, vol. 34, Supplement_2, pp. S251–S257, 2011.

[15] N. B. Jørgensen, S. H. Jacobsen, C. Dirksen et al., "Acute and long-term effects of Roux-en-Y gastric bypass on glucose metabolism in subjects with type 2 diabetes and normal glucose tolerance," *American Journal of Physiology-Endocrinology and Metabolism*, vol. 303, no. 1, pp. E122–E131, 2012.

[16] M. E. Doyle and J. M. Egan, "Glucagon-like peptide-1," *Recent Progress in Hormone Research*, vol. 56, no. 1, pp. 377–400, 2001.

[17] L. S. Gasbjerg, M. B. N. Gabe, B. Hartmann et al., "Glucose-dependent insulinotropic polypeptide (GIP) receptor antagonists as anti-diabetic agents," *Peptides*, vol. 100, pp. 173–181, 2018.

[18] B. A. Whitson, D. B. Leslie, T. A. Kellogg et al., "Entero-endocrine changes after gastric bypass in diabetic and non-diabetic patients: a preliminary study," *Journal of Surgical Research*, vol. 141, no. 1, pp. 31–39, 2007.

[19] B. Laferrère, J. Teixeira, J. McGinty et al., "Effect of weight loss by gastric bypass surgery versus hypocaloric diet on glucose and incretin levels in patients with type 2 diabetes," *The Journal of Clinical Endocrinology & Metabolism*, vol. 93, no. 7, pp. 2479–2485, 2008.

[20] C. de Jonge, S. S. Rensen, F. J. Verdam et al., "Endoscopic duodenal-jejunal bypass liner rapidly improves type 2 diabetes," *Obesity Surgery*, vol. 23, no. 9, pp. 1354–1360, 2013.

[21] P. Koehestanie, K. Dogan, F. Berends et al., "Duodenal-jejunal bypass liner implantation provokes rapid weight loss and improved glycemic control, accompanied by elevated fasting ghrelin levels," *Endoscopy International Open*, vol. 2, no. 01, pp. E21–E27, 2014.

[22] U. Rohde, C. A. Federspiel, P. Vilmann et al., "The impact of EndoBarrier gastrointestinal liner in obese patients with normal glucose tolerance and in patients with type 2 diabetes," *Diabetes, Obesity & Metabolism*, vol. 19, no. 2, pp. 189–199, 2017.

[23] B. Stratmann, Y. Krepak, E. Schiffer et al., "Beneficial metabolic effects of duodenal jejunal bypass liner for the treatment of adipose patients with type 2 diabetes mellitus: analysis of responders and non-responders," *Hormone and Metabolic Research*, vol. 48, no. 10, pp. 630–637, 2016.

[24] N. C. Penney, J. Kinross, R. C. Newton, and S. Purkayastha, "The role of bile acids in reducing the metabolic complications of obesity after bariatric surgery: a systematic review," *International Journal of Obesity*, vol. 39, no. 11, pp. 1565–1574, 2015.

[25] M. E. Patti, S. M. Houten, A. C. Bianco et al., "Serum bile acids are higher in humans with prior gastric bypass: potential contribution to improved glucose and lipid metabolism," *Obesity*, vol. 17, no. 9, pp. 1671–1677, 2009.

[26] M. Mraz, P. Kavalkova, P. Trachta et al., "Ten months of treatment with endoscopic duodeno-jejunal bypass liner reduce glycaemic variability and partially restore the incretin effect in obese type 2 diabetic subjects," in *75th Annual Meeting of the American Diabetes Association*, American Diabetes Association (ADA), 2014.

[27] A. Vrieze, E. Van Nood, F. Holleman et al., "Transfer of intestinal microbiota from lean donors increases insulin sensitivity in individuals with metabolic syndrome," *Gastroenterology*, vol. 143, no. 4, pp. 913–916.e7, 2012.

[28] R. E. Ley, P. J. Turnbaugh, S. Klein, and J. I. Gordon, "Microbial ecology: human gut microbes associated with obesity," *Nature*, vol. 444, no. 7122, pp. 1022-1023, 2006.

[29] J. P. Furet, L. C. Kong, J. Tap et al., "Differential adaptation of human gut microbiota to bariatric surgery-induced weight loss: links with metabolic and low-grade inflammation markers," *Diabetes*, vol. 59, no. 12, pp. 3049–3057, 2010.

[30] P. J. Turnbaugh, M. Hamady, T. Yatsunenko et al., "A core gut microbiome in obese and lean twins," *Nature*, vol. 457, no. 7228, pp. 480–484, 2008.

[31] J. V. Li, H. Ashrafian, M. Bueter et al., "Metabolic surgery profoundly influences gut microbial-host metabolic cross-talk," *Gut*, vol. 60, no. 9, pp. 1214–1223, 2011.

[32] L. C. Kong, J. Tap, J. Aron-Wisnewsky et al., "Gut microbiota after gastric bypass in human obesity: increased richness and associations of bacterial genera with adipose tissue genes," *The American Journal of Clinical Nutrition*, vol. 98, no. 1, pp. 16–24, 2013.

[33] H. Zhang, J. K. DiBaise, A. Zuccolo et al., "Human gut microbiota in obesity and after gastric bypass," *Proceedings of the National Academy of Sciences*, vol. 106, no. 7, pp. 2365–2370, 2009.

[34] E. G. H. de Moura, G. S. Lopes, B. da Costa Martins et al., "Effects of duodenal-jejunal bypass liner (EndoBarrier®) on gastric emptying in obese and type 2 diabetic patients," *Obesity Surgery*, vol. 25, no. 9, pp. 1618–1625, 2015.

[35] B. Betzel, J. Homan, E. O. Aarts et al., "Weight reduction and improvement in diabetes by the duodenal-jejunal bypass liner: a 198 patient cohort study," *Surgical Endoscopy*, vol. 31, no. 7, pp. 2881–2891, 2017.

[36] N. Riedel, K. Laubner, A. Lautenbach et al., "Longitudinal evaluation of efficacy, safety and nutritional status during one-year treatment with the duodenal-jejunal bypass liner," *Surgery for Obesity and Related Diseases*, vol. 14, no. 6, pp. 769–779, 2018.

[37] B. Ryder and Association of British Clinical Diabetologists (ABCD), "Duodenal jejunal bypass liner for diabesity - the risk benefit ratio from the world wide Endobarrier registry," *European Association for Study of Diabetes*, 2018.

[38] P. M. Forner, T. Ramacciotti, J. E. Farey, and R. V. Lord, "Safety and effectiveness of an endoscopically placed duodenal-jejunal bypass device (EndoBarrier®): outcomes in 114 patients," *Obesity Surgery*, vol. 27, no. 12, pp. 3306–3313, 2017.

[39] GID Release, "GI Dynamics touts no complications, lowered insulin in EndoBarrier reimplantation trial," 2017, https://www.massdevice.com/gi-dynamics-touts-no-complications-lowered-insulin-in-reimplantation-trial/.

[40] N. Quezada, R. Muñoz, C. Morelli et al., "Safety and efficacy of the endoscopic duodenal-jejunal bypass liner prototype in severe or morbidly obese subjects implanted for up to 3 years," *Surgical Endoscopy*, vol. 32, no. 1, pp. 260–267, 2018.

19

Perioperative Care of Patients with Inflammatory Bowel Disease: Focus on Nutritional Support

Patrick L. Stoner,[1] **Amir Kamel**,[2] **Fares Ayoub**,[1] **Sanda Tan**,[3] **Atif Iqbal**,[3] **Sarah C. Glover**,[1] **and Ellen M. Zimmermann**[1]

[1]*Department of Medicine, Division of Gastroenterology, University of Florida, 2000 SW Archer Rd, Gainesville, FL 32610, USA*
[2]*Department of Pharmacotherapy, College of Pharmacy, University of Florida, 2000 SW Archer Rd, Gainesville, FL 32610, USA*
[3]*Department of Surgery, Division of Colorectal Surgery, College of Medicine, University of Florida, 2000 SW Archer Rd, Gainesville, FL 32610, USA*

Correspondence should be addressed to Patrick L. Stoner; patrick.stoner@medicine.ufl.edu

Academic Editor: Martin Hubner

Patients with inflammatory bowel disease (IBD) commonly require surgery despite the availability of an increasingly large repertoire of powerful immunosuppressive medications for the treatment of IBD. Optimizing patients' care preoperatively is crucial to obtaining good surgical outcomes. This review discusses preoperative assessment and management principles including assessing disease location and activity with cross-sectional or endoscopic imaging, addressing modifiable risk factors (i.e., stopping smoking, weaning steroids, and correcting anemia), and properly managing medications. The major focus of our literature review is the evaluation for malnutrition, a common finding that affects up to 70% of patients with IBD and a well-known, independent risk factor for adverse postoperative outcomes. Our review confirms that whenever feasible, oral or enteral nutrition (EN) is the preferred method of nutritional support; parenteral nutrition (PN) should be reserved for nutritionally deficient IBD patients unable to tolerate EN. In selected patients, recent data demonstrated that the use of preoperative PN resulted in improved nutritional status, fewer postoperative complications, and reduced disease severity. Our review highlights the need for well-designed, prospective trials investigating perioperative nutritional support in patients with IBD. Future studies should perform modern nutritional assessment, standardize for diet, and include patients with UC since this subset of patients is underrepresented in existing studies. In addition, relevant outcome of interest specific to Crohn's disease (CD) patients such as length of small bowel resected, number of anastomoses, and need for an ostomy should be included as these patients may require repeated small bowel resections.

1. Introduction

Inflammatory bowel disease (IBD), including Crohn's disease (CD) and ulcerative colitis (UC), is characterized by chronic relapsing gastrointestinal (GI) inflammation. Though the underlying cause of IBD remains unknown, important insights into the pathogenesis have been gained through studies of immune mechanisms, genetics, and the microbiome [1]. In addition, an explosion of new therapeutics has revolutionized our approach to treatment. While new therapies have helped decrease hospital admission rates, incidence rates for surgery remain high. Indeed, the risk of surgery in patients with Crohn's disease is approximately 50% at a 10-year disease duration [2], while 40% of patients with ulcerative colitis requiring inpatient care will ultimately require proctocolectomy [3]. Postoperative endoscopic recurrence of CD is near 90% at one year. In ulcerative colitis, a disease that has historically been considered curative with surgery, significant rates of postoperative transition to CD, difficult to control pouchitis, and systemic inflammatory manifestations remind us that the disease has an immunologic basis that persists even after proctocolectomy [3].

An explanation for the persistently high surgical rates in CD even in the era of aggressive use of potent anti-inflammatory medications eludes the field. The answer can likely be found in the molecular mechanisms that underlie the progression from inflammation to fibrosis causing end organ dysfunction and structural damage such as strictures that often require surgery. Pathogenically, it seems that inflammatory mechanisms trigger fibrotic pathways that march on despite our potent therapeutics. In certain patients, aggressive disease appears to predispose patients to multiple surgeries such that 35% of patients requiring one resection will require a second resection within 10 years [2].

Identifying patients destined to have aggressive IBD can help clinicians tailor therapy and set a strategy for monitoring disease progression. Discussing these risks with patients can help improve patient understanding of their disease and improve their adherence to medication and testing regimens. Understanding the consequences can help patients modify risk factors such as smoking in patients with CD. Predictors of aggressive CD are shown in Table 1 [4–7].

Preoperative assessment and management are key to good outcomes in IBD. Imaging is fundamental to the planning of both medical and surgical strategies as it highlights the sites and severity of inflammation and identifies complications. Colonoscopy has been the primary modality for recognition of dysplasia in IBD, especially ulcerative colitis as the inflamed sites are within the reach of the colonoscope. In CD, ileocolonic disease can be assessed by colonoscopy. In patients with more proximal disease, cross-sectional imaging such as computed tomography enterography (CTE) and magnetic resonance enterography (MRE) can evaluate bowel proximal to the reach of the colonoscope and also evaluate for extraluminal disease [8]. Perioperative assessment and management principles in CD are shown in Table 2 and recently reviewed [9].

Malnutrition is an independent risk factor for adverse postoperative outcomes and affects up to 70% of the IBD population [10, 11]. Malnourished patients undergoing surgery are at a particularly increased risk for postoperative complications given their systemic illness and the many other risk factors for poor surgical outcomes they may possess. This review will focus on perioperative nutritional support in IBD patients, with a particular emphasis on parenteral nutrition.

2. Surgical Techniques and Perioperative Medical Management

The cornerstone for elective surgical management of UC is a restorative total proctocolectomy with ileal pouch-anal anastomosis (IPAA). For patients with severe UC requiring urgent or emergent surgery who have been on high-dose steroids, a three-stage procedure is recommended with subtotal abdominal colectomy and end ileostomy performed initially, with a subsequent completion of proctectomy with IPAA [12]. In CD, surgery may be indicated for the treatment of refractory disease or for complications including strictures, obstruction, fistulae, abscesses, perforation, or dysplasia/cancer. Resection of a diseased segment of small or large bowel is often needed, with ileocecal resection being the most common surgery performed in CD. Alternatives to surgical resection such as stricturoplasty and occasionally endoscopic dilation are employed in the treatment of strictures in attempts to preserve bowel [13].

The optimal protocol for use of IBD therapies in the preoperative setting remains incompletely defined; however, several solid principles have emerged. Most importantly, steroids have a serious negative impact on postoperative

Table 1: Predictors of aggressive Crohn's disease [4–7].

(i) Clinical risk factors
(a) Young age at presentation
(b) Steroids required at first presentation or within 6 months
(c) Perianal disease
(d) Upper tract disease
(e) >2 steroid courses
(f) Current smokers
(g) Multiple admissions
(h) Early resection
(ii) Increased number of positive antibodies identified children at risk for complicated disease
(a) ANCA, ASCA, and anti-CBir 1
(iii) One or more NOD2 mutations associated with aggressive fibrostenotic course
(iv) Presence of a stricture on CTE, MRE, or colonoscopy risk factor for future complications (fistula, abscess, perforation, and obstruction)

ANCA: antineutrophil cytoplasmic antibodies; ASCA: anti-Saccharomyces cerevisiae antibodies; anti-CBir 1: bacterial flagellin antibodies; NOD2: nucleotide-binding oligomerization domain-containing protein 2; CTE: computed tomography enterography; MRE: magnetic resonance enterography.

Table 2: Preoperative assessment and management in CD patients [9].

(i) Preoperative cross-sectional imaging
(a) Identify sites of inflammation and assess for abscess, fistula, and stricture
(ii) Address modifiable risk factors
(a) Smoking—stop preoperatively, even 4 weeks prior shows benefit
(b) Steroids—wean preoperatively (ideally 4 weeks preoperatively)
(c) Anemia—IV iron often needed, transfusion not usually indicated
(iii) Optimize nutritional status when indicated
(a) Weight loss > 10–15% within 6 months
(b) Body mass index < 18.5 kg/m^2
(c) Serum albumin < 3 g/dl (with no evidence of hepatic or renal dysfunction)
(iv) Preoperative colonoscopy (typically but not uniformly needed)
(v) Medical therapy through surgery
(a) Thiopurines—no change
(b) Anti-TNFs—assess levels and antibodies, try not to interrupt
(c) Other biologics—little or no data
(d) Thromboembolism prophylaxis—inpatient

IV: intravenous; anti-TNF: tumor necrosis factor inhibitors.

outcomes [14]. In a meta-analysis by Subramanian et al. [15], patients on steroids have an increased risk of all postoperative complications (infectious and noninfectious) that was dose related. Zangenberg et al. [14] recommend a gradual withdrawal of steroids be attempted so that patients are steroid free for 1 week prior to surgery and recommend against adding additional "stress doses" of steroids for patients who remain on preoperative steroids. Some immunosuppressive medications, such as cyclosporine, are strongly associated with impairments in postoperative wound healing and therefore have higher rates of wound dehiscence, infections, and hernia formation [16]. The more commonly used thiopurines (azathioprine and 6-mercaptopurine) have minimal impact on postoperative complications [17, 18]. Studies investigating the impact of antitumor necrosis factors (anti-TNFs) on surgical outcomes have yielded mixed results, but more recent studies indicate that surgery can be safely performed on both CD and UC patients on biologic therapy [19, 20]. Further, preoperative anti-TNF therapy may have advantages such as decreasing operative times and decreasing the length of resection [21, 22].

Both the American Gastroenterological Association (AGA) and the American College of Gastroenterology (ACG) have published recent guidelines addressing medical therapy in the postoperative setting [23, 24]. While evidence is rapidly emerging, preoperative medical therapy remains institution or surgeon specific. These issues are particularly important to consider in CD because they can influence surgical approach and outcomes, complication rates, and postoperative disease recurrence rates. Addressing modifiable risk factors such as smoking and steroid use in CD is particularly important to achieve good outcomes [9, 14].

3. Identifying and Addressing Malnutrition in the Preoperative Period

Patients with active IBD are at a significantly increased risk for malnutrition, with prevalence rates ranging from 25 to 69% in this population [10]. Malnutrition can occur in UC but is a more common problem in CD since CD can affect any part of the GI tract and UC is restricted to the colon, which has few direct malabsorptive effects [25]. Depending on disease severity, 65% to 76% of CD patients experience weight loss in comparison to 18% to 62% of UC patients [26, 27]. Reasons for malnutrition in IBD patients are multiple and include: increased nutritional requirements from the associated hypermetabolic state seen in systemic inflammation, diarrhea, increased nutrient losses, reduced dietary intake, anorexia, drug-nutrient interactions, and nutrient malabsorption related to intestinal inflammation or reduced intestinal absorptive area from surgical resection [28, 29]. The European Society for Clinical Nutrition and Metabolism (ESPEN) therefore recommends that these patients be screened for malnutrition at the time of diagnosis and thereafter on a regular basis [30]. In addition, IBD patients, even those who appear well nourished, are vulnerable to micronutrient deficiencies (particularly vitamin D, iron, zinc, vitamin C, vitamin B12, and vitamin B6) and regular screening and deficit correction are recommended [28, 30, 31].

Defining malnutrition is difficult, especially in IBD patients, and a gold-standard test of malnutrition has not been identified [32]. Body mass index (BMI), unintentional weight loss, reduced dietary intake, nitrogen balance, and body fat percentage are commonly used clinical measures in the determination of nutritional status [28]. Wagner and Rombeau [32] arbitrarily defined malnutrition in perioperative patients as a serum albumin level of less than 3.5 g/dl and/or unintentional weight loss of 15% of a patient's usual weight over 3 to 4 months. In addition to serum albumin, prealbumin, transferrin, total cholesterol, and triiodothyronine (T3) have all been used as surrogate serologic markers to determine nutritional status but these markers are considered negative acute-phase reactants and are not specific for malnutrition, making them unreliable [32, 33]. Nevertheless, serum albumin of <3 g/dl is included as one of the best indicators of severe malnutrition in CD in the recent guidelines by ESPEN, in addition to a BMI < 18.5 kg/m^2 and weight loss > 10–15% within six months [11, 20, 30, 34].

In hospitalized patients, malnutrition is an independent risk factor for venous thromboembolism, nonelective surgery, longer admission, and increased mortality [30]. Malnutrition is also a well-known risk factor for adverse postoperative outcomes in all surgical patients [11]. Up to 50% of patients with CD will require surgery at some point, and it is estimated that up to 85% of patients awaiting surgery are malnourished. Malnourished IBD patients may also possess several other risk factors for poor surgical outcomes. A recent meta-analysis by Huang et al. [35] identified steroid use, low albumin level, prior surgical history, and preoperative abscess (all common in CD) as risk factors for adverse surgical outcomes in CD patients. "Intra-abdominal septic complications" (anastomotic leaks, intra-abdominal abscesses, and enterocutaneous fistulae), one of the most dreaded complications in CD patients undergoing surgery, can occur in up to 20% of patients and frequently require reoperation or percutaneous drainage [11, 36]. Therefore, optimizing preoperative nutritional status in IBD patients is crucial for good surgical outcomes.

4. Preoperative Nutritional Support

4.1. Oral and Enteral Nutrition. In the preoperative period as in general, oral nutrition is preferred if patients can meet their energy and/or protein needs from normal food by mouth. The caloric need can be high due to malnutrition and the desire to enhance nutritional status before surgery. In addition, symptoms including nausea, abdominal pain, and diarrhea or high-volume fistula output can limit the ability to effectively utilize the gut. If patients are unable to meet their needs, oral nutritional supplements (ONS) that are high in protein and supplemented with vitamins and minerals can be added as a first step; however, they are generally a minor supportive therapy, providing a supplementary intake of only up to 600 kcal/day [30]. If caloric needs are not met through oral intake and/or oral feeding is not possible, enteral nutrition (EN) typically through a nasogastric or nasoenteric tube is indicated. Updated nutritional guidelines for patients with IBD were put forth by ESPEN in 2016 [30]. In these guidelines, most of the recommendations for preoperative nutritional support were based on consensus among experts or extrapolated from the considerable evidence of nutritional support in the general gastrointestinal surgical population and in critically ill patients [11].

Enteral nutrition is administered in either polymeric, semielemental, or elemental formulas depending on the presence of malabsorption [29]. The general consensus is that enteral nutrition (EN) is recommended for IBD patients undergoing surgery if they are able meet their metabolic demands, but if EN is not feasible (e.g., intestinal obstruction or high output fistula) or if metabolic needs are not met by EN alone, parenteral nutrition (PN) should be employed according to the established guidelines for use in the general population [11, 30, 37]. Compared to PN, EN carries decreased infectious risks, is less costly, and is more physiologic given that it promotes gastrointestinal growth and function [32, 38].

When EN is used to meet 100% of a patient's dietary requirements, it is termed exclusive enteral nutrition (EEN). There is an emerging body of literature demonstrating the role of EEN for primary therapy of Crohn's disease, particularly in the pediatric population. EEN has been shown to induce mucosal healing and have a direct anti-inflammatory effect by decreasing proinflammatory cytokines [11, 39]. In the pediatric CD population, EEN is the treatment of choice for induction of remission because it is as effective as corticosteroids in this regard (up to 80% of patients achieve remission) and sparing the detrimental side effects of corticosteroids (i.e., bone loss and growth retardation) [40, 41]. Studies demonstrating this effect in adult CD patients have been less conclusive due to issues with EEN compliance in this population [40].

Studies evaluating EEN use in the preoperative setting in CD patients have yielded promising results. Li et al. [42] demonstrated that preoperative EEN in patients with fistulizing CD is associated with a significantly decreased risk of intra-abdominal septic complications and may result in an accelerated recovery and ability to return to work sooner. A 2017 retrospective case-control study by Heerasing et al. [41] found that preoperative EEN frequently downstages the need for surgery in CD patients with stricturing or penetrating complications and is associated with reductions in systemic inflammation, operative times, and incidence of postoperative abscess or anastomotic leak. Wang et al. [43] observed that 4 weeks of preoperative EEN in CD patients led to significant reductions in both infectious and noninfectious complications and significant improvements in nutritional and inflammatory status. At 6 months postoperatively, significant reductions in endoscopic recurrence rates were seen in the EEN group; however, during the 2-year follow-up, this significance was lost. In addition, incidence of clinical recurrence was similar in the EEN and non-EEN groups during the 2-year follow-up [43]. A retrospective study of 83 patients by Zhu et al. [44] in 2017 found that for CD patients with percutaneously undrainable abscesses, the use of EEN was associated with a decreased need for surgery. In those patients who did require surgery, EEN was associated with increased albumin levels, decreased ESR and CRP levels, a lower risk of postoperative intra-abdominal septic complications, and a shorter duration of postoperative hospitalization compared to the group who did not receive EEN [44]. In a large retrospective 2015 study by Li et al. [45], the addition of EEN to a preoperative immunosuppressant-free interval led to lower rates of stoma creation, decreased postoperative complications, decreased urgent operation requirement, and extended preoperative immunosuppressant-free interval.

With regard to the optimal EN formula in CD, there are no significant differences between elemental, semielemental, and polymeric formulas in active CD [46]. Prior studies have shown that low-fat formulas may offer improved efficacy compared to formulas with high amounts of long-chain triglycerides but formulas with increased amounts of medium-chain triglycerides provided remission rates that were the same as those of low-fat formulas [47, 48]. A recent systematic review of 29 clinical trials [49] concurred that formulas with relatively low total long-chain triglyceride content and proportionately high medium-chain triglyceride content offer the most optimal approach for attaining remission in active CD. In addition, this study also concluded that ideal EN formulas were ones with relatively low amounts of monounsaturated fatty acids (MUFA) and high omega-6 : omega-3 fatty acid ratios [49].

In contrast to CD, there is no evidence that EEN alters the inflammatory response in UC, and therefore, it is not used in the treatment of active UC, nor in the maintenance of remission in UC [50]. However, according to ESPEN, EN has not been adequately evaluated in active UC and its efficacy needs to be tested in larger cohorts of patients [30]. EN can be used to treat or prevent malnutrition in UC patients and is safe to use as nutritional support during severe UC exacerbations and in the perioperative phase [30, 50].

There are certain clinical scenarios in which EN (or EEN) is not feasible. Poor tolerability of EN and poor palatability of formulations are major hindrances to patient compliance, and about 50% of patients relapse within 6 months and revert to a normal diet [39, 51]. In these cases, PN may be the next best alternative. PN is necessary when there is bowel obstruction and placement of a feeding tube beyond this obstruction is not possible. It is also required in patients with short bowel with severe malnutrition and/or fluid and electrolyte loss that is unable to be managed enterally [30]. High-output fistulae, inability to maintain enteral access, intractable nausea and vomiting, paralytic ileus, and inability to meet >60% of energy needs via the enteral route are also indications for PN [11, 29, 38].

4.2. Parenteral Nutrition. Only a few studies have examined the effect that perioperative PN has on postoperative outcomes. Table 3 shows summaries and comparisons of these studies. Overall, the literature indicates that perioperative PN does not increase postoperative complications and that there is a general trend towards improvement in postoperative outcomes associated with perioperative PN use in IBD patients. However, the evidence supporting perioperative PN use is based on studies with small sample sizes that are limited with high degrees of heterogeneity with respect to study interventions, controls, measures, and outcomes.

Table 3: Characteristics of primary studies investigating the use of perioperative PN in IBD patients.

Author and year	Patient population and interventions	Measured outcomes	Results	Conclusions	Study strengths	Study limitations
Rombeau et al. [52] 1982 retrospective cohort study	Patients with IBD undergoing abdominal surgery; group 1: 11 patients with 0–5 days preoperative PN versus group 2: 22 patients with ≤5 days of preoperative PN	Postoperative complications and length of hospital stay	(i) Group 2 (≤5 days preoperative PN) had significantly fewer postoperative complications ($p < 0.05$); no statistically significant difference in length of hospital stay (ii) All patients with postoperative complications had either a preoperative serum albumin level <3.5 g/dl or a serum transferrin level < 150 mg/dl	Preoperative PN for at least 5 days is strongly recommended in patients with IBD who have severe protein deficiency	(i) Study groups comparable with respect to demographic data, diagnoses, and types of surgery (ii) Preoperative nutritional status was comparable in the two groups	(i) Small sample size (ii) Lack of PN composition data (iii) Lack of control for diet in group 1 patients who did not receive PN
Lashner et al. [55] 1989 retrospective cohort study	103 patients with CD undergoing bowel resection (segmental small bowel resection, ileocecectomy, or segmental or total colectomy). Preoperative PN vs control groups compared between surgery types	Length of resected bowel and length of hospital stay	(i) Preoperative PN associated with reduced length of small bowel resection (20.4 ± 14.3 cm less bowel resected in those undergoing segmental small bowel resection and 11.2 ± 4.2 cm less in those undergoing ileocecectomy) that was independent of length of disease determined preoperatively (ii) No difference in length of large bowel resected between the PN and non-PN groups (iii) PN associated with a longer hospitalization (13.5 ± 2.6 days longer for the PN group)	Preoperative PN for CD patients is beneficial for those undergoing small bowel resection but was of little benefit for those undergoing colectomy	Controlling for confounding variables with the multivariate regression model did not change the results	(i) Lack of PN composition data (ii) Lack of control for diet in non-PN groups (iii) Patient selection bias (criteria for patient selection varied among attending physicians and no standardized criteria were established)

Table 3: Continued.

Author and year	Patient population and interventions	Measured outcomes	Results	Conclusions	Study strengths	Study limitations
Yao et al. [53] 2005 nonrandomized controlled trial	32 severely malnourished CD patients (BMI $< 15.0\,kg/m^2$) undergoing abdominal surgery; 16 patients received 1 week of preoperative PN and 3 weeks of postoperative PN versus 16 patients in the control group received intravenous fluids with an isocaloric diet "comparable in energy to PN"	Serum immunoglobulins, BMI, weight change, liver function, postoperative complications, and return to work	(i) No significant differences in postoperative complications between groups (ii) BMI significantly increased in the PN group (from 13.9 ± 0.6 to $15.3 \pm 0.7\,kg/m^2$, $p = 0.02$) and did not change significantly in the control group (14.1 ± 0.7 to $14.5 \pm 0.5\,kg/m^2$, $p = 0.81$) (iii) Serum IgM levels in the PN group declined to normal value (139 ± 41 to 105 ± 29 mg/dl, $p = 0.04$), whereas no statistically significant change is seen in control group's IgM levels (from 133 ± 16 to 129 ± 13 mg/dl, $p = 0.34$) (iv) More patients in the study group returned to work than in the control group	Perioperative PN possibly ameliorates the humoral immunity, reverses malnutrition, and facilitates rehabilitation	(i) Novel study measures able to show objective improvement in nutritional status and humoral immunity with preoperative PN (ii) Equal number of patients in the study vs control groups (important in studies with small number of patients)	(i) Small sample size (ii) Limited description of results (iii) Methods for controlling for diet were not specified
Grivceva Stardelova et al. [26] 2008 retrospective/ prospective cohort study	90 patients with IBD undergoing abdominal surgery; 29 patients (16 CD, 13 UC) received an average duration of 19.1 ± 18.5 days of preoperative PN and 61 patients (50 CD, 11 UC) did not receive PN	BMI, disease activity index (CDAI/AI), laboratory indices, and length of hospital stay	(i) CDAI scores decreased in the PN group more than in the control group and BMI increased more in the PN group than in the control group; however, neither of these findings was statistically significant (no p values provided)	Patients in the PN group had more severe baseline disease (lower BMIs and higher CDAI scores of statistical significance). Although improvements in BMI and CDAI are not statistically	(i) First study that investigated the effect of PN on disease activity scores	(i) Relatively small sample size (ii) Lack of PN composition data (iii) Lack of control for diet in the non-PN group (iv) Inconsistent reporting of statistical significances and vague explanations

Table 3: Continued.

Author and year	Patient population and interventions	Measured outcomes	Results	Conclusions	Study strengths	Study limitations
			(ii) No statistically significant difference in length of hospital stay	significant, PN aided improvement in clinical status to the level of the healthier controls. Authors estimate that duration of effective PN should be at least 7–14 days		of the significant differences in laboratory indices
Jacobson [33] 2012 nonrandomized controlled trial	120 patients with moderate to severe CD undergoing intestinal resection. 15 patients received preoperative PN versus 105 patients not given PN preoperatively	Early (within 30 days) postoperative complications	(i) A significant reduction in early postoperative complications ($p < 0.05$) was seen in the PN group (0 patients with complications) versus the control group (29 patients with complications) (ii) Results suggested that preoperative PN increased body weight, serum albumin, and serum triiodothyronine, which reflected an improved nutritional state as well as a lowered risk of postoperative complications. (iii) PN also decreased serum haptoglobin and white blood cell count which suggested decreased inflammatory activity	Patients with moderate to severe CD undergoing intestinal resection should be treated with at least 18 days of preoperative PN to lower the risk of early surgical complications	(i) PN solution composition provided (ii) Lab markers for nutrition and inflammation were measured, and authors were able to show that improvements in these measures were associated with preoperative PN use	(i) Small sample size (ii) Lack of control for nutrient intake in the control group (iii) Average CDAI for control subjects was not calculated (iv) Sevenfold matching based on baseline characteristics (v) Controls were historical rather than contemporaneous (vi) PN compositions varied widely

Table 3: Continued.

Author and year	Patient population and interventions	Measured outcomes	Results	Conclusions	Study strengths	Study limitations
Salinas et al. [54] 2012 retrospective cohort study	235 UC patients undergoing abdominal surgery. 56 patients received preoperative PN and 179 did not	Early (within 30 days) postoperative complications	(i) PN was associated with more total postoperative complications (50% vs 35.2% in the control group, $p = 0.047$); however, when line infections were excluded, total complications were comparable (37.5% vs 35.2%, $p = 0.753$)	Routine preoperative PN for the general population of UC patients undergoing surgeries is not indicated	(i) Larger sample size compared to other studies (ii) Total and individual postoperative complications were compared between groups	(i) Statistically significant disparities in baseline nutritional status and disease severity between groups (ii) Lack of control for diet in the non-PN group (iii) Lack of PN duration and composition
Ayoub et al. [20] 2018 retrospective cohort study	144 CD patients undergoing major abdominal surgery; 55 received preoperative PN and 89 did not	30-day postoperative complications	(i) No statistical differences were seen in infectious complications (18.2% in the PN group, 12.3% in the non-PN group, $p = 0.34$) or noninfectious complications (14.5% in the PN group, 16.8% in the non-PN group, $p = 0.71$) (ii) Patients receiving preoperative PN for >60 days had significantly lower odds of developing noninfectious complications (OR 0.07, 95% CI 0.01–0.80, $p = 0.03$) with no associated increase in infectious complications (iii) Weight loss of >10% in the past 6 months was a significant predictor of postoperative complications	In a subset of malnourished CD patients, PN is safe and allows comparable postoperative outcomes to controls	(i) Largest study to date on preoperative PN in CD patients (ii) Detailed description and comparison of baseline patient characteristics, including disease and surgical characteristics between groups (iii) Authors provided a detailed description of rationale for initiation of PN	(i) Lack of a validated preoperative nutritional assessment for all patients

PN: parenteral nutrition; IBD: inflammatory bowel disease; CD: Crohn's disease; BMI: body mass index; UC: ulcerative colitis; CDAI: Crohn's disease activity index.

Therefore, as with preoperative medical therapy for CD, use of preoperative PN in this patient population is largely institution and surgeon specific.

Table 3 highlights details of the studies on the use of perioperative PN. Postoperative complications measured in these articles included: infections, perforation with free peritonitis, wound dehiscence, intestinal obstruction, fistulas, intra-abdominal abscess, anastomotic leak, intra-abdominal bleeding, and death. Of the seven studies reviewed in Table 3, two [33, 52] found statistically significant reductions in postoperative complications. Another study, the largest study to date to study perioperative PN in CD patients, found that preoperative PN for >60 days was associated with significantly lower odds of developing noninfectious complications (OR 0.07, 95% CI 0.01–0.80, $p = 0.03$) with no associated increase in infectious complications [20]. An additional study [53] did not find any significant differences in postoperative complications; however, statistical significances were observed with decreases in serum IgM ($p = 0.04$) and increases in BMI ($p = 0.02$) in the PN group when compared to the control group. One study [54] of exclusively UC patients saw more total postoperative complications in the PN group (50% vs 35.2% in the control group, $p = 0.047$); however, when line infections were taken out of the analysis, total complications were comparable (37.5% vs 35.2%, $p = 0.753$). The main outcome of interest in the study by Lashner et al. [55] was not postoperative complications, but complication rates were nearly identical in the two groups (49 total patients in PN groups with 10 complications, 54 total patients in control groups with 11 complications), indicating no increased risk of postoperative complications.

In general, measures of nutritional status and disease severity improved in patients receiving perioperative PN. More considerable BMI increases were noted with perioperative PN as compared with control groups in 2 studies [26, 53], with one observing statistical significance in this outcome [53]. Additionally, Jacobson [33] reported increases in BMI in the PN group but did not comment on BMIs in the control group. Jacobson [33] also stated that the PN group in their study had reductions in CDAI to the point of clinical remission by time of surgery; however, CDAI scores were not calculated in the control groups, and therefore, statistical significance could not be determined. Grivceva Stardevola et al. [26] saw that CDAI scores improve more in the PN group versus the control group but the results were not statistically significant.

Lashner et al. [52] found that preoperative PN was associated with reduced length of small bowel resection (albeit at the expense of a longer hospital stay). Since up to 70% of CD patients will require surgery at some point in their disease course, any interventions that can spare functional bowel and prevent short bowel syndrome are of the upmost importance. However, the referenced study is almost 30 years old and it does not appear that this specific measure has been studied in IBD patients receiving or not receiving PN preoperatively since then. Future studies should aim to measure the effect of perioperative PN on the length of bowel resection if possible in attempts to validate and possibly expand on the findings of this earlier study.

Regarding limitations, common themes were found among the studies and articles in this review. Small sample sizes were seen in all the studies. None of the studies controlled for diet, which is a significant limitation. Four of the seven research articles lacked PN composition data, which is also a significant limitation because it limits the ability to associate specific PN components with outcomes. Study designs were also understandably hindered for several reasons. Disease severity necessitating PN likely precluded the ability to randomize nutritional support in these patients. In addition, as shown by many of these studies, patients requiring PN are sicker at baseline, and therefore, directly comparing postoperative outcomes in this subset of patients to outcomes of control groups would be inherently flawed. Only a small number of studies used propensity matching or other statistical techniques to control for disease severity and other differences between groups. Also, blinding is obviously difficult when comparing PN to EN or oral nutritional intake.

PN can be given through peripheral lines, but since either increased fluid provision or limited nutrient content in the solution to maintain an osmolarity ≤ 900 mOsm/l is needed, it is usually given through a central venous catheter [28]. Central venous catheters have historically carried a higher risk of bloodstream infections, which has led to significant healthcare costs as well as patient morbidity and mortality. In a 2005 study, Beghetto et al. [56] asserted that PN was an independent risk factor for central venous catheter-related infection in nonselected hospitalized adult patients. PN has been associated with noninfectious complications as well, such as refeeding syndrome, hyperglycemia, hypertriglyceridemia, hepatic steatosis, intrahepatic cholestasis, biliary sludge, and bone demineralization [57]. However, as Cotogni [58] points out, the incidence of PN-related complications has markedly decreased in recent years due to proven, standardized policies that reduce catheter-related bloodstream infections. In addition, other provisions including appropriate blood glucose control, use of olive oil- and fish oil-based lipid emulsions rather than soybean oil-based ones, and the adoption of insertion and care bundles for central venous access devices have moved the field closer to the goal of "near-zero" PN complications [58, 59]. Also, there is increased awareness of the association between overfeeding and infectious complications [60]. Two recent randomized controlled trials (the CALORIES trial [61] and NUTRIREA-2 [62]) studying early nutritional support in critically ill patients found no statistically significant differences in infectious complications between the EN and PN groups. In the 2018 study by Ayoub et al. from our group at the University of Florida [20], there were no statistical differences seen in infectious complications between preoperative IBD patients on PN and control patients (18.2% in the PN group, 12.3% in the non-PN group, $p = 0.34$). In our study, a subset of malnourished patients benefited from PN in the preoperative period. Our findings concur with Schwartz [28] who proposed that IBD patients with underlying severe malnutrition may be the better candidates for perioperative PN since the benefit of preoperative nitrogen balance optimization may outweigh any infectious risks incurred by placing a central venous catheter for PN.

Omega-3 fatty acids (contained in fish oil) have anti-inflammatory activity via their ability to regulate inflammatory processes and cellular responses [63]. Given this, its use in IBD has warranted investigation. In a rat model of experimental colitis, omega-3-enriched parenteral lipid emulsions decreased colonic concentrations of proinflammatory mediators and attenuated the inflammatory consequences of colitis [63]. The ICU lipid study [64] showed that parenteral administration of a lipid emulsion containing 10% fish oil reduced the risk of nosocomial infections in critically ill medical and surgical patients, although it did not have an effect on ICU, hospital, or 6-month mortality. While two recent Cochrane reviews [65, 66] failed to show any evidence to support the use of oral omega-3 fatty acids for maintenance of remission in CD or UC, studies investigating the use of omega-3-enriched parenteral lipid emulsions in the human IBD population are lacking. Further studies are needed before fish oil in PN can be routinely recommended in the IBD population.

Home PN is sometimes indicated in select patients with CD, such as those with chronic intestinal failure from short bowel syndrome (which is usually a consequence of repeated small bowel resections), prolonged incomplete bowel obstruction, high-output stomas, and persistent fistulas [25, 27]. Home PN has not been associated with significant increases in body weight or reductions in the frequency of further CD-related surgeries. However, increased quality of life, higher serum albumin and transferrin levels, and a reduction in oral steroid requirements have been noted [25]. Complications of home PN are the same as those of hospital-administered PN and include catheter-related infections, cholestasis, refeeding syndrome, and bone demineralization [27]. While the benefits of perioperative PN illustrated in this review could theoretically be applied to home perioperative PN use, home PN use in the perioperative period has not been studied, and therefore, there is insufficient evidence either for or against its use.

5. Preoperative Optimization

Optimizing nutritional status preoperatively is crucial to mitigating postoperative complications. According to ESPEN guidelines [30] published in 2017, surgical intervention in IBD patients should ideally be delayed for 7–14 days whenever possible if malnutrition is identified, during which time-intensive artificial feeding (EN preferably) should be initiated [30]. When surgery cannot be delayed or emergency surgery is needed, ESPEN [30] recommends that nutritional support (preferably EN over PN if possible) be initiated without delay in patients who are malnourished and even in patients without significant malnutrition if it is expected that the patient will be unable to eat for more than seven days perioperatively. Nutritional support should also be provided in patients who cannot maintain oral intake above 60–75% of recommended intake for more than 10 days. In cases where EN is initiated in hospitalized patients, additional supplemental PN should be introduced if after 7–10 days of EN, the patient is unable to meet >60% of energy and/or protein requirements. There is evidence that adding supplemental PN prior to this 7–10-day period in those patients already receiving EN does not improve outcomes and may actually be detrimental [67].

The timing of surgery in patients with malnutrition deserves additional comment. While the optimal duration for preoperative PN is not certain, one could argue that a surgical delay of 7–14 days cited by ESPEN [30] is not long enough to optimize IBD patients preoperatively with PN. Patel et al. [9] continue PN until albumin levels are >3 g/dl, CRP levels are <5 mg/l, and BMI improves; in the only study reporting these improved outcomes [33], this approach took a minimum of 18 days and a mean of 46 days of PN treatment. Our group [20] showed that PN for >60 days preoperatively in CD patients was associated with lower odds of developing noninfectious complications with no associated increase in infectious complications. To our knowledge, the optimal duration of preoperative PN in UC patients has not been studied. Clearly, a balance of contributing factors exists, and, in the absence of convincing evidence to guide decision making, this remains institution specific with good opportunities for additional investigation. Since universal recommendations favor the use of EN over PN whenever possible, it is not surprising that patients in need of PN are those with the most complicated and severe disease [30]. This was corroborated in several studies in this review [20, 26, 33, 52, 54] showing that patients requiring PN were more malnourished with higher disease activity and lower albumin levels at baseline compared to control groups. For this reason, all possible steps to improve these patients' preoperative conditions should be taken. The concept of preoperative optimization has shown promising data in IBD [11, 14, 68, 69]. This concept is based on a multimodal approach (including nutritional strategies) to optimize a patient's preoperative condition and to reduce the risk of unfavorable postoperative outcomes.

Studies on preoperative optimization have demonstrated favorable outcomes. Zerbib et al. [69] reported retrospectively on the results of preoperative optimization for patients undergoing ileocecal resection for penetrating CD, with focus on rates of major postoperative complications and need for fecal diversion. 50 of the 74 total patients (64%) received two weeks of preoperative nutritional support with either EN (5 patients) or PN (45 patients) in combination with bowel rest, two weeks of intravenous antibiotics, withdrawal from steroids and immunosuppressants, and/or abscess drainage. The postoperative morbidity rate was low (18%), with only six temporary fecal diversions and no deaths. Similarly, Bellolio et al. [68] compared surgical outcomes of CD patients with perforating versus nonperforating disease following ileocolic resection. In this study of 434 patients, 56 received preoperative PN because of septic complications or malnourishment. Patients with perforating disease were more likely to be the ones receiving preoperative PN (17.1% vs 4.3%, $p < 0.001$). They found that PN in combination with antibiotics, abscess drainage, and postponed surgery in patients with perforating disease led to similar complication rates compared with that in patients with nonperforating disease (13% vs 11%). A systematic review of 50 studies by Zangenberg et al. [14] examined preoperative optimization in IBD patients undergoing gastrointestinal surgery and recommended weaning of steroids if possible, avoidance of stress dose of steroids, percutaneous drainage of abscesses if present, smoking cessation, appropriate thromboembolism prophylaxis, administration of prophylactic IV antibiotics, and screening for malnutrition with appropriate nutritional support. They concluded, however, that large prospective studies comparing different types and duration of preoperative nutrition are needed, especially in UC patients since most studies deal with CD.

6. Conclusion

Addressing nutritional needs of IBD patients in the perioperative period can improve patient outcomes. Nutritional assessment and perioperative nutritional support are often neglected components of good disease management. When providing nutritional support, the enteral route is favored over the parenteral route in most cases. In certain severe IBD cases, PN seems to reduce postoperative complications, improve nutritional status, and reduce disease severity. Our recommendation is that the current use of perioperative PN in IBD patients should be in line with the ESPEN guidelines for PN in the general surgical population [37]. That is, PN should be considered preoperatively only if metabolic needs are not met by EN alone or if disease presentation at the time of surgery impedes the use of EN (e.g., high-output fistula or intestinal obstruction) [11]. Additional, well-controlled studies of EN and PN in the perioperative setting are warranted.

References

[1] C. Abraham and R. Medzhitov, "Interactions between the host innate immune system and microbes in inflammatory bowel disease," *Gastroenterology*, vol. 140, no. 6, pp. 1729–1737, 2011.

[2] M. Regueiro, F. Velayos, J. B. Greer et al., "American Gastroenterological Association Institute technical review on the management of Crohn's disease after surgical resection," *Gastroenterology*, vol. 152, no. 1, pp. 277–295.e3, 2017.

[3] P. Hindryckx, V. Jairath, and G. D'Haens, "Acute severe ulcerative colitis: from pathophysiology to clinical management," *Nature Reviews. Gastroenterology & Hepatology*, vol. 13, no. 11, pp. 654–664, 2016.

[4] L. Beaugerie, P. Seksik, I. Nion–Larmurier, J.–. P. Gendre, and J. Cosnes, "Predictors of Crohn's disease," *Gastroenterology*, vol. 130, no. 3, pp. 650–656, 2006.

[5] M. C. Dubinsky, S. Kugathasan, L. Mei et al., "Increased immune reactivity predicts aggressive complicating Crohn's disease in children," *Clinical Gastroenterology and Hepatology*, vol. 6, no. 10, pp. 1105–1111, 2008.

[6] J. Seiderer, F. Schnitzler, S. Brand et al., "Homozygosity for theCARD15frameshift mutation 1007fs is predictive of early onset of Crohn's disease with ileal stenosis, entero-enteral fistulas, and frequent need for surgical intervention with high risk of re-stenosis," *Scandinavian Journal of Gastroenterology*, vol. 41, no. 12, pp. 1421–1432, 2009.

[7] N. A. Chaudhry, M. Riverso, J. R. Grajo et al., "A fixed stricture on routine cross-sectional imaging predicts disease-related complications and adverse outcomes in patients with Crohn's disease," *Inflammatory Bowel Diseases*, vol. 23, no. 4, pp. 641–649, 2017.

[8] D. H. Bruining, E. M. Zimmermann, E. V. Loftus Jr et al., "Consensus recommendations for evaluation, interpretation, and utilization of computed tomography and magnetic resonance enterography in patients with small bowel Crohn's disease," *Gastroenterology*, vol. 154, no. 4, pp. 1172–1194, 2018.

[9] K. V. Patel, A. A. Darakhshan, N. Griffin, A. B. Williams, J. D. Sanderson, and P. M. Irving, "Patient optimization for surgery relating to Crohn's disease," *Nature Reviews. Gastroenterology & Hepatology*, vol. 13, no. 12, pp. 707–719, 2016.

[10] D. D. Mijač, G. L. J. Janković, J. Jorga, and M. N. Krstić, "Nutritional status in patients with active inflammatory bowel disease: prevalence of malnutrition and methods for routine nutritional assessment," *European Journal of Internal Medicine*, vol. 21, no. 4, pp. 315–319, 2010.

[11] F. Grass, B. Pache, D. Martin, D. Hahnloser, N. Demartines, and M. Hübner, "Preoperative nutritional conditioning of Crohn's patients-systematic review of current evidence and practice," *Nutrients*, vol. 9, no. 6, 2017.

[12] L. Hancock, A. C. Windsor, and N. J. Mortensen, "Inflammatory bowel disease: the view of the surgeon," *Colorectal Disease*, vol. 8, Supplement 1, pp. 10–14, 2006.

[13] J. M. Hwang and M. G. Varma, "Surgery for inflammatory bowel disease," *World Journal of Gastroenterology*, vol. 14, no. 17, pp. 2678–2690, 2008.

[14] M. S. Zangenberg, N. Horesh, U. Kopylov, and A. el-Hussuna, "Preoperative optimization of patients with inflammatory bowel disease undergoing gastrointestinal surgery: a systematic review," *International Journal of Colorectal Disease*, vol. 32, no. 12, pp. 1663–1676, 2017.

[15] V. Subramanian, S. Saxena, J. Y. Kang, and R. C. G. Pollok, "Preoperative steroid use and risk of postoperative complications in patients with inflammatory bowel disease undergoing abdominal surgery," *The American Journal of Gastroenterology*, vol. 103, no. 9, pp. 2373–2381, 2008.

[16] R. R. Cima, "Surgical outcomes in inflammatory bowel disease patients and the potential impact of biologic therapies," *Seminars in Colon and Rectal Surgery*, vol. 23, no. 2, pp. 89–93, 2012.

[17] V. Subramanian, R. C. G. Pollok, J. Y. Kang, and D. Kumar, "Systematic review of postoperative complications in patients with inflammatory bowel disease treated with immunomodulators," *British Journal of Surgery*, vol. 93, no. 7, pp. 793–799, 2006.

[18] U. Ahmed Ali, S. T. Martin, A. D. Rao, and R. P. Kiran, "Impact of preoperative immunosuppressive agents on postoperative outcomes in Crohn's disease," *Diseases of the Colon and Rectum*, vol. 57, no. 5, pp. 663–674, 2014.

[19] L. Ferrari, M. K. Krane, and A. Fichera, "Inflammatory bowel disease surgery in the biologic era," *World Journal of Gastrointestinal Surgery*, vol. 8, no. 5, pp. 363–370, 2016.

[20] F. Ayoub, A. Y. Kamel, A. Ouni et al., "Preoperative total parenteral nutrition improves postoperative outcomes in a subset

of Crohn's disease patients undergoing major abdominal surgery," *Gastroenterology Report*, 2018.

[21] P. G. Kotze, S. Ghosh, W. A. Bemelman, and R. Panaccione, "Preoperative use of anti-tumor necrosis factor therapy in Crohn's disease: promises and pitfalls," *Intestinal Research*, vol. 15, no. 2, pp. 160–165, 2017.

[22] A. Y. Kamel, F. Ayoub, D. Banerjee et al., "Effects of preoperative use of biologic agents on operative outcomes in Crohn's disease patients," *The American Surgeon*, 2018.

[23] G. C. Nguyen, E. V. Loftus Jr, I. Hirano et al., "American Gastroenterological Association Institute guideline on the management of Crohn's disease after surgical resection," *Gastroenterology*, vol. 152, no. 1, pp. 271–275, 2017.

[24] G. R. Lichtenstein, E. V. Loftus, K. L. Isaacs, M. D. Regueiro, L. B. Gerson, and B. E. Sands, "ACG clinical guideline: management of Crohn's disease in adults," *The American Journal of Gastroenterology*, vol. 113, no. 4, pp. 481–517, 2018.

[25] J. Goh and C. A. O'Morain, "Nutrition and adult inflammatory bowel disease," *Alimentary Pharmacology and Therapeutics*, vol. 17, no. 3, pp. 307–320, 2003.

[26] K. Grivceva Stardelova, P. Misevska, M. Zdravkovska, D. Trajkov, and V. Serafimoski, "Total parenteral nutrition in treatment of patients with inflammatory bowel disease," *Prilozi*, vol. 29, no. 1, pp. 21–43, 2008.

[27] J. K. Triantafillidis and A. E. Papalois, "The role of total parenteral nutrition in inflammatory bowel disease: current aspects," *Scandinavian Journal of Gastroenterology*, vol. 49, no. 1, pp. 3–14, 2014.

[28] E. Schwartz, "Perioperative parenteral nutrition in adults with inflammatory bowel disease: a review of the literature," *Nutrition in Clinical Practice*, vol. 31, no. 2, pp. 159–170, 2016.

[29] A. Wędrychowicz, A. Zając, and P. Tomasik, "Advances in nutritional therapy in inflammatory bowel diseases: review," *World Journal of Gastroenterology*, vol. 22, no. 3, pp. 1045–1066, 2016.

[30] A. Forbes, J. Escher, X. Hébuterne et al., "ESPEN guideline: clinical nutrition in inflammatory bowel disease," *Clinical Nutrition*, vol. 36, no. 2, pp. 321–347, 2017.

[31] S. Massironi, R. E. Rossi, F. A. Cavalcoli, S. Della Valle, M. Fraquelli, and D. Conte, "Nutritional deficiencies in inflammatory bowel disease: therapeutic approaches," *Clinical Nutrition*, vol. 32, no. 6, pp. 904–910, 2013.

[32] I. J. Wagner and J. L. Rombeau, "Nutritional support of surgical patients with inflammatory bowel disease," *Surgical Clinics of North America*, vol. 91, no. 4, pp. 787–803, 2011, viii.

[33] S. Jacobson, "Early postoperative complications in patients with Crohn's disease given and not given preoperative total parenteral nutrition," *Scandinavian Journal of Gastroenterology*, vol. 47, no. 2, pp. 170–177, 2012.

[34] A. Spinelli, M. Allocca, M. Jovani, and S. Danese, "Review article: optimal preparation for surgery in Crohn's disease," *Alimentary Pharmacology & Therapeutics*, vol. 40, no. 9, pp. 1009–1022, 2014.

[35] W. Huang, Y. Tang, L. Nong, and Y. Sun, "Risk factors for postoperative intra-abdominal septic complications after surgery in Crohn's disease: a meta-analysis of observational studies," *Journal of Crohn's & Colitis*, vol. 9, no. 3, pp. 293–301, 2015.

[36] L. Zuo, Y. Li, H. Wang et al., "A practical predictive index for intra-abdominal septic complications after primary anastomosis for Crohn's disease: change in C-reactive protein level before surgery," *Diseases of the Colon and Rectum*, vol. 58, no. 8, pp. 775–781, 2015.

[37] M. Braga, O. Ljungqvist, P. Soeters et al., "ESPEN guidelines on parenteral nutrition: surgery," *Clinical Nutrition*, vol. 28, no. 4, pp. 378–386, 2009.

[38] T. Nickerson and A. Merchea, "Perioperative considerations in Crohn disease and ulcerative colitis," *Clinics in Colon and Rectal Surgery*, vol. 29, no. 2, pp. 80–84, 2016.

[39] D. L. Nguyen, B. Limketkai, V. Medici, M. Saire Mendoza, L. Palmer, and M. Bechtold, "Nutritional strategies in the management of adult patients with inflammatory bowel disease: dietary considerations from active disease to disease remission," *Current Gastroenterology Reports*, vol. 18, no. 10, p. 55, 2016.

[40] A. MacLellan, J. Connors, S. Grant, L. Cahill, M. Langille, and J. Van Limbergen, "The impact of exclusive enteral nutrition (EEN) on the gut microbiome in Crohn's disease: a review," *Nutrients*, vol. 9, no. 5, 2017.

[41] N. Heerasing, B. Thompson, P. Hendy et al., "Exclusive enteral nutrition provides an effective bridge to safer interval elective surgery for adults with Crohn's disease," *Alimentary Pharmacology & Therapeutics*, vol. 45, no. 5, pp. 660–669, 2017.

[42] G. Li, J. Ren, G. Wang et al., "Preoperative exclusive enteral nutrition reduces the postoperative septic complications of fistulizing Crohn's disease," *European Journal of Clinical Nutrition*, vol. 68, no. 4, pp. 441–446, 2014.

[43] H. Wang, L. Zuo, J. Zhao et al., "Impact of preoperative exclusive enteral nutrition on postoperative complications and recurrence after bowel resection in patients with active Crohn's disease," *World Journal of Surgery*, vol. 40, no. 8, pp. 1993–2000, 2016.

[44] Y. Zhu, L. Xu, W. Liu, W. Qi, Q. Cao, and W. Zhou, "Safety and efficacy of exclusive enteral nutrition for percutaneously undrainable abdominal abscesses in Crohn's disease," *Gastroenterology Research and Practice*, vol. 2017, Article ID 6360319, 8 pages, 2017.

[45] Y. Li, L. Zuo, W. Zhu et al., "Role of exclusive enteral nutrition in the preoperative optimization of patients with Crohn's disease following immunosuppressive therapy," *Medicine (Baltimore)*, vol. 94, no. 5, article e478, 2015.

[46] A. M. Griffiths, A. Ohlsson, P. M. Sherman, and L. R. Sutherland, "Meta-analysis of enteral nutrition as a primary treatment of active Crohn's disease," *Gastroenterology*, vol. 108, no. 4, pp. 1056–1067, 1995.

[47] M. A. Gassull, F. Fernández-Bañares, E. Cabré et al., "Fat composition may be a clue to explain the primary therapeutic effect of enteral nutrition in Crohn's disease: results of a double blind randomised multicentre European trial," *Gut*, vol. 51, no. 2, pp. 164–168, 2002.

[48] T. Sakurai, T. Matsui, T. Yao et al., "Short-term efficacy of enteral nutrition in the treatment of active Crohn's disease: a randomized, controlled trial comparing nutrient formulas," *Journal of Parenteral and Enteral Nutrition*, vol. 26, no. 2, pp. 98–103, 2002.

[49] S. M. Ajabnoor and A. Forbes, "Effect of fat composition in enteral nutrition for Crohn's disease in adults: a systematic review," *Clinical Nutrition*, 2017.

[50] C. Dragomir and I. Grigoras, "Role of nutrition in the management of inflammatory bowel disease-current status," *Annals of Gastroenterology*, vol. 20, no. 4, pp. 246–250, 2007.

[51] E. Richman and J. M. Rhodes, "Review article: evidence-based dietary advice for patients with inflammatory bowel disease," *Alimentary Pharmacology & Therapeutics*, vol. 38, no. 10, pp. 1156–1171, 2013.

[52] J. L. Rombeau, L. R. Barot, C. E. Williamson, and J. L. Mullen, "Preoperative total parenteral nutrition and surgical outcome in patients with inflammatory bowel disease," *American Journal of Surgery*, vol. 143, no. 1, pp. 139–143, 1982.

[53] G. X. Yao, X. R. Wang, Z. M. Jiang, S. Y. Zhang, and A. P. Ni, "Role of perioperative parenteral nutrition in severely malnourished patients with Crohn's disease," *World Journal of Gastroenterology*, vol. 11, no. 36, pp. 5732–5734, 2005.

[54] H. Salinas, A. Dursun, I. Konstantinidis et al., "Does preoperative total parenteral nutrition in patients with ulcerative colitis produce better outcomes?," *International Journal of Colorectal Disease*, vol. 27, no. 11, pp. 1479–1483, 2012.

[55] B. A. Lashner, A. A. Evans, and S. B. Hanauer, "Preoperative total parenteral nutrition for bowel resection in Crohn's disease," *Digestive Diseases and Sciences*, vol. 34, no. 5, pp. 741–746, 1989.

[56] M. G. Beghetto, J. Victorino, L. Teixeira, and M. J. de Azevedo, "Parenteral nutrition as a risk factor for central venous catheter-related infection," *Journal of Parenteral and Enteral Nutrition*, vol. 29, no. 5, pp. 367–373, 2005.

[57] W. H. Hartl, K. W. Jauch, K. Parhofer, P. Rittler, and Working Group for Developing the Guidelines for Parenteral Nutrition of the German Association for Nutritional Medicine, "Complications and monitoring-guidelines on parenteral nutrition, Chapter 11," *German Medical Science*, vol. 7, 2009.

[58] P. Cotogni, "Management of parenteral nutrition in critically ill patients," *World Journal of Critical Care Medicine*, vol. 6, no. 1, pp. 13–20, 2017.

[59] N. P. O'Grady, M. Alexander, L. A. Burns et al., "Guidelines for the prevention of intravascular catheter-related infections," *American Journal of Infection Control*, vol. 39, no. 4, pp. S1–34, 2011.

[60] M. Opilla, "Epidemiology of bloodstream infection associated with parenteral nutrition," *American Journal of Infection Control*, vol. 36, no. 10, pp. S173.e5–S173.e8, 2008.

[61] S. E. Harvey, F. Parrott, D. A. Harrison et al., "Trial of the route of early nutritional support in critically ill adults," *The New England Journal of Medicine*, vol. 371, no. 18, pp. 1673–1684, 2014.

[62] J. Reignier, J. Boisramé-Helms, L. Brisard et al., "Enteral versus parenteral early nutrition in ventilated adults with shock: a randomised, controlled, multicentre, open-label, parallel-group study (NUTRIREA-2)," *The Lancet*, vol. 391, no. 10116, pp. 133–143, 2018.

[63] S. Klek, "Omega-3 fatty acids in modern parenteral nutrition: a review of the current evidence," *Journal of Clinical Medicine*, vol. 5, no. 3, 2016.

[64] T. Grau-Carmona, A. Bonet-Saris, A. García-de-Lorenzo et al., "Influence of n-3 polyunsaturated fatty acids enriched lipid emulsions on nosocomial infections and clinical outcomes in critically ill patients: ICU lipids study," *Critical Care Medicine*, vol. 43, no. 1, pp. 31–39, 2015.

[65] R. Lev-Tzion, A. M. Griffiths, O. Ledder, D. Turner, and Cochrane IBD Group, "Omega 3 fatty acids (fish oil) for maintenance of remission in Crohn's disease," *Cochrane Database of Systematic Reviews*, 2014.

[66] D. Turner, P. S. Shah, A. H. Steinhart, S. Zlotkin, and A. M. Griffiths, "Maintenance of remission in inflammatory bowel disease using omega-3 fatty acids (fish oil): a systematic review and meta-analyses," *Inflammatory Bowel Diseases*, vol. 17, no. 1, pp. 336–345, 2011.

[67] S. A. McClave, J. K. DiBaise, G. E. Mullin, and R. G. Martindale, "ACG clinical guideline: nutrition therapy in the adult hospitalized patient," *The American Journal of Gastroenterology*, vol. 111, no. 3, pp. 315–334, 2016, quiz 335.

[68] F. Bellolio, Z. Cohen, H. M. MacRae et al., "Outcomes following surgery for perforating Crohn's disease," *The British Journal of Surgery*, vol. 100, no. 10, pp. 1344–1348, 2013.

[69] P. Zerbib, D. Koriche, S. Truant et al., "Pre-operative management is associated with low rate of post-operative morbidity in penetrating Crohn's disease," *Alimentary Pharmacology & Therapeutics*, vol. 32, no. 3, pp. 459–465, 2010.

Cyclooxygenase-2 Expression Is a Predictive Marker for Late Recurrence in Colorectal Cancer

Sung Hoo Kim,[1] Byung Kyu Ahn,[1] Seung Sam Paik,[2] and Kang Hong Lee[1]

[1]*Department of Surgery, Hanyang University College of Medicine, Seoul, Republic of Korea*
[2]*Department of Pathology, Hanyang University College of Medicine, Seoul, Republic of Korea*

Correspondence should be addressed to Kang Hong Lee; leekh@hanyang.ac.kr

Academic Editor: Gianluca Pellino

Introduction. Cyclooxygenase-2 (COX-2) expression is elevated in colorectal cancer (CRC). However, data about the relation between COX-2 expression and the impact on the biologic behavior of recurrent disease are inconclusive as yet. The aim of this study is to investigate the relationship between the status of COX-2 expression in the primary CRC and the characteristics of recurrence after curative resection of stage I to III CRC. *Materials and Methods.* Ninety-eight patients with recurrence in 376 CRC patients, who underwent curative surgery between January 1991 and August 2001, were retrospectively assessed. Immunohistochemical staining, performed for the presence of COX-2 on tissue microarrays, was analyzed. *Results.* Forty-six patients showed elevated COX-2 expression, and 52 patients did not. The mean time to recurrence was significantly longer in the positive group than in the negative group (34.1 months ± 30.0 versus 21.9 months ± 17.4; $P = 0.019$). Positive COX-2 expression was correlated with late recurrence (>3 years after surgery) [43.5% versus 13.5%; $P = 0.001$]. In multivariate analysis, COX-2 expression was an independent factor associated with late recurrence (OR 4.656; 95% CI, 1.696 to 12.779; $P = 0.003$). Recurrence pattern and postrecurrence survival were not different between the two groups. *Conclusions.* Elevated COX-2 expression in itself is not a prognostic factor, but COX-2 expression in tumor tissue may be an independent predictive marker of late recurrence for patients with stage I to III CRC.

1. Introduction

The mainstay of colorectal cancer (CRC) treatment is curative resection, and tumor recurrence is a major concern after surgery. There have been several attempts to identify molecular markers that can predict recurrence and survival rates, but still, none is approved for clinical application.

Cyclooxygenase-2 (COX-2) is a rate-limiting enzyme involved in the conversion of arachidonic acid to prostaglandins and thromboxanes. These products play crucial roles in cell proliferation, immune response, angiogenesis, and inflammatory reaction, which may involve tumor development and progression [1, 2]. Previous studies have reported that COX-2 overexpression is detected in colorectal, gastric, breast, pulmonary, esophageal, and pancreatic cancer [3–7]. Increased COX-2 gene expression has been reported in human colorectal adenocarcinoma and in carcinogen-induced rat colonic tumors [8–12]. However, the molecular mechanisms by which COX-2 contributes to CRC progression and metastasis remain unclear. In addition, it remains controversial whether COX-2 expression is a prognostic factor for the survival of CRC patients or not [13–15].

The aim of this study is to investigate the relationship between the status of COX-2 expression and the characteristics of recurrent disease in stage I–III CRC patients after curative resection.

2. Methods

2.1. Selection of Patients. We retrospectively reviewed, between January 1991 and August 2001, 492 patients with the diagnosis of CRC and treated in one tertiary care center. 44 patients were excluded by the inclusion criteria. The inclusion criteria were stage I–III patients with curative resection

(R_0). Patients with (a) distant metastasis ($n = 29$), (b) incomplete resection ($n = 2$), and (c) metachronous cancers ($n = 3$) were excluded. The patients who expired due to other causes ($n = 10$) were also excluded. As a result, formalin-fixed paraffin-embedded samples from 376 patients were available. Patients with lymph node-positive disease received 5-FU-based adjuvant chemotherapy, and none of the patients received preoperative chemotherapy or radiotherapy. The median follow-up period was 56 months (range, 3 to 192 months). Of the 376 patients, COX-2 expression was elevated in 211 patients (56.0%, 211 patients), and the overall recurrence rate was 26.0% (98/376 patients).

2.2. Tissue Microarrays (TMAs). After the histological examination of H&E-stained samples by an experienced pathologist, parts containing a high proportion of tumor cells were assembled. TMAs were constructed with a tissue arrayer (AccuMac Arrayer, ISU ABXIS Co. Ltd., Seoul, Korea). The assembled TMAs were held in an X-Y position guide with 1 mm increments between individual samples and a 3 mm punch-depth stop device. Briefly, this instrument was utilized to make holes in a recipient block with defined array cores, and a solid stylet, which fitted the needle closely, was used to transfer the tissue cores into the recipient block. Due to the limited size of representative areas of the tumors, triplicate 1 mm diameter tissue cores were made from each donor block.

2.3. Immunohistochemical Staining. We obtained multiple 4 μm cut sections using a Leica microtome in immunohistochemical staining. The obtained sections were shifted to adhesive-coated slides. Dewaxing was performed with the TMA slides by heating at 55°C for 30 min and by three washes, of 5 min each, with xylene. Rehydration was done with the tissues by 5 min washes in 100%, 90%, and 70% ethanol and phosphate-buffered saline (PBS). Antigen was retrieved by heating the samples for 4 min 20 s in a microwave at full power in 250 ml 10 mM sodium citrate (pH 6.0). Endogenous peroxidase activity was blocked with 0.3% hydrogen peroxidase for 20 min. The sections were incubated with primary goat polyclonal anti-COX-2 antibody (N-20; Santa Cruz Biotechnology, Santa Cruz, CA, USA) diluted 1 : 100 in goat serum at room temperature for 1 h. After three washes of 2 min each with PBS, the sections were incubated with biotinylated anti-goat secondary antibody for 30 min (DAKO, Carpinteria, CA, USA). After three further washes with PBS, horseradish peroxidase streptavidin (DAKO) was added to the section for 30 min, followed by another three washes. The samples were developed for 1 min with 3,3′-diaminobenzidine substrate (Vector Laboratories, Burlington, Ontario, Canada) and counterstained with Mayer's hematoxylin. They were dehydrated according to standard procedures and closed with coverslips.

2.4. Interpretation of COX-2 Expression. COX-2 expression was interpreted independently by two experienced pathologists (SS Paik and SH Jang) on the basis of staining intensity and extent. Three punches per case were evaluated and considered a whole. Staining intensity was scored as 0 to 3 (0 = negative; 1 = weak; 2 = moderate; and 3 = strong) (Figure 1). Staining extent was scored as 0 to 4 based on the percentage of positive-stained cells (0 = 0%; 1 = 1–25%; 2 = 26–50%; 3 = 51–75%; and 4 = 76–100%). The final staining score was determined with a sum of the intensity and extent score. We divided all cases into four expression groups based on their sum of scores (0 = negative; 1–3 = low; 4-5 = moderate; and 6-7 = high). If the sum of scores was ≥4, we classified the cases as elevated COX-2 expression (positive). If the sum of scores was ≤3, we classified the cases as COX-2 negative. When there was a disagreement between the two pathologists, reinvestigation of the slide was performed with a multi-headed microscope and the final agreement was achieved.

2.5. Statistical Analysis. Statistical analysis was conducted with SPSS ver. 19.0 (SPSS Inc., Chicago, IL, USA). The chi-square test and Student's t-test were used to examine the association between COX-2 expression and clinical and pathological features including age, gender, tumor location, tumor size, gross type, cell type, differentiation, lymphatic invasion, vascular invasion, T category, N category, AJCC stage, and time to recurrence. Survival curves were constructed using the Kaplan-Meier method, and survival differences were analyzed by the log-rank test. P values < 0.05 were considered statistically significant.

3. Results

3.1. COX-2 Expression Is Related with Time to Recurrence. The clinical and pathological characteristics of the 376 patients are described in Table 1 according to the COX-2 expression status. In univariate analysis, the COX-2-positive group was different from the COX-2-negative group in terms of differentiation, lymphatic invasion, N category, AJCC stage, and recurrence rate. The clinical and pathologic findings of the 98 patients with tumor recurrence are included in Table 2. There were no statistically significant differences in terms of age, gender, tumor location, tumor size, gross type, cell type, differentiation, lymphatic invasion, vascular invasion, T category, N category, or AJCC stage between the two groups except for the time to recurrence. This was significantly longer in the COX-2-positive group than in the COX-2-negative group (34.1 months ± 30.0 versus 21.9 months ± 17.4, $P = 0.019$).

71 out of 98 patients with recurrence experienced early recurrence (72.4%), and 27 patients had late recurrence (27.6%). In univariate analysis, lymphatic invasion and positive COX-2 expression were significantly different between the two groups ($P = 0.012$ and $P = 0.001$, resp.) (Table 3). Positive lymphatic invasion was significantly correlated with early recurrence ($P = 0.012$), while positive COX-2 expression was significantly related with late recurrence ($P = 0.001$). Multivariate analysis revealed that lymphatic invasion was an independent factor for the early recurrence (OR 0.309; 95% CI, 0.103 to 0.924; $P = 0.036$), and positive COX-2 expression was an independent factor for the late recurrence (OR 4.656; 95% CI, 1.696 to 12.779; $P = 0.003$) (Table 3).

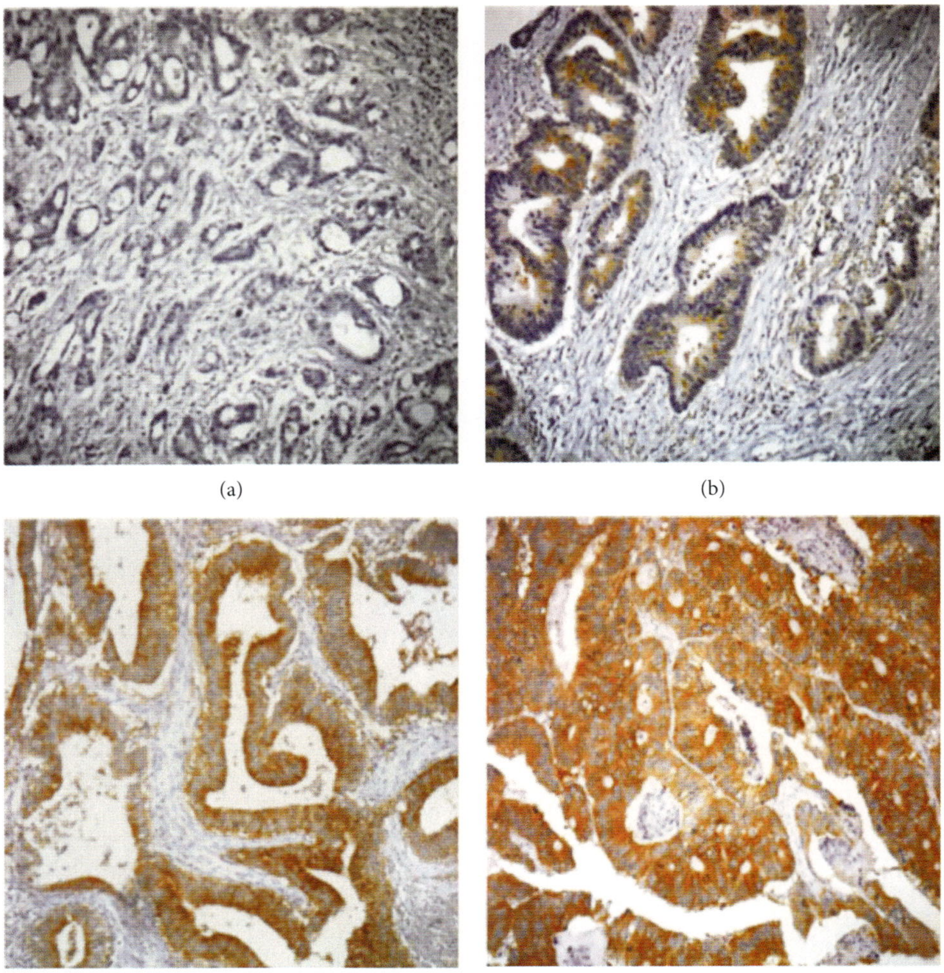

(a) (b) (c) (d)

FIGURE 1: The microphotographs of COX-2 immunostaining by intensity in colorectal cancer: (a) negative, (b) weak, (c) moderate, and (d) strong.

3.2. Recurrence Patterns and Postrecurrence Survival according to the COX-2 Expression Status. Thirty-two (8.5%) of the 376 patients experienced local recurrence, and 66 (17.5%) had distant metastasis. The most common site of distant metastasis was the liver ($n = 25$, 6.6%) followed by the lung ($n = 19$, 5.1%). The patterns of recurrence in the positive and the negative COX-2 expression groups were not different (Table 4). In the 98 patients with recurrence, there was no relation on postrecurrence survival according to the COX-2 expression status (Figure 2).

4. Discussion

Our results suggest that COX-2 expression in CRC is associated with late recurrence (>3 years after surgery) during the postsurgery follow-up period, which may not mean that COX-2 expression prevents early recurrence. In this study, lymphatic invasion was a significant factor for the early recurrence but COX-2 expression was a significant factor for the late recurrence. We assumed that positive COX-2 expression do not prevent early recurrence but induce late recurrence. Maybe there are other mechanisms which contribute to recurrence in the positive COX-2 expression group different from the lymphatic invasion group. A number of mechanisms may be involved in the process of late recurrence. COX-2 overexpression increases the migration and proliferation of intestinal epithelial cell and inhibits programmed cell death, so prolonging the survival of abnormal cells [16]. Interestingly, another study found that COX-2 overexpression was correlated with elevated intracellular telomerase and reduced apoptosis [17]. In nonsmall cell lung cancer, COX-2 overexpression has been shown to stabilize survivin, an inhibitor of apoptosis [18]. In breast cancer, the presence of cytoplasmic survivin positively correlates with COX-2 expression [19]. COX-2 and survivin are overexpressed and positively correlated in endometrial adenocarcinoma [20]. Although our data do not have a bearing on molecular mechanisms, we suspect that the relation between COX-2 overexpression and late recurrence may be due to a decreased rate of apoptosis of surviving tumor cells. We suspect that surviving tumor cells in the stromal compartment may grow and migrate to other organs, and time may be required for surviving tumor cells to acquire resistance to adjuvant treatment.

TABLE 1: Clinical and pathological characteristics according to COX-2 expression in 376 patients with R0 resection.

Variable	Total patient ($n = 376$)	COX-2 negative ($n = 165$)	COX-2 positive ($n = 211$)	P value
Age (yr)				0.496
<70	311 (82.7%)	134 (81.2%)	177 (83.9%)	
≥70	65 (17.3%)	31 (18.8%)	34 (16.1%)	
Gender				0.436
Male	208 (55.3%)	95 (57.6%)	113 (53.6%)	
Female	168 (44.7%)	70 (42.4%)	98 (46.4%)	
Tumor location				0.209
Right colon	82 (21.8%)	34 (20.6%)	48 (22.7%)	
Left colon	113 (30.1%)	43 (26.1%)	70 (33.2%)	
Rectum	181 (48.1%)	88 (53.3%)	93 (44.1%)	
Tumor size				0.961
<5 cm	118 (31.4%)	52 (31.5%)	66 (31.3%)	
≥5 cm	258 (68.6%)	113 (68.5%)	145 (68.7%)	
Gross type				0.297
Fungating	180 (44.9%)	83 (50.3%)	97 (46.0%)	
Infiltrative	170 (46.9%)	69 (41.8%)	101 (47.8%)	
Unknown	26 (8.2%)	13 (7.9%)	13 (6.2%)	
Cell type				0.303
Nonmucinous	356 (94.7%)	154 (93.3%)	202 (95.7%)	
Mucinous	20 (5.3%)	11 (6.7%)	9 (4.3%)	
Differentiation				0.032
WD	10 (2.7%)	5 (3.0%)	5 (2.4%)	
MD	301 (80.1%)	141 (85.5%)	160 (75.8%)	
PD	65 (17.3%)	19 (11.5%)	46 (21.8%)	
Lymphatic invasion				0.004
Absent	180 (47.9%)	65 (39.4%)	115 (54.5%)	
Present	196 (52.1%)	100 (60.6%)	96 (45.5%)	
Vascular invasion				0.634
Absent	372 (98.9%)	164 (99.4%)	208 (98.6%)	
Present	4 (1.1%)	1 (0.6%)	3 (1.4%)	
T category				0.089
T1	7 (1.9%)	1 (0.6%)	6 (2.8%)	
T2	32 (8.5%)	9 (5.5%)	23 (10.9%)	
T3	330 (87.8%)	152 (92.1%)	178 (84.4%)	
T4	7 (1.9%)	3 (1.8%)	4 (1.9%)	
N category				0.019
N0	185 (49.2%)	69 (41.8%)	116 (55.0%)	
N1	90 (23.9%)	41 (24.8%)	49 (23.2%)	
N2	101 (26.9%)	55 (33.3%)	46 (21.8%)	
Stage				0.003
I	31 (8.2%)	7 (4.2%)	24 (11.4%)	
II	158 (42.0%)	62 (37.6%)	96 (45.5%)	
III	187 (49.7%)	96 (58.2%)	91 (43.1%)	
Recurrence				0.001
Early (≤3 yrs)	71 (18.9%)	45 (27.4%)	26 (12.3%)	
Late (>3 yrs)	27 (7.2%)	7 (4.3%)	20 (9.4%)	
No	278 (73.9%)	112 (67.9%)	166 (78.7%)	

Table 2: Clinical and pathological characteristics according to COX-2 expression in patients with recurrence.

Variable	Total patient ($n = 98$)	COX-2 negative ($n = 52$)	COX-2 positive ($n = 46$)	P value
Age (yr)				0.200
<70	80 (81.6%)	40 (76.9%)	40 (87.0%)	
≥70	18 (18.4%)	12 (23.1%)	6 (13.0%)	
Gender				0.267
Male	56 (57.1%)	27 (51.9%)	29 (63.0%)	
Female	42 (42.9%)	25 (48.1%)	17 (37.0%)	
Tumor location				0.725
Right colon	25 (25.5%)	13 (25.0%)	12 (26.1%)	
Left colon	16 (16.3%)	9 (17.3%)	7 (15.2%)	
Rectum	57 (58.2%)	30 (57.7%)	26 (58.7%)	
Tumor size				0.286
<5 cm	33 (33.7%)	20 (38.5%)	13 (28.3%)	
≥5 cm	65 (66.3%)	32 (61.5%)	33 (71.7%)	
Gross type				0.680
Fungating	44 (44.9%)	22 (42.3%)	22 (47.8%)	
Infiltrative	46 (46.9%)	25 (48.0%)	21 (45.6%)	
Unknown	8 (8.2%)	5 (9.6%)	3 (6.5%)	
Cell type				1.000
Nonmucinous	93 (94.9%)	49 (94.2%)	44 (95.7%)	
Mucinous	5 (5.1%)	3 (5.8%)	2 (4.3%)	
Differentiation				0.291
WD	4 (4.1%)	2 (3.8%)	2 (4.3%)	
MD	75 (76.5%)	43 (82.7%)	32 (69.6%)	
PD	19 (19.4%)	7 (13.5%)	12 (26.1%)	
Lymphatic invasion				0.190
Absent	20 (20.4%)	8 (15.4%)	12 (26.1%)	
Present	78 (79.6%)	44 (84.6%)	34 (73.9%)	
Vascular invasion				1.000
Absent	98 (100%)	52 (100%)	46 (100%)	
Present	0 (0%)	0 (0%)	0 (0%)	
T category				0.840
T1	0 (0%)	0 (0%)	0 (0%)	
T2	3 (3.1%)	1 (1.9%)	2 (4.3%)	
T3	92 (93.9%)	49 (94.2%)	43 (93.5%)	
T4	3 (3.1%)	2 (3.8%)	1 (2.2%)	
N category				0.479
N0	22 (22.4%)	11 (21.2%)	11 (23.9%)	
N1	27 (27.6%)	17 (32.7%)	10 (21.7%)	
N2	49 (50.0%)	24 (46.2%)	25 (54.3%)	
Stage				0.713
I	1 (1%)	0 (0%)	1 (2.2%)	
II	22 (22.4%)	11 (21.2%)	11 (23.9%)	
III	75 (76.6%)	41 (78.8%)	34 (73.9%)	
Time to recurrence (month)	27.6 ± 24.8	21.9 ± 17.4	34.1 ± 30.0	0.019
Recurrence type				0.001
Early (≤3 yrs)	71 (72.4%)	45 (86.5%)	26 (56.5%)	
Late (>3 yrs)	27 (27.6%)	7 (13.5%)	20 (43.5%)	

TABLE 3: Univariate and multivariate analysis of independent risk factors associated with late recurrence.

Variable	Early recurrence (<3 yr) ($n = 71$)	Late recurrence (≥3 yr) ($n = 27$)	Univariate analysis (P value)	Multivariate analysis (OR, 95% CI, P value)
Age (yr)			0.382	
<70	56 (78.9%)	24 (88.9%)		
≥70	15 (21.1%)	3 (11.1%)		0.726 (0.174–3.024) 0.660
Gender			0.473	
Male	39 (54.9%)	17 (63.0%)		0.996 (0.361–2.747) 0.993
Female	32 (45.1%)	10 (37.0%)		
Tumor location			1.000	
Right colon	18 (25.3%)	7 (25.9%)		
Left colon	12 (16.9%)	4 (14.8%)		
Rectum	41 (57.7%)	16 (59.3%)		
Tumor size			0.965	
<5 cm	24 (33.8%)	9 (33.3%)		
≥5 cm	47 (66.2%)	18 (66.7%)		
Gross type			0.280	
Fungating	30 (42.3%)	14 (51.9%)		
Infiltrative	36 (50.7%)	10 (37.0%)		
Unknown	5 (7.0%)	3 (11.1%)		
Cell type			0.614	
Nonmucinous	68 (95.8%)	25 (92.6%)		
Mucinous	3 (4.2%)	2 (7.4%)		
Differentiation			0.818	
WD	3 (4.2%)	1 (3.7%)		
MD	53 (74.6%)	22 (81.5%)		
PD	15 (21.1%)	4 (14.8%)		
Lymphatic invasion			0.012	
Absent	10 (14.1%)	10 (37.0%)		
Present	61 (85.9%)	17 (63.0%)		0.309 (0.103–0.924) 0.036
Vascular invasion			1.000	
Absent	71 (100%)	27 (100%)		
Present	0 (0%)	0 (0%)		
T category			0.193	
T1	0 (0%)	0 (0%)		
T2	1 (1.4%)	2 (7.4%)		
T3	67 (94.4%)	25 (92.6%)		
T4	3 (4.2%)	0 (0%)		
N category			0.102	
N0	12 (16.9%)	10 (37.0%)		
N1	21 (29.6%)	6 (22.3%)		
N2	38 (53.5%)	11 (40.7%)		
Stage			0.051	
I	0 (0%)	1 (3.7%)		
II	13 (18.3%)	9 (33.3%)		
III	58 (81.7%)	17 (63.0%)		1.315 (0.256–6.753) 0.743
COX-2 expression			0.001	
Negative	45 (63.4%)	7 (25.9%)		
Positive	26 (36.6%)	20 (74.1%)		4.656 (1.696–12.779) 0.003

Table 4: Recurrence pattern according to the status of COX-2 expression in the 98 patients with recurrence.

	COX-2 negative ($n = 52$)	COX-2 positive ($n = 46$)	P value
			0.256
Local recurrence	14 (26.9%)	18 (39.1%)	
Liver	13 (25.0%)	12 (26.1%)	
Lung	9 (17.3%)	10 (21.7%)	
Peritoneal seeding	5 (9.6%)	3 (6.5%)	
Others (brain, bone, skin)	11 (21.2%)	3 (6.5%)	

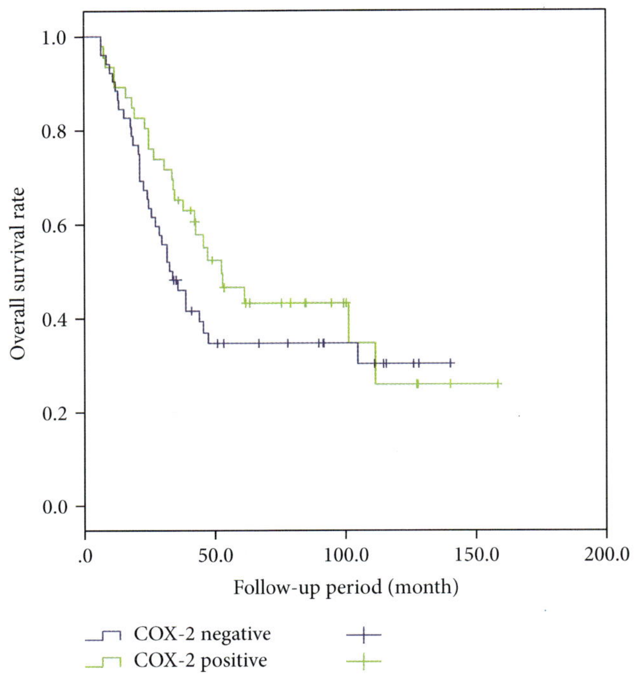

Figure 2: Postrecurrence survival was not significantly different according to the COX-2 status of the 98 patients with recurrence ($P = 0.230$).

Some studies have suggested that elevated COX-2 expression of CRC patients is related with reduced survival [15, 21]. However, others found that the elevated expression of COX-2 protein had no significant impact on disease-specific survival and overall survival in CRC patients [22, 23]. We observed no significant postrecurrence survival difference according to COX-2 expression status. Thus, COX-2 expression is not likely a prognostic factor for postrecurrence in CRC.

After curative surgery, CRC patients with positive COX-2 expression have an increased probability of late tumor recurrence based on the result of this study. Therefore, the positive COX-2 patients should be considered candidates for more frequent testing after 3 years of follow-up and extend follow-up period longer than 5 years after surgery. In protocols for postsurgery surveillance, there is a tendency for the frequency of follow-up and testing to be reduced after 3 years. We suggest that since COX-2 expression may be a marker for late recurrence, the frequency of follow-up and testing should not be reduced after 3 years. Furthermore, suspending follow-up after 5 years from the initial operation may be inappropriate especially in COX-2-positive patients. A further prospective randomized study is required to identify optimal surveillance methods and follow-up intervals.

As smoking habit and body mass index may modify the risk of CRC in COX-2 genotype, this bias could affect our conclusions regarding the predictive marker [24]. A further well-designed, large, sample-sized study is mandatory.

A limitation of this study was its retrospective design, which is subject to selection bias. Also, the cases were all from a single institution. As no molecular biological study was performed, it was not clear how COX-2 expression contributed to late recurrence. But it is meaningful that the study revealed a novel finding about the relationship between elevated COX-2 expression and late recurrence of CRC: we were able to demonstrate the possibility of COX-2 expression as a biologic marker predicting late recurrence in CRC patients.

5. Conclusions

Elevated COX-2 expression in itself is not a prognostic factor, but COX-2 expression in tumor tissue may be an independent predictive marker of late recurrence for patients with stage I to III CRC. A further well-designed study is required to demonstrate the regulatory mechanism of COX-2 expression on CRC recurrence.

Authors' Contributions

Sung Hoo Kim contributed to the collection of data, analysis, interpretation, and writing the article. Byung Kyu Ahn contributed to the critical revision of the article. Seung Sam Paik contributed to the critical revision of the article. Kang Hong Lee contributed to the conceiving of the design and approved the final version of the manuscript.

References

[1] J. R. Vane, Y. S. Bakhle, and R. M. Botting, "Cyclooxygenases 1 and 2," *Annual Review of Pharmacology and Toxicology*, vol. 38, no. 1, pp. 97–120, 1998.

[2] K. Subbaramaiah and A. J. Dannenberg, "Cyclooxygenase-2: a molecular target for cancer prevention and treatment," *Trends in Pharmacological Sciences*, vol. 24, no. 2, pp. 96–102, 2003.

[3] A. Ristimäki, N. Honkanen, H. Jänkälä, P. Sipponen, and M. Härkönen, "Expression of cyclooxygenase-2 in human gastric carcinoma," *Cancer Research*, vol. 57, no. 7, pp. 1276–1280, 1997.

[4] T. Hida, Y. Yatabe, H. Achiwa et al., "Increased expression of cyclooxygenase 2 occurs frequently in human lung cancers, specifically in adenocarcinomas," *Cancer Research*, vol. 58, no. 17, pp. 3761–3764, 1998.

[5] D. Hwang, J. Byrne, D. Scollard, and E. Levine, "Expression of cyclooxygenase-1 and cyclooxygenase-2 in human breast

cancer," *Journal of the National Cancer Institute*, vol. 90, no. 6, pp. 455–460, 1998.

[6] K. C. Zimmermann, M. Sarbia, A. A. Weber, F. Borchard, H. E. Gabbert, and K. Schrör, "Cyclooxygenase-2 expression in human esophageal carcinoma," *Cancer Research*, vol. 59, no. 1, pp. 198–204, 1999.

[7] O. N. Tucker, A. J. Dannenberg, E. K. Yang et al., "Cyclooxygenase-2 expression is up-regulated in human pancreatic cancer," *Cancer Research*, vol. 59, no. 5, pp. 987–990, 1999.

[8] J. Dimberg, A. Samuelsson, A. Hugander, and P. Soderkvist, "Differential expression of cyclooxygenase 2 in human colorectal cancer," *Gut*, vol. 45, no. 5, pp. 730–732, 1999.

[9] C. E. Eberhart, R. J. Coffey, A. Radhika, F. M. Giardiello, S. Ferrenbach, and R. N. Dubois, "Up-regulation of cyclooxygenase 2 gene expression in human colorectal adenomas and adenocarcinomas," *Gastroenterology*, vol. 107, no. 4, pp. 1183–1188, 1994.

[10] H. Sano, Y. Kawahito, R. L. Wilder et al., "Expression of cyclooxygenase-1 and -2 in human colorectal cancer," *Cancer Research*, vol. 55, no. 17, pp. 3785–3789, 1995.

[11] R. N. DuBois, A. Radhika, B. S. Reddy, and A. J. Entingh, "Increased cyclooxygenase-2 levels in carcinogen-induced rat colonic tumors," *Gastroenterology*, vol. 110, no. 4, pp. 1259–1262, 1996.

[12] P. de Heer, M. J. E. M. Gosens, E. C. de Bruin et al., "Cyclooxygenase 2 expression in rectal cancer is of prognostic significance in patients receiving preoperative radiotherapy," *Clinical Cancer Research*, vol. 13, no. 10, pp. 2955–2960, 2007.

[13] E. Rahme, A. N. Barkun, Y. Toubouti, and M. Bardou, "The cyclooxygenase-2-selective inhibitors rofecoxib and celecoxib prevent colorectal neoplasia occurrence and recurrence," *Gastroenterology*, vol. 125, no. 2, pp. 404–412, 2003.

[14] T. Fujita, M. Matsui, K. Takaku et al., "Size- and invasion-dependent increase in cyclooxygenase 2 levels in human colorectal carcinomas," *Cancer Research*, vol. 58, no. 21, pp. 4823–4826, 1998.

[15] M. Rao, W. Yang, A. M. Seifalian, and M. C. Winslet, "Role of cyclooxygenase-2 in the angiogenesis of colorectal cancer," *International Journal of Colorectal Disease*, vol. 19, no. 1, pp. 1–11, 2004.

[16] A. J. Dannenberg, N. K. Altorki, J. O. Boyle et al., "Cyclo-oxygenase 2: a pharmacological target for the prevention of cancer," *The Lancet Oncology*, vol. 2, no. 9, pp. 544–551, 2001.

[17] Z. H. Zhuang, S. W. Tsao, W. Deng et al., "Early upregulation of cyclooxygenase-2 in human papillomavirus type 16 and telomerase-induced immortalization of human esophageal epithelial cells," *Journal of Gastroenterology and Hepatology*, vol. 23, no. 10, pp. 1613–1620, 2008.

[18] K. Krysan, H. Dalwadi, S. Sharma, M. Põld, and S. Dubinett, "Cyclooxygenase 2-dependent expression of survivin is critical for apoptosis resistance in non-small cell lung cancer," *Cancer Research*, vol. 64, no. 18, pp. 6359–6362, 2004.

[19] N. Barnes, P. Haywood, P. Flint, W. F. Knox, and N. J. Bundred, "Survivin expression in in situ and invasive breast cancer relates to COX-2 expression and DCIS recurrence," *British Journal of Cancer*, vol. 94, no. 2, pp. 253–258, 2006.

[20] S. Erkanli, F. Bolat, F. Kayaselcuk, B. Demirhan, and E. Kuscu, "COX-2 and survivin are overexpressed and positively correlated in endometrial carcinoma," *Gynecologic Oncology*, vol. 104, no. 2, pp. 320–325, 2007.

[21] L. T. Soumaoro, H. Uetake, T. Higuchi, Y. Takagi, M. Enomoto, and K. Sugihara, "Cyclooxygenase-2 expression: a significant prognostic indicator for patients with colorectal cancer," *Clinical Cancer Research*, vol. 10, no. 24, pp. 8465–8471, 2004.

[22] K. Zafirellis, G. Agrogiannis, and A. Zachaki, "Prognostic value of COX-2 immunohistochemical expression evaluated by quantitative image analysis in colorectal cancer," *APMIS*, vol. 116, no. 10, pp. 912–922, 2008.

[23] R. Fux, M. Schwab, K. P. Thon, C. H. Gleiter, and P. Fritz, "Cyclooxygenase-2 expression in human colorectal cancer is unrelated to overall patient survival," *Clinical Cancer Research*, vol. 11, no. 13, pp. 4754–4760, 2005.

[24] L. L. Xing, Z. N. Wang, L. Jiang et al., "*Cyclooxygenase 2* polymorphism and colorectal cancer: -765G>C variant modifies risk associated with smoking and body mass index," *World Journal of Gastroenterology*, vol. 14, no. 11, pp. 1785–1789, 2008.

21

Ingesting Self-Grown Produce and Seropositivity for Hepatitis E in the United States

Thomas M. Diehl[1] **Daniel J. Adams,**[2] **and Cade M. Nylund**[3]

[1]*McGill University, Faculty of Medicine, Montreal, QC, Canada H3G 2M1*
[2]*Department of Pediatrics, Naval Medical Center Portsmouth, Portsmouth, VA 23708, USA*
[3]*Department of Pediatrics, F. Edward Hébert School of Medicine, Uniformed Services University of the Health Sciences, Bethesda, MD 20814, USA*

Correspondence should be addressed to Cade M. Nylund; cade.nylund@usuhs.edu

Academic Editor: Paul Enck

Background. Hepatitis E virus (HEV) is a major cause of hepatitis in developing and industrialized countries worldwide. The modes of HEV transmission in industrialized countries, including the United States, remain largely unknown. This study is aimed at evaluating the association between HEV seropositivity and consumption of self-grown foods in the United States. *Methods.* Cross-sectional data was extracted from the 2009–2012 National Health and Nutrition Examination Survey (NHANES). Data from the dietary interview and the serum HEV IgG and IgM enzyme immunoassay test results were linked and examined. Univariate and multivariable logistic regression models were used to evaluate the significance and effect size of an association between self-grown food consumption and hepatitis E seropositivity. *Results.* The estimated HEV seroprevalence in the civilian, noninstitutionalized US population was 6.6% in 2009–2012, which corresponds to an estimated hepatitis E national seroprevalence of 17,196,457 people. Overall, 10.9% of participants who ingested self-grown foods had positive HEV antibodies versus 6.1% of participants who did not consume self-grown foods ($P < 0.001$; odds ratio (OR) 1.87; 95% CI 1.41–2.48). In the age-stratified multivariable analysis, the correlation between ingesting self-grown foods and HEV seropositivity was significant for participants 40–59 years old, but not overall, or for those < 40 years or ≥60 years. *Conclusions.* Ingesting self-grown food, or simply the process of gardening/farming, may be a source of zoonotic HEV transmission.

1. Introduction

HEV is an enterically transmitted acute viral hepatitis and major cause of sporadic and epidemic hepatitis worldwide [1–3]. Infection by HEV is typically self-limited and resolves within 4–6 weeks; however, the severity of infection ranges from subclinical to fulminate hepatitis [2, 4, 5]. Hepatitis E is unique in its severity among pregnant women, who may face up to a 28% mortality rate, and the immunocompromised, who frequently progress to chronic hepatitis E without antiviral treatment [6–8]. Although identified clinical cases are rare, asymptomatic hepatitis E infection is now known to be widespread in industrialized nations [1, 4].

HEV transmission is linked to fecally contaminated drinking water [9, 10]. These cases are usually reported as part of a large-scale outbreak, often following a flood or another natural disaster in developing countries [5, 11]. The modes of HEV transmission in industrialized countries, including the United States, remain largely unknown. For years, it was suspected that HEV infections diagnosed in industrialized nations stemmed from travel to hyperendemic regions, especially in South Asia and North Africa [2]. Recent studies have demonstrated autochthonous (locally acquired) infection in several industrialized countries [12–14]. Unlike hepatitis A virus, HEV is not readily transmitted by person-to-person contact; therefore, it is postulated that these autochthonous infections originate from a zoonotic source [15].

Hepatitis E is recognized as a zoonotic disease [16]. Swine are a known HEV reservoir and many wild and domestic animals have been connected to transmission [5, 10, 16]. People whose occupations involve working with animals, especially livestock, have higher rates of HEV seropositivity [17, 18]. More recent studies support zoonotic transmission of HEV from domestic and pet animals [16]. Foodborne transmission has also been clearly described as a mode of sporadic zoonotic transmission in industrialized countries. Reports highlight consumption of raw or undercooked pork products (wild and domestic), game meats, shellfish, and produce as possible sources of human HEV infection [4, 10, 19–21]. We propose that humans may be exposed to HEV through self-grown foods, such as fruits and vegetables from a home garden contaminated by a zoonotic source. Our aim is to use cross-sectional data to evaluate the association between HEV seropositivity and consumption of self-grown foods.

2. Materials and Methods

Using data collected in the 2009–2012 National Health and Nutrition Examination Survey (NHANES), we performed a cross-sectional study to assess whether ingesting self-grown foods is associated with detection of HEV-specific IgM and IgG. The NHANES sample is a stratified multistage probability cluster designed to represent the total civilian noninstitutionalized US population. Probability sampling weights are applied to collected data to account for oversampling and nonparticipation and are used to calculate national estimates. Standardized interviewers, physical examinations, and tests of biologic samples are used to collect data in five major categories: demographics, dietary information, physical and dental examinations, laboratory tests, and questionnaires. Additional details concerning NHANES sampling and survey design can be found in the NHANES section of the Centers for Disease Control and Prevention (CDC) website [22].

The NHANES questionnaire asks participants to report demographics including age, gender, race/ethnicity, and birthplace. The race/ethnicity is reported in five categories: Mexican American, other Hispanic, non-Hispanic White, non-Hispanic Black, or other/multiracial. As for the dietary questionnaire, two dietary interviews were administered to all participants. The first interview was administered in person at the designated NHANES site. The second interview was administered over the phone 3–10 days later. Proxy interviews were administered for children 1–11 years old and for individuals unable to reliably answer questions themselves. During each dietary interview, participants were asked to report the types and sources of each food item eaten over the previous 24-hour period. Food items grown, caught, or hunted by the participant or someone the participant knew were categorized as self-grown foods. The recorded self-grown foods were then subcategorized into groups, which included fruits, vegetables, meat products, dairy, and grains.

HEV-specific IgM and IgG serologic tests were performed on all participants ≥ 6 years using enzyme immunoassay (EIA) kits provided by DSI—Diagnostics System Italy of Saronno, Italy. The CDC reported the IgM assay (DS-EIA-ANTI-HEV-M) as having 98% sensitivity and 95.2% specificity, and the manufacturer reported the IgG assay (DS-EIA-ANTI-HEV-G) as having 100% sensitivity and 97.5% specificity [13]. Detailed specimen collection and processing protocols can be found in the NHANES Laboratory Procedures Manual [23]. Further information concerning the anti-HEV EIA kits can be found in the CDC Laboratory Procedure Manuals for HEV testing [24, 25].

2.1. Statistical Methods. The raw number of survey participants is reported to describe the inclusion and exclusion of subjects from combining data from the demographic questionnaire, dietary interview, and laboratory NHANES datasets. The NHANES demographic and dietary questionnaires are available online [25–27]. All further analyses and seroprevalence estimates accounted for the NHANES survey design and included appropriate survey weights, which accounted for the differential probabilities of selection, nonresponse, and oversampling. Univariate analysis of the respective variables and seroprevalence was conducted first with standard errors estimated by the Taylor series linearization. Comparison of continuous variables was performed using Student's t-statistic. Univariate and multivariable logistic regression evaluated the significance and effect size of investigated independent variables with hepatitis E seropositivity (either IgG or IgM positive) as the dependent variable. The independent variables evaluated include: ingestion of self-grown food, sex, race/ethnicity, and foreign versus US born. The NHANES race/ethnicity categories were used with the modification that "Mexican–American" and "other Hispanic" categories were combined.

The seroprevalence by age was calculated and used to estimate a force of infection method as described by Shkedy et al. [28]. Rates of both self-grown food consumption and hepatitis E seropositivity were evaluated to identify whether self-grown food was significantly associated with hepatitis E seropositivity among various age groups. These age groups were based on the force of infection curve. An alpha level of 0.05 was utilized to determine statistical significance. Analyses were conducted using SAS 9.3 (SAS Institute, Cary, NC). The study was reviewed and deemed exempt by the responsible institutional review board because the data is deidentified and publicly available online.

3. Results

20,293 individuals participated in the 2009–2012 NHANES survey; 16,984 were ≥ 6 years old and therefore eligible to participate. Out of all eligible individuals, 14,951 had recorded HEV serologies. Participants with insufficient blood drawn and incomplete laboratory exams do not have recorded HEV serologies. Serum analysis showed that 894 (6.0%) individuals were positive for HEV-specific IgG and 146 (1.0%) were positive for HEV-specific IgM. Evaluating participants positive for either HEV-specific IgG or HEV-specific IgM yielded a seroprevalence of 6.6% (95% confidence interval (CI) 5.8%–7.4%), which corresponds to an estimated national HEV seroprevalence of 17,196,457 people (95% CI 14,561,770–19,831,144) in the civilian, noninstitutionalized US population.

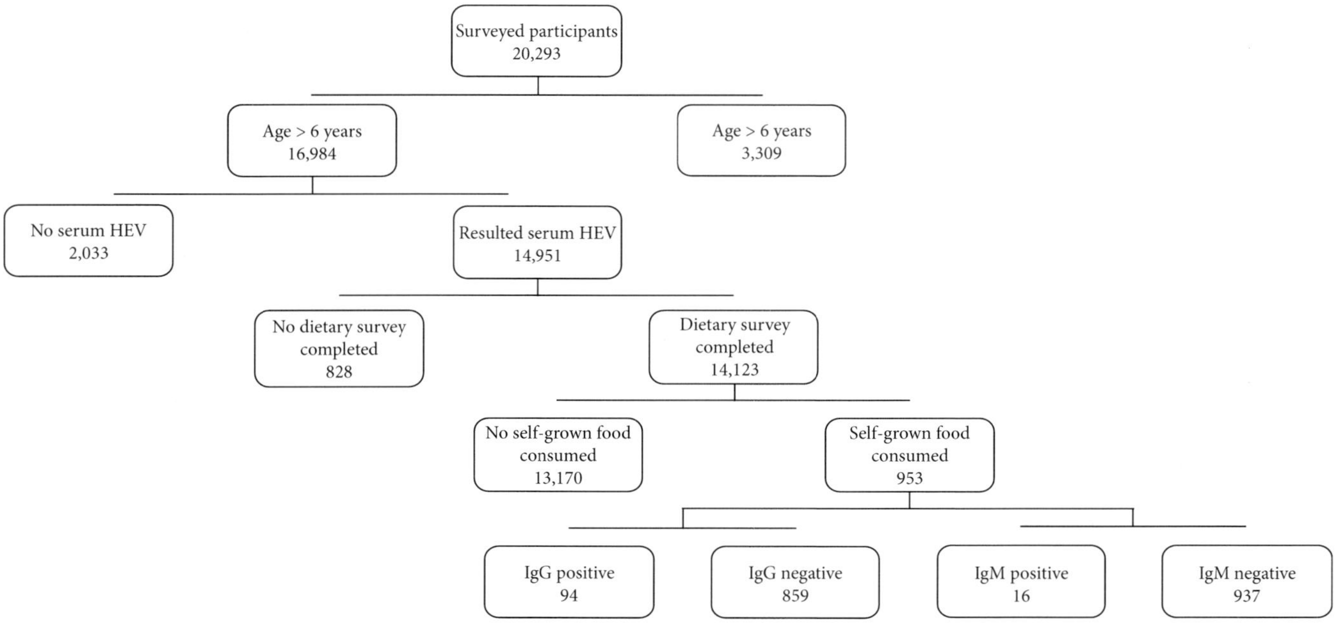

FIGURE 1: Participant analysis flow diagram, NHANES 2009–2012.

As for the nutritional component, 18,273 out of 20,293 survey participants completed the dietary interview. Approximately 7.3% (95% CI 6.2%–8.5%) of participants reported eating self-grown food, which represents an estimated 24,091,324 (95% CI 19,339,036–28,843,612) people nationally. Those who reported eating self-grown foods were older (median age 52.0; interquartile range (IQR) 36.5–66.0) than the remainder of the population (median 39.1; IQR 22.3–55.1; $P < 0.001$). All participants with both completed dietary interview and HEV serologies (14,123 out of 14,951) were included for further analysis (Figure 1).

The dietary interviews of participants with resulted HEV serologies included 317,416 foods. A total of 1833 items were reported in the self-grown food category. Self-grown foods reported by HEV-seropositive participants included fruits (45%), vegetables (23%), meat products (15%), dairy products (9%), honey/sweeteners (5%), and grains (3%).

Approximately 9.7% (standard error of percent (SEP) 1.2) of participants who ingested self-grown foods had detectable HEV-specific IgG compared to 5.4% (SEP 0.2) of participants who did not consume self-grown food ($P < 0.001$; OR 1.89; 95% CI 1.46–2.44). HEV-specific IgM was detected in 1.7% (SEP 0.52) of those who reported consuming self-grown food, versus 1.0% (SEP 0.2) in those who did not ($P = 0.21$; OR 1.66; 95% CI 0.76–3.66). When evaluating for any HEV antibodies (IgG or IgM), participants who reported eating self-grown foods had 10.9% seropositivity versus 6.1% in participants who did not consume self-grown foods ($P < 0.001$; OR 1.87; 95% CI 1.41–2.48). In the age-stratified multivariable analysis, however, the correlation between ingesting self-grown foods and HEV seropositivity was significant for participants 40–59 years old (OR 1.70; 95% CI 1.06–2.74), but not overall, or for those < 40 years or ≥60 years.

In addition to consuming self-grown foods, several other factors were found to be associated with HEV seropositivity. HEV-seropositive individuals were found to be older, with a median age of 57.6 years (IQR 45.0–69.0), compared to a median age of 40.7 years (IQR 23.7–56.3; $P < 0.001$) in the overall serum-tested population. This finding is consistent with previous reports [29, 30]. Furthermore, the estimated seropositivity steadily increases throughout life, with a maximum force of infection peaking at 36 per 100,000 in the 6th decade of life. The prevalence and force of infection by age are presented in Figure 2.

Univariate and multivariable-adjusted odds ratios for HEV seropositivity by selected characteristics are shown in Table 1, with multivariable-adjusted odds ratios further stratified by age in Table 2. Birth country was a significant associative factor, as the seroprevalence of participants born outside of the Unites States (9.3%; SEP 0.88; OR 1.78; 95% CI 1.23–2.58) was higher than that of US-born participants (6.0%; SEP 0.45). In gender comparisons, young females (6–39 years) were found to have higher HEV seropositivity compared to males of the same age group (OR 1.44, 95% CI 1.03–2.02). Finally, non-Hispanic Black participants had lower rates of HEV infection than White participants (OR 0.60, 95% CI 0.46–0.79). Other race/ethnicity comparisons were not statistically significant.

4. Discussion

This study demonstrates an association between ingesting self-grown food and seropositivity for HEV. Based on the 2009–2012 National Health and Nutrition Survey (NHANES), the estimated HEV seroprevalence of the US civilian and noninstitutionalized population is 17.2 million people (6.6%). Since the best-characterized modes of HEV transmission—drinking fecally contaminated water and working with infected swine—are relatively rare in the US, exploring other modes of transmission is critical to understanding HEV epidemiology. HEV

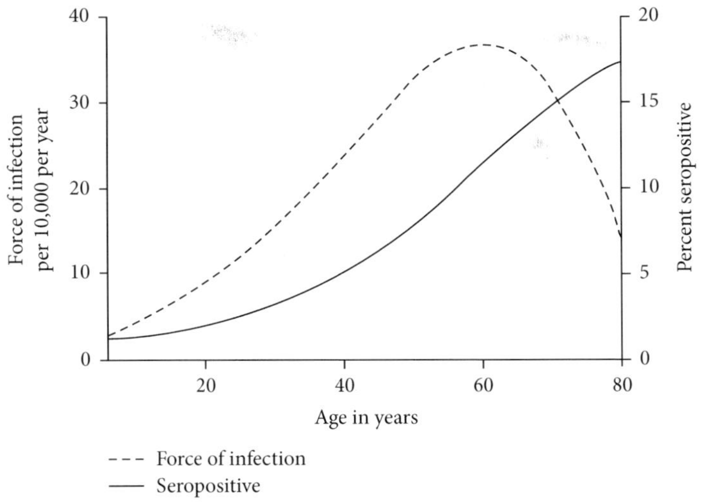

Figure 2: HEV-estimated force of infection and seropositivity by age for 2009–2012 NHANES participants.

Table 1: Odds ratios and adjusted odds ratios with 95 percent confidence intervals (CI) for HEV seropositivity by selected characteristics, NHANES 2009–2012.

	Odds ratio (95% CI)	Adjusted odds ratio (95% CI)
Self-grown food	1.87 (1.41–2.48)	1.32 (0.96–1.81)
Foreign born	1.61 (1.24–2.10)	1.78 (1.23–2.58)
Female versus male	1.13 (0.96–1.34)	1.08 (0.91–1.29)
Age	1.50 (1.44–1.57)	1.50 (1.43–1.57)
Race/ethnicity		
Non-Hispanic Black versus White	0.48 (0.38–0.61)	0.60 (0.46–0.79)
Hispanic versus White	0.81 (0.63–1.04)	0.91 (0.65–1.27)
Other versus White	1.21 (0.93–1.58)	1.21 (0.86–1.70)

transmission through contaminated self-grown produce is plausible based on the ever-expanding range of identified zoonotic hosts and identification of HEV on agricultural products [19, 20, 31].

A mounting body of evidence has demonstrated that other animal species play a major role in HEV transmission to humans [10, 16, 32]. Despite documentation of cross-species HEV transmission to humans, the mechanisms of infection remain unclear [33]. Swine are a well-known reservoir, as multiple studies have reported positive HEV serologies in swine worldwide [5, 34]. Recent reports have expanded the range of possible zoonotic hosts after finding similar strains of HEV in cattle, deer, rabbits, wild boar, birds, rats, and several other animals [16, 33].

As the list of identified zoonotic sources has expanded, so have the possible modes of transmission. Consuming raw or uncooked meats has been linked to cases of human HEV in multiple countries [4, 10, 21, 35]. Occupations that require frequent contact with livestock are known to increase the likelihood of HEV infection [17, 18, 36, 37]. Gardeners who work with, or live near, these animals may be spreading HEV through irrigation runoffs, or transferring the virus directly from animal feces to garden products. Therefore, even the process of gardening (planting, weeding, and preparing soil) may be a cause of HEV exposure.

Recent North American and European studies have demonstrated that HEV can be found on agricultural products such as raspberries, strawberries, lettuce, and other vegetables at the primary production level and point of sale [19, 20, 31]. Teshale and Hu reported an increased HEV prevalence in Americans who consumed more green leafy vegetables or lettuce salad [3]. In our study, fruits and vegetables comprised two-thirds of all reported self-grown foods, with tomatoes, cucumbers, and apples representing the most commonly reported self-grown food items among seropositive participants. Still, it is important to bear in mind that the NHANES nutritional survey is a brief snapshot of participant-reported foods ingested by individuals. The behavior of gardening, farming, and ingesting self-grown foods is likely a pattern that persists across all seasons and types of produce.

In our univariate analysis, consuming self-grown food was found to be significantly associated with HEV seropositivity in all age ranges. The multivariable logistic model, however, found ingesting self-grown food to be significantly associated with positive HEV serologies only for participants

Table 2: Adjusted odds ratios with 95 percent confidence intervals (CI) for HEV seropositivity using age-stratified multivariable logistic regression, NHANES 2009–2012.

	Age 6–39 years	Age 40–59 years	Age ≥ 60 years
Self-grown food	1.43 (0.50–4.10)	1.70 (1.06–2.74)	1.15 (0.79–1.67)
Foreign born	4.46 (3.09–6.44)	1.14 (0.62–2.08)	1.49 (0.96–2.33)
Female versus male	1.44 (1.03–2.02)	0.94 (0.65–1.36)	1.07 (0.82–1.41)
Race/ethnicity			
Non-Hispanic Black versus White	0.49 (0.28–0.83)	0.83 (0.54–1.28)	0.50 (0.33–0.76)
Hispanic versus White	0.74 (0.44–1.23)	1.35 (0.84–2.17)	0.67 (0.43–1.04)
Other versus White	1.23 (0.69–2.17)	1.74 (0.92–3.31)	0.80 (0.43–1.47)

aged 40–59 years (not participants < 40 years or ≥60 years). This finding is consistent with the force of infection, which peaks within the same age range. These results suggest that people aged 40–59 years may be at increased risk for acquiring HEV infection, although the reason for this remains unclear.

This study identified other factors associated with HEV seropositivity. As expected, increasing age corresponded with increased HEV seroprevalence. Gender played a role in HEV infection in the younger population (6–39 years), as females were found to have higher HEV seroprevalence than males. Among all races/ethnic groups, our results, in concordance with other reports [12, 29], found the highest rates of HEV seroprevalence in the non-Hispanic White population. Finally, foreign birth was significantly associated with positive HEV serologies only for participants in the youngest age category (6–39 years). This finding is consistent with the epidemiology of HEV infection in developing nations, where young adults have the highest rates of HEV detection and disease [38–40]. Unfortunately, travel history was not included in the NHANES survey and we are therefore unable to determine whether patients have travelled outside of the United States to endemic regions.

This study is one of few nationally representative studies looking at HEV transmission in the United States. Furthermore, NHANES' standardized sampling methods, questionnaires, and protocols make it a reliable and powerful source for national epidemiological studies. It is important, however, to interpret our findings in the context of their limitations. First, this is a cross-sectional study and therefore cannot demonstrate self-grown food consumption as a cause of HEV infection. Second, the data may be subject to recall bias, as participants were asked to remember foods eaten during two 24-hour periods. Third, past studies have detected HEV-specific IgG in the blood up to 14 years after infection [5, 41], which helps explain why HEV seroprevalence rises throughout life, but may also mask associations, as there could be a lag between exposure to HEV and detection of HEV-specific antibodies. Finally, it is possible that there are other confounding factors that should be considered, such as geography (i.e., urban versus rural region), occupation, and genotype data that are not reported by NHANES. These confounding variables could be useful in describing HEV epidemiology and associated factors. Documenting the distribution of HEV genotypes could be particularly helpful in clarifying the proportions of travel-related and autochthonous HEV infections in the United States.

In conclusion, hepatitis E virus is prevalent in the United States, with an estimated national seroprevalence of 6.6%. Middle-aged participants (40–59 years) in the 2009–2012 NHANES dietary survey who reported consuming self-grown foods, such as vegetables from a home garden, were more likely to be seropositive for HEV. Self-grown foods exposed to HEV-contaminated animal feces may be a source of zoonotic transmission to humans in industrialized countries. In addition, the process of growing produce and working in HEV-contaminated soil may be a mode of zoonotic HEV transmission to humans. As with all foods, self-grown foods should be carefully cleaned before consumption, especially for people at high risk for HEV-related complications, such as pregnant women and immunosuppressed patients. Further investigation concerning HEV transmission is an essential step toward developing effective preventive measures against hepatitis E infection.

Disclosure

The views expressed in this article are those of the author(s) and do not necessarily reflect the official policy or position of the Department of the Navy, Department of the Air Force, Department of Defense, or the United States Government. An abstract with preliminary research was presented in poster form at the Digestive Disease Week in Chicago, Illinois, in May 2014.

Acknowledgments

The authors would like to thank Ms. Apryl Susi for providing biomedical statistical review of this manuscript prior to publication.

References

[1] H. R. Dalton, S. D. Pas, R. G. Madden, and A. A. van der Eijk, "Hepatitis e virus: current concepts and future perspectives," *Current Infectious Disease Reports*, vol. 16, no. 4, p. 399, 2014.

[2] N. Kamar, R. Bendall, F. Legrand-Abravanel et al., "Hepatitis E," *The Lancet*, vol. 379, no. 9835, pp. 2477–2488, 2012.

[3] E. H. Teshale and D. J. Hu, "Hepatitis E: epidemiology and prevention," *World Journal of Hepatology*, vol. 3, no. 12, pp. 285–291, 2011.

[4] H. R. Dalton, R. Bendall, S. Ijaz, and M. Banks, "Hepatitis E: an emerging infection in developed countries," *The Lancet Infectious Diseases*, vol. 8, no. 11, pp. 698–709, 2008.

[5] M. T. Perez-Gracia, B. Suay, and M. L. Mateos-Lindemann, "Hepatitis E: an emerging disease," *Infection, Genetics and Evolution*, vol. 22, pp. 40–59, 2014.

[6] N. Kamar, C. Garrouste, E. B. Haagsma et al., "Factors associated with chronic hepatitis in patients with hepatitis E virus infection who have received solid organ transplants," *Gastroenterology*, vol. 140, no. 5, pp. 1481–1489, 2011.

[7] U. Navaneethan, M. Al Mohajer, and M. T. Shata, "Hepatitis E and pregnancy: understanding the pathogenesis," *Liver International*, vol. 28, no. 9, pp. 1190–9, 2008.

[8] R. H. Purcell and S. U. Emerson, "Hepatitis E: an emerging awareness of an old disease," *Journal of Hepatology*, vol. 48, no. 3, pp. 494–503, 2008.

[9] R. Aggarwal and S. Naik, "Epidemiology of hepatitis E: current status," *Journal of Gastroenterology and Hepatology*, vol. 24, no. 9, pp. 1484–1493, 2009.

[10] D. M. Yugo and X. J. Meng, "Hepatitis E virus: foodborne, waterborne and zoonotic transmission," *International Journal of Environmental Research and Public Health*, vol. 10, no. 10, pp. 4507–4533, 2013.

[11] H. Zhuang, X. Y. Cao, C. B. Liu, and G. M. Wang, "Epidemiology of hepatitis E in China," *Gastroenterologia Japonica*, vol. 26, Supplement 3, pp. 135–138, 1991.

[12] J. Drobeniuc, T. Greene-Montfort, N. T. le et al., "Laboratory-based surveillance for hepatitis E virus infection, United States, 2005–2012," *Emerging Infectious Diseases*, vol. 19, no. 2, pp. 218–222, 2013.

[13] J. Drobeniuc, J. Meng, G. Reuter et al., "Serologic assays specific to immunoglobulin M antibodies against hepatitis E virus: pangenotypic evaluation of performances," *Clinical Infectious Diseases*, vol. 51, no. 3, pp. e24–e27, 2010.

[14] M. F. Faramawi, E. Johnson, S. Chen, and P. R. Pannala, "The incidence of hepatitis E virus infection in the general population of the USA," *Epidemiology & Infection*, vol. 139, no. 8, pp. 1145–1150, 2011.

[15] R. H. Purcell, "Hepatitis viruses: changing patterns of human disease," *Proceedings of the National Academy of Sciences of the United States of America*, vol. 91, no. 7, pp. 2401–2406, 1994.

[16] C. Spahr, T. Knauf-Witzens, T. Vahlenkamp, R. G. Ulrich, and R. Johne, "Hepatitis E virus and related viruses in wild, domestic and zoo animals: a review," *Zoonoses and Public Health*, vol. 65, no. 1, pp. 11 29, 2018.

[17] X. J. Meng, B. Wiseman, F. Elvinger et al., "Prevalence of antibodies to hepatitis E virus in veterinarians working with swine and in normal blood donors in the United States and other countries," *Journal of Clinical Microbiology*, vol. 40, no. 1, pp. 117–122, 2002.

[18] B. J. Wilhelm, A. Rajić, J. Greig et al., "A systematic review/meta-analysis of primary research investigating swine, pork or pork products as a source of zoonotic hepatitis E virus," *Epidemiology & Infection*, vol. 139, no. 8, pp. 1127–1144, 2011.

[19] J. Brassard, M. J. Gagné, M. Généreux, and C. Côté, "Detection of human food-borne and zoonotic viruses on irrigated, field-grown strawberries," *Applied and Environmental Microbiology*, vol. 78, no. 10, pp. 3763–3766, 2012.

[20] P. Kokkinos, I. Kozyra, S. Lazic et al., "Harmonised investigation of the occurrence of human enteric viruses in the leafy green vegetable supply chain in three European countries," *Food and Environmental Virology*, vol. 4, no. 4, pp. 179–191, 2012.

[21] C. G. Teo, "Much meat, much malady: changing perceptions of the epidemiology of hepatitis E," *Clinical Microbiology and Infection*, vol. 16, no. 1, pp. 24–32, 2010.

[22] Centers for Disease Control and Prevention, "National Health and Nutrition Examination Survey," November 2016, http://www.cdc.gov/nchs/nhanes/index.htm.

[23] NHANES, "Laboratory Procedures Manual," July 2009, http://www.cdc.gov/nchs/data/nhanes/nhanes_09_10/lab.pdf.

[24] Centers for Disease Control and Prevention, "It is the detailed lab procedure for the anti-HEV EIA kits used in NHANES 2009-2012," January 2012, http://www.cdc.gov/nchs/data/nhanes/nhanes_09_10/HEPE_F_met_IgG_antibody.pdf.

[25] NHANES, "Demographics information," 2012, https://wwwn.cdc.gov/nchs/data/nhanes/2011-2012/questionnaires/dmq.pdf.

[26] National Health and Nutrition Examination Survey, "2011–2012 data documentation, codebook, and frequencies, dietary interview - total nutrient intakes, first day(DR1TOT_G)," September 2014, https://wwwn.cdc.gov/Nchs/Nhanes/2011-2012/DR1TOT_G.htm.

[27] US Department of Agriculture, Agricultural Research Service, "The USDA food and nutrient database for dietary studies 2011-2012: documentation and user guide," September 2014, https://www.ars.usda.gov/ARSUserFiles/80400530/pdf/fndds/fndds_2011_2012_doc.pdf.

[28] Z. Shkedy, M. Aerts, G. Molenberghs, P. Beutels, and P. van Damme, "Modelling age-dependent force of infection from prevalence data using fractional polynomials," *Statistics in Medicine*, vol. 25, no. 9, pp. 1577–1591, 2006.

[29] I. Ditah, F. Ditah, P. Devaki, C. Ditah, P. S. Kamath, and M. Charlton, "Current epidemiology of hepatitis E virus infection in the United States: low seroprevalence in the National Health and Nutrition Evaluation Survey," *Hepatology*, vol. 60, no. 3, pp. 815–822, 2014.

[30] E. H. Teshale, M. M. Denniston, J. Drobeniuc, S. Kamili, C. G. Teo, and S. D. Holmberg, "Decline in hepatitis E virus antibody prevalence in the United States from 1988-1994 to 2009-2010," *The Journal of Infectious Diseases*, vol. 211, no. 3, pp. 366–373, 2015.

[31] P. Ward, P. Müller, A. Letellier et al., "Molecular characterization of *hepatitis E* virus detected in swine farms in the province

of Quebec," *Canadian Journal of Veterinary Research*, vol. 72, no. 1, pp. 27–31, 2008.

[32] X. J. Meng, "Zoonotic and foodborne transmission of hepatitis E virus," *Seminars in Liver Disease*, vol. 33, no. 1, pp. 41–49, 2013.

[33] X. J. Meng, "Expanding host range and cross-species infection of hepatitis E virus," *PLoS Pathogens*, vol. 12, no. 8, article e1005695, 2016.

[34] Y. Sato, H. Sato, K. Naka et al., "A nationwide survey of hepatitis E virus (HEV) infection in wild boars in Japan: identification of boar HEV strains of genotypes 3 and 4 and unrecognized genotypes," *Archives of Virology*, vol. 156, no. 8, pp. 1345–1358, 2011.

[35] P. Colson, P. Borentain, B. Queyriaux et al., "Pig liver sausage as a source of hepatitis E virus transmission to humans," *The Journal of Infectious Diseases*, vol. 202, no. 6, pp. 825–834, 2010.

[36] J. Hartl, B. Otto, R. Madden et al., "Hepatitis E seroprevalence in Europe: a meta-analysis," *Viruses*, vol. 8, no. 8, 2016.

[37] Y. V. Karetnyi, M. J. Gilchrist, and S. J. Naides, "Hepatitis E virus infection prevalence among selected populations in Iowa," *Journal of Clinical Virology*, vol. 14, no. 1, pp. 51–55, 1999.

[38] R. Aggarwal, "Hepatitis E: clinical presentation in disease-endemic areas and diagnosis," *Seminars in Liver Disease*, vol. 33, no. 1, pp. 30–40, 2013.

[39] V. A. Arankalle, S. A. Tsarev, M. S. Chadha et al., "Age-specific prevalence of antibodies to hepatitis A and E viruses in Pune, India, 1982 and 1992," *The Journal of Infectious Diseases*, vol. 171, no. 2, pp. 447–450, 1995.

[40] A. S. F. Lok, R. T. Chan, C.-L. Lai et al., "Seroepidemiological survey of hepatitis E in Hong Kong by recombinant-based enzyme immunoassays," *The Lancet*, vol. 340, no. 8829, pp. 1205–1208, 1992.

[41] M. S. Khuroo and M. S. Khuroo, "Seroepidemiology of a second epidemic of hepatitis E in a population that had recorded first epidemic 30 years before and has been under surveillance since then," *Hepatology International*, vol. 4, no. 2, pp. 494–499, 2010.

Risk Factors for Acute Hemorrhagic Rectal Ulcer Syndrome and Its Prognosis: A Density Case-Control Study

Toshihiko Komai,[1,2] Fumio Omata,[1] Yasutoshi Shiratori,[1] Daiki Kobayashi,[1] and Hiroko Arioka[1]

[1]*Department of Internal Medicine, St. Luke's International University, 9-1 Akashi-cho, Chuo-ku, Tokyo 104-8560, Japan*
[2]*Department of Allergy and Rheumatology, Graduate School of Medicine, The University of Tokyo, 7-3-1 Hongo, Bunkyo-ku, Tokyo 113-8655, Japan*

Correspondence should be addressed to Fumio Omata; omataf@icloud.com

Academic Editor: Paul Enck

Acute hemorrhagic rectal ulcer syndrome (AHRUS) can cause fatal gastrointestinal bleeding. However, there have been few epidemiological studies investigating risk factors of AHRUS. To determine the risk factors and predict one-year survival after onset of AHRUS, we conducted a retrospective density case-control study in a tertiary referral hospital. Patients with hematochezia, bloody stool, and rectal ulcer confirmed by colonoscopy between 2003 and 2011 were diagnosed as AHRUS ($n = 38$). Patients with malignancies, infectious colitis, ulcerative colitis, or solitary rectal ulcer syndrome were excluded. Control subjects ($n = 123$) without rectal ulcer were selected by risk set sampling for each AHRUS. Multivariate logistic regression analyses revealed that the significant adjusted odds ratio (95% confidence interval) of hospitalization, antithrombotic drug use, and one gram increase of serum albumin was 15.7 (2.25–108.9), 12.1 (1.53–94.4), and 0.11 (0.02–0.52), respectively. Endoscopic hemostasis for rectal bleeding was performed in 8 cases (21%). Seventeen percent of patients died within one year after the episode of AHRUS from non-AHRUS causes. This study revealed that hospitalization, antithrombotic drug use, and lower serum albumin value were significant risk factors for AHRUS, and that AHRUS was an unfavorable prognostic condition. This information could be helpful in recognizing high-risk patients of rectal bleeding and applying preventive measures.

1. Introduction

Rectal ulcer, unrelated to malignancy, inflammatory bowel diseases (IBD), or infectious colitis includes two distinct disease entities: solitary rectal ulcer syndrome (SRUS) [1, 2] and acute hemorrhagic rectal ulcer syndrome (AHRUS) [3]. SRUS is a chronic benign disorder, most common in young adults, often associated with bowel disturbances, abnormal defecation, and mucosal prolapse [4, 5]. AHRUS is characterized by sudden massive rectal bleeding, most often in elderly patients with underlying comorbidities [6, 7]. AHRUS has been reported to be the most common cause of acute lower gastrointestinal bleeding in hospitalized patients with comorbidities [3, 6, 7].

Fecal evacuation disorder was reported to be a potential risk factor for SRUS [8–10], and gut-directed biofeedback therapy is an effective behavioral intervention [8, 9]. However, there have been few studies investigating risk factors and prophylactic interventions of life-threatening AHRUS. This lack of information may contribute to delay in making the diagnosis and in instituting preventive measures. In addition, there has been no report of survival analysis of the patients suffering from AHRUS. The aims of our study were to determine risk factors of AHRUS and to predict its one-year survival.

2. Materials and Methods

2.1. Study Population. A total of 23,988 colonoscopies were performed in a tertiary referral hospital in Tokyo, Japan, from 2003 to 2011. Thirty-eight cases with the diagnosis of AHRUS [3, 6] were identified after excluding associated

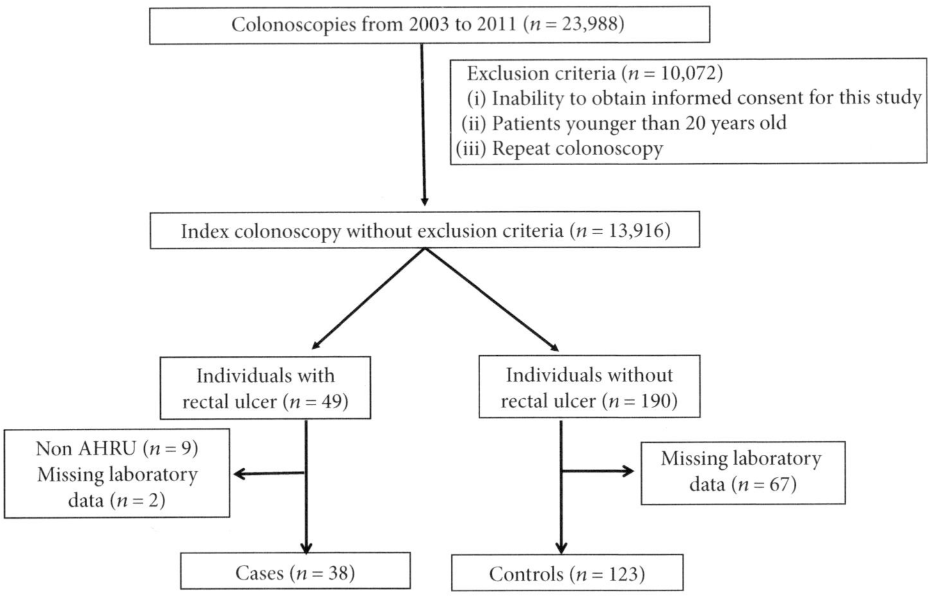

Figure 1: Study flow diagram depicting selection of cases and controls. 13,916 index colonoscopies out of 23,988 were performed in the patients older than 20 years of age in a tertiary medical center in Tokyo, Japan. Thirty-eight acute hemorrhagic rectal ulcer syndrome patients were diagnosed. From the same database of index colonoscopies, 123 patients without rectal ulcer were selected as a control group by risk set sampling.

ulcerative colitis ($n = 3$), infectious colitis ($n = 1$), rectal ulcer with no gastrointestinal bleeding ($n = 4$), SRUS ($n = 1$), and lack of laboratory data ($n = 2$). Subjects who had not given informed consent for use of their electronic records and subjects under 20 years of age were also excluded. We waived informed consent from patients who were included in our study.

One hundred twenty-three subjects without rectal ulcer and with adequate laboratory values were selected as controls by risk set sampling [11, 12] (Figure 1). When the laboratory values of controls were missing on the same day of colonoscopy, their laboratory values within 6 months after colonoscopy were imputed. This study was approved by St. Luke's International University Research Ethics Committee (authorization number: 11-R162).

2.2. Data Availability. The data of this study were handled with all of the authors under strict control, and availability was restricted for ethical reasons. However, anonymized data could be available for other researchers upon request with the permission of our ethical committee.

2.3. Diagnosis of Rectal Ulcer. The diagnosis of rectal ulcer in cases and confirmation of no rectal ulcer in controls were established with colonoscopy. AHRUS was defined as ulcer associated with hematochezia or bloody stool, whereas rectal ulcer was present at colonoscopy after excluding other diseases which might cause rectal ulcer [3, 6]. The location of ulcers in the rectum was classified like that used for colorectal cancer: rectosigmoid (Rs), rectum above the peritoneal reflection (Ra), or rectum below the peritoneal reflection (Rb).

2.4. Candidate Risk Factors for AHRUS. We investigated whether age, gender, comorbidities, laboratory values, hospitalization, and antithrombotic use were associated with AHRUS.

2.5. Statistical Analyses. Fisher's exact test was applied for proportion. Student's t-test or Wilcoxon rank sum test was used for continuous variables. Bivariate and multivariate logistic regressions were used to calculate odds ratio (OR). Variables with P value less than 0.2 in bivariate logistic regression were used in multivariate analyses. P value less than 0.05 was considered statistically significant. Kaplan-Meier estimates were used for survival analysis. All 95% confidence intervals were two-sided. All analyses were conducted with JMP® version 13 statistical software (SAS Institute, Cary, NC). In conducting this study, we followed the checklist of items for case-control study described in strengthening the reporting of observational studies in epidemiology (STROBE) statement [13].

3. Results

3.1. Characteristics of Patients with AHRUS. Table 1 presents patients' characteristics, candidate risk factors for AHRUS, laboratory data, and the results of bivariate analyses. Age, hospitalization, antithrombotic drug use, comorbidities (hypertension, ischemic heart disease, and cerebrovascular disease), and laboratory findings (serum albumin, serum creatinine, white blood cell count, and hemoglobin levels) were significantly different between cases and controls. Enemas were not used in the enrolled participants.

More than half of the rectal ulcer was located in Rb (Figure 2). We performed biopsy in eleven patients. The histological findings of all these patients were nonspecific and did not show any finding suggesting SRUS or IBD.

TABLE 1: Patients' characteristics and bivariate analyses.

Variable	Cases	Controls	P value
Age (years), mean (SD)	76 (12)	60 (15)	<0.0001
Sex, male, n (%)	18 (47.4)	62 (50.4)	0.85
Hospitalization, n (%)	32 (84.2)	14 (11.4)	<0.0001
Hospitalization period (day), mean (SD)	19.0 (24.4)	1.0 (4.9)	<0.0001
Usage of antithrombotic drugs, n (%)	25 (65.8)	16 (13.0)	<0.0001
Comorbidity			
Hypertension, n (%)	23 (60.5)	45 (36.6)	0.014
Diabetes mellitus, n (%)	10 (26.3)	19 (15.5)	0.15
Ischemic heart disease, n (%)	13 (34.2)	5 (4.1)	<0.0001
Cerebral vascular disease, n (%)	17 (44.7)	8 (6.5)	<0.0001
Under hemodialysis, n (%)	4 (10.5)	3 (2.44)	0.054
Malignancies, n (%)	6 (15.8)	30 (24.4)	0.37
Laboratory findings			
Serum albumin (mg/dl), mean (SD)	2.67 (0.60)	4.09 (0.52)	<0.0001
Serum Cr (mg/dl), mean (SD)	1.35 (1.50)	1.16 (2.21)	0.63
Serum AST (U/l), mean (SD)	26.0 (14.6)	22.8 (9.9)	0.13
Serum ALT (U/l), mean (SD)	25.3 (19.9)	23.3 (21.8)	0.62
White blood cell count (cells/μl), mean (SD)	8013 (4757)	5959 (2047)	0.0002
Hemoglobin (g/dl), mean (SD)	9.51 (2.09)	12.7 (2.06)	<0.0001
Platelet count (thousand cells/μl), mean (SD)	247.3 (132.4)	236.7 (90.8)	0.58

SD: standard deviation; AST: aspartate aminotransferase; ALT: alanine aminotransferase.

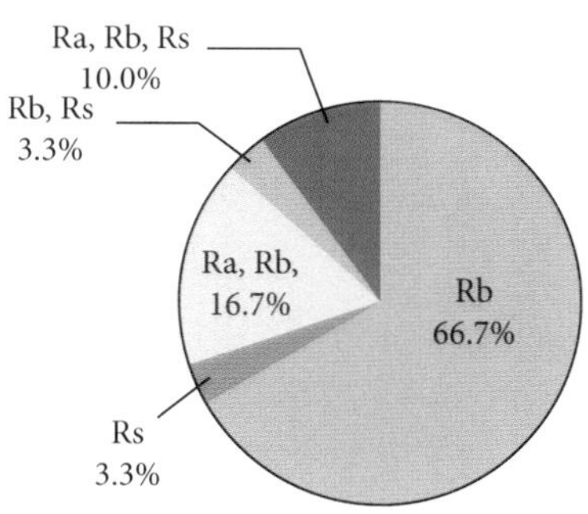

FIGURE 2: Pie chart depicting the location of rectal ulcer in 30 of 38 patients with acute hemorrhagic rectal ulcer syndrome (in 8 cases, rectal ulcer location was not described in endoscopy report). Rs: rectosigmoid; Ra: rectum above the peritoneal reflection; Rb: rectum below the peritoneal reflection.

3.2. Density Case-Control Analysis for the Identification of Risk Factors for AHRUS. In bivariate logistic regression analyses, age, hospitalization, antithrombotic drug use; the comorbidities of ischemic heart disease, cerebrovascular disease, and chronic kidney disease under hemodialysis; and the laboratory findings of white blood cell count, hemoglobin, and serum albumin values were significantly associated with AHRUS.

In multivariate logistic regression analyses, hospitalization (adjusted OR 15.65, 95% CI 2.25–108.9), antithrombotic drug use (adjusted OR 12.05, 95% CI 1.53–94.4), and one gram decrease of serum albumin (adjusted OR 0.11, 95% CI 0.02–0.52) were significantly associated with AHRUS. On the other hand, neither of age, the indicated comorbidities were not significant risk factors (Table 2).

3.3. Outcome and Long-Term Survival of Rectal Bleeding. Endoscopic treatment for attempted control of bleeding (clipping or band ligation) was performed in 8 of the 38 patients (21%), as listed in Table 3. Rebleeding occurred in two patients and was treated successfully with reclipping. Sixteen of the 38 patients (42%; 95% CI 28–58%) needed blood transfusion. All patients received hydration and restriction of oral intake. We did not use sucralfate enema in any patient.

Survival analysis showed that 17% of patients died within one year after their rectal bleeding episode from causes not related to their AHRUS (Figure 3). These results collectively indicated that AHRUS could be an unfavorable prognostic condition, and the preventive intervention based on the risk factors would be necessary.

Among 33 survivors at one year, follow-up colonoscopy at least 30 days after rectal bleeding was performed in four patients; complete rectal ulcer healing was confirmed in all these patients.

4. Discussion

This study is the first case-control study that we are aware of about risk factors for AHRUS. We found that hospitalization, antithrombotic drug use, and hypoalbuminemia were significant risk factors for developing AHRUS. Seventeen percent of AHRUS patients died within one year of causes not related to the AHRUS.

Table 2: Bivariate and multivariate logistic regression analyses.

Variable	Crude OR	95% CI	*P* value	Adjusted OR	95% CI	*P* value
Age	1.10	1.06–1.14	<0.0001	1.03	0.96–1.11	0.36
Hospitalization	41.52	14.8–116.8	<0.0001	15.65	2.25–108.9	0.006
Antithrombotic drug use	12.86	5.49–30.13	<0.0001	12.05	1.53–94.4	0.018
Comorbidity						
Hypertension	2.66	1.26–5.61	0.0093	0.51	0.08–3.18	0.47
Diabetes mellitus	0.13	0.82–4.68	0.141	1.33	0.12–14.8	0.82
Ischemic heart disease	12.27	4.01–37.53	<0.0001	8.44	0.89–80.3	0.063
Cerebral vascular disease	11.64	4.45–30.40	<0.0001	2.41	0.42–13.7	0.32
On hemodialysis	4.71	1.00–22.05	0.049	0.66	0.01–33.5	0.84
Laboratory findings						
White blood cell count	1.26	1.09–1.46	0.0004	1.24	0.94–1.63	0.11
Hemoglobin	0.53	0.43–0.66	<0.0001	0.97	0.59–1.60	0.9
Serum AST	1.02	0.99–1.05	0.145	0.98	0.92–1.05	0.64
Serum albumin	0.036	0.01–0.10	<0.0001	0.11	0.02–0.52	0.006

OR: odds ratio; AST: aspartate aminotransferase.

Table 3: Endoscopic hemostatic procedure.

Procedures and rebleeding rate	Cases
Hemostatic procedure, *n* (%)	8 (21)
Band ligation, *n*	2
Clipping, *n*	6
Rebleeding after hemostatic procedure, *n* (%)	2 (25)

Rectal ulcers with massive hemorrhage in critically ill patients have long been recognized [6, 14, 15], but the infrequency and fatal clinical course has precluded clinical studies about its risk factors and establishing this condition as an independent clinical disease. Recently, however, rectal ulcers with massive hemorrhage have been recognized as an emerging clinical entity, AHRUS [3, 6, 7, 16].

Previous observational studies have reported the characteristics of AHRUS patients, such as older age, immobility, antithrombotic drug use, and comorbidities such as diabetes mellitus, coronary artery diseases, cerebrovascular attacks, sepsis, liver failure [3], hypoalbuminemia [17–19], and chronic renal failure with hemodialysis [15]. The characteristics of cases in our research were compatible with those in observational studies and supported etiological assumptions except for older age [17–20]. Like others [6, 7], we found that AHRUS patients often require hemostatic procedures and blood transfusion. We did not use sucralfate enemas in our patients, although a case series [21] reported it effective.

Several studies have shown that serum hypoalbuminemia can be an independent risk factor for decreased microperfusion and pressure ulcers because albumin helps maintain oncotic pressure and vascular refilling [22–24]. Our results were compatible with the results of the previous observational study, which suggested that hypoalbuminemia and high blood urea nitrogen levels were risk factors for lower gastrointestinal bleeding, mainly due to ischemic colitis and rectal ulcer in critically ill patients [19].

It seems reasonable that immobility during hospitalization, hypoperfusion of local rectal blood flow in the elderly, and hypoalbuminemia could lead to the formation of rectal ulcer; previous epidemiological studies suggested that these could be risk factors of SRUS or stercoral ulcer [2, 9, 10]. Our endoscopic findings indicated that more than 90% of rectal ulcers were located in Rb, which implied specific local vascular flow disturbance.

Baseline blood flow in the rectal mucosa, measured by laser Doppler flowmetry, has been found significantly below normal in patients with SRUS [9] or AHRUS [25], and the blood flow is significantly reduced in the horizontal supine position at bed rest. Baroreceptor-mediated vasoconstriction in hypovolemic conditions [26] or in bedridden, elderly, or hospitalized patients has been reported to cause ischemic proctitis [27].

Although ischemia might be involved in both SRUS and AHRUS, the pathogenesis of the two clinical entities seems different. Comparing with patients with SRUS associated with fecal evacuation disorders [10], the higher prevalence of AHRUS among immobilized older patients with cardiovascular risks [6, 7] suggests that nutrient blood flow is disturbed in AHRUS, rather than there is local or direct pressure in the rectum as in SRUS.

Our study has limitations and strengths. First, we did not assess the possible role of constipation or overactivity of the anal sphincter in causing rectal ulceration or ischemia because of retrospective design. Second, there could be selection bias by excluding subjects with missing laboratory values; this bias might have an effect toward the null on the odds ratio of hospitalization for AHRS. Despite these factors, our study was valuable because this was the first density case-control study in Japan to explore the comprehensive risk factors for the occurrence of AHRUS and patients' survival after AHRUS.

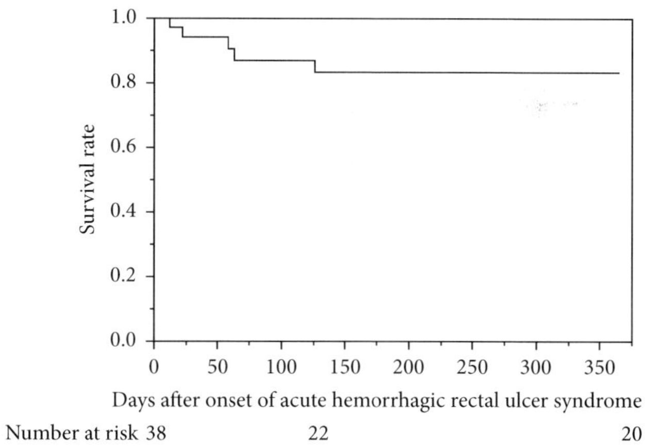

FIGURE 3: Kaplan-Meier estimates after onset of acute rectal hemorrhagic rectal ulcer. 17 percent of patients with acute hemorrhagic rectal ulcer syndrome (AHRUS) died of non-AHRUS problem in one year.

5. Conclusions

Hospitalization, antithrombotic drug use, and hypoalbuminemia were significant risk factors for AHRUS. Knowledge of these risk factors could make clinicians more alert to the possibility of AHRUS being the cause of lower gastrointestinal bleeding, to take measures to prevent it and to perform proctoscopy or colonoscopy promptly to diagnose it. Onset of AHRUS has an unfavorable prognosis.

Acknowledgments

The authors thank Professor Emeritus William R. Brown, University of Colorado School of Medicine, USA, for a critical review of the manuscript.

References

[1] N. R. Womack, N. S. Williams, J. H. Holmfield, and J. F. Morrison, "Pressure and prolapse-the cause of solitary rectal ulceration," *Gut*, vol. 28, no. 10, pp. 1228-1233, 1987.

[2] Q. C. Zhu, R. R. Shen, H. L. Qin, and Y. Wang, "Solitary rectal ulcer syndrome: clinical features, pathophysiology, diagnosis and treatment strategies," *World Journal of Gastroenterology*, vol. 20, no. 3, pp. 738–744, 2014.

[3] C. A. Tseng, L. T. Chen, K. B. Tsai et al., "Acute hemorrhagic rectal ulcer syndrome: a new clinical entity? Report of 19 cases and review of the literature," *Diseases of the Colon and Rectum*, vol. 47, no. 6, pp. 895–905, 2004.

[4] A. I. Sharara, C. Azar, S. S. Amr, M. Haddad, and M. A. Eloubeidi, "Solitary rectal ulcer syndrome: endoscopic spectrum and review of the literature," *Gastrointestinal Endoscopy*, vol. 62, no. 5, pp. 755–762, 2005.

[5] J. J. Tjandra, V. W. Fazio, J. M. Church, I. C. Lavery, J. R. Oakley, and J. W. Milsom, "Clinical conundrum of solitary rectal ulcer," *Diseases of the Colon and Rectum*, vol. 35, no. 3, pp. 227–234, 1992.

[6] C. K. Lin, C. C. Liang, H. T. Chang, F. M. Hung, and T. H. Lee, "Acute hemorrhagic rectal ulcer: an important cause of lower gastrointestinal bleeding in the critically ill patients," *Digestive Diseases and Sciences*, vol. 56, no. 12, pp. 3631–3637, 2011.

[7] K. Takeuchi, Y. Tsuzuki, T. Ando et al., "Clinical characteristics of acute hemorrhagic rectal ulcer," *Journal of Clinical Gastroenterology*, vol. 33, no. 3, pp. 226–228, 2001.

[8] S. S. C. Rao, R. Ozturk, S. De Ocampo, and M. Stessman, "Pathophysiology and role of biofeedback therapy in solitary rectal ulcer syndrome," *The American Journal of Gastroenterology*, vol. 101, no. 3, pp. 613–618, 2006.

[9] M. E. Jarrett, A. V. Emmanuel, C. J. Vaizey, and M. A. Kamm, "Behavioural therapy (biofeedback) for solitary rectal ulcer syndrome improves symptoms and mucosal blood flow," *Gut*, vol. 53, no. 3, pp. 368–370, 2004.

[10] A. Sharma, A. Misra, and U. C. Ghoshal, "Fecal evacuation disorder among patients with solitary rectal ulcer syndrome: a case-control study," *Journal of Neurogastroenterology and Motility*, vol. 20, no. 4, pp. 531–538, 2014.

[11] B. Langholz and L. Goldstein, "Risk set sampling in epidemiologic cohort studies," *Statistical Science*, vol. 11, no. 1, pp. 35–53, 1996.

[12] K. J. Rothman, *Epidemiology. An Introduction*, Boson: Oxford University Press, 2002.

[13] E. von Elm, D. G. Altman, M. Egger, S. J. Pocock, P. C. Gøtzsche, and J. P. Vandenbroucke, "The strengthening the reporting of observational studies in epidemiology (STROBE) statement: guidelines for reporting observational studies," *The Lancet*, vol. 370, no. 9596, pp. 1453–1457, 2007.

[14] M. Goldberg, G. C. Hoffman, and D. G. Wombolt, "Massive hemorrhage from rectal ulcers in chronic renal failure," *Annals of Internal Medicine*, vol. 100, no. 3, p. 397, 1984.

[15] F. Kanwal, G. Dulai, D. M. Jensen et al., "Major stigmata of recent hemorrhage on rectal ulcers in patients with severe hematochezia: endoscopic diagnosis, treatment, and outcomes," *Gastrointestinal Endoscopy*, vol. 57, no. 4, pp. 462–468, 2003.

[16] S. B. Almadani and M. Brown, "Acute hemorrhagic rectal ulcer syndrome (AHRUS): an under-recognized condition," *The American Journal of Gastroenterology*, vol. 108, p. S362, 2013.

[17] T. Hotta, K. Takifuji, S. Tonoda et al., "Risk factors and management for massive bleeding of an acute hemorrhagic rectal ulcer," *The American Surgeon*, vol. 75, no. 1, pp. 66–73, 2009.

[18] B. C. Kim, J. H. Cheon, T. I. Kim, and W. H. Kim, "Risk factors and the role of bedside colonoscopy for lower gastrointestinal hemorrhage in critically ill patients," *Hepato-Gastroenterology*, vol. 55, no. 88, pp. 2108–2111, 2008.

[19] J. H. Jung, J. W. Kim, H. W. Lee et al., "Acute hemorrhagic rectal ulcer syndrome: comparison with non-hemorrhagic rectal ulcer lower gastrointestinal bleeding," *Journal of Digestive Diseases*, vol. 18, no. 9, pp. 521–528, 2017.

[20] T. Oku, M. Maeda, H. Ihara et al., "Clinical and endoscopic features of acute hemorrhagic rectal ulcer," *Journal of Gastroenterology*, vol. 41, no. 10, pp. 962–970, 2006.

[21] S. A. Zargar, M. S. Khuroo, and R. Mahajan, "Sucralfate retention enemas in solitary rectal ulcer," *Diseases of the Colon and Rectum*, vol. 34, no. 6, pp. 455–457, 1991.

[22] S. Iizaka, H. Sanada, Y. Matsui et al., "Serum albumin level is a limited nutritional marker for predicting wound healing in patients with pressure ulcer: two multicenter prospective cohort studies," *Clinical Nutrition*, vol. 30, no. 6, pp. 738–745, 2011.

[23] E. Mistrík, S. Dusilová-Sulková, V. Bláha, and L. Sobotka, "Plasma albumin levels correlate with decreased microcirculation and the development of skin defects in hemodialyzed patients," *Nutrition*, vol. 26, no. 9, pp. 880–885, 2010.

[24] R. Serra, S. Caroleo, G. Buffone et al., "Low serum albumin level as an independent risk factor for the onset of pressure ulcers in intensive care unit patients," *International Wound Journal*, vol. 11, no. 5, pp. 550–553, 2014.

[25] S. Nakamura, K. Okawa, J. Hara et al., "Etiology of acute hemorrhagic rectal ulcer laser Doppler analysis of rectal mucosal blood flow in lateral and horizontal supine position at bed rest," *Gastroenterological Endoscopy*, vol. 38, pp. 1481–1487, 1996.

[26] A. Thorén, S. E. Ricksten, S. Lundin, B. Gazelius, and M. Elam, "Baroreceptor-mediated reduction of jejunal mucosal perfusion, evaluated with endoluminal laser Doppler flowmetry in conscious humans," *Journal of the Autonomic Nervous System*, vol. 68, no. 3, pp. 157–163, 1998.

[27] A. E. Bharucha, W. J. Tremaine, C. D. Johnson, and K. P. Batts, "Ischemic proctosigmoiditis," *The American Journal of Gastroenterology*, vol. 91, no. 11, pp. 2305–2309, 1996.

Adherence to CRC Screening and Surveillance Guidelines when Using Split-Dose Bowel Preparation

Stacy B. Menees,[1,2] H. Myra Kim,[2] Grace H. Elta,[1] Sheryl Korsnes,[1] and Philip Schoenfeld[3]

[1]*Division of Gastroenterology, University of Michigan Health System, Ann Arbor, MI, USA*
[2]*Division of Gastroenterology, Ann Arbor Veterans' Administration Health Care System, Ann Arbor, MI, USA*
[3]*John D. Dingell VA Medical Center, Detroit, MI, USA*

Correspondence should be addressed to Stacy B. Menees; sbartnik@med.umich.edu

Academic Editor: Leticia Moreira

Goal. To prospectively assess physician recommendations for repeat colonoscopy in an average-risk screening cohort. *Background.* Endoscopists' adherence to colorectal cancer screening and surveillance guidelines for repeat colonoscopy have not been well characterized. Furthermore, little is known about patient and colonoscopy factors that are associated with endoscopists' nonadherence to guideline recommendation. *Study.* This is a prospective cohort of average-risk patients undergoing colonoscopy for colorectal cancer screening between August 2011 and January 2013. The primary outcome was assessment of physician recommendations for repeat colonoscopy. *Results.* 462 participants were prospectively enrolled. 13.6% (62) had guideline-inconsistent recommendations. 89% of the guideline-inconsistent recommendations were for an earlier interval. Endoscopists' reports cited suboptimal bowel preparation as the most common reason for earlier repeat colonoscopy. On multivariable analysis, patient split-dose preparation noncompliance was significantly associated with guideline-inconsistent recommendation ($OR = 2.7$) even after adjusting for other patient or bowel preparation-related characteristics. Additionally, increased odds of guideline-inconsistent recommendation were associated with older age (>70 years old), higher BMI, having 3 or more polyps, having had at least two previous colonoscopies, suboptimal bowel preparation, and having taken at least 12 hours till clear bowel movement. *Conclusions.* Gastroenterologists are adherent to CRC screening and surveillance guidelines. Suboptimal bowel preparation is the most frequently cited factor in endoscopy reports leading to deviation from guidelines. Continued emphasis on optimization of bowel preparation, particularly patient compliance to split-dose regimen, is needed.

1. Introduction

Colonoscopy is an effective colorectal cancer (CRC) screening test, but it may be overused [1, 2]. This overuse is partly defined as recommending a repeat colonoscopy sooner than 10 years after a normal screening colonoscopy in an average-risk individual aged ≥50 or recommending repeat colonoscopy sooner than 5 years after finding 1-2 nonadvanced adenomas in an average-risk individual [3]. Minimizing overuse of colonoscopy for CRC screening and colon polyp surveillance is a worthy goal because it minimizes patients' exposure to the risks, inconvenience, and cost of colonoscopy. Also, the importance of making guideline-consistent recommendations will only increase. First, the 2015 multisociety position statement on quality indicators in colonoscopy [4] now recommends that guideline-consistent recommendations should be made in at least 90% of cases. Second, recommendation for timing of repeat colonoscopy in an average-risk patient after a normal CRC screening colonoscopy or after finding 1-2 nonadvanced adenomas is an approved quality indicator for the Physician Quality Reporting System (PQRS) instituted by the Centers for Medicare and Medicaid Services (CMS). Third, this quality indicator is also likely to be incorporated into a value-based index of colonoscopy quality by 2017, which will further impact reimbursement for colonoscopy by CMS.

Suboptimal bowel preparation is frequently associated with overuse [5, 6]. Our retrospective review of 1387 average-risk individuals aged ≥50 years with a normal screening colonoscopy found that 24% received recommendations for repeat colonoscopy that were inconsistent with guideline recommendations, and these guideline-inconsistent recommendations were always to have a repeat colonoscopy sooner than recommended by guidelines [5]. We also found that "fair" bowel preparation, as defined by the Aronchick scale, was highly associated with guideline-inconsistent recommendations compared to "excellent" bowel preparation of patients (OR = 18; 95% CI: 12–28). Specifically, only 15% of patients with "excellent" preps received guideline-inconsistent recommendations while 75% of patients with "fair" preps received this type of recommendation. These findings were supported by our second retrospective database study of over 16,000 patients which found that repeat colonoscopy within 5 years was recommended for 70% of average-risk patients with a normal screening colonoscopy and a "fair" prep [7]. This recommendation is understandable since our study also found an adenoma miss rate of 28% when these patients had repeat colonoscopy within 3 years.

Our previously reported data was performed in cohorts that used PM-only bowel preparation as opposed to split-dose bowel preparation, which is superior for bowel cleansing [8–13]. Institution of split-dose bowel preparation could minimize guideline-inconsistent recommendations for timing of repeat colonoscopy by increasing the frequency of optimal bowel cleansing. However, other factors associated with guideline-inconsistent recommendations should be identified in the split-dose bowel preparation era in order to facilitate quality improvement. Therefore, the aim of our study is to assess these issues in a prospective study. With this information, future research can assess interventions to minimize the frequency of guideline-inconsistent recommendations.

Table 1: Guideline recommendations (2006, 2008) utilized for follow-up colonoscopy intervals after screening colonoscopy in average-risk patient.

Colonoscopy finding	Follow-up interval (years)
No polyps	10
Any colonoscopy with poor/inadequate bowel prep	≤1
Small (<10 mm) hyperplastic polyps in rectum or sigmoid	10
1-2 small (<10 mm) tubular adenomas	5–10
3–10 tubular adenomas	3
>10 tubular adenomas	<3
One or more tubular adenomas ≥10 mm	3
One or villous adenomas	3
Adenoma with high-grade dysplasia	3
Poor/inadequate bowel preparation	≤1
Piecemeal resection of adenoma, if question of resection of completeness	≤1

2. Materials and Methods

2.1. Study Design. Eligible patients were average-risk 50–74-year-old individuals undergoing colonoscopy for CRC screening at an ambulatory endoscopy center or a hospital-based endoscopy unit. Exclusion criteria included patients unable to read, comprehend, or consent for their involvement in the study; patients undergoing colonoscopy for abdominal pain, hematochezia, change in bowel habits, or other gastrointestinal symptoms; and patients with a family history of CRC in first-degree relative or previous history of polyps or colon cancer.

Split-dose bowel preparation for all laxative regimens in all patients was instituted uniformly at the study sites in 2010 [14]. At our institution, the standard tool for assessing the quality of bowel preparation is the Aronchick scale (excellent, good, fair, and poor) [15]. For this prospective trial, endoscopists also graded bowel preparation with the Boston bowel preparation scale (BBPS), a valid and reliable instrument [16, 17]. BPPS score can range from 0–9. In BBPS, cleanliness of the right colon, transverse colon, and left colon is assessed separately on a 0–3 scale. BBPS scores were collected after washing and suctioning of residual stool per usual protocol. Colon preparation quality was considered adequate if BBPS was ≥6 [18]. All endoscopists were trained in the BBPS through a didactic session at a mandatory faculty meeting utilizing an instructional video [19]. Additionally, posters of the BBPS scale were posted in every endoscopy room. Endoscopy nurses and study personnel insured proper completion of the BPPS.

After obtaining informed consent from eligible patients before colonoscopy, the following data was collected: age, race/ethnicity, sex, body mass index (BMI), concurrent medical illnesses including presence/absence of diabetes, concurrent medication use including narcotics and tricyclic antidepressant (TCA) usage, marital status, education, employment, income, use of Medicaid insurance, type of bowel preparation agent used, time of colonoscopy, time of first bowel movement after starting bowel preparation, time to first clear bowel movement after starting the bowel preparation (options included: less than 4 hours, between 4–8 hrs, between 9–12 hrs, more than 12 hrs, and never had clear bowel movement), time that bowel preparation was started, and completed for split-dose bowel regimen. Split-dose bowel regimen compliance was assessed with the following survey question: "Please pick the sentence below that best describes how you took the liquid/pill laxative prep." The participants were given the following choices: (a) "I took all of the liquid/pill laxative prep yesterday"; (b) "I took some of the liquid/pill laxative prep yesterday and some of it today"; (c) "I took all of the liquid/pill laxative prep today"; or (d) "I never took my liquid/pill laxative prep." Participants who chose "I took some of the liquid/pill laxative prep yesterday and some of it today" were considered compliant with the split-dose bowel regimen.

Colonoscopy data about GI fellow participation, endoscopists' categorization of procedural difficulty, time of day when colonoscopy was performed, number of previous screening colonoscopies performed on the patient, location

TABLE 2: Study participant characteristics by whether physician recommendation was guideline compliant or not ($N = 456$).

Patient characteristic	Compliant ($n = 394$; 86%)	Noncompliant ($n = 62$; 14%)	Total ($N = 456$)	p value[a]
Demographic characteristics				
Age in years, mean (SD)	56.6 (6.6)	57.7 (8.2)	56.7 (6.8)	0.22
Male	196 (49.9)	33 (53.2)	229 (50.3)	0.62
White	340 (86.3)	54 (87.1)	394 (86.4)	0.86
Married	286 (72.6)	41 (66.1)	327 (71.7)	0.29
BMI[b], kg/m^2, mean (SD)	28.7 (5.7)	30.3 (6.0)	28.9 (5.7)	0.04
Full-time employment	232 (58.9)	31 (50.0)	263 (57.7)	0.19
On Medicaid or no insurance	16 (4.2)	3 (5.0)	19 (4.3)	0.76
≤75K annual income	153 (40.4)	29 (50.9)	182 (41.7)	0.13
Health-related measures				
Very good or excellent health	264 (67.9)	35 (56.5)	299 (66.3)	0.08
History of stroke	10 (2.6)	2 (3.2)	12 (2.7)	0.67
On prescription pain pills	23 (5.9)	7 (11.3)	30 (6.6)	0.16
On tricyclic antidepressant[c]	5 (1.3)	1 (1.6)	6 (1.3)	0.58
History of constipation	69 (17.8)	12 (19.4)	81 (18.0)	0.77

All values are N (% of split-dose compliant or % of split-dose noncompliant), unless otherwise specified. The total number of patients for each characteristic may not add to the total ($N = 462$) due to missing data. [a]From testing differences in the distribution of the patient characteristics between patient compliant versus noncompliant to split-dose guideline, based on t-test for continuous variables and chi-square test or Fisher's exact test for categorical variables. No adjustments for multiple testing were done as the tests were not meant to be inferential, but to identify variables that are potentially associated with guideline-compliant physician recommendation. [b]Body mass index [c]on any of Tofranil, Elavil, Norpramin, Sinequan, and Pamelor.

of procedure (ambulatory endoscopy center versus academic hospital endoscopy unit), number/location/size of polyps, and pathology reports was also collected.

This prospective study was approved by the Institutional Review Board of the University of Michigan.

2.2. Endoscopists' Recommendation Intervals. Endoscopists' recommendation for follow-up screening colonoscopy was abstracted from patient colonoscopy reports and follow-up pathology letters. The IRB did not permit the collection of data about specific endoscopists' characteristics so endoscopists could not be singled out, such as by sex or endoscopy site. Follow-up recommendations were labeled as either consistent or inconsistent with guidelines (Table 1). At our institution, if a patient had poor bowel preparation by the Aronchick scale, then the standard recommendation is to repeat colonoscopy within 12 months. This is consistent with the 2012 multisociety guidelines [3]. Failure to provide a recommendation for repeat screening colonoscopy was also considered inconsistent with guideline recommendations.

2.3. Statistical Analysis. Recommended follow-up interval colonoscopy was recorded as a dichotomous variable defined as consistent with versus inconsistent with guideline recommendations. Chi-square tests and student t-tests were used to assess study population differences in sociodemographic characteristics, bowel preparation quality-related variables, and whether the recommendation was consistent with guidelines. Logistic regression modeling was used to determine independent predictors of follow-up recommendations inconsistent with guidelines. The models were adjusted for bowel preparation type, number of polyps, compliance with split-dose bowel preparation, endoscopy site, sex, race, and concurrent medical illnesses and medications. All models were adjusted for sex and race regardless of statistical significance. Adjusted odds ratios and 95% confidence limits were derived from the final model estimates.

In order to assess for an association between inadequate/poor bowel preparation versus suboptimal bowel preparation versus optimal bowel preparation, the BBPS score was categorized into BBPS 0–4, BBPS = 5, and BBPS = 6–9. Similar analyses were performed for inadequate bowel preparation for a single segment of colon (BBPS = 0-1) or adequate (BBPS 2-3). Also, the Aronchick scale was used to compare poor bowel preparation versus fair bowel preparation versus good/excellent bowel preparation. Database management and statistical analyses were performed using Stata 12.0 (StataCorp LP, College Station, TX).

3. Results

Four hundred and sixty-two individuals meeting eligibility were prospectively enrolled. Complete data about bowel preparation quality based on BBPS was missing in six subjects, leaving 456 individuals for inclusion. Mean age of participants was 56.8 years (SD = 6.9), and 50% was male (Table 2). Based on the Aronchick scale, 79% (362/456) had good/excellent bowel cleansing, 14% (63/456) had fair bowel cleansing, 5% (21/456) had poor bowel cleansing, and 2% (10/456) had missing data (Table 3). Based on the BBPS scale, 93.4% (426/526) had an adequate bowel preparation with BBPS ≥ 6 with 2.1% (10/456) having BBPS = 5 and 4.3% (20/456) having BBPS < 5.

Among the 456 eligible patients, 13.6% (62/456) had guideline-inconsistent recommendations. The majority (89%, $N = 55/62$) instructed the patient to get repeat

Table 3: Distribution of bowel preparation-related variables by whether physician recommendation was guideline compliant or not ($N = 456$).

Bowel preparation characteristics	Compliant ($n = 394$)	Noncompliant ($n = 62$)	Total ($N = 456$)	p value[a]
BBPS total score				
BBPS ≥ 6	374 (94.9)	52 (83.9)	426 (93.4)	
BBPS = 5	3 (0.76)	7 (11.3)	10 (2.1)	
BBPS < 5	17 (4.3)	3 (4.8)	20 (4.3)	<0.001
BBPS segment score				
2 or greater for each segment	371 (94.2)	45 (72.6)	416 (91.2)	
0/1 in any segment	23 (5.8)	17 (27.4)	40 (8.8)	<0.001
Aronchick scale				
Excellent/good prep quality	333 (86.7)	29 (49.2)	362 (79.3)	
Fair prep quality	35 (9.1)	28 (47.5)	63 (13.8)	
Inadequate/poor prep quality	16 (4.2)	2 (3.4)	18 (3.9)	<0.001
Noncompliance to split-dose preparation	54 (13.7)	17 (27.4)	385 (84.4)	0.006
Number of polyps				
0	207 (52.5)	28 (45.2)	235 (51.5)	
1	95 (24.1)	8 (12.9)	103 (22.6)	
2	43 (10.9)	6 (9.7)	49 (10.8)	
3	19 (4.8)	8 (12.9)	27 (5.9)	
4	12 (3.1)	5 (8.1)	17 (3.7)	
≥5	18 (4.6)	7 (11.3)	25 (5.5)	0.004
Endoscopy suite				
Ambulatory surgery centers	184 (46.7)	24 (38.7)	208 (45.6)	
Academic hospital unit	210 (53.3)	38 (61.3)	248 (54.4)	0.24
First colonoscopy	250 (63.8)	36 (58.1)	286 (63.0)	0.39
Had ≥2 previous colonoscopies	29 (7.4)	14 (22.6)	43 (9.5)	<0.001
Followed laxative instructions exactly	264 (67.0)	37 (60.0)	301 (66.0)	0.26
Bowel prep type				
PEG	143 (36.5)	24 (38.7)	167 (36.8)	
MiraLAX®/Gatorade®	226 (57.7)	37 (59.7)	263 (57.9)	
Other[b]	23 (5.9)	1 (1.6)	24 (5.3)	0.38
Colonoscopy appointment was before 10:30 am.	193 (49.0)	22 (35.5)	215 (47.2)	0.05
>12 hours or never till clear BM	139 (35.6)	30 (49.2)	169 (37.5)	0.04

All values are N (% of split-dose compliant or % of split-dose noncompliant), unless otherwise specified. [a]Please see footnote under Table 2. [b]Includes sodium phosphate/Osmoprep, Half-Lytely, Moviprep, and 2-day prep.

colonoscopy earlier than recommended by guidelines with 6% advising patients to get repeat colonoscopy longer than recommended intervals, and 5% (3/62) of patients did not get any specific recommendation. In bivariate analysis of colonoscopy-associated factors (Table 3), "fair" bowel preparation by the Aronchick scale ($p < 0.001$), BBPS of 0-1 for any colon segment ($p < 0.001$), BBPS total score of 5 ($p < 0.001$), noncompliance with split-dose preparation ($p = 0.006$), and presence of 3 or more polyps ($p = 0.004$), having had at least two prior colonoscopies (<0.001), and having >12 hours or never between starting bowel preparation and first clear bowel movement ($p = 0.04$), were each associated with guideline-inconsistent recommendations (Table 3). In bivariate analyses of patient-associated factors, higher body mass index, ≤high school education, and Medicare eligible status were each associated with guideline-inconsistent physician recommendations (Table 3).

In adjusted multivariable logistic regression analysis, two factors that may be amenable to intervention were independently associated with guideline-inconsistent recommendations: noncompliance with split-dose preparation (OR = 3.6; 95% CI: 1.7–7.7) and having required >12 hours or never till clear stool (OR = 3.4; 95% CI: 1.4–6.6) (Table 4). In addition, multiple patient-related characteristics not amenable to intervention were associated with guideline-inconsistent recommendations: older age (>70 years old), BMI ≥ 3 polyps, and having had ≥2 previous colonoscopies (Table 4).

When bowel preparation quality measured by the Aronchick scale, total BBPS score, or BBPS score for individual colon segments were added separately to the model, a fair bowel preparation on the Aronchick scale (8.89; 4.31–18.39), a BBPS = 5 (OR 15.26; 95% CI: 2.67–87.17), or having any colon segment with BBPS = 0-1 (5.62; 2.42–13.03) were

TABLE 4: Adjusted odds ratios (95% confidence intervals) based on logistic regression models for guideline-compliant physician recommendation.

Patient characteristic	Model 1			Model 2 with BBPS Total score			Model 3 with BBPS segment score			Model 4 with Aronchick		
	AOR	95% CI	p value	AOR	95% CI	p value	AOR	95% CI	p value	AOR	95% CI	p value
Noncompliant to split-dose preparation	3.6	(1.7–7.7)	0.001	2.9	(1.3–6.5)	0.01	2.4	(1.1–5.4)	0.03	2.5	(1.1–5.9)	0.03
BBPS total												
≥6	—	—	—	1.0	Reference	—	—	—	—	—	—	—
=5	—	—	—	15.26	(2.7–87.2)	0.00	—	—	—	—	—	—
<5	—	—	—	1.35	(0.3–5.8)	0.68	—	—	—	—	—	—
BBPS segment												
≥2	—	—	—	—	—	—	1.0	Reference	—	—	—	—
0/1	—	—	—	—	—	—	5.62	(2.4–13.0)	0.00	—	—	—
Aronchick												
≥Good	—	—	—	—	—	—	—	—	—	1.0	Reference	—
Fair	—	—	—	—	—	—	—	—	—	8.9	(4.3–18.3)	0.00
Poor	—	—	—	—	—	—	—	—	—	1.4	(0.3–7.7)	0.70
Age > 70 years old	3.6	(1.2–10.6)	0.02	3.4	(1.3–11.2)	0.02	3.7	(1.2–11.6)	0.02	4.9	(1.4–16.6)	0.01
Male	1.2	(0.6–2.2)	0.59	1.1	(0.6–2.2)	0.58	1.2	(0.6–2.2)	0.6	1.2	(0.6–2.3)	0.59
White	1.4	(0.6–3.5)	0.48	1.5	(0.6–3.7)	0.41	1.8	(0.7–4.9)	0.24	1.4	(0.5–3.8)	0.53
Endoscopy at hospital a	1.2	(0.7–2.2)	0.54	1.3	(0.7–2.5)	0.37	1.2	(0.7–2.3)	0.51	1.3	(0.6–2.4)	0.51
Number of polyps: 0	1.0	Reference		1.0	Reference		1.0	Reference		1.0		
1	0.7	(0.3–1.6)	0.35	0.7	(0.3–1.6)	0.36	0.7	(0.3–1.6)	0.34	0.7	(0.3–2.0)	0.54
2	1.0	(0.4–2.7)	0.98	1.0	(0.3–2.7)	0.94	0.9	(0.3–2.7)	0.87	1.2	(0.4–3.6)	0.77
3	3.0	(1.4–6.3)	0.005	3.2	(1.5-6.9)	0.003	3.3	(1.5–7.0)	0.00	4.4	(2.0–10)	0.00
Had ≥2 previous colonoscopies	3.7	(1.6–8.7)	0.003	3.3	(1.4–8.0)	0.007	3.0	(1.2–7.3)	0.02	2.5	(0.9–6.5)	0.07
>12 hours or never till clear BM	3.4	(1.8–6.6)	<0.001	3.1	(1.6–6.1)	0.002	2.8	(1.4-5.4)	0.00	2.6	(1.3–5.4)	0.01
Body mass index	1.1	(1.0-1.1)	0.03	1.1	(1.0-1.1)	0.04	1.1	(1.0-1.1)	0.02	1.1	(1.0-1.1)	0.10

AOR: adjusted odds ratio; CI: confidence interval; BM: bowel movement. a versus ambulatory surgery centers.

associated with guideline-inconsistent recommendation. Also, noncompliance with split-dose preparation (OR = 2.4–2.9) and >12 hours or never between starting bowel preparation and the first clear bowel movement (OR = 2.6–3.1) remained significantly associated with guideline-inconsistent recommendation in all models (Table 4).

4. Discussion

Overuse of colonoscopy for CRC screening and colon polyp surveillance, defined as recommending repeat colonoscopy sooner than recommended by guidelines, has been described in multiple studies [1, 2, 4]. Minimizing this practice minimizes patients' exposure to the risks, inconvenience, and cost of colonoscopy. Furthermore, performing colonoscopy every 10 years after normal screening exams is necessary to maintain the cost-effectiveness of colonoscopy [3, 4]. In our study, the frequency of guideline-inconsistent recommendations was 13.6% and suboptimal bowel preparation was associated with guideline-inconsistent recommendations in adjusted multivariate logistic regression analysis. Specifically, fair bowel preparation by the Aronchick scale (OR = 8.89; 95% CI: 4.31–18.34) and BBPS = 5 (OR = 15.26; 95% CI: 2.67–87.17) were associated with recommendations to return early for colonoscopy. Our study also identified modifiable patient-related factors that were associated with guideline-inconsistent recommendations: noncompliance with split-dose preparation (OR = 2.89; 95% CI: 1.29–6.45) and requiring >12 hours to have the first clear bowel movement or never having a clear stool (OR = 3.13; 95% CI: 1.6–6.10). These findings, which have not been assessed in prior prospective studies after institution of split-dose bowel preparation, may guide potential interventions for quality improvement programs and future research.

Other patient-related and colonoscopy-related factors associated with guideline-inconsistent recommendations include patients >70, increasing BMI, ≥3 polyps, and ≥2 previous colonoscopies. These associations seem to be clinically intuitive from an endoscopist's perspective. Advancing age and increasing BMI are both associated with a higher likelihood of adenomas; endoscopists, therefore, may place these subjects in higher risk categories [20, 21]. Patients with ≥3 polyps found at colonoscopy may also elevate the endoscopist's index of suspicion for missed adenomas or future adenoma recurrence. The NCI Pooling Project found a linear increase in risk for advanced and nonadvanced neoplasia with each additional adenoma while the VA cooperative study 380 showed an increased risk of advanced neoplasia with the multiplicity of adenomas [22, 23]. While some or all of these factors might heighten endoscopists' suspicions or increase their level of concern, these concerns should not supersede evidence-based guideline recommendations in most patients. Conversely, endoscopists should remember that 100% adherence to these recommendations is not expected. The ACG/ASGE position statement on quality indicators for colonoscopy [4] targets 90% adherence, so endoscopists can individualize care for 10% of patients.

In our study, adherence was 86.4%. In order to improve adherence, interventions need to be identified and implemented. Split-dose noncompliance or requiring >12 hours to produce a clear bowel movement or never having a clear liquid stool during bowel preparation is potentially a modifiable factor. Therefore, future research may assess efficacy of having patients consume additional laxatives if they have not passed clear liquid stool within 12 hours of starting their bowel preparation. Multiple interventions improve patient compliance with bowel preparation including educational videos, phone calls, and education booklets [24–28], so quality improvement programs may consider implementing these interventions. Following implementation, QI programs could then track quality of bowel preparation and adherence to guideline recommendations.

Our study has significant strengths and limitations. Our findings are congruent with other retrospective studies demonstrating that suboptimal bowel preparation is associated with nonadherence to guideline recommendations [5–7, 29, 30]. It is a prospective study that utilized the BBPS, a validated bowel preparation quality measure for colonoscopy-oriented research, in addition to the commonly used Aronchick scale. Although Medicare claims database studies of overuse of colonoscopy can assess a much larger sample of patients, these studies may not be able to fully account for bowel preparation quality as a contributing factor [2, 31]. This study also was performed after institution of split-dose bowel preparation. However, this research was performed at an academic center, which may limit the generalizability of our findings for endoscopists, patients, and practice settings. Our sample size is relatively small, so this research need to be replicated in other settings in order to confirm or refute our findings.

In conclusion, gastroenterologists in this study were adherent with guidelines for timing of repeat colonoscopy in more than 85% of patients, but did not attain the recommended target of 90% adherence. Suboptimal bowel preparation is associated with guideline-inconsistent recommendations, and patient-modifiable factors were identified that may minimize this outcome while also improving quality of bowel preparation. Since this is a reportable quality indicator in PQRS and will probably be incorporated into CMS value-based index for reimbursement of colonoscopy, this issue is likely to garner closer scrutiny. Therefore, additional research about modifiable factors that are associated with guideline-inconsistent recommendations and research about interventions to minimize this outcome will be helpful to maximize the quality of CRC screening with colonoscopy.

Abbreviations

CRC: Colorectal cancer screening
GI: Gastrointestinal.

Authors' Contributions

Stacy B. Menees did the data acquisition, statistical analysis, analysis and interpretation of data, drafting of manuscript, and draft revision; H. Myra Kim did the statistical analysis and draft revision; Sheryl Korsnes did the data acquisition; Grace H. Elta did the survey design and draft revision; Philip Schoenfeld did the study concept and design, analysis and interpretation of data, critical revision of the manuscript for important intellectual content, obtained the funding, and study supervision.

Acknowledgments

Dr. Schoenfeld is supported by NIH Mid-Career Mentoring Award (1K24DK084208-01A1) and is a research scientist in the Ann Arbor VAHCS Center of Clinical Management Research. Dr. Menees was supported by the Michigan Institute for Clinical and Health Research MICHR T2 Translational Science Award Program Application (MICHR T2), Grant no. UL1RR024986.

References

[1] R. E. Schoen, P. F. Pinsky, J. L. Weissfeld et al., "Utilization of surveillance colonoscopy in community practice," *Gastroenterology*, vol. 138, no. 1, pp. 73–81, 2010.

[2] K. M. Sheffield, Y. Han, Y. F. Kuo, T. S. Riall, and J. S. Goodwin, "Potentially inappropriate screening colonoscopy in Medicare patients: variation by physician and geographic region," *JAMA Internal Medicine*, vol. 173, no. 7, pp. 542–550, 2013.

[3] D. A. Lieberman, D. K. Rex, S. J. Winawer, F. M. Giardiello, D. A. Johnson, and T. R. Levin, "Guidelines for colonoscopy surveillance after screening and polypectomy: a consensus update by the US multi-society task force on colorectal cancer," *Gastroenterology*, vol. 143, no. 3, pp. 844–857, 2012.

[4] D. K. Rex, P. S. Schoenfeld, J. Cohen et al., "Quality indicators for colonoscopy," *The American Journal of Gastroenterology*, vol. 110, no. 1, pp. 72–90, 2015.

[5] S. B. Menees, E. Elliott, S. Govani et al., "The impact of bowel cleansing on follow-up recommendations in average-risk patients with a normal colonoscopy," *The American Journal of Gastroenterology*, vol. 109, no. 2, pp. 148–154, 2014.

[6] S. B. Menees, E. Elliott, S. Govani, C. Anastassiades, and P. Schoenfeld, "Adherence to recommended intervals for surveillance colonoscopy in average-risk patients with 1 to 2 small (<1 cm) polyps on screening colonoscopy," *Gastrointestinal Endoscopy*, vol. 79, no. 4, pp. 551–557, 2014.

[7] S. B. Menees, H. M. Kim, E. E. Elliott, J. L. Mickevicius, B. B. Graustein, and P. S. Schoenfeld, "The impact of fair colonoscopy preparation on colonoscopy use and adenoma miss rates in patients undergoing outpatient colonoscopy," *Gastrointestinal Endoscopy*, vol. 78, no. 3, pp. 510–516, 2013.

[8] A. Parra-Blanco, D. Nicolas-Perez, A. Gimeno-Garcia et al., "The timing of bowel preparation before colonoscopy determines the quality of cleansing, and is a significant factor contributing to the detection of flat lesions: a randomized study," *World Journal of Gastroenterology*, vol. 12, no. 38, pp. 6161–6166, 2006.

[9] E. Aoun, H. Abdul-Baki, C. Azar et al., "A randomized single-blind trial of split-dose PEG-electrolyte solution without dietary restriction compared with whole dose PEG-electrolyte solution with dietary restriction for colonoscopy preparation," *Gastrointestinal Endoscopy*, vol. 62, no. 2, pp. 213–218, 2005.

[10] J. Park, C. Sohn, S. Hwang et al., "Quality and effect of single dose versus split dose of polyethylene glycol bowel preparation for early-morning colonoscopy," *Endoscopy*, vol. 39, no. 7, pp. 616–619, 2007.

[11] S. S. Park, D. H. Sinn, Y. H. Kim et al., "Efficacy and tolerability of split-dose magnesium citrate: low-volume (2 liters) polyethylene glycol vs. single- or split-dose polyethylene glycol bowel preparation for morning colonoscopy," *The American Journal of Gastroenterology*, vol. 105, no. 6, pp. 1319–1326, 2010.

[12] A. Rostom, E. Jolicoeur, C. Dubé et al., "A randomized prospective trial comparing different regimens of oral sodium phosphate and polyethylene glycol-based lavage solution in the preparation of patients for colonoscopy," *Gastrointestinal Endoscopy*, vol. 64, no. 4, pp. 544–552, 2006.

[13] A. M. A. El Sayed, Z. A. Kanafani, F. H. Mourad et al., "A randomized single-blind trial of whole versus split-dose polyethylene glycol-electrolyte solution for colonoscopy preparation," *Gastrointestinal Endoscopy*, vol. 58, no. 1, pp. 36–40, 2003.

[14] System, University of Michigan Health System, "Colonoscopy," 2010, September 2013, http://www.med.umich.edu/1libr/aha/umcolon.htm.

[15] C. A. Aronchick, W. H. Lipshutz, S. H. Wright, F. DuFrayne, and G. Bergman, "Validation of an instrument to assess colon cleansing," *The American Journal of Gastroenterology*, vol. 94, no. 9, p. 2667, 1999.

[16] E. J. Lai, A. H. Calderwood, G. Doros, O. K. Fix, and B. C. Jacobson, "The Boston bowel preparation scale: a valid and reliable instrument for colonoscopy-oriented research," *Gastrointestinal Endoscopy*, vol. 69, no. 3, pp. 620–625, 2009.

[17] S. Mittal, "The Boston bowel preparation scale: reliable not only for colonoscopy-oriented research but clinical practice also," *Gastrointestinal Endoscopy*, vol. 71, no. 1, p. 221, 2010.

[18] A. H. Calderwood, P. C. Schroy III, D. A. Lieberman, J. R. Logan, M. Zurfluh, and B. C. Jacobson, "Boston bowel preparation scale scores provide a standardized definition of adequate for describing bowel cleanliness," *Gastrointestinal Endoscopy*, vol. 80, no. 2, pp. 269–276, 2014.

[19] August 2014, http://www.bmc.org/gastroenterology/research.htm.

[20] A. R. Williams, B. A. Balasooriya, and D. W. Day, "Polyps and cancer of the large bowel: a necropsy study in Liverpool," *Gut*, vol. 23, no. 10, pp. 835–842, 1982.

[21] Q. Ben, W. An, Y. Jiang et al., "Body mass index increases risk for colorectal adenomas based on meta-analysis," *Gastroenterology*, vol. 142, no. 4, pp. 762–772, 2012.

[22] M. E. Martínez, J. A. Baron, D. A. Lieberman et al., "A pooled analysis of advanced colorectal neoplasia diagnoses after

colonoscopic polypectomy," *Gastroenterology*, vol. 136, no. 3, pp. 832–841, 2009.

[23] D. A. Lieberman, D. G. Weiss, W. V. Harford et al., "Five-year colon surveillance after screening colonoscopy," *Gastroenterology*, vol. 133, no. 4, pp. 1077–1085, 2007.

[24] A. H. Calderwood, E. J. Lai, O. K. Fix, and B. C. Jacobson, "An endoscopist-blinded, randomized, controlled trial of a simple visual aid to improve bowel preparation for screening colonoscopy," *Gastrointestinal Endoscopy*, vol. 73, no. 2, pp. 307–314, 2011.

[25] S. R. Prakash, S. Verma, J. McGowan et al., "Improving the quality of colonoscopy bowel preparation using an educational video," *Canadian Journal of Gastroenterology*, vol. 27, no. 12, pp. 696–700, 2013.

[26] B. M. R. Spiegel, J. Talley, P. Shekelle et al., "Development and validation of a novel patient educational booklet to enhance colonoscopy preparation," *The American Journal of Gastroenterology*, vol. 106, no. 5, pp. 875–883, 2011.

[27] T.-Y. Shieh, M.-J. Chen, C.-W. Chang et al., "Effect of physician-delivered patient education on the quality of bowel preparation for screening colonoscopy," *Gastroenterology Research and Practice*, vol. 2013, Article ID 570180, 5 pages, 2013.

[28] J. W. Tae, J. C. Lee, S. J. Hong et al., "Impact of patient education with cartoon visual aids on the quality of bowel preparation for colonoscopy," *Gastrointestinal Endoscopy*, vol. 76, no. 4, pp. 804–811, 2012.

[29] E. R. Kim, D. H. Sinn, J. Y. Kim et al., "Factors associated with adherence to the recommended postpolypectomy surveillance interval," *Surgical Endoscopy*, vol. 26, no. 6, pp. 1690–1695, 2012.

[30] D. F. Ransohoff, B. Yankaskas, Z. Gizlice, and L. Gangarosa, "Recommendations for post-polypectomy surveillance in community practice," *Digestive Diseases and Sciences*, vol. 56, no. 9, pp. 2623–2630, 2011.

[31] J. S. Goodwin, A. Singh, N. Reddy, T. S. Riall, and Y. F. Kuo, "Overuse of screening colonoscopy in the Medicare population," *Archives of Internal Medicine*, vol. 171, no. 15, pp. 1335–1343, 2011.

24

Long-Term Outcomes of Caustic Esophageal Stricture with Endoscopic Balloon Dilatation in Chinese Children

Lan-Lan Geng,[1] Cui-Ping Liang,[1] Pei-Yu Chen,[1] Qiang Wu,[1] Min Yang,[1] Hui-Wen Li,[1] Zhao-Hui Xu,[1] Lu Ren,[1] Hong-Li Wang,[1] Shunxian Cheng,[1] Wan-Fu Xu,[1] Yang Chen,[1] Chao Zhang,[1] Li-Ying Liu,[1] Ding-You Li,[2] and Si-Tang Gong[1]

[1]*Department of Gastroenterology, Guangzhou Women and Children's Medical Center, 9 Jinsui Road, Guangzhou 510623, China*
[2]*Division of Gastroenterology, Children's Mercy Hospital, 2401 Gillham Road, Kansas City, MO 64108, USA*

Correspondence should be addressed to Ding-You Li; dyli@cmh.edu and Si-Tang Gong; sitangg@126.com

Lan-Lan Geng and Cui-Ping Liang contributed equally to this work.

Academic Editor: Alfred Gangl

Caustic esophageal stricture (CES) in children still occurs frequently in developing countries. We aimed to evaluate the long-term outcomes of endoscopic balloon dilatation (EBD) in treating CES in children and the influencing factors associated with outcome. We retrospectively reviewed the data of all patients who had a diagnosis of CES and underwent EBD from August 1, 2005, to December 31, 2014. The primary outcome was EBD success, which was defined as the maintenance of dysphagia-free status for at least 12 months after the last EBD. The secondary outcome was to analyze influencing factors associated with EBD success. Forty-three patients were included for analysis (29 males; mean age at first dilatation 44 months with range 121 months). 26 (60.5%) patients had long segment (>2 cm) stricture. A total of 168 EBD procedures were performed. Twenty-six (60.5%) patients were considered EBD success. Seventeen (39.5%) patients failed EBD and required stent placement and/or surgery. Patients in the EBD success group had significantly shorter stricture segments when compared to the EBD failure group ($t = 2.398$, $P = 0.018$, $OR = 3.206$, 95% OR: 1.228–8.371). Seven (4.4%) esophageal perforations occurred in 6 patients after EBD. Stents were placed in 5 patients, and gastric tube esophagoplasty was performed in 14 patients. In conclusion, 26 (60.5%) of 43 children with CES had EBD success. Length of stricture was the main influencing factor associated with EBD treatment outcome.

1. Introduction

Caustic esophageal stricture (CES) in children still occurs frequently in developing countries, due to accidental ingestion of caustic substances including strong alkalis and acids [1, 2]. Because of inadequate public education and lack of law enforcement for child-proof containers in China, caustic substances are dispensed and sold in ordinary bottles that can be easily opened by children, resulting in accidental caustic substance ingestion. The rate of esophageal stricture formation after caustic ingestion is reported to be between 2% and 63% [3–5].

Current management for CES includes esophageal dilatation, retrievable stent placement, surgical resection of short segment stricture, and esophageal replacement. The foremost goal of treatment for CES is to preserve the esophagus and restore its function. Dilatation has been considered as the treatment of choice for CES and can be performed endoscopically or fluoroscopically, using a balloon dilator or rigid dilator [6]. The major disadvantage of fluoroscopically guided dilatation is repeat exposures to radiation because of the requirement for multiple dilatation treatment sessions. Several case series reports have shown that endoscopic balloon dilatation (EBD) is a safe and effective treatment for children with CES [7, 8]. However, there is still a lack of a well-established consensus on when and how to optimize dilatation in children with CES. Esophageal stent placement or surgery is indicated when dilatation is not successful. In our center, the prerequisite for esophageal stent placement is that the diameter of a stricture can be dilated at least to 1 cm, which is the smallest stent diameter available commercially. Surgery is usually performed when dilatation fails, esophageal perforation occurs with dilatation, or stent placement is contraindicated. Gastric tube esophagoplasty (GTE) has become the most commonly used operation for esophageal replacement in pediatric surgery [9, 10]. The aim of this study was to evaluate the long-term outcomes of endoscopic balloon dilatation (EBD) in treating CES in children and the influencing factors associated with EBD treatment outcome.

2. Patients and Methods

A retrospective case-series analysis was carried out in a tertiary children's hospital in Guangzhou, China. We included all patients who had a diagnosis of CES and underwent EBD from August 1, 2005, to December 31, 2014. Patients were followed up until December 31, 2015. We excluded patients who had previous dilatation or surgery for stricture in other hospitals or who were lost for follow-up. The medical records were reviewed to obtain each patient's demographic and clinical data including age, gender, grade of dysphagia, stricture site and length, stricture diameter, type of caustic substance, type and number of treatments, the date and duration of treatments, and adverse events.

Dysphagia was graded according to the patient's ability to swallow at initial presentation: 0, no dysphagia; 1, intermittent solid food dysphagia; 2, unable to swallow solids; 3, unable to swallow pureed food; and 4, unable to swallow liquids [6].

EBD is considered the treatment of choice for CES [6–8]. An esophageal stent placement is indicated for refractory esophageal stricture [11], which refers to those that do not respond to repeated esophageal dilatations at an up to 4-week interval and continues to anatomic stricture and persistent dysphagia [12]. Surgery is indicated if a severe esophageal stricture was not suitable for dilatation or refractory to repeated EBD and/or stent placement, or if esophageal perforation occurred during dilatation [13].

2.1. Endoscopic Balloon Dilatation. Initial dilatation was performed at ≥2 weeks after caustic ingestion. Dilatation was repeated every 2 to 4 weeks in the first few months and as needed depending upon the degree of dysphagia. Various types of gastroscopes (standard or high-definition, with 4.9–9.8 mm diameters; Olympus, Fujinon, or Pentax), balloon dilators (Boston Scientific, USA), and force pump (Alliance, Boston Scientific, USA) were used.

Under general anesthesia with endotracheal intubation, the gastroscope was inserted and advanced just above the stricture area. A balloon dilatation catheter (Boston Scientific, USA) of appropriate size (6–18 mm) was chosen according to the initial endoscopic estimation of stricture or previous dilatations and inserted and inflated for 2 minutes, followed by deflation for 2 minutes and repeated inflation for 2 times based on our own experience and others [14]. For strictures longer than 5 cm, dilatation begun from the upper section and then moved down to the lower section. For a stricture diameter less than 5 mm after dilatation, a nasogastric tube was inserted to prevent esophagus closure. Antibiotics were routinely administered for 48 h after the procedure.

Table 1: Characteristics of patients with caustic esophageal stricture.

Variable	Statistics
Total number of patients	43
Boy	29 (67.4%)
Girl	14 (32.6%)
Mean age (range)	44 months (18–121)
Dysphagia score	
Grade 1	1 (2.3%)
Grade 2	11 (25.6%)
Grade 3	30 (69.8%)
Grade 4	1 (2.3%)
Length of stricture (cm)	
Short stricture (≤2 cm)	17 (39.5%)
Long stricture (>2 cm)	26 (60.5%)
Stricture location	
Upper esophagus	4 (9.3%)
Middle esophagus	31 (72.1%)
Lower esophagus	3 (7.0%)
Middle and low esophagus	4 (9.3%)
All esophagus	1 (2.3%)

2.2. Esophageal Stent Placement. Under general anesthesia with endotracheal intubation, the stricture was dilated to 1 cm and then a guide wire was inserted through the scope's biopsy channel and pushed out the scope. A stent conveyer was inserted through the guide wire and positioned using a standard protocol. With the supplied delivery system, a stainless steel stent (Sigma Jiangsu, China; type Z with diameter 1–1.4 cm) was placed. Endoscopy was performed after stent placement to make sure that the upper side of the stent was 2 cm above the stricture margin. Routine X-ray was used to check for stent migration every 2 weeks. Antibiotics were routinely administered for 48 h after the procedure. The stent was left in place for up to 3 months.

2.3. Surgery. Gastric tube esophagoplasty (GTE) was performed for long stricture whereas a narrow segment resection was performed for short strictures [13].

2.4. Outcomes. The primary outcome of this study was EBD success, which was defined as the maintenance of dysphagia-free status for at least 12 months after last EBD. EBD failure was defined as persistent or worsening dysphagia after EDB or requirement for further interventions including stent placement and/or surgery. The secondary outcomes included influencing factors associated with EBD success, serious adverse events such as perforation, bleeding, infection, mortality, and the percentage of patients requiring stent placement and/or surgery.

2.5. Statistical Analysis. The SPSS version 24.0 (IBM SPSS Statistics for Windows; IBM Corporation, Somers, NY) was

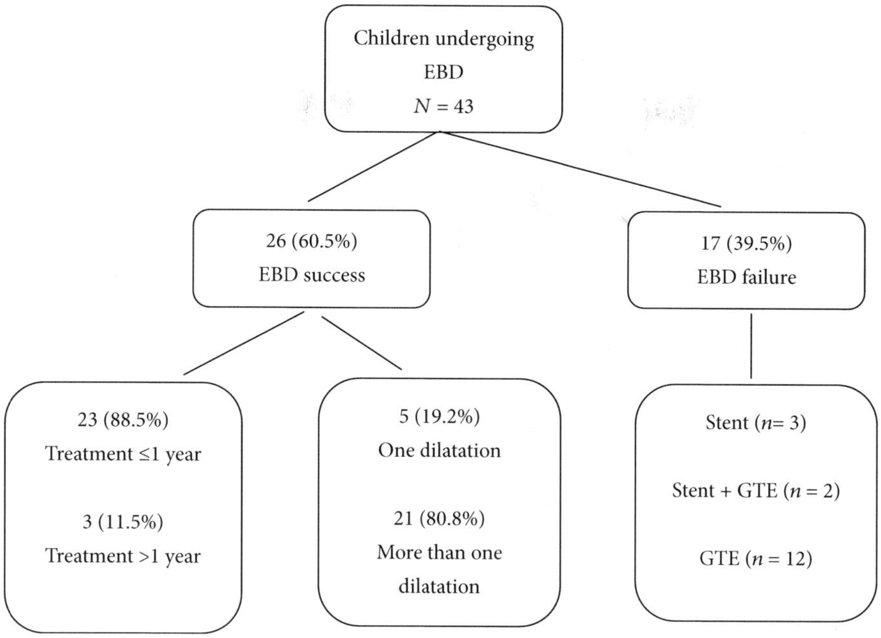

FIGURE 1: Flowchart of treatment outcomes of children with caustic esophageal strictures. EBD: esophageal balloon dilatation; GTE: gastric tube esophagoplasty.

used for data analysis. Categorical data were expressed as percentages and compared by using the Fisher exact test or the chi-square test. Continuous variables were expressed as mean, standard deviation, range, maximum, and minimum, based on the data characteristics. Quantitative data were assessed for normality by the Kolmogorov-Smirnov test and compared by using the Student t-test, and abnormality quantitative data was compared with the rank-sum test. Because treatment variable (EBD or surgery) is categorical data, and the same subject might had more than one treatment, a recently available generalized linear mixed model procedure was applied to include both fixed effects and a random effect to account for within-subject correlations due to repeated observations of the same patients. This analysis was used to fit the multilevel logistic regression model to our data with hierarchical structure.

3. Results

3.1. Patients. The institutional ethics committee of Guangzhou Women and Children's Medical Center approved this study protocol (approval number 2017102414).

A total of 46 patients met inclusion criteria, but 3 patients were excluded due to loss to follow-up. Thus, 43 patients (29 males) were included for analysis (Table 1). Mean age at first dilatation was 44 months (range 18–121 month). Only 3 patients were admitted to our hospital immediately after caustic substance ingestion, and all others were referred to our hospital for dysphagia after the acute phase. The mean time for referral was 49.7 days after caustic ingestion (range 1–140 days).

As shown in Table 1, dysphagia scores of patients were as follows: grade 1 ($n = 1$), grade 2 ($n = 11$), grade 3 ($n = 30$), and grade 4 ($n = 1$). The lengths of the strictures, as assessed by endoscopic and/or radiologic measurements, were as follows: 9 (20.9%) patients ≤2 cm and 34 (79.1%) patients >2 cm. Locations of esophageal strictures were in the upper esophagus in 4 (9.3%), in the middle esophagus in 31 (72.1%) patients, in the lower esophagus in 3 (7.0%) patients, in the middle-lower esophagus in 4 (9.3%) patients, and in the whole esophagus in one case (2.3%).

3.2. Endoscopic Balloon Dilatation (EBD). A total of 168 EBD sessions were performed in 43 patients (Figure 1). Twenty-six (60.5%) patients were considered EBD success. 17 (39.5%) patients were considered EBD failures and underwent stent placement and/or surgery. In the EBD success group, 23 (88.5%) patients achieved dysphagia-free status within 12 months and another 3 (11.5%) patients achieved dysphagia-free status between 12 to 18 months; 21 (80.8%) patients required more than one dilatation, and 5 (19.2%) patients required only one dilatation.

As shown in Table 2, univariate analysis showed that patients in the EBD failure group had significantly longer stricture segments when compared to the EBD success group ($t = 4.622$, $P < 0.001$). Between the two groups, there were no statistical differences in stricture diameter, time of first EBD, number of EBD, and interval between EBD sessions. No differences were observed among different caustic substances ($\chi^2 = 0.251$, $P = 0.999$). In addition, effectiveness of EBD treatment did not differ among different dysphagia scores ($\chi^2 = 2.125$, $P = 0.999$). In multivariate analyses with generalized linear mixed models, the length of stricture in the EBD failure group was higher than that in the EBD success group ($t = 2.398$, $P = 0.018$, OR = 3.206, 95% OR: 1.228–8.371), but other variables were not associated with the different treatment outcomes.

Seven (4.4%) esophageal perforations occurred in 6 (13.6%) patients. No dilatation-related mortality, massive hemorrhage, or severe infections were observed. Four

Table 2: Comparison between esophageal balloon dilatation (EBD) clinical resolution and failure groups. Values are expressed as mean ± SD (range).

Variable	EBD success $N = 26$ mean ± SD (range) or N	EBD failure $N = 17$ mean ± SD (range) or N	Univariate analysis Statistics	Univariate analysis P	Multivariate analyses (generalized linear mixed models) Coefficient	t	P	OR	95% OR LCI	95% OR UCI
Diameter of stricture (mm)	3.4 ± 1.5 (6)	2.7 ± 1.2 (5)	1.69[a]	0.099	−0.24	−0.539	0.59	0.787	0.326	1.896
Length of stricture (cm)	4.0 ± 1.9 (7)	7.6 ± 3.2 (13)	4.622[a]	**<0.001**	1.165	2.398	**0.018**	3.206	1.228	8.371
Time of first EBD (weeks)	7.6 ± 3.3 (16)	6.6 ± 2.9 (12)	0.952[a]	0.347	0.045	0.491	0.624	1.046	0.872	1.033
Number of EBD	3.0 ± 1.8 (7)	5.2 ± 4.6 (15)	1.443[b]	0.149	—	—	—	—	—	—
Interval of EBD (months)	2.3 ± 2.3 (9.7)	1.9 ± 1.5 (4.9)	0.623[a]	0.536	−0.003	−0.009	0.993	0.997	0.445	2.182
Median follow-up time (months)	77.0 ± 27.0 (97)	64.0 ± 13.0 (44)	1.628[b]	0.104	−0.054	−1.235	0.219	0.948	0.87	1.033
Age	46 ± 29 (121)	40 ± 23 (83)	0.698[a]	0.489	−0.044	−0.449	0.654	0.957	0.787	1.163
Gender (female/male (reference))	7/19	7/10	0.951[c]	0.329	1.908	0.878	0.381	6.74	0.092	493.12
Caustic substance										
Alkali	16	10			−2.091	−0.849	0.397	0.124	0.001	16.025
Acids	5	4			1.154	−0.404	0.687	3.171	0.011	896.717
Detergents and bleach (reference)	5	3	0.251[c]	0.999	—	—	—	—	—	—
Dysphagia score										
Grade 1	1	0			−21,567	−0.003	0.999	0	0	—
Grade 2	7	4			−8.608	−0.003	0.999	0	0	—
Grade 3	18	12	2.125[c]	0.811	−10.309	−0.003	0.999	0	0	—
Grade 4 (reference)	0	1			—	—	—	—	—	—
Stricture location										
Upper esophagus	2	2			−18.338	−0.014	0.993	0	0	—
Middle esophagus	19	12			−21.503	−0.017	0.991	0	0	—
Lower esophagus	3	0	3.664	0.552	−21.61	−0.017	0.991	0	0	—
Middle and low esophagus	2	2			−32.553	−0.013	0.993	0	0	—
All esophagus (reference)	0	1			—	—	—	—	—	

[a]*t*-test; [b]rank-sum test; [c]chi-square test or Fisher exact method. Values are expressed as mean ± SD (range) in EBD clinical resolution and EBD failure.

patients were managed initially with fasting, intravenous antibiotics, and parenteral nutrition, and two patients required gastrostomy placement. After 10–14 days of treatment, radiologic studies revealed perforation closure but esophageal strictures were severe and long (4–10 cm). All six patients had GTE later.

3.3. Esophageal Stent Placement. Five stents were placed in 4 patients because of persistent dysphagia after repeated EBD (8, 10, 12, and 15 times, resp.). All 4 patients had long segment strictures. Two patients ingested alkali and two ingested acids. Stents were removed after 2–3 months. Three patients had clinical resolution after stent placement 1-2 times. Two patients failed stenting and subsequently had surgery.

3.4. Gastric Tube Esophagoplasty (GTE). GTE was performed in 14 patients. All of them had long strictures. Nine patients ingested alkali and 5 ingested acids. Two patients developed an anastomotic fistula which closed after 10–14 days of conservative management including intravenous antibiotics and nasogastric feeding. Two patients developed an anastomotic stricture which resolved after EBD 1-2 times.

4. Discussion

Esophageal balloon dilatation has been recommended as the choice of treatment for esophageal stricture in children. Patients with caustic substance-induced strictures have less satisfactory outcome and require a significantly higher number of dilatation sessions for improvement as compared with noncaustic strictures [3, 4, 6–8, 15]. However, there is still lack of a well-established consensus on when and how to optimize dilatation in children with CES, such as the best time to begin dilatation, the dilatation interval, the maximum number of dilatations to be considered failure, and the time to consider other treatment options. In our series, 60% of patients had clinical resolution with EBD and 40% failed EBD. Only length of stricture segment was statistically different between the EBD success group and the failure group. Initial dysphagia scores were not associated with the outcome of EBD. We did not observe any difference in time of the first EBD between EBD clinical resolution and failure groups.

The EBD success rate of 60% in our study is lower than that reported by others [8, 16] and may be due to several factors: (1) Most of our patients had long segment strictures. (2) Most of our patients were referred to our hospital more than 4 weeks after caustic substance ingestion. Uygun et al. [16] reported that earlier (7–25 days after ingestion of caustic substances) balloon dilatation was more effective with significantly shorter dilatation duration and less dilatation sessions when compared to late (26–60 days) dilatation. Alshammari et al. [8] waited at least 3 weeks between EBDs. A decision to consider balloon dilatation as failure is still debatable. Some studies suggest that esophageal strictures require 6 months to 3 years for stabilization [17–19]. In our study, the interval in EBD was between 3 and 40 weeks with an average of 8 weeks. In our EBD success group, the majority of patients (88.5%) were resolved within the first year.

With repeated EBD, 40% of our patients did not have clinical resolution and required stent placement and/or GTE. In our study, 7 (4.4%) esophageal perforations occurred in 6 (13.6%) patients, which is consistent with the observation reported by Contini et al. [18], who showed that delayed dilatation (>6 weeks after caustic ingestion) in children carried a higher risk of perforation and a higher recurrence rate in comparison to timely (<6 weeks) dilatation.

In conclusion, we report here our experience of 43 children with caustic esophageal stricture treated with EBD in the past ten years. Twenty-six (60.5%) patients considered EBD success, which correlated with stricture length. However, about 40% of our patients did not have clinical improvement after EBD and required stent placement and/or GTE. Optimization of EBD is needed for the treatment of caustic esophageal stricture in children.

Ethical Approval

This study was approved by the Institutional Ethics Committee of the Guangzhou Women and Children's Medical Center.

Disclosure

The work was presented as an abstract in the 51st Annual Meeting of ESPGHAN in Geneva, Switzerland, May 9–12, 2018.

Acknowledgments

The authors thank Dr. Craig Friesen from Children's Mercy Hospital, Kansas City, Missouri, USA, for the critical reading of the manuscript.

References

[1] M. Elshabrawi and H. H. A-Kader, "Caustic ingestion in children," *Expert Review of Gastroenterology & Hepatology*, vol. 5, no. 5, pp. 637–645, 2011.

[2] S. Contini and C. Scarpignato, "Caustic injury of the upper gastrointestinal tract: a comprehensive review," *World Journal of Gastroenterology*, vol. 19, no. 25, pp. 3918–3930, 2013.

[3] A. L. de Jong, R. Macdonald, S. Ein, V. Forte, and A. Turner, "Corrosive esophagitis in children: a 30-year review," *International Journal of Pediatric Otorhinolaryngology*, vol. 57, no. 3, pp. 203–211, 2001.

[4] Y. C. Huang, Y. H. Ni, H. S. Lai, and M. H. Chang, "Corrosive esophagitis in children," *Pediatric Surgery International*, vol. 20, no. 3, pp. 207–210, 2004.

[5] D. Baskın, N. Urgancı, L. Abbasoğlu et al., "A standardised protocol for the acute management of corrosive ingestion in children," *Pediatric Surgery International*, vol. 20, no. 11-12, pp. 824–828, 2004.

[6] J. S. Scolapio, T. M. Pasha, C. J. Gostout et al., "A randomized prospective study comparing rigid to balloon dilators for benign esophageal strictures and rings," *Gastrointestinal Endoscopy*, vol. 50, no. 1, pp. 13–17, 1999.

[7] L. C. L. Lan, K. K. Y. Wong, S. C. L. Lin et al., "Endoscopic balloon dilatation of esophageal strictures in infants and children: 17 years' experience and a literature review," *Journal of Pediatric Surgery*, vol. 38, no. 12, pp. 1712–1715, 2003.

[8] J. Alshammari, S. Quesnel, S. Pierrot, and V. Couloigner, "Endoscopic balloon dilatation of esophageal strictures in children," *International Journal of Pediatric Otorhinolaryngology*, vol. 75, no. 11, pp. 1376–1379, 2011.

[9] S. H. Ein, B. Shandling, and C. A. Stephens, "Twenty-one year experience with the pediatric gastric tube," *Journal of Pediatric Surgery*, vol. 22, no. 1, pp. 77–81, 1987.

[10] W. Liu, J. H. Liang, J. H. Zeng, and J. Tang, "Preliminary study on gastric tube esophagoplasty for corrosive strictures of the esophagus in children," *Zhonghua Wei Chang Wai Ke Za Zhi*, vol. 15, no. 9, pp. 954–956, 2012.

[11] C. Best, B. Sudel, J. E. Foker, T. C. K. Krosch, C. Dietz, and K. M. Khan, "Esophageal stenting in children: indications, application, effectiveness, and complications," *Gastrointestinal Endoscopy*, vol. 70, no. 6, pp. 1248–1253, 2009.

[12] A. Tringali, M. Thomson, J. M. Dumonceau et al., "Pediatric gastrointestinal endoscopy: European Society of Gastrointestinal Endoscopy (ESGE) and European Society for Paediatric Gastroenterology Hepatology and Nutrition (ESPGHAN) Guideline Executive summary," *Endoscopy*, vol. 49, no. 1, pp. 83–91, 2017.

[13] S. T. Schettini and J. Pinus, "Gastric-tube esophagoplasty in children," *Pediatric Surgery International*, vol. 14, no. 1-2, pp. 144–150, 1998.

[14] O. Wallner and B. Wallner, "Balloon dilation of benign esophageal rings or strictures: a randomized clinical trial comparing two different inflation times," *Diseases of the Esophagus*, vol. 27, no. 2, pp. 109–111, 2014.

[15] A. Temiz, P. Oguzkurt, S. S. Ezer, E. Ince, and A. Hicsonmez, "Long-term management of corrosive esophageal stricture with balloon dilation in children," *Surgical Endoscopy*, vol. 24, no. 9, pp. 2287–2292, 2010.

[16] I. Uygun, M. S. Arslan, B. Aydogdu, M. H. Okur, and S. Otcu, "Fluoroscopic balloon dilatation for caustic esophageal stricture in children: an 8-year experience," *Journal of Pediatric Surgery*, vol. 48, no. 11, pp. 2230–2234, 2013.

[17] A. Kukkady and P. Pease, "Long-term dilatation of caustic strictures of the oesophagus," *Pediatric Surgery International*, vol. 18, no. 5-6, pp. 486–490, 2002.

[18] S. Contini, M. Garatti, A. Swarray-Deen, N. Depetris, S. Cecchini, and C. Scarpignato, "Corrosive oesophageal strictures in children: outcomes after timely or delayed dilatation," *Digestive and Liver Disease*, vol. 41, no. 4, pp. 263–268, 2009.

[19] O. Mutaf, "Treatment of corrosive esophageal strictures by long-term stenting," *Journal of Pediatric Surgery*, vol. 31, no. 5, pp. 681–685, 1996.

Tumor Location Correlates with Clinicopathological Features and Prognosis of the Solid Pseudopapillary Neoplasm

Zibo Meng,[1] Mingsi Cao,[2] Feiyang Wang,[1] Yushun Zhang,[1] and Heshui Wu[1]

[1]*Department of Pancreatic Surgery, Union Hospital, Tongji Medical College, Huazhong University of Science and Technology, Wuhan 430022, China*
[2]*Institute of Cardiology, Union Hospital, Tongji Medical College, Huazhong University of Science and Technology, Wuhan 430022, China*

Correspondence should be addressed to Feiyang Wang; 1335528702@qq.com and Heshui Wu; heshuiwu@hust.edu.cn

Academic Editor: Alessandro Zerbi

Background. Solid pseudopapillary neoplasms (SPNs) of the pancreas are rare neoplasms with low malignant behavior. These neoplasms can be aggressive and cause bad ending of SPN patients. The purpose of this article is to identify certain prognostic factors. *Method.* We retrospectively evaluated 196 patients from our hospital and SEER database. We identified that tumor location was an independent prognostic indicator of SPN patients. *Results.* DSS and OS of pancreatic head SPNs (HOP) were significantly shorter than those of other locations (OOP). Operation methods and age were different between HOP and OOP groups. Compared to OOP group, patients in HOP group were younger. Operation time was longer, and hospital stays were longer. *Conclusion.* This work suggests that pancreatic head SPNs have distinct clinicopathological features and clinical outcome. It is urgent to optimize the treatment of SPN patients and identify effective prognostic indicators of SPN.

1. Introduction

Solid pseudopapillary neoplasms (SPNs) of the pancreas are uncommon, constituting 1%-2% of all pancreatic tumors [1]. It was first reported by Frantz in 1959 and classified as solid pseudopapillary tumors by the World Health Organization (WHO) in 1996 and redefined in 2010 [2]. SPNs are low, yet unpredictable, malignant potential tumors which always occur in young female [3]. The disease among most of the patients is localized, only 9–15% occurring with metastasis or local invasion [4]. At present, surgical treatment is the primary treatment for SPN. After complete margin-negative resection of the SPN, most of the patients are cured, with a low recurrence rate ranging from 2% to 9.4% according to several published SPN case series [5–10]. And the 5-year survival is favorable about 94%–97% [3, 11].

Although most SPN patients have excellent prognosis, some SPNs still exhibit malignant features, leading to recurrence and death of SPN patients. Articles reported that age, gender, tumor diameter, Ki-67 index, extrahepatic metastasis, complete resection of metastases, and recurrence might relate to the aggressive behaviors of the SPNs [12, 13]. However, the cases of SPN are relatively rare and above conclusions are based on small-sample case series and case reports. Reliable prognostic indicators need to be further identified and verified through large sample data analysis.

We know that different tumor sites of the same kind of tumor lead to distinct tumor invasion, relapse, and metastasis states. Khashab et al. report that the head location of pancreatic serous cystic neoplasms (SCNs), which are considered premalignant neoplasms, predicts the tumor aggressive behavior [14]. The degree of malignancy and slow progression between SPN and SCN are similar. Compared with other locations (OOP), the pancreatic head SPNs (HOP) have different clinicopathological features and clinical outcomes. Therefore, we collected 196 SPN cases to explore these clinical features of pancreatic head SPNs.

2. Materials and Methods

2.1. Patients and Data Collection. SPN cases were from our hospital and SEER database. From April 2012 to September 2016, 55 cases of SPN were diagnosed and received surgical treatment in our hospital. We retrospectively evaluated these patients and included all the eligible cases. Data including age, gender, race, symptoms, location, tumor size, surgical options, operation time, complication, number of lymph nodes removed, postoperative diet recovery time, postoperative hospital stay, total hospital stay, and survival information were extracted from medical records in our hospital. Survival period was measured from the time of diagnosis to the time of death or until January 15, 2018. This study was approved by the ethics committee of Union Hospital, Tongji Medical College, Huazhong University of Science and Technology. The written informed consent was obtained from all 55 participants in our institution.

For the cases from SEER database, we used SEER*Stat software (version 8.3.4) to obtain the SPN cohort. We identified SPNs according to ICD-O-3 histology code (code: 8452). Patients were included if (1) diagnostic confirmation was positive histology or/and cytology; (2) SPN was the first tumor; (3) surgical procedure was applied; and (4) prognostic information was available. We extracted the available clinicopathological data which was mentioned above (including age, gender, race, location, tumor size, surgical options, number of lymph nodes removed, and outcome) from the SPN data list. Patients were followed up until December 2014. Since SEER data were from the public database, no ethical consent was needed for this part.

We divided the SPNs into the pancreas head originated group (HOP) and other parts originated group (OOP) in order to further analyze the clinicopathological features and prognostic character of the pancreatic head SPNs.

2.2. Statistical Analysis. We used chi-square test or Fisher's exact test to process qualitative variables. Two-sided Student's t-test or Wilcoxon test was applied to calculate the quantitative parameters. We applied Kaplan-Meier analyses with the log-rank test to examine the statistical differences in survival and portray the patient survival curves (disease-specific survival (DSS) and overall survival (OS)). We also used Cox proportional hazards regression analyses to calculate the hazard ratios with 95% CIs and to exhibit the effects on DSS and OS of the location of the SPNs. All p values were 2-sided, and p values < 0.05 were considered statistically significant. All the analyses were conducted using SPSS software version 20.0 (SPSS Inc., USA).

3. Results

3.1. Clinicopathological Features of Extracted SPN Cases. In total, 196 cases including 55 cases from our institution and 141 SEER cases were selected into our study. Most of the patients were female. The age of the patients ranged from 8 to 90 years (mean, 34.5 years) for all patients in two cohorts. In SEER group, 101 (71.6%), 16 (11.3%), 20 (14.2%), and 4 (2.8%) patients were white, yellow, black, and other races, respectively. All patients in our department were yellow. In our cases, 24 SPNs (42.9%) occurred in pancreatic head, 9 (16.1%) SPNs in pancreatic body, 11 (19.6%) SPNs in the pancreatic tail, and 11 (19.6%) SPNs were in other locations. Similar proportion was also shown in SEER cohort. The median tumor size was 5.0 cm and 5.4 cm, respectively, in our cases and SEER cases. We defined operation methods into four categories: OP1: local excision of tumor; OP2: partial pancreatectomy and partial or local pancreatectomy and duodenectomy without distal/partial gastrectomy; OP3: Whipple's procedure and extended pancreatoduodenectomy; and OP4: other operation methods. In total, 8 patients underwent OP1 procedure; 114 patients underwent OP2 procedure; and 40 and 30 patients, respectively, performed OP3 and OP4 surgeries. Mean number of resected lymph nodes was 8 (ranged 0 to 52) during the surgery. Clinical data of SPN patients in our hospital was more detailed. The most common initial presentation was found by accident (26/55, 47.3%), followed by abdominal pain (22/55, 40.0%), abdominal mass (5/55, 9.1%), and other symptoms (2/55, 3.6%). 31 patients (31/54, 57.4%) experienced postoperative complications including biliary fistula, infection, hemorrhage, intestinal fistula, and pancreatic fistula. Median operation time took was about 330 minutes, and restoration of oral feeding time was about 6 days. Median postoperative discharged time was about 12 days, and the total hospital stay was about 17 days. All the clinicopathological details were summarized in Table 1.

3.2. Disease-Specific Survival and Overall Survival for Different SPN Locations. Survival information of pancreas head-originated SPNs were listed in Table 2. We analyzed survival data of 188 patients including 47 cases from our hospital and 141 SEER cases. The average follow-up time was 33.7 months in our department and 58.3 months in SEER database. In all patients, 5 cases suffered from SPN-related death and 14 patients died from all causes. In SEER cohort, 1-, 3-, and 5-year DSS rates were 98.5%, 97.8%, and 97.1%, respectively, and the 1-, 3-, and 5-year OS rates were 97.8%, 97.2%, and 95.7%, respectively. In our cohort, the HOP group had lower 1- and 3-year overall survival rates compared to the OOP group. For the small number of SPN patients in our hospital, we only used SEER cohort to analyze the prognostic factor. Table 3 shows the prognostic factors of the DSS and OS. Multivariate analysis showed that only tumor location ($p = 0.028$) was statistically related to DSS. Tumor location ($p = 0.022$) influenced the OS of SPN patients. The DSS and OS K-M curves according to the classification of location are shown in Figure 1.

3.3. Comparison of Clinicopathological Parameters between HOP and OOP. Analyzed results are given in Table 4. Chi-square test or Fisher's exact test results showed that operation methods ($p < 0.001$) were statistically distinct between HOP and OOP in both cohorts. However, there were no differences between HOP and OOP in gender, symptom ($p = 0.979$), and complication ($p = 0.667$). Student's t-test or Wilcoxon test exhibited that age, operation time ($p < 0.001$), and hospital stay ($p = 0.05$) were different between HOP and

Table 1: Clinicopathological features of the SPN patients in our study.

Characteristics	Our cohort Numbers (percentage)	Characteristics	SEER cohort Numbers (percentage)
Age	29 (16–45)	Age	33 (22–45)
Sex		Sex	
Male	12 (21.8)	Male	23 (16.3)
Female	43 (78.2)	Female	118 (83.7)
Location		Location	
Head	24 (42.9)	Head	35 (24.8)
Body	9 (16.1)	Body	19 (13.5)
Tail	11 (19.6)	Tail	69 (48.9)
Others	11 (19.6)	Others	18 (12.8)
Size	5.0 (4.0–7.0)	Size	5.4 (3.5–9.5)
Operation category		Operation category	
1	3	1	5 (3.5)
2	33	2	81 (57.4)
3	18	3	22 (15.6)
4	1	4	29 (20.6)
Symptom		Race	
Pain	22 (40)	White	101 (71.6)
Asymptomatic	26 (47.3)	Yellow	16 (11.3)
Mass	5 (9.1)	Black	20 (14.2)
Others	2 (3.6)	Lymph nodes examined	
Complication arise	31 (57.4)	≤5	65 (47.8)
Operation time	330 (270–435)	>5	71 (52.2)
Postoperative diet days	6 (3.5–9)		
Discharge days	12 (10.5–19)		
Hospital stay, days	17 (13.5–31)		

Values are expressed as number (percentage) or median (Q1–Q3). Operation category: 1: local excision of tumor; 2: partial pancreatectomy and partial or local pancreatectomy and duodenectomy without distal/partial gastrectomy; 3: Whipple's procedure and extended pancreatoduodenectomy; and 4: other operation methods.

Table 2: Survival data of 188 SPN cases in our study.

Our cohort Survival characteristics	Parameter	SEER cohort Survival characteristics	Parameter
Follow-up time		Follow-up time	
Mean (m ± SD)	33.7 ± 18.7	Mean (m ± SD)	58.3 ± 51.3
Median (m, range)	28 (9–65)	Median (m, range)	50 (2–152)
Survival data		Survival data	
All-cause deaths	5	SPN-related deaths	5
Survival rates (%)		All-cause deaths	9
1/3 OS	95.7/89.4	Survival rates (%)	
1/3 HOP-OS	92.3/88.5	1/3/5 DSS	98.5/97.8/97.1
1/3 OOP-OS	100/90.5	1/3/5 OS	97.8/97.2/95.7

OOP, while size, restoration of oral feeding time, and postoperative discharged time were not different between the two groups. We further investigated the data of 5 patients who died in our hospital; tumors of these patients had bigger sizes than the average level (mean size, 8.6 cm versus 6.1 cm). There was no significant difference in other data including ki67, β-catenin, vimentin, CD56, and CD10.

4. Discussion

SPNs are rare pancreatic cystic neoplasms which account for 1% of all pancreatic tumors and 3% of all cystic pancreas neoplasms [15]. With the continuous improvement of multi-detector computed tomography (CT) technology, there has been a remarkable increase in the number of incidentally

Table 3: Prognostic factors for DSS and OS in SEER cohort according to univariate and multivariate analysis.

Survival	Univariate analysis				Multivariate analysis			
DSS	HR	Down	Up	p value	HR	Down	Up	p value
Race	0.54	0.10	2.89	0.47				
Age	1.02	0.96	1.08	0.62				
Gender	1.22	0.14	11.04	0.86				
Location	13.99	1.56	125.33	0.02	12.75	1.31	124.21	0.028
Size	1.009	0.959	1.063	0.719				
Operation methods	1.49	0.58	3.78	0.41				
Lymph nodes examined	1.04	0.98	1.11	0.23				
OS	HR	Down	Up	p value	HR	Down	Up	p value
Race	0.78	0.29	0.78	0.63				
Age	1.03	0.99	1.08	0.17				
Gender	1.35	0.28	6.55	0.71				
Location	4.04	1.08	15.07	0.038	6.08	1.29	28.66	0.022
Size	1.01	0.94	1.08	0.89				
Operation methods	1.42	0.70	2.87	0.33				
Lymph nodes examined	1.03	0.97	1.09	0.31				

DSS: disease-specific survival; OS: overall survival; HR: hazard ratio.

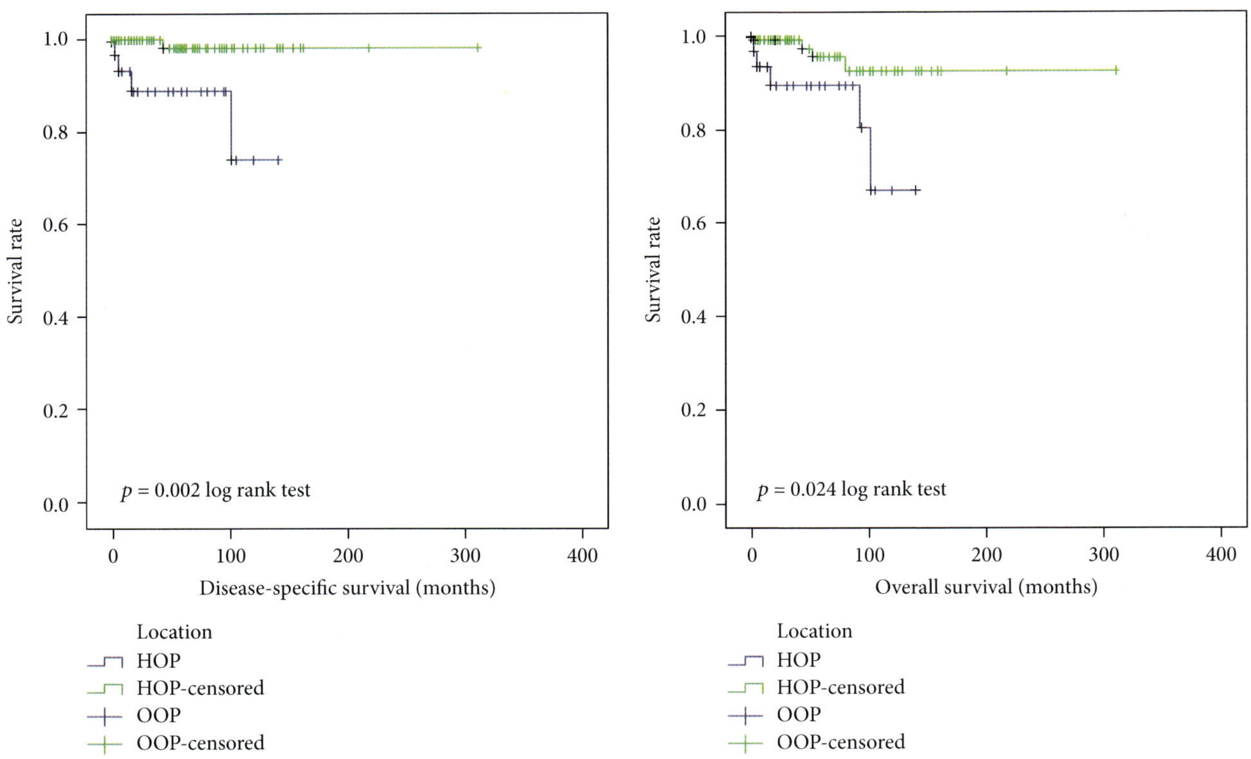

Figure 1: The DSS and OS K-M curves of SEER cohort according to the classification of location.

detected pancreatic cysts over the last decade [16]. It is not difficult to understand why the number of SPN cases reported throughout the literature was also increasing. Therefore, identifying SPNs that have the potential for malignancy seems particularly important. Considering the rarity of SPN, we collected 55 SPN cases surgically treated at our hospital and 141 SPN cases from SEER database to identify the potential factors which need to be considered when making treatment plan.

In our analysis, the majority of patients were young women, and SPNs often showed nonspecific symptoms, such as pain and discomfort. Patients' prognosis was excellent, with a 97.1% 5-year DSS rate and a 95.7% 5-year OS rate in SEER cohort. These data basically consisted of the information

TABLE 4: Comparison of selected clinicopathological parameters between the HOP group and the OOP group.

Character	Our cohort HOP	OOP	*p* value	Character	SEER cohort HOP	OOP	*p* value
Gender			0.069	Gender			0.496
Male	15	20		Male	7	16	
Female	44	117		Female	28	90	
Operation			<0.001	Operation			<0.001
1	0	3		1	3	2	
2	5	28		2	11	70	
3	18	0		3	15	7	
4	1	0		4	5	24	
Age			0.007	Age			0.647
Juvenile	11	4		Juvenile	3	12	
Adult	13	27		Adult	32	94	
Symptom			0.979	Race			0.152
Pain	9	13		White	25	76	
By accident	12	14		Yellow	6	10	
Mass	2	3		Black	2	18	
Others	1	1					
Complication			0.667				
No	11	12					
Yes	13	18					
Age (year)	26.21 (18.08)	36.61 (16.89)	0.03	Age (year)	30.57 (12.94)	37.01 (15.77)	0.03
Size (cm)	5.50 (3.05)	6.50 (3.72)	0.29	Size (cm)	6.54 (3.29)	7.64 (10.09)	0.55
Operation time (minute)	371.74 (121.61)	228.87 (71.62)	<0.001	Examined lymph nodes	11.74 (9.53)	7.10 (8.17)	0.01
Examined lymph nodes	8.20 (5.02)	6.27 (5.53)	0.36				
Restoration oral feeding (day)	7.93 (6.40)	4.82 (2.70)	0.10				
Postoperative discharge (day)	18.96 (16.98)	13.52 (5.70)	0.10				
Hospital stay (day)	27.46 (18.58)	19.03 (7.89)	0.05				

reported in the former literature [11, 17]. In comparison to tumors located in other sites, patients in the HOP group were younger than those in the OOP group. Tumor location determined the surgical approach and also influenced the number of resected lymph nodes. Compared with the OOP group, HOP patients had longer operation time and hospital stay. What is more, patients with tumors which developed in the head of the pancreas had a worse prognosis according to our survival analysis. To our knowledge, this is the first study to identify the clinicopathological characteristics related to pancreatic head SPNs.

In public mind, SPN is a kind of cystic, solid, and localized tumor with an excellent prognosis [2]. The treatment of SPN is complete resection no matter with or without metastasis. Local resection or enucleation is employed for small tumors with complete capsule; pancreatic head tumor is treated with pancreatoduodenectomy (Whipple procedure); distal pancreatectomy is performed for pancreatic body and/or tail tumors [18]. For SPN patients in different situations, in addition to these location-related basic rules, there are no clear rules and differences for surgical methods and follow-up examinations. However, there are still some SPNs which may behave aggressively and lead to poor ending. Yin et al. reported that large tumor size, pancreatic tail localization, and disrupted capsule were viewed as the malignant SPN phenotype [19]. Mao considered that SPNs in older and male patients were more aggressive [20]. In our research, tumor size, gender, pancreatic tail location, and age have no significant correlation to the patients' prognosis. Pancreatic head location seems more worthy of our attention. Goh et al. reported that age, sex, tumor size, elevated CEA, and elevated CA-199 could not predict the malignancy of SPN before surgery, and our results were largely similar to the conclusion of Goh's data [21]. Researchers supposed that pancreatic head SPNs could lead to the apparent clinical symptoms which increased the chances of early detection and thus avoid further tumor progression [19]. However, in our study, there was no significant difference in the clinical symptoms between different tumor sites ($p = 0.979$) and the prognosis was worse in pancreatic head SPN patients which did not support the abovementioned theory. We infer poor prognosis of SPNs in the pancreatic head may be due to the following reasons.

From the anatomical standpoint, the head of the pancreas is rich in blood supply and surrounded by many lymph nodes, which facilitates the early metastasis of SPN. Pancreatic head and descendant duodenum are closely linked, which provides the direction for the invasion of SPN. From the perspective of embryonic development, pancreatic head originates from the ventral pancreas, and the other parts originate from the dorsal pancreas. It can also partly explain the differences in the clinicopathological features and outcomes of SPNs at different tumor locations. In terms of surgical treatment, pancreatic head SPNs are primarily treated by pancreatoduodenectomy. Due to the difficulty of its operation procedures, the probability of intraoperative tumor implantation and postoperative complications would be increased, and the prognosis of patients will be influenced accordingly.

For the above reason, the treatment and follow-up of pancreatic head SPNs should be more cautious. Complete surgical resection, with negative surgical margins, needs to be applied in these patients. Appropriate lymphadenectomy is necessary to prevent the nodal metastases, and the follow-up period of these patients should be extended appropriately. The limitations to this study include the small number of cases and the retrospective nature. Long-term follow-up is necessary because of the indolent character of SPN. The patients are predominantly yellow and white, and extensive multicenter studies with more races are needed to identify the risk factors associated with the SPN patients' outcome. What is more, due to the reason of data collection, the roles of pathology results, radiotherapy, and chemotherapy have not been identified in our study. More prognostic factors such as tumor calcification, solid component, capsule integrity, and IHC markers need to be explored in further research.

5. Conclusion

SPNs are rare tumors with good prognosis. Tumor sites are associated with the prognosis of SPN patients. Patients with pancreatic head SPNs have worse outcome and accompany distinct clinicopathological features.

Authors' Contributions

Zibo Meng, Mingsi Cao, and Feiyang Wang contributed equally to this work.

Acknowledgments

This work was supported by the National Natural Science Foundation of China (Grant no. 81372261).

References

[1] R. C. G. Martin, D. S. Klimstra, M. F. Brennan, and K. C. Conlon, "Solid-pseudopapillary tumor of the pancreas: a surgical enigma?," *Annals of Surgical Oncology*, vol. 9, no. 1, pp. 35–40, 2002.

[2] S. Suzuki, T. Hatori, T. Furukawa, K. Shiratori, and M. Yamamoto, "Clinical and pathological features of solid pseudopapillary neoplasms of the pancreas at a single institution," *Digestive Surgery*, vol. 31, no. 2, pp. 143–150, 2014.

[3] T. Papavramidis and S. Papavramidis, "Solid pseudopapillary tumors of the pancreas: review of 718 patients reported in english literature," *Journal of the American College of Surgeons*, vol. 200, no. 6, pp. 965–972, 2005.

[4] J. K. Law, A. Ahmed, V. K. Singh et al., "A systematic review of solid-pseudopapillary neoplasms: are these rare lesions?," *Pancreas*, vol. 43, no. 3, pp. 331–337, 2014.

[5] T. Morikawa, T. Onogawa, S. Maeda et al., "Solid pseudopapillary neoplasms of the pancreas: an 18-year experience at a single japanese institution," *Surgery Today*, vol. 43, no. 1, pp. 26–32, 2013.

[6] N. Lubezky, M. Papoulas, Y. Lessing et al., "Solid pseudopapillary neoplasm of the pancreas: management and long-term outcome," *European Journal of Surgical Oncology*, vol. 43, no. 6, pp. 1056–1060, 2017.

[7] J. S. Lee, H. J. Han, S. B. Choi, C. W. Jung, T. J. Song, and S. Y. Choi, "Surgical outcomes of solid pseudopapillary neoplasm of the pancreas: a single institution's experience for the last ten years," *The American Surgeon*, vol. 78, no. 2, pp. 216–219, 2012.

[8] A. El Nakeeb, M. Abdel Wahab, W. F. Elkashef, M. Azer, and T. Kandil, "Solid pseudopapillary tumour of the pancreas: incidence, prognosis and outcome of surgery (single center experience)," *International Journal of Surgery*, vol. 11, no. 6, pp. 447–457, 2013.

[9] M. J. Kim, D. W. Choi, S. H. Choi, J. S. Heo, and J. Y. Sung, "Surgical treatment of solid pseudopapillary neoplasms of the pancreas and risk factors for malignancy," *The British Journal of Surgery*, vol. 101, no. 10, pp. 1266–1271, 2014.

[10] Y. Cai, X. Ran, S. Xie et al., "Surgical management and long-term follow-up of solid pseudopapillary tumor of pancreas: a large series from a single institution," *Journal of Gastrointestinal Surgery*, vol. 18, no. 5, pp. 935–940, 2014.

[11] S. Reddy, J. L. Cameron, J. Scudiere et al., "Surgical management of solid-pseudopapillary neoplasms of the pancreas (Franz or Hamoudi tumors): a large single-institutional series," *Journal of the American College of Surgeons*, vol. 208, no. 5, pp. 950–957, 2009.

[12] N. Vassos, A. Agaimy, P. Klein, W. Hohenberger, and R. S. Croner, "Solid-pseudopapillary neoplasm (spn) of the pancreas: case series and literature review on an enigmatic entity," *International Journal of Clinical and Experimental Pathology*, vol. 6, no. 6, pp. 1051–1059, 2013.

[13] M. Xu, X. Shi, T. Wan et al., "Treatment and prognosis of solid pseudopapillary neoplasms with metastases or recurrence," *Zhonghua Wai Ke Za Zhi*, vol. 53, no. 9, pp. 685–689, 2015.

[14] M. A. Khashab, E. J. Shin, S. Amateau et al., "Tumor size and location correlate with behavior of pancreatic serous cystic neoplasms," *American Journal of Gastroenterology*, vol. 106, no. 8, pp. 1521–1526, 2011.

[15] F. Yang, D. L. Fu, C. Jin et al., "Clinical experiences of solid pseudopapillary tumors of the pancreas in China," *Journal of Gastroenterology and Hepatology*, vol. 23, no. 12, pp. 1847–1851, 2008.

[16] T. A. Laffan, K. M. Horton, A. P. Klein et al., "Prevalence of unsuspected pancreatic cysts on MDCT," *AJR. American Journal of Roentgenology*, vol. 191, no. 3, pp. 802–807, 2008.

[17] S. Ozkara, F. Vardar Aker, A. Yitik et al., "Solid pseudopapillary tumor of the pancreas: a case series of 9 patients," *The Turkish Journal of Gastroenterology*, vol. 23, no. 6, pp. 727–735, 2012.

[18] P. F. Yu, Z. H. Hu, X. B. Wang et al., "Solid pseudopapillary tumor of the pancreas: a review of 553 cases in chinese literature," *World Journal of Gastroenterology*, vol. 16, no. 10, pp. 1209–1214, 2010.

[19] Q. Yin, M. Wang, C. Wang et al., "Differentiation between benign and malignant solid pseudopapillary tumor of the pancreas by MDCT," *European Journal of Radiology*, vol. 81, no. 11, pp. 3010–3018, 2012.

[20] C. Mao, M. Guvendi, D. R. Domenico, K. Kim, N. R. Thomford, and J. M. Howard, "Papillary cystic and solid tumors of the pancreas: a pancreatic embryonic tumor? Studies of three cases and cumulative review of the world's literature," *Surgery*, vol. 118, no. 5, pp. 821–828, 1995.

[21] B. K. P. Goh, Y. M. Tan, P. C. Cheow et al., "Solid pseudopapillary neoplasms of the pancreas: an updated experience," *Journal of Surgical Oncology*, vol. 95, no. 8, pp. 640–644, 2007.

Blood Ammonia Level Correlates with Severity of Cirrhotic Portal Hypertensive Gastropathy

Feriel El-Kalla,[1] Loai Mansour,[1] Abdelrahman Kobtan,[1] Asmaa Elzeftawy,[1] Lobna Abo Ali,[1] Sherief Abd-Elsalam,[1] Sahar Elyamani,[1] Mohamed Yousef,[1] I. Amer,[2] H. Mourad,[3] and Mohamed Elhendawy[1]

[1]*Tropical Medicine and Infectious Diseases Department, Faculty of Medicine, Tanta University, Tanta, Egypt*
[2]*Hepatology and Gastroenterology Department, Faculty of Medicine, Kafrelsheikh University, Kafr Elsheikh, Egypt*
[3]*Clinical Pathology Department, Faculty of Medicine, Tanta University, Tanta, Egypt*

Correspondence should be addressed to Abdelrahman Kobtan; aakobtan@yahoo.com

Academic Editor: Mario Pirisi

Background. Portal hypertensive gastropathy (PHG) is a common anomaly with potential for bleeding found in portal hypertension. Blood ammonia levels correlate well with liver disease severity and existence of portosystemic shunts. Increased ammonia results in vasodilation and hepatic stellate cell activation causing and exacerbating portal hypertension. *Objective.* To assess the relation of blood ammonia to the presence and severity of portal hypertensive gastropathy in cirrhosis. *Methods.* This cross-sectional study included 381 cirrhotics undergoing screening for esophageal varices (EV) divided into a portal hypertensive gastropathy group (203 patients with EV and PHG), esophageal varix group (41 patients with EV but no PHG), and control group (137 patients with no EV or PHG). A full clinical examination, routine laboratory tests, abdominal ultrasonography, child score calculation, and blood ammonia measurement were performed for all patients. *Results.* Blood ammonia, portal vein, splenic vein, and splenic longitudinal diameters were significantly higher and platelet counts lower in patients with EV and EV with PHG than controls. Patients having EV with PHG had significantly higher bilirubin and ammonia than those with EV but no PHG. Severe PHG was associated with significantly higher ammonia, EV grades, and superior location and a lower splenic longitudinal diameter than mild PHG. The PHG score showed a positive correlation with blood ammonia and a negative correlation with splenic longitudinal diameter. *Conclusions.* Blood ammonia levels correlate with the presence, severity, and score of portal hypertensive gastropathy in cirrhosis suggesting a causal relationship and encouraging trials of ammonia-lowering treatments for the management of severe PHG with a tendency to bleed.

1. Introduction

Portal hypertensive gastropathy (PHG) is a gastric mucosal anomaly commonly found in patients with portal hypertension [1]. It is more common and more aggressive in patients with cirrhosis than in those with portal hypertension due to noncirrhotic conditions [2].

The key element for the development of PHG is portal hypertension causing vascular congestion of the gastric mucosa with a resultant activation of cytokines, growth factors, and hormones that maintain and further the pathology which is characterized by capillary and venule dilatation, as well as congestion and tortuosity of the submucosal venules together with possible lamina propria stromal fibrosis and edema [3–5].

The endoscopic appearance is characterized by a mosaic or snake-skin-like appearance most commonly at the gastric body and fundus which may be associated with the presence of red spots [6].

PHG has been classified into mild and severe forms by different classification systems with the mild form in general having an appearance of mosaic-like pattern, scarlatiniform rash, superficial reddening, and snake-skin pattern, and the severe form displaying added red marks of variable diameter, with or without bleeding [7, 8]. The Baveno scoring system also classifies PHG into mild and severe using a score calculation that incorporates the presence or absence of gastric antral vascular ectasia (GAVE) [9]. This system has been found to be accurate in reflection of the bleeding risk from PHG among cirrhotic patients [10].

PHG is accountable for approximately 8% of nonvariceal upper gastrointestinal bleeding in hepatic patients [11]. Acute bleeding may infrequently complicate PHG especially when severe, yet chronic gastric mucosal bleeding leading to recurrent iron deficiency anemia is much more common and occurs in around 11–25% of cases [6, 7, 12, 13].

The major risk factors for PHG bleeding are increased duration, extent, and severity together with advanced cirrhosis, and eradication of esophageal varices by sclerotherapy or band ligation [3, 14].

Blood ammonia levels have been found to correlate well with the severity of liver disease and existence of portosystemic shunts, especially esophageal varices [15]. Accumulation of ammonia in splanchnic vessels in cases of liver function impairment results in vasodilatation and increased portal blood flow bringing about portal hypertension [16, 17]. There are indications that ammonia also affects endoplasmic reticulum dynamics and induces oxidative stress, both of which result in hepatic stellate cell (HSC) activation with production of multiple proinflammatory, contractile, and profibrogenic genes and proteins. A trial involving removal of ammonia in vitro, and lowering ammonia in vivo, has documented a downregulation of HSC activation markers with resulting reestablishment of HSC biology, suggesting that ammonia is a possible target for therapy directed at lowering portal hypertension [18].

PHG is a common manifestation of portal hypertension, and therefore, we aimed at finding out if blood ammonia levels correlate with the presence and severity of portal hypertensive gastropathy in cirrhotic patients.

2. Patients and Methods

This cross-sectional study was conducted on 381 cirrhotic patients positive for HCV or HBV attending the Tropical Medicine Endoscopy Unit, Tanta University, for endoscopic screening of esophageal varices. The study was conducted during the period from 7/1/2017 to 2/28/2018, 2018. The sample size of 381 was calculated based on a previous study by Kumar et al., who found the prevalence of portal hypertensive gastropathy in patients with cirrhosis to be 55%, with 5% precision and 95% confidence level [19]. Patients were excluded from the study if they had cardiac or kidney failure, hepatic encephalopathy or coma, active gastrointestinal bleeding, a history of bleeding during the previous two weeks to inclusion in the study, hepatocellular carcinoma, or portal vein thrombosis or were taking lactulose. Patients with factors affecting the portal pressure and gastric mucosal vascularity and blood flow such as those taking beta blockers and those for whom a previous intervention for varices (sclerotherapy, endoscopic band ligation, or scleroligation) or PHG (argon plasma coagulation or gastric mucosal band ligation) had been performed were also excluded.

A total of 381 patients were enrolled in the study. They were divided into three groups: (1) the portal hypertensive gastropathy group—203 patients with esophageal varices (EV) and PHG, (2) the esophageal varix group—41 patients with EV but no PHG, and (3) the control group—137 patients with no EV or PHG.

A detailed history was taken; a full clinical examination, routine laboratory tests, and pelvic-abdominal ultrasonography were performed for all participating patients after obtaining an informed written consent. Child-Pugh scores were calculated for each patient.

To overcome potential bias of results, study collaborators who were not involved in the upper endoscopy procedures screened and enrolled the participants, and all endoscopists were blinded to the study outcome.

2.1. Upper GI Endoscopy. Upper GI endoscopy was performed for all the patients. Classification of varices was performed according to the Japanese classification [20]. This involved recording of location (L), form (F), color (C), and red color signs (RC) of the varices. Classification and scoring of portal hypertensive gastropathy were performed according to the Baveno II scoring system; the mild mucosal mosaic pattern was given 1 point, and the severe pattern, 2 points. Isolated red markings were given 1 point, and confluent markings, 2. The presence of gastric antral vascular ectasia (GAVE) was noted and a further 2 points added to the score when flat or slightly raised, red stripes were seen radiating from the pylorus to the antrum and body of the stomach. PHG is considered mild when the score is ≤ 3 and severe at a score ≥ 4 [9].

2.2. Measurement of Blood Ammonia Level. A venous blood sample was collected from each patient after a minimum of 6 hours of fasting and 9 hours of abstinence from smoking. All patients had been instructed not to perform any physical exercise the day before.

The samples were taken at the laboratory, put in EDTA-containing sterile specimen tubes, and separated within 15 minutes of collection to be analyzed immediately. These precautions are necessary as the ammonia content of standing blood increases spontaneously due to generation and release of ammonia from red blood cells and due to deamination of amino acids by enzymes in the blood. Analysis was performed by the enzymatic method using reagents manufactured by BIOLABO SAS, Maizy, France.

2.3. Statistical Analysis. Statistical analysis was carried out using SPSS, version 15 for Microsoft Windows (SPSS, Chicago, Illinois, USA). The statistical data were reported as mean ± SD, frequencies (number), and percentages when appropriate. A comparison of numerical variables between the study groups was performed using one-way analysis of variance test followed by post hoc Tukey's multiple comparison test when data were normally distributed. Student's *t*-test was used to compare independent samples from two groups when the samples were normally distributed. Pearson's correlation was used to quantify the association between continuous variables. To compare categorical

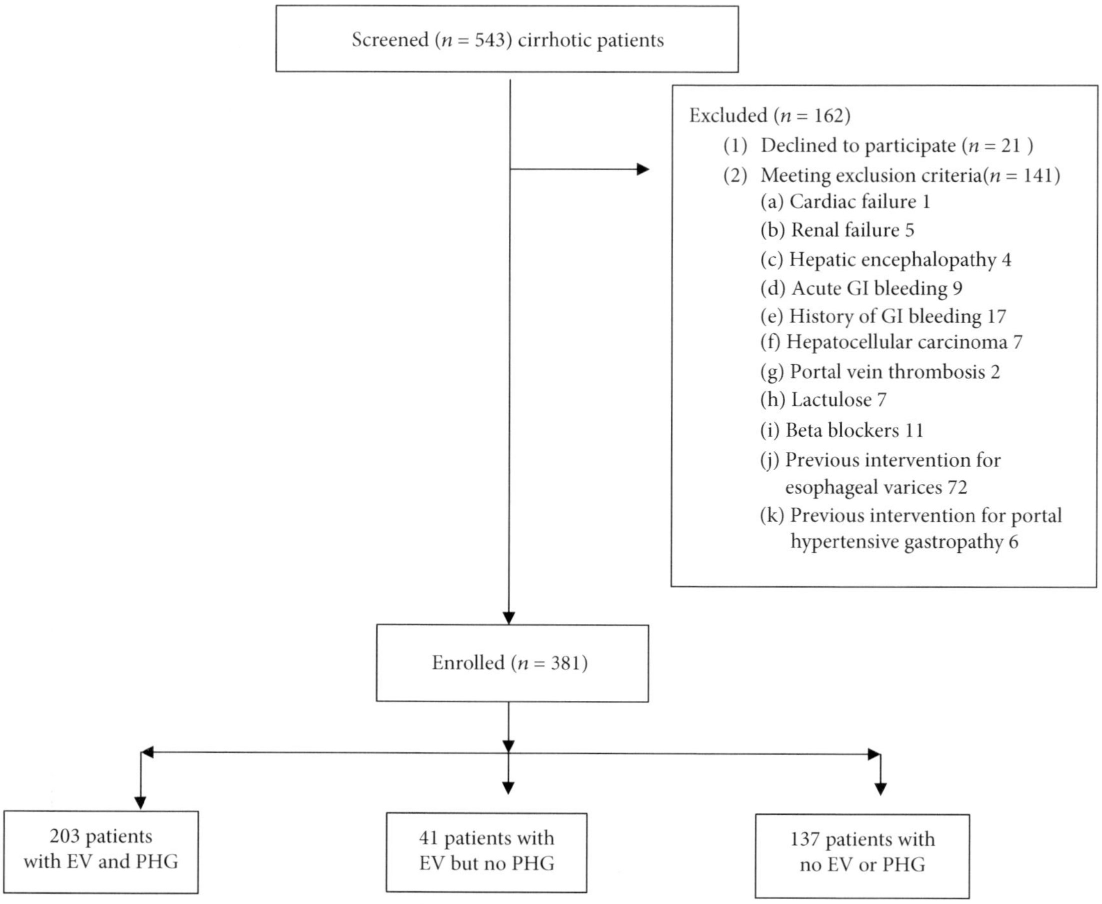

FIGURE 1: Study analysis population. *n*: number of patients; EV: esophageal varices; PHG: portal hypertensive gastropathy.

data, the χ^2 test was performed. P values less than 0.05 (two-tailed) were considered statistically significant.

2.4. Ethical Considerations. All participating subjects provided written informed consents. The study protocol conforms to the ethical guidelines of the 1975 Declaration of Helsinki as reflected in a prior approval by the institution's human research committee. The study was approved by the Ethics Committee of the Faculty of Medicine, Tanta University (approval code 31588/06/17).

3. Results

In total, 543 cirrhotic patients attending the Tropical Medicine Endoscopy Unit, Tanta University, were screened for participation in this study. 162 were excluded due to the presence of exclusion criteria in 141 patients and refusal to participate by 21. Thus, 381 cirrhotic patients were enrolled in this cross-sectional study; they were 258 males (67.7%) and 123 females (32.3%) (Figure 1). Testing for HCV RNA was positive for 377, whereas only 4 patients were HBV DNA positive. The participants were divided into three groups with no significant differences regarding distribution of age, sex, or Child-Pugh class: (1) the portal hypertensive gastropathy group—203 (53.28%) patients with EV and PHG, (2) the esophageal varices group—41 (10.76%) patients with EV but no PHG, and (3) the control group—137 (35.96%) patients with neither EV nor PHG (Table 1).

Patient baseline characteristics and demographic data are presented in Table 1. Platelet counts were significantly lower among patients with EV and PHG as well as those with EV only than in controls ($P < 0.001$). We found the group with EV and PHG to have significantly higher serum bilirubin levels than either controls or patients with EV only ($P = 0.007$) (Table 1).

Blood ammonia was significantly higher among patients with EV than controls and among patients with EV and PHG than among those with EV only as well as controls ($P = 0.001$) (Table 1).

The portal vein, splenic vein, and splenic longitudinal diameters were significantly higher in patients with EV and PHG as well as those with EV only than in controls ($P < 0.001$) (Table 1).

By using the Baveno II PHG scoring system to classify our 203 patients with PHG, we found that 149 (73.4%) had mild PHG (score ≤ 3) and 54 (26.6%) had severe PHG (score ≥ 4) (Table 2).

There was a significant difference between mild and severe PHG patients regarding the grading of the accompanying EV ($P = 0.002$), with a higher percentage of EV grades 1, 3, and 4 among the severe cases. Of interest was the

TABLE 1: Patient baseline characteristics.

Parameter	PHG ($n = 203$)	EV ($n = 41$)	Controls ($n = 137$)	P value
Age, years (mean, SD)	53.57 ± 6.61	55 ± 8.72	52.33 ± 11.06	0.923
Sex: male, n (%)	142 (69.95)	31 (75.61)	85 (62.04)	0.456
Etiology of cirrhosis, n (%)				
Hepatitis C virus	199 (98.03)	41 (100)	137 (100)	0.471
Hepatitis B virus	4 (1.97)	0 (0)	0(0)	
Ascites, n (%)	90 (44.33)	17 (41.46)	39 (28.47)	0.063
History of hepatic encephalopathy, n (%)	28 (13.79)	4 (9.76)	6 (4.38)	0.089
Hemoglobin (g/dL)	11.15 ± 1.81	10.99 ± 1.52	11.31 ± 2.53	0.726
WBCs ($\times 10^9$/L)	5.23 ± 2.22	5.15 ± 2.09	5.93 ± 2.60	0.180
Platelets ($\times 10^9$/L)	101.70 ± 31.34^{a}	100 ± 30.61^{c}	125.54 ± 36.25	<0.001*
ALT (U/L)	43.34 ± 17.49	35.54 ± 15.69	39.28 ± 23.34	0.129
AST (U/L)	62.20 ± 26.62	53.34 ± 30.71	56.64 ± 29.67	0.308
Serum albumin (g/dL)	3.03 ± 0.56	3.05 ± 0.42	3.24 ± 0.61	0.086
Total serum bilirubin (mg/dL)	1.83 ± 1.24^{a,b}	1.29 ± 0.55	1.31 ± 0.92	0.007*
International normalized ratio	1.29 ± 0.24	1.22 ± 0.19	1.24 ± 0.30	0.449
Creatinine (mg/dL)	0.97 ± 0.21	0.94 ± 0.27	0.96 ± 0.24	0.781
Blood ammonia (μg/dL)	162.12 ± 58.17^{a,b}	153.04 ± 59.41^{c}	103.23 ± 72.76	<0.001*
Child-Pugh class, n (%)				
Class A	97 (47.79)	22 (53.66)	77 (56.20)	0.067
Class B	66 (32.51)	17 (41.46)	44 (32.12)	
Class C	40 (19.70)	2 (4.88)	16 (11.68)	
Portal vein diameter (mm)	13.64 ± 1.81^{a}	13.42 ± 1.49^{c}	11.75 ± 2.11	<0.001*
Splenic longitudinal diameter (cm)	15.84 ± 1.69^{a}	15.75 ± 1.74^{c}	14.28 ± 2.65	<0.001*
Splenic vein diameter (mm)	11.19 ± 1.20^{a}	11.10 ± 0.92^{c}	8.55 ± 1.91	<0.001*
Esophageal varices, n (%)	203 (100)	41 (100)	—	—

*Statistically significant at $P < 0.05$; $^{a}P < 0.05$ when compared with controls; $^{b}P < 0.05$ when compared with esophageal varices; $^{c}P < 0.05$ when compared with controls. ALT: alanine aminotransferase; AST: aspartate aminotransferase: WBCs, white blood cells; EV: esophageal varices; PHG: portal hypertensive gastropathy.

absence of grade 4 EV among the patients with mild PHG (Table 2).

A significant difference in EV location was noticed between mild and severe PHG patients ($P = 0.013$), with severe cases having higher percentages of association with locus superior EV than their counterparts with mild PHG (14.82% versus 3.36%, resp.) (Table 2).

We compared between mild and severe cases of PHG with regard to multiple variables and found no difference between them in respect to patient age, blood count, liver function tests, Child-Pugh scores, or portal vein diameter. On the other hand, cases with severe PHG had significantly higher levels of blood ammonia (192.69 ± 59.87 versus 151.39 ± 54.37 μg/dL) ($P = 0.026$) and significantly lower splenic longitudinal diameters ($P = 0.001$) (Table 3).

The PHG score itself was significantly higher with higher locations of the varices ($P = 0.046$) (Table 4).

We further studied the correlation between the PHG score and differential variables which revealed a significant positive correlation with blood ammonia and hemoglobin levels, and a significant negative correlation with the splenic longitudinal diameter ($P < 0.05$) (Table 5).

4. Discussion

Portal hypertensive gastropathy (PHG) is a common gastric mucosal anomaly in patients with cirrhosis and portal hypertension [1]. The condition carries a potential risk of acute and chronic gastrointestinal bleeding among these patients [13]. Evidence suggests that the key factor for the development of PHG is portal hypertension [3].

Increased blood ammonia in cases of liver function impairment is a pathogenetic factor for the production of portal hypertension and has been suggested as a possible target for portal hypertension lowering therapy [16–18]. In the light of this data, we aimed at finding out if blood ammonia levels correlate with severity of portal hypertensive gastropathy in cirrhotic patients.

Platelet counts were significantly lower among patients with EV and PHG as well as those with EV alone than in controls ($P < 0.001$). It has been found by other recent studies that low platelet counts are associated with the presence of varices in viral cirrhotic patients [21–23].

Patients with EV and PHG in our study were found to have significantly higher serum bilirubin levels than either

Table 2: Relationship of PHG severity with demographic, clinical, and endoscopic characteristics.

Parameter	Portal hypertensive gastropathy severity ($n = 203$) Mild ($n = 149$) n	(%)	Severe ($n = 54$) n	(%)	P value
Sex					
Male	105	70.47	37	68.52	0.965
Female	44	29.53	17	31.48	
Child-Pugh class					
Class A	76	51.01	21	38.89	
Class B	41	27.52	25	46.29	0.539
Class C	32	21.47	8	14.82	
EV grading					
Grade 1	56	37.58	25	46.29	
Grade 2	68	45.64	13	24.07	0.002*
Grade 3	25	16.78	12	22.22	
Grade 4	0	0.00	4	7.41	
EV red color sign (RC)					
RC0 (none)	84	56.38	38	70.37	
HCS (hematocystic spots)	20	13.42	0	0.00	0.063
CRS (cherry red spots)	8	5.37	4	7.41	
RWM (red wale markings)	37	24.83	12	22.22	
EV form (F)					
F1	84	56.38	29	53.70	
F2	44	29.53	16	29.63	0.973
F3	21	14.09	9	16.67	
Risk signs					
No	93	62.42	38	70.37	0.578
Yes	56	37.58	16	29.63	
EV location (L)					
LI (inferior)	96	64.43	25	46.29	
LM (medialis)	48	32.22	21	38.89	0.013*
LS (superior)	5	3.36	8	14.82	
EV color (C)					
Cw (white varices)	101	67.78	41	75.93	0.535
Cb (blue varices)	48	32.22	13	24.07	
PHG mosaic pattern					
No	20	13.42	0	0.00	
Mild	121	81.21	16	29.63	<0.001*
Severe	8	5.37	38	70.37	
PHG red markings					
No	121	81.21	8	14.82	
Isolated	28	18.79	13	24.07	<0.001*
Confluent	0	0.00	33	61.11	
GAVE					
No	133	89.26	46	85.19	0.729
Yes	16	10.74	8	14.81	

*Statistically significant at $P < 0.05$. EV: esophageal varices; PHG: portal hypertensive gastropathy; GAVE: gastric antral vascular ectasia.

controls or patients with EV only ($P = 0.007$) indicating that the presence of PHG is related to severity of the hepatic disease. This finding is similar to that of the HALT-C Trial in 2006, which recorded that bilirubin was significantly higher among PHG patients than those without [24]. However, contrary to the HALT-C Trial,

TABLE 3: Relationship of portal hypertensive gastropathy severity with different variables.

Parameter	Portal hypertensive gastropathy severity ($n = 203$) Mild ($n = 149$) Mean ± SD	Severe ($n = 54$) Mean ± SD	P value
Age, years	53.43 ± 7.71	58.00 ± 8.15	0.076
Hemoglobin (g/dL)	10.86 ± 1.62	11.97 ± 2.11	0.055
Platelets ($\times 10^9$/L)	103.68 ± 32.44	96.08 ± 28.44	0.458
WBCs ($\times 10^9$/L)	5.05 ± 2.22	5.74 ± 2.23	0.341
AST (U/L)	63.59 ± 29.48	58.23 ± 16.26	0.538
ALT (U/L)	43.16 ± 17.54	43.85 ± 18.03	0.905
Serum albumin (g/dL)	3.06 ± 0.59	2.95 ± 0.52	0.578
Total serum bilirubin (mg/dL)	1.92 ± 1.35	1.59 ± 0.89	0.413
International normalized ratio	1.33 ± 0.26	1.18 ± 0.17	0.056
Creatinine (mg/dL)	0.98 ± 0.20	0.95 ± 0.26	0.672
Child-Pugh score	7.19 ± 2.17	7.31 ± 1.93	0.863
Blood ammonia (μg/dL)	151.39 ± 54.37	192.69 ± 59.87	0.026*
Portal vein diameter (mm)	13.85 ± 1.68	13.07 ± 2.11	0.184
Splenic longitudinal diameter (cm)	16.31 ± 1.59	14.51 ± 1.26	0.001*
Splenic vein diameter (mm)	11.39 ± 1.08	10.64 ± 1.39	0.052

*Statistically significant at $P < 0.05$. ALT: alanine aminotransferase; AST: aspartate aminotransferase; WBCs: white blood cells.

we did not record any significant worsening in albumin or INR levels.

Several authors have found a correlation between the presence of PHG and Child-Pugh stage [2, 6, 25]. In this study, there were no significant differences in Child class between the cases with or without PHG. This is congruent with the results of Spina et al., Primignani et al., Merkel et al., and Bellis et al. [8, 13, 26, 27].

Blood ammonia was significantly higher among patients with EV than controls ($P = 0.001$). Other studies have found this relation between the presence of varices and elevated blood ammonia and even suggested a blood ammonia cutoff value for prediction of variceal presence [15, 28–30]. This can be explained by the role ammonia plays in production of portal hypertension and hence development of varices [18].

Blood ammonia levels were significantly higher among patients with EV and PHG ($162.12 \pm 58.17\,\mu$g/dL) than among those with EV but no PHG as well as the cirrhotic controls (153.04 ± 59.41 and $103.23 \pm 72.76\,\mu$g/dL, resp.) ($P = 0.001$). It is known that PHG pathogenesis is associated with a hyperdynamic state brought about by portal hypertension in which there is an increased splanchnic and total gastric blood flow and most probably a decreased gastric mucosal blood flow [31]. Ammonia has been postulated to be part of a vicious circle in which elevation of ammonia results from the presence of portal hypertension and portosystemic collaterals and then leads to a further increase in portal hypertension [32]. It has also been suggested that PHG is associated with increased portal hypertension [24]. This could explain the higher levels of ammonia in cases with both PHG and EV and suggests a causal relationship.

The portal vein, splenic vein, and splenic longitudinal diameters were significantly higher in patients with EV and PHG as well as those with EV only than in controls ($P < 0.001$), which is expected as these are indicators of raised portal pressure; however, we found no difference in these parameters between patients having PHG and those without PHG in contrary to the HALT-C Trial [24]. Zardi et al. concluded their study in 2015 with there being no relation between splenic vein diameter and PHG [25].

By using the Baveno II PHG scoring system to classify our 203 patients with PHG, we found that 149 (73.4%) had mild PHG (score ≤ 3) and 54 (26.6%) had severe PHG (score ≥ 4). This more frequent pattern of mild PHG is consistent with the recorded prevalence range of mild PHG (29%–57%) and of severe PHG (9%–46%) among patients with portal hypertension [1].

There was no difference between mild or severe PHG regarding Child-Pugh class as also recorded by Abbasi et al. and Primignani et al. [13, 33]. Esophageal varix form, color, red color signs, or presence of risky bleeding signs were also not significantly different between the two PHG forms. This is the opposite to the findings of Taranto et al. who reported that PHG severity was closely related to the hemorrhagic risk of esophageal varices and Child-Pugh criteria [34].

A significant difference was recorded between mild and severe PHG patients regarding the grading of the accompanying EV ($P = 0.002$), with a higher percentage of large EV (grades 3 and 4) with the severe form of PHG than with the mild form (29.9% versus 16.78%). Of interest was the absence of grade 4 EV among the patients with mild PHG pointing to the relationship between severity of both PHG and portal hypertension and the similar mechanism for development of EV and PHG in response to increased portal pressure. Multiple previous studies have also reached this same interpretation which is supported by the strong correlation

Table 4: Relationship of portal hypertensive gastropathy score with demographic, clinical, and endoscopic characteristics.

Parameter	Portal hypertensive gastropathy score ($n = 203$)		P value
	n	Mean ± SD	
Sex			
Male	142	1.89 ± 1.05	0.954
Female	61	1.87 ± 1.13	
Hepatitis C virus			
No	4	1.00 ± 0.83	0.408
Yes	199	1.89 ± 1.07	
Hepatitis B virus			
No	199	1.89 ± 1.08	0.611
Yes	4	1.50 ± 0.71	
Ascites			
No	133	1.75 ± 1.04	0.334
Yes	90	2.05 ± 1.09	
History of hepatic encephalopathy			
No	175	1.84 ± 1.02	0.486
Yes	28	2.14 ± 1.35	
Child-Pugh class			
Class A	97	1.75 ± 0.99	
Class B	66	2.00 ± 1.27	0.716
Class C	40	2.00 ± 0.94	
EV grading			
Grade 1	81	1.85 ± 1.27	
Grade 2	81	1.75 ± 0.85	0.616
Grade 3	37	2.11 ± 1.05	
Grade 4	4	3.00 ± 0.95	
EV red color sign (RC)			
RC0 (none)	122	1.93 ± 1.17	
HCS (hematocystic spots)	20	1.60 ± 0.55	0.912
CRS (cherry red spots)	12	1.67 ± 1.16	
RWM (red wale markings)	49	1.92 ± 0.99	
EV form (F)			
F1	113	1.82 ± 1.19	
F2	60	1.87 ± 0.83	0.780
F3	30	2.14 ± 1.07	
EV risk signs			
No	131	1.88 ± 1.16	0.965
Yes	72	1.89 ± 0.90	
EV location (L)			
LI (inferior)	121	1.77 ± 0.94	
LM (medialis)	69	1.82 ± 1.13	0.046*
LS (superior)	13	3.33 ± 1.16	
EV color (C)			
Cw (white varices)	142	1.89 ± 1.13	0.954
Cb (blue varices)	61	1.87 ± 0.92	

*Statistically significant at $P < 0.05$. EV: esophageal varices; GAVE: gastric antral vascular ectasia.

Table 5: Correlation between portal hypertensive gastropathy score and different variables.

Parameter	Portal hypertensive gastropathy score ($n = 203$)	
	R	P value
Age (years)	0.187	0.194
Hemoglobin (g/dL)	0.325	0.021*
Platelets ($\times 10^9$/L)	−0.127	0.378
WBCs ($\times 10^9$/L)	0.114	0.431
AST (U/L)	−0.066	0.651
ALT (U/L)	−0.014	0.922
Serum albumin (g/dL)	−0.072	0.620
Total serum bilirubin (mg/dL)	−0.080	0.581
International normalized ratio (INR)	−0.137	0.342
Creatinine (mg/dL)	0.086	0.555
Child-Pugh score	−0.228	0.111
Blood ammonia (μg/dL)	0.295	0.037*
Portal vein diameter (mm)	−0.142	0.325
Splenic longitudinal diameter (cm)	−0.383	0.006*
Splenic vein diameter (mm)	−0.233	0.104

*Statistically significant at $P < 0.05$. WBCs: white blood cells; ALT: alanine aminotransferase; AST: aspartate aminotransferase.

between severity of PHG and hepatic venous pressure gradient (HVPG) [13, 24, 26, 33, 35]. Kim et al. in their study on 331 cirrhotic patients noted that patients with severe PHG had significantly raised HVPG than those with either mild or no gastropathy [35].

Regarding the location of the EV ($P = 0.013$), severe PHG cases had higher percentages of association with locus superior EV than their counterparts with mild PHG (14.82% versus 3.36%, resp.) ($P = 0.013$), and the PHG score itself was significantly higher with higher locations of the varices ($P = 0.046$), a further indication of the relation with increased portal pressure.

Severe PHG can cause acute or chronic bleeding in cirrhotic patients, yet we found no significant decrease in hemoglobin levels among patients with severe PHG. The reason may be the exclusion of patients with active gastrointestinal bleeding or a history of bleeding during the previous two weeks to the study to eliminate the effect on blood ammonia levels.

Child-Pugh class and liver function tests were no different statistically in cases with severe PHG than in those with mild PHG indicating that worsening and progression of the condition is not affected by worsening of the liver condition. Primignani et al. also reported an unexpected low prevalence of severe gastropathy in patients with Child C class [13]. Taranto et al. in 1994 concluded that the severity of the mosaic-like appearance correlated with the severity of liver dysfunction yet made no such conclusion regarding the presence or appearance of the gastric mucosal red spots [34].

Cases with severe PHG had significantly higher levels of blood ammonia than those with mild PHG (192.69 ±

59.87 μg/dL versus 151.39 ± 54.37 μg/dL, resp.) ($P = 0.026$). We recorded a significant positive correlation between PHG scores and blood ammonia levels ($P = 0.037$). Increased ammonia in splanchnic vessels in cases of liver function impairment results in vasodilatation and increased portal blood flow bringing about portal hypertension [16, 17]. The increased levels may also cause such an increase in the gastric blood flow aggravating the vascular congestion characteristic of PHG and provoking cytokines, growth factors, and hormones to further worsen the condition. Ammonia is also known to affect endoplasmic reticulum dynamics and induce oxidative stress [18]. To our knowledge, no other studies have been performed to study the relationship between ammonia levels and severity of PHG; therefore, we could not compare our results with any others.

Significantly lower splenic longitudinal diameters were recorded among our patients with severe PHG than those with mild PHG ($P = 0.001$). This is in disagreement with the results recorded by Kim et al. whose patients with severe PHG had higher splenic diameters than those with mild PHG or no PHG [35].

A significantly negative correlation of the PHG score was found with the splenic longitudinal diameter ($P = 0.006$). This may be due to the effect of factors other than portal hypertension that maintain and further the pathology of PHG such as cytokines, growth factors, and hormones [3–5]. Even though the development of PHG is related to the presence of portal hypertension, there is generally no direct correlation with the level of the portal pressure [36].

Another study from Egypt by Nashaat et al. found that mean splenic bipolar diameter (MSBD) showed a significantly positive correlation with the presence of OV but not with PHG [37].

There is controversy regarding the correlation of splenic size with portal pressure as Nedredal et al. [38] state that spleen size does not correlate well with portal venous pressure in contrary to splenic stiffness which may be another explanation for our finding.

We recorded an unexpected significant positive correlation between PHG scores and serum hemoglobin levels; this may be related to the lower spleen size and therefore to lower phagocytic activity resulting in a decreased incidence of anemia among our patients with severe PHG having no present or recent related gastric mucosal bleeding.

The limitation of this study was the absence of a patient group with portal hypertensive gastropathy and no esophageal varices.

5. Conclusions

Blood ammonia levels correlate with the presence, severity, and score of portal hypertensive gastropathy in cirrhosis suggesting a causal relationship and encouraging trials of ammonia-lowering treatments for the management of severe PHG with a tendency to bleed.

References

[1] P. J. Thuluvath and H. Y. Yoo, "Portal hypertensive gastropathy," *The American Journal of Gastroenterology*, vol. 97, no. 12, pp. 2973–2978, 2002.

[2] S. K. Sarin, D. V. Sreenivas, D. Lahoti, and A. Saraya, "Factors influencing development of portal hypertensive gastropathy in patients with portal hypertension," *Gastroenterology*, vol. 102, no. 3, pp. 994–999, 1992.

[3] R. Cubillas and D. C. Rockey, "Portal hypertensive gastropathy: a review," *Liver International*, vol. 30, no. 8, pp. 1094–1102, 2010.

[4] B. K. De and T. K. Das, "Color Doppler and laser velocimetry studies in the assessment of portal hemodynamics and severity of chronic liver disease," *Indian Journal of Gastroenterology*, vol. 21, no. 5, pp. 173–175, 2002.

[5] M. Ohta, S. Yamaguchi, N. Gotoh, and M. Tomikawa, "Pathogenesis of portal hypertensive gastropathy: a clinical and experimental review," *Surgery*, vol. 131, no. 1, pp. S165–S170, 2002.

[6] M. Merli, G. Nicolini, S. Angeloni, F. Gentili, A. F. Attili, and O. Riggio, "The natural history of portal hypertensive gastropathy in patients with liver cirrhosis and mild portal hypertension," *The American Journal of Gastroenterology*, vol. 99, no. 10, pp. 1959–1965, 2004.

[7] T. T. McCormack, J. Sims, I. Eyre-Brook et al., "Gastric lesions in portal hypertension: inflammatory gastritis or congestive gastropathy?," *Gut*, vol. 26, no. 11, pp. 1226–1232, 1985.

[8] G. P. Spina, R. Arcidiacono, J. Bosch et al., "Gastric endoscopic features in portal hypertension: final report of a consensus conference, Milan, Italy, September 19, 1992," *Journal of Hepatology*, vol. 21, no. 3, pp. 461–467, 1994.

[9] S. K. Sarin, "Diagnostic issues: portal hypertensive gastropathy and gastric varices," in *Portal Hypertension II. Proceedings of the Second Baveno International Consensus Workshop on Definitions, Methodology and Therapeutic Strategies*, pp. 30–54, Baveno, Italy, 1996.

[10] C. A. Stewart and A. J. Sanyal, "Grading portal gastropathy: validation of a gastropathy scoring system," *The American Journal of Gastroenterology*, vol. 98, no. 8, pp. 1758–1765, 2003.

[11] C. J. Gostout, T. R. Viggiano, and R. K. Balm, "Acute gastrointestinal bleeding from portal hypertensive gastropathy: prevalence and clinical features," *The American Journal of Gastroenterology*, vol. 88, no. 12, pp. 2030–2033, 1993.

[12] G. D'Amico, L. Montalbano, M. Traina et al., "Natural history of congestive gastropathy in cirrhosis," *Gastroenterology*, vol. 99, no. 6, pp. 1558–1564, 1990.

[13] M. Primignani, L. Carpinelli, P. Preatoni et al., "Natural history of portal hypertensive gastropathy in patients with liver cirrhosis," *Gastroenterology*, vol. 119, no. 1, pp. 181–187, 2000.

[14] S. K. Sarin, H. M. Shahi, M. Jain, A. K. Jain, S. K. Issar, and N. S. Murthy, "The natural history of portal hypertensive gastropathy: influence of variceal eradication," *The American Journal of Gastroenterology*, vol. 95, no. 10, pp. 2888–2893, 2000.

[15] G. Tarantino, V. Citro, P. Esposito et al., "Blood ammonia levels in liver cirrhosis: a clue for the presence of portosystemic collateral veins," *BMC Gastroenterology*, vol. 9, no. 1, article 21, 2009.

[16] J. N. Benoit, J. A. Barrowman, S. L. Harper, P. R. Kvietys, and D. N. Granger, "Role of humoral factors in the intestinal hyperemia associated with chronic portal hypertension," *American Journal of Physiology-Gastrointestinal and Liver Physiology*, vol. 247, no. 5, pp. G486–G493, 1984.

[17] J. N. Benoit and D. N. Granger, "Splanchnic hemodynamics in chronic portal hypertension," *Seminars in Liver Disease*, vol. 6, no. 04, pp. 287–298, 1986.

[18] R. Jalan, F. de Chiara, V. Balasubramaniyan et al., "Ammonia produces pathological changes in human hepatic stellate cells and is a target for therapy of portal hypertension," *Journal of Hepatology*, vol. 64, no. 4, pp. 823–833, 2016.

[19] A. Kumar, S. R. Mishra, P. Sharma, B. C. Sharma, and S. K. Sarin, "Clinical, laboratory, and hemodynamic parameters in portal hypertensive gastropathy: a study of 254 cirrhotics," *Journal of Clinical Gastroenterology*, vol. 44, no. 4, pp. 294–300, 2010.

[20] Y. Idezuki and Japanese Research Society for Portal Hypertension, "General rules for recording endoscopic findings of esophagogastric varices (1991)," *World Journal of Surgery*, vol. 19, no. 3, pp. 420–422, 1995.

[21] F. Schepis, C. Cammà, D. Niceforo et al., "Which patients with cirrhosis should undergo endoscopic screening for esophageal varices detection?," *Hepatology*, vol. 33, no. 2, pp. 333–338, 2001.

[22] L. Nada, E. F. Samira, B. Bahija, I. Adil, and A. Nourdine, "Noninvasive predictors of presence and grade of esophageal varices in viral cirrhotic patients," *The Pan African Medical Journal*, vol. 20, p. 145, 2015.

[23] S. Abd-Elsalam, E. Habba, W. Elkhalawany et al., "Correlation of platelets count with endoscopic findings in a cohort of Egyptian patients with liver cirrhosis," *Medicine*, vol. 95, no. 23, article e3853, 2016.

[24] R. J. Fontana, A. J. Sanyal, S. Mehta et al., "Portal hypertensive gastropathy in chronic hepatitis C patients with bridging fibrosis and compensated cirrhosis: results from the HALT-C Trial," *The American Journal of Gastroenterology*, vol. 101, no. 5, pp. 983–992, 2006.

[25] E. M. Zardi, G. Ghittoni, D. Margiotta, F. T. Viera, F. di Matteo, and S. Rossi, "Portal hypertensive gastropathy in cirrhotics without varices: a case-control study," *European Journal of Gastroenterology & Hepatology*, vol. 27, no. 1, pp. 91–96, 2015.

[26] C. Merkel, M. Schipilliti, R. Bighin et al., "Portal hypertension and portal hypertensive gastropathy in patients with liver cirrhosis: a haemodynamic study," *Digestive and Liver Disease*, vol. 35, no. 4, pp. 269–274, 2003.

[27] L. Bellis, S. Nicodemo, A. Galossi et al., "Hepatic venous pressure gradient does not correlate with the presence and the severity of portal hypertensive gastropathy in patients with liver cirrhosis," *Journal of Gastrointestinal and Liver Diseases*, vol. 16, no. 3, pp. 273–277, 2007.

[28] N. El-Hefny, M. Hareedy, and R. Abdel-Aal, *Blood ammonia level and other non invasive parameters as indicators of portosystemic collaterals in cirrhotic patients. Thesis submitted for partial fulfillment of MSC degree in internal medicine*, Assiut University, 2013.

[29] M. F. Montasser, H. M. Abdella, and A. H. Samy, "Evaluation of venous ammonia level, splenic longitudinal diameter, portal vein and splenic vein diameters as non-invasive indicators for the presence of portosystemic collaterals in Egyptian cirrhotic patients," *Open Journal of Gastroenterology*, vol. 04, no. 06, pp. 265–274, 2014.

[30] A. A. Ali, A. M. Badawy, A. A. Sonbol, and M. E. Ayad, "Study of the relationship between blood ammonia level and esophageal varices in patients with liver cirrhosis," *Afro-Egyptian Journal of Infectious and Endemic Diseases*, vol. 5, pp. 78–85, 2015.

[31] M. Gjeorgjievski and M. S. Cappell, "Portal hypertensive gastropathy: a systematic review of the pathophysiology, clinical presentation, natural history and therapy," *World Journal of Hepatology*, vol. 8, no. 4, pp. 231–262, 2016.

[32] J. G. Bode, T. Peters-Regehr, A. M. Gressner, and D. Häussinger, "De novo expression of glutamine synthetase during transformation of hepatic stellate cells into myofibroblast-like cells," *The Biochemical Journal*, vol. 335, no. 3, pp. 697–700, 1998.

[33] A. Abbasi, A. R. Bhutto, N. Butt, S. M. Munir, and A. K. Dhillo, "Frequency of portal hypertensive gastropathy and its relationship with biochemical, haematological and endoscopic features in cirrhosis," *Journal of the College of Physicians and Surgeons–Pakistan*, vol. 21, no. 12, pp. 723–726, 2011.

[34] D. Taranto, R. Suozzo, M. Romano et al., "Gastric endoscopic features in patients with liver cirrhosis: correlation with esophageal varices, intra-variceal pressure, and liver dysfunction," *Digestion*, vol. 55, no. 2, pp. 115–120, 2004.

[35] M. Y. Kim, H. Choi, S. K. Baik et al., "Portal hypertensive gastropathy: correlation with portal hypertension and prognosis in cirrhosis," *Digestive Diseases and Sciences*, vol. 55, no. 12, pp. 3561–3567, 2010.

[36] F. Wong, "Portal hypertensive gastropathy," *Gastroenterology & Hepatology*, vol. 3, no. 6, pp. 428–473, 2007.

[37] E. H. Nashaat, H. Abd- Elaziz, M. Sabry, and A. A. Ibrahim, "Non-endoscopic predictors of esophageal varices and portal hypertensive gastropathy," *Nature and Science*, vol. 8, no. 6, pp. 43–50, 2010.

[38] G. I. Nedredal, M. Yin, T. McKenzie et al., "Portal hypertension correlates with splenic stiffness as measured with MR elastography," *Journal of Magnetic Resonance Imaging*, vol. 34, no. 1, pp. 79–87, 2011.

Comparison of Anthropometric Parameters after Ultralow Anterior Resection and Abdominoperineal Resection in Very Low-Lying Rectal Cancers

Jun Woo Bong, Seok-Byung Lim, Jong Lyul Lee, Chan Wook Kim, Yong Sik Yoon, In Ja Park, Chang Sik Yu, and Jin Cheon Kim

Department of Surgery, Asan Medical Center, University of Ulsan College of Medicine, 88 Olympic-ro 43-gil, Songpa-gu, Seoul 05505, Republic of Korea

Correspondence should be addressed to Seok-Byung Lim; sblim@amc.seoul.kr

Academic Editor: Per Hellström

Background and Aim. Ultralow anterior resection (uLAR) is a sphincter-saving procedure for very low-lying rectal cancers. This procedure, however, has complications related to defecation which can aggravate the patient's quality of life postoperatively. In this study, we compared the anthropometric and nutritional parameters after uLAR and abdominoperineal resection (APR). *Methods.* We retrospectively reviewed the data of patients who underwent either uLAR or APR in 2012 for rectal cancers within 3 cm from the anal verge. Data including body weight, body mass index (BMI), levels of total protein, albumin, and hemoglobin and lymphocyte count were analyzed. We compared the changes of these parameters before operations to 3 years after discharge between uLAR and APR groups by ANOVA for repeated measures and Bonferroni comparison method. *Results.* After 3 years of discharge, the body weight and BMI of the APR group were fully recovered to the preoperative levels; however, those of the uLAR group did not. The hemoglobin level in the APR group was recovered to the preoperative level within 3 months of discharge; however, that in the uLAR group was recovered after 1 year of discharge. *Conclusions.* Recovery of anthropometric and nutritional status of patients was more stable after APR than after uLAR. These findings might indirectly reflect the low anterior syndrome effect of uLAR and help colorectal surgeons in selecting better surgical methods and in better counseling patients with very low-lying rectal cancer.

1. Introduction

The main goals in the surgical treatment of rectal cancer are complete resection with total mesorectal excision and conservation of the sphincter function. However, in cases in which a tumor-free distal resection margin is not achievable, a locally far-advanced tumor is present, and the patient shows severely decreased anal function preoperatively, surgeons should perform abdominoperineal resection (APR) requiring a permanent colostomy. Permanent colostomy can lead to psychological problems. Colostomy was reported to be associated with depression, low self-esteem, and low rates of social participation [1]. However, there is controversy about the patients' quality of life (QoL) with a permanent colostomy. Some authors reported that patients undergoing APR tended to show better physical, emotional, and social function and reported less fatigue and gastrointestinal symptoms than patients undergoing low anterior resection [2, 3].

Ultralow anterior resection (uLAR), as a sphincter-saving procedure, has been developed for the treatment of very low-lying rectal cancers. Recently, surgeons have been encouraged to perform uLAR with a better understanding of the distal surgical margin, adaptation of preoperative chemoradiation therapy (PCRT), and development of surgical techniques such as intersphincteric resection [4, 5]. However, the lower the anastomotic level after uLAR, the greater the likelihood of functional disorder development, the so-called low anterior resection syndrome (LARS) [6, 7]. LARS includes symptoms of incontinence for flatus, urgency, and frequent bowel movements and has been associated with a negative impact on the QoL [8, 9]. The main causes of LARS are poor function of the neorectum, sphincter damage, and surgical denervation of the rectum or anal sphincter [10].

In general, patients complain of sleeplessness, diarrhea, and difficulty in controlling stools and eventual loss of appetite with decreased body weight at the outpatient clinic during the follow-up period after uLAR. However, there is a paucity of studies on the effects on anthropometric status, including body weight change of LARS, after uLAR. Therefore, the main objective of the present study was to compare the postoperative changes in the patients' anthropometric and nutritional status after APR and uLAR for the treatment of low rectal cancer and to identify the factors predicting the clinical and nutritional changes postoperatively.

2. Materials and Methods

2.1. Patients and Data. A total of 749 patients underwent surgery for rectal cancer from January to December 2012 at Asan Medical Center and had a minimum follow-up of 36 months. The data were extracted from a prospectively collected colorectal cancer registry in our division of colorectal surgery and analyzed retrospectively. Of the 749 patients, 132 had a very low-lying rectal cancer ($\leq$3 cm from the anal verge). The inclusion criteria are shown in Figure 1. Finally, 35 patients were included in our study and were divided into two groups according to the type of operation they underwent for rectal cancer: 17 patients were categorized into the APR group and 18 patients into the uLAR group.

We reviewed and compared the data of each group. The preoperative variables were age at operation, sex, PCRT, location of tumor from the anal verge, clinical T/N categories, and time interval from PCRT to the operation. Operative factors such as method of ligation of the inferior mesenteric artery (high versus low ligation) and surgical approach (open versus minimally invasive) and pathologic findings including histological differentiation and pathological T/N categories were reviewed. Whether patients received adjuvant chemotherapy or radiotherapy was also recorded.

Body weight and hematological/biochemical parameters were investigated to assess the nutritional status of the patients. The hematological/biochemical parameters included the levels of total protein, albumin, and hemoglobin and the lymphocyte count. Preoperative body weight was measured at the time of admission for surgery, and body weight was measured again at discharge. Body mass index (BMI) was calculated using the standard formula: weight (kg)/height (m^2). When patients visited the outpatient clinic after discharge according to their regular follow-up schedules, all these parameters were measured. All parameters were assessed preoperatively; at discharge; at 1, 2, and 3 months after discharge; and at 1, 2, and 3 years after discharge. The changes in body weight and other nutritional parameters were measured by calculating the proportion of change at the designated time after discharge compared with the preoperative value (proportion of change = [(value at the designated time after discharge − preoperative value)/preoperative value] × 100%). To investigate the risk factors of weight loss at 3 years after discharge, we analyzed the clinicopathologic variables mentioned above. We defined weight loss as a weight reduction at 3 years after discharge compared with the preoperative weight. This study was approved by the Institutional Review Board of Asan Medical Center (IRB approval number: S2017-2246-0001).

2.2. Operation. All surgeries were performed by colorectal surgeons who have at least a 5-year experience in treating rectal cancer. All patients in both groups underwent total mesorectal excision including radical resection of the primary tumor and regional lymph nodes and preservation of autonomic nerves in the pelvis. The decision on performing APR or uLAR was made by the surgeon according to intraoperative findings such as distal resection margin and invasion of the sphincter muscle. End-to-end anastomosis was constructed in all patients in the uLAR group with either the hand-sewn ($n = 6$) or double-stapling method ($n = 12$). All patients in the uLAR group received a loop ileostomy for diversion, and ileostomy closure was performed at about 6 months (5.7 ± 1.1 months) after the operation.

2.3. Statistical Analysis. Data were analyzed using SPSS software version 21.0 (SPSS, Chicago, IL, USA). Discrete values such as sex, clinical stages, and surgical approaches were compared using Pearson's χ^2 test. Student's t-test was used to compare continuous values such as age, weight, and biochemical parameters. Data are presented as mean ± standard deviation. Analysis of variance (ANOVA) for repeated measures analysis was used to compare the patterns of changes in the anthropometric and nutritional data at discharge between the two groups, 1, 2, and 3 months after discharge and 1, 2, and 3 years after discharge. Bonferroni post hoc analysis was performed to compare the changes of variables at each time between the two groups. Univariate and multivariate analyses were performed using a logistic regression model for risk factors of weight loss at 3 years after discharge. Statistical significance was set at $p < 0.05$.

3. Results

3.1. Clinicopathologic Characteristics of Patients. The demographic and preoperative characteristics did not differ between the two groups except for the tumor location from the anal verge (Table 1). The mean distance of the tumor from the anal verge was shorter in the APR group ($p < 0.001$). The proportion of patients who received PCRT was not different between the two groups: 16 (94.1%) in the APR group and 16 (88.9%) in the uLAR group. There was also no difference in clinical stages. Parameters related to baseline nutritional status such as body weight; BMI; protein, albumin, and hemoglobin levels; and lymphocyte count did not differ between the two groups. The operative and pathologic results of the two groups also showed no significant difference (Table 2). Most operations were performed through an open approach, 16 cases (94.1%) in the APR group and 13 cases (72.2%) in the uLAR group, with no significant difference. All patients in the APR group and 16 patients (88.9%) in the uLAR group received adjuvant chemotherapy.

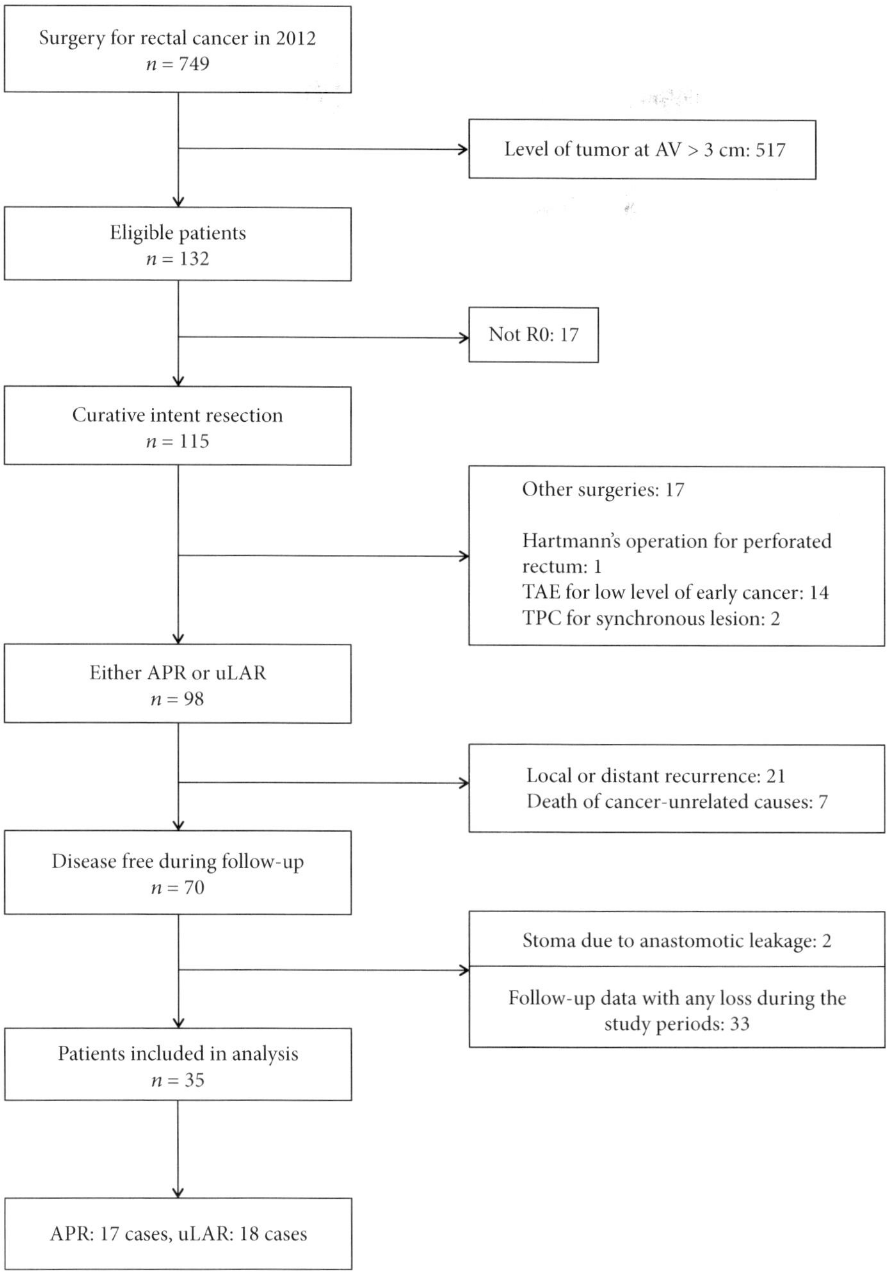

FIGURE 1: Flowchart of patient selection. AV: anal verge; APR: abdominoperineal resection; uLAR: ultralow anterior resection; TAE: transanal excision; TPC: total proctocolectomy.

3.2. Evaluation of Postoperative Nutritional Status. The analysis of body weight revealed that the patterns of body weight change at discharge; 1, 2, and 3 months after discharge; and 1, 2, and 3 years after discharge compared with the preoperative values had a significant difference between the two groups ($p = 0.001$, Figure 2(a)). The body weight change at 3 years after discharge was $+5.30 \pm 5.42\%$ of the preoperative value in the APR group but $-1.41 \pm 7.31\%$ in the uLAR group ($p = 0.004$). According to the results of Bonferroni comparison at each time, there were significant differences between the two groups in the weight changes at 1, 2, and 3 years after discharge ($p < 0.001$, $p = 0.001$, and $p = 0.004$, resp.). The patterns of BMI change during the same periods were also different between the two groups ($p < 0.001$, Figure 2(b)). The changes of BMI at 1, 2, and 3 years after discharge were also statistically different between the two groups after Bonferroni comparison at each time, ($p < 0.001$, $p = 0.001$, and $p = 0.003$, resp.). The BMI change at 3 years after discharge was $+1.25 \pm 1.30\ \mathrm{kg/m^2}$ of the preoperative BMI in the APR group but $-0.36 \pm 1.61\ \mathrm{kg/m^2}$ in the uLAR group ($p = 0.003$). The proportion of patients who experienced weight loss at 3 years compared with the preoperative weight was higher in the uLAR group: 13 patients (72.2%) in the uLAR group and 3 patients (17.6%) in the ARP group ($p = 0.001$). In univariate analysis, uLAR and a low tumor location from the anal verge were significant risk factors of weight loss

Table 1: Demographics and preoperative data.

	Total ($n = 35$)	APR ($n = 17$)	uLAR ($n = 18$)	p value
Age at operation, years	57.9 ± 10.3	56.6 ± 10.9	59.0 ± 9.8	0.495
Sex: male, n (%)	19 (54.3)	11 (64.7)	8 (44.4)	0.229
BMI, kg/m^2	23.3 ± 2.3	23.7 ± 2.5	23.0 ± 2.3	0.423
Body weight, kg	60.6 ± 7.7	61.0 ± 7.8	60.2 ± 7.7	0.572
Protein, g/dL	7 ± 0.59	7.0 ± 0.7	7.0 ± 0.48	0.912
Albumin, g/dL	4.1 ± 0.4	4.1 ± 0.5	4.2 ± 0.29	0.458
Hemoglobin, g/dL	12.3 ± 1.0	12.0 ± 1.1	12.6 ± 0.9	0.07
Lymphocytes, mm^3	1183 ± 425	1206 ± 501	1162 ± 352	0.766
PCRT, n (%)	32 (91.4)	16 (94.1)	16 (88.9)	0.581
Tumor location from AV, cm	2.2 ± 0.77	1.62 ± 0.63	2.72 ± 0.43	<0.001
Clinical T category, n (%)				0.684
1-2	9 (25.7)	5 (29.4)	4 (22.2)	
3-4	26 (74.3)	12 (70.6)	14 (77.8)	
Clinical N category, n (%)				0.318
0	8 (22.9)	3 (17.6)	5 (27.8)	
1	11 (31.4)	4 (23.5)	7 (38.9)	
2	16 (45.7)	10 (58.8)	6 (33.3)	

APR: abdominoperineal resection; uLAR: ultralow anterior resection; BMI: body mass index; PCRT: preoperative chemoradiation therapy; AV: anal verge.

Table 2: Operative and pathologic results, n (%).

	Total ($n = 35$)	APR ($n = 17$)	uLAR ($n = 18$)	p value
Interval from PCRT to operation, weeks[a]	7.0 ± 0.91	6.85 ± 0.85	7.12 ± 0.97	0.46
Surgical approach				0.086
Open	29 (82.9)	16 (94.1)	13 (72.2)	
Minimally invasive	6 (17.1)	1 (5.9)	5 (27.8)	
Ligation of IMA (high)	14 (55.6)	7 (53.8)	8 (57.1)	0.863
Pathologic T category				0.779
1-2	11 (32.4)	4 (23.5)	7 (38.9)	
3-4	25 (68.6)	13 (76.5)	11 (61.1)	
Pathologic N category				0.486
0	30 (85.6)	14 (82.3)	16 (88.8)	
1	4 (11.5)	3 (17.7)	1 (5.6)	
2	1 (2.9)	0	1 (5.6)	
Adjuvant chemotherapy	33 (94.3)	17 (100)	16 (88.9)	0.157
Adjuvant radiation therapy	2 (8)	1 (8.3)	1 (7.7)	0.953

[a]Data from 32 patients who underwent preoperative chemoradiation therapy. APR: abdominoperineal resection; uLAR: ultralow anterior resection; PCRT: preoperative chemoradiation therapy; IMA: inferior mesenteric artery.

after 3 years ($p = 0.003$ and 0.02, respectively; Table 3). uLAR was the only independent risk factor in multivariate analysis ($p = 0.049$).

Analysis of the hematologic and biochemical parameters showed that the pattern of changes in total hemoglobin level significantly differed during the same time intervals ($p < 0.001$, Figure 3(a)). There were significant differences between the two groups in hemoglobin changes at 1 and 3 years after discharge according to Bonferroni comparison at each time ($p = 0.001$ and $p = 0.006$, resp.). However, the changes in the levels of total protein and albumin and the lymphocyte count did not show a different pattern (Figures 3(b)–3(d)). Additionally, these variables showed no significant difference in changes at each time.

4. Discussion

With the acceptable oncologic outcomes and increased sphincter-saving rates, uLAR has recently replaced APR, and APR now tends to be performed in limited cases for the treatment of patients with rectal cancer. In our study, the uLAR group tended to recover their preoperative body

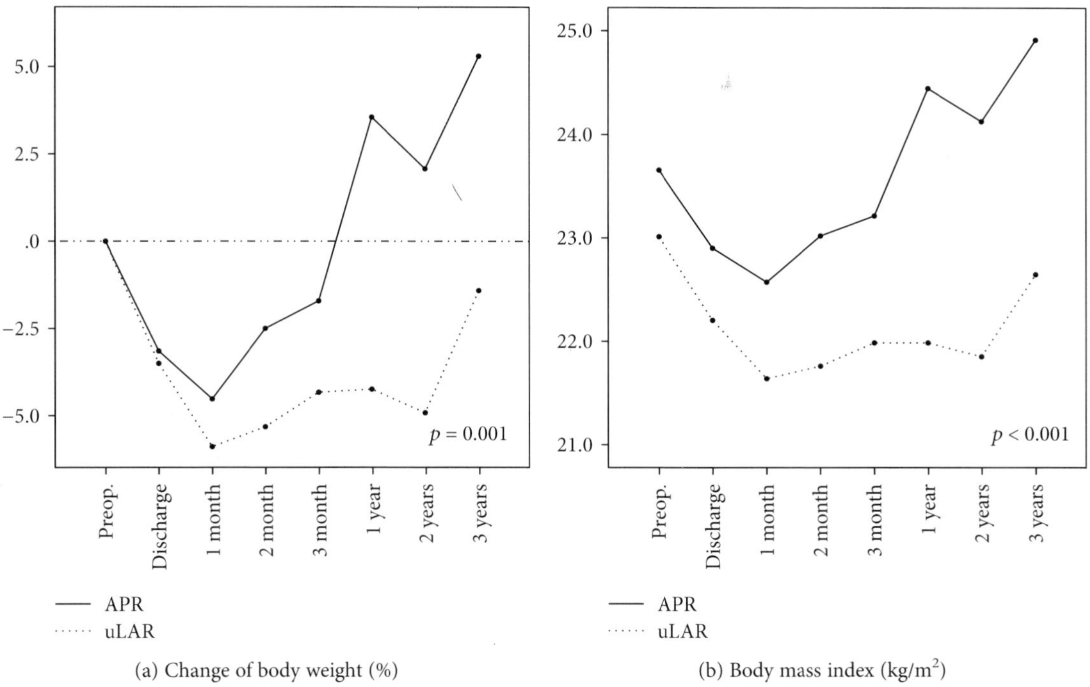

FIGURE 2: Changes in anthropometric parameters. Proportion of changed (a) body weight and (b) body mass index. APR: abdominoperineal resection; uLAR: ultralow anterior resection.

TABLE 3: Risk factors of weight loss at 3 years after the operation compared with the preoperative body weight.

Parameters	Univariate analysis β-Coefficient (95% CI)	p value	Multivariate analysis[a] β-Coefficient (95% CI)	p value
Age	1.04 (0.97–1.11)	0.31		
Sex: female	1.16 (0.30–4.40)	0.831		
PCRT[a]	0.39 (0.03-4.74)	0.46		
Ligation of IMA (high)	3.03 (0.75–12.21)	0.12		
Adjuvant chemotherapy	0.83 (0.05–14.48)	0.9		
Adjuvant radiation therapy	1.20 (0.07–20.85)	0.9		
Clinical T category	1.07 (0.23–4.92)	0.93		
Type of surgery (uLAR)	12.13 (2.41–61.20)	0.003	10.147 (1.01–101.8)	0.049
Length from AV	3.57 (1.22–10.42)	0.02	1.2 (0.25–5.61)	0.835

[a] $R^2 = 0.459$. PCRT: preoperative chemoradiation therapy; IMA: inferior mesenteric artery; uLAR: ultralow anterior resection; AV: anal verge.

weight more slowly than the APR group. Rather, the mean weight change at 3 years after discharge in the uLAR group was −1.41% of the preoperative value. Although we did not examine the changes of QoL of the two groups, we assumed that the difference in anthropometric and nutritional status might come from LARS. Many reports mentioned that patients with very low anastomoses are susceptible to the development of LARS, which could also severely impair the QoL, and recent studies showed the QoL after sphincter-saving surgery was not better than that after APR [11]. Konanz et al. [12] reported that uLAR also showed worse scores especially in appetite loss and weight loss than APR. Appetite and weight loss can result from LARS because many patients with this syndrome tend to worry about bowel habit changes or discomfort after eating. This can affect the postoperative nutritional status if the patient feels that consuming food is a burden and thus continuously avoids eating. Assessment of nutritional status is necessary in the long-term care of patients, and careful monitoring of nutritional status leads to an individualized plan of care. Patients undergoing major gastrointestinal surgery are frequently at a risk of developing malnutrition, not only due to the disease itself but also to the treatment processes and postoperative functional deterioration of the gastrointestinal tract [13]. The risk of malnutrition remains after surgery if postoperative gastrointestinal problems and limitation of dietary intake continue, which can also influence the QoL.

Generally, weight loss is the most prominent outcome during the period from 4 to 12 weeks after gastrointestinal tract surgeries [14]. However, the time to reach the

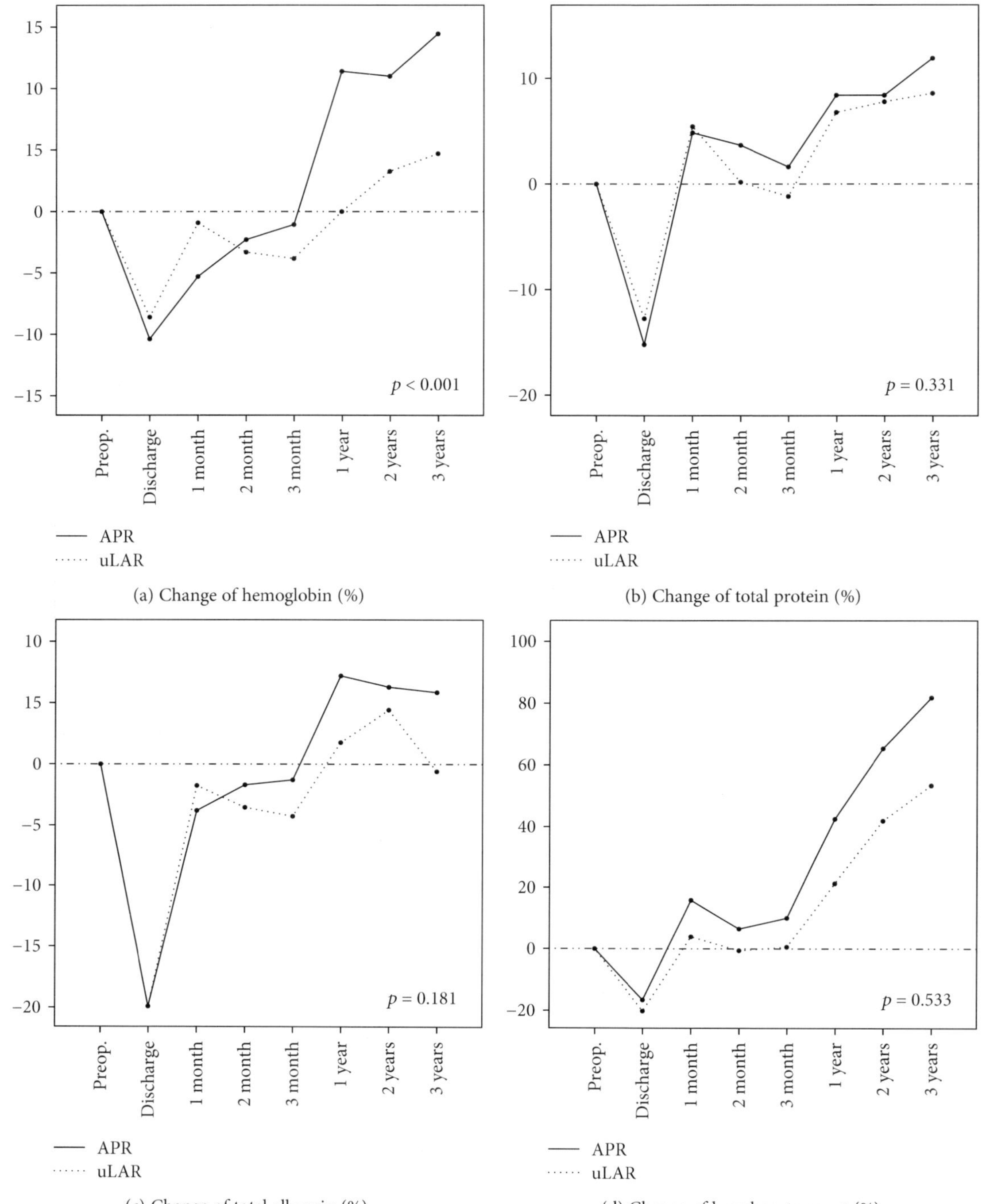

(a) Change of hemoglobin (%)

(b) Change of total protein (%)

(c) Change of total albumin (%)

(d) Change of lymphocyte count (%)

FIGURE 3: Changes in nutritional parameters. Proportion of changed (a) hemoglobin, (b) total protein, (c) total albumin, and (d) lymphocyte count. APR: abdominoperineal resection; uLAR: ultralow anterior resection.

preoperative weight mostly depends on how long it takes for patients to recover their preoperative QoL with a normal functioning body [13]. In this study, weight change was measured at monthly intervals until 12 weeks after discharge to evaluate the immediate body weight changes and at 1-year interval until 3 years after discharge to analyze the long-term weight changes. According to the ANOVA analysis, the body weights of patients in the APR and uLAR groups changed differently during the 3 years after discharge ($p = 0.001$). Patients in the APR group tended to recover their preoperative weight by 1 year after discharge, and their body weights seemed to continue to increase thereafter. However, it was difficult to conclude that the uLAR group showed a prominent recovery of body weight until 1 year after discharge. Their body weight seemed to have begun to increase in the third year, although their preoperative weight has not been recovered on average. Additionally, although the statistical difference was marginal ($p = 0.049$), uLAR was the only risk factor for weight loss at 3 years after discharge in the multivariate analysis.

The slow weight recovery rate of uLAR patients until 3 months after surgery may be attributable to the effect of ileostomy. Most nutrients are absorbed by the duodenum and jejunum; however, the ileum also absorbs a significant amount of nutrients including vitamins and electrolytes. As the bowel transit time of food is shortened in patients with an ileostomy, the absorption capacity of these patients can be decreased [15]. However, considering that all patients in our study underwent ileostomy closure at 6 months after surgery, ileostomy cannot be considered a factor affecting the weight change 1 year later. As there was no significant difference in the clinical courses between the two groups after 1 year of discharge, it could be inferred that the difference in body weight change between the two groups was due to LARS-induced changes in dietary habits. The change of body weight in the uLAR group was, however, not a clinicallysignificant involuntary weight loss, which is defined as a loss of 4.5 kg or >5% of the usual body weight during a period of 6–12 months [16]. Moreover, there was no statistical difference between the two groups in the change of total protein and albumin levels and the total lymphocyte count during 3 years after discharge. None of the parameters in both groups decreased to the level indicating a malnutrition status during the follow-up periods. Those parameters were recovered to the preoperative levels within 3 months after discharge and increased continuously. In low rectal surgery, the absorption capacity of the small intestine is almost the same as before surgery. Thus, the recovery rates of these parameters were almost same between the two groups. However, the recovery rates of hemoglobin level showed a different pattern between the two groups. The hemoglobin level in the APR group was recovered to the preoperative level within 3 months of discharge; that in the uLAR group tended to be recovered to their preoperative level after 1 year of discharge. The slow recovery of hemoglobin level in the uLAR group seems to be attributable to the effect of ileostomy. Vitamin B12 and iron deficiencies are common problems in patients with an ileostomy [17, 18]. Although the exact level of vitamin B12 or iron was not analyzed in this study, the decreased absorption capacity of those nutrients could have affected the recovery of hemoglobin in the uLAR group before ileostomy closure.

This study has several limitations owing to its retrospective nature. First, to continuously analyze changes in patients during 3 years, we had to exclude some patients with loss of data owing to irregular follow-up, and this may have caused a selection bias in the results. In addition, the parameters used in our study were selected to monitor the postoperative status of rectal cancer patients; more sensitive and accurate markers reflecting nutritional status, such as the levels of prealbumin, retinol-binding protein, transferrin, and iron could not be measured [13]. In this study, some patients with local or distant recurrences were also excluded to compare the nutritional effect after surgeries, not the outcome of the disease itself.

We also excluded cases that needed a permanent stoma for the treatment of postoperative complications after uLAR because those cases were not suitable for the evaluation of LARS. There was no prophylactic procedure for LARS before ileostomy closure. After ileostomy closure, nutritional counseling or medical supports were provided to the patients who complained about frequent defecation or urgency over 10 times per day. The biofeedback therapy was recommended to the patient who showed intractable low anterior syndromes that persisted at least 1 year after ileostomy closure. The biofeedback therapy in our institute included coordination training, sensory training, and strength training and was performed once weekly for 10 consecutive weeks. Five (27.8%) patients in the uLAR groups had underwent biofeedback therapy and two of them reported improved symptoms. One patient did not show any change after therapy, and the other two patients refused to continue the biofeedback therapy. We could not include the results after these measures for patients in this study, because of the lack of medical records that came from the limitation of the retrospective study.

A study including those cases might find a relationship between nutritional and oncological status after uLAR and APR. Additionally, in order to observe when patients in the uLAR group completely restored their preoperative weight and when a plateau of the nutritional parameters was formed in the two groups, it seems necessary to conduct a study with a follow-up period of 3 years or more. According to the results of other studies, patients who underwent uLAR tended to adapt to their defecation problems over time, and if the patients are free of cancer after 5 years, the presence of an abdominal stoma impairs the QoL to a greater extent than do LARS-related problems [19, 20]. It is also unclear that weight gain of the APR group was not associated with increased food intake with limited activities and mood disorders after APR. Therefore, a more long-term investigation of nutritional status and QoL including the patients' defecation and eating habits, with a questionnaire survey conducted concurrently, will better clarify the association between LARS after uLAR and the nutritional status over time.

5. Conclusions

In conclusion, although the capacity of recovering the preoperative body weight in patients who underwent uLAR was not low to the extent of aggravating the patients' nutritional status, it was slower than that in patients who underwent APR. LARS might be one of the primary causes of this difference, but more studies are required to clarify this relationship. Even so, the results of this study might indirectly reflect the low anterior syndrome effect of uLAR and help colorectal surgeons in selecting better surgical methods and in better counseling patients with very low-lying rectal cancer.

References

[1] L. D. MacDonald and H. R. Anderson, "The health of rectal cancer patients in the community," *European journal of surgical oncology*, vol. 11, no. 3, pp. 235–241, 1985.

[2] L. F. de Campos-Lobato, A.–. F. PC, I. C. Lavery, and R. P. Kiran, "Abdominoperineal resection does not decrease quality of life in patients with low rectal cancer," *Clinics*, vol. 66, no. 6, pp. 1035–1040, 2011.

[3] P. How, S. Stelzner, G. Branagan et al., "Comparative quality of life in patients following abdominoperineal excision and low anterior resection for low rectal cancer," *Diseases of the Colon & Rectum*, vol. 55, no. 4, pp. 400–406, 2012.

[4] M. R. Weiser, H. M. Quah, J. Shia et al., "Sphincter preservation in low rectal cancer is facilitated by preoperative chemoradiation and intersphincteric dissection," *Annals of Surgery*, vol. 249, no. 2, pp. 236–242, 2009.

[5] P. Campelo and E. Barbosa, "Functional outcome and quality of life following treatment for rectal cancer," *Journal of Coloproctology*, vol. 36, no. 4, pp. 251–261, 2016.

[6] T. Juul, M. Ahlberg, S. Biondo et al., "Low anterior resection syndrome and quality of life: an international multicenter study," *Diseases of the Colon and Rectum*, vol. 57, no. 5, pp. 585–91, 2014.

[7] A. Sturiale, J. Martellucci, L. Zurli et al., "Long-term functional follow-up after anterior rectal resection for cancer," *International Journal of Colorectal Disease*, vol. 32, no. 1, pp. 83–88, 2017.

[8] K. J. Emmertsen and S. Laurberg, "Low anterior resection syndrome score: development and validation of a symptom-based scoring system for bowel dysfunction after low anterior resection for rectal cancer," *Annals of Surgery*, vol. 255, no. 5, pp. 922–928, 2012.

[9] C. Keane, C. Wells, G. O'Grady, and I. P. Bissett, "Defining low anterior resection syndrome: a systematic review of the literature," *Colorectal disease*, vol. 19, no. 8, pp. 713–722, 2017.

[10] C. L. C. Bryant, P. J. Lunniss, C. H. Knowles, M. A. Thaha, and C. L. H. Chan, "Anterior resection syndrome," *The Lancet Oncology*, vol. 13, no. 9, pp. e403–e408, 2012.

[11] J. Pachler and P. Wille-Jørgensen, "Quality of life after rectal resection for cancer, with or without permanent colostomy," *Cochrane Database of Systematic Reviews*, no. 12, 2012.

[12] J. Konanz, F. Herrle, C. Weiss, S. Post, and P. Kienle, "Quality of life of patients after low anterior, intersphincteric, and abdominoperineal resection for rectal cancer—a matched-pair analysis," *International Journal of Colorectal Disease*, vol. 28, no. 5, pp. 679–688, 2013.

[13] S. H. Kong, J. S. Park, I. K. Lee et al., "Postoperative oral nutritional supplementation after major gastrointestinal surgery: a randomized controlled clinical trial," *Asia Pacific Journal of Clinical Nutrition*, vol. 26, no. 5, pp. 811–819, 2017.

[14] F. Smedley, T. Bowling, M. James et al., "Randomized clinical trial of the effects of preoperative and postoperative oral nutritional supplements on clinical course and cost of care," *British Journal of Surgery*, vol. 91, no. 8, pp. 983–990, 2004.

[15] J. Nightingale and J. M. Woodward, "Guidelines for management of patients with a short bowel," *Gut*, vol. 55, Supplement 4, pp. iv1–iv12, 2006.

[16] N. Collins, "Protein-energy malnutrition and involuntary weight loss: nutritional and pharmacological strategies to enhance wound healing," *Expert Opinion on Pharmacotherapy*, vol. 4, no. 7, pp. 1121–1140, 2003.

[17] D. Owczarek, T. Rodacki, R. Domagala-Rodacka, D. Cibor, and T. Mach, "Diet and nutritional factors in inflammatory bowel diseases," *World Journal of Gastroenterology*, vol. 22, no. 3, pp. 895–905, 2016.

[18] T. S. Schiergens, V. Hoffmann, T. N. Schobel et al., "Long-term quality of life of patients with permanent end ileostomy: results of a nationwide cross-sectional survey," *Diseases of the Colon & Rectum*, vol. 60, no. 1, pp. 51–60, 2017.

[19] C. Fucini, R. Gattai, C. Urena, L. Bandettini, and C. Elbetti, "Quality of life among five-year survivors after treatment for very low rectal cancer with or without a permanent abdominal stoma," *Annals of Surgical Oncology*, vol. 15, no. 4, pp. 1099–1106, 2008.

[20] L. Sideris, F. Zenasni, D. Vernerey et al., "Quality of life of patients operated on for low rectal cancer: impact of the type of surgery and patients' characteristics," *Diseases of the Colon & Rectum*, vol. 48, no. 12, pp. 2180–2191, 2005.

Neutrophil to Lymphocyte Ratio as a Predictor of Poor Prognosis in Metastatic Pancreatic Cancer Patients Treated with Nab-Paclitaxel plus Gemcitabine: A Propensity Score Analysis

J. Ventriglia,[1] A. Petrillo,[2] M. Huerta Alváro,[3] M. M. Laterza,[2] B. Savastano,[4] V. Gambardella,[3] G. Tirino,[2] L. Pompella,[2] A. Diana,[2] F. Iovino,[5] T. Troiani,[2] E. Martinelli,[2] F. Morgillo,[2] M. Orditura,[2] A. Cervantes,[3] F. Ciardiello,[2] and F. De Vita[2]

[1]*Uro-Gynaecological Department, INT G. Pascale, Via Mariano Semmola, 80131 Naples, Italy*
[2]*U.O.C. Medical Oncology, School of Medicine, Università della Campania L. Vanvitelli, c/o II Policlinico, Via Pansini 5, 80131 Naples, Italy*
[3]*Department Hematology and Medical Oncology, INCLIVA Biomedical Research Institute, University of Valencia, Blasco Ibáñez 17, 46010 Valencia, Spain*
[4]*Breast Department, INT G. Pascale, Via Mariano Semmola, 80131 Naples, Italy*
[5]*Department of Cardiothoracic and Respiratory Sciences, School of Medicine, Università della Campania L. Vanvitelli, c/o II Policlinico, Via Pansini 5, 80131 Naples, Italy*

Correspondence should be addressed to J. Ventriglia; j.ventriglia@hotmail.it

Academic Editor: Alessandro Passardi

Background. High neutrophil to lymphocyte ratio (NLR) has shown to be a predictor of poor outcomes in various malignancies, including pancreatic cancer. *Methods.* We assessed 70 consecutive pts with histologically confirmed mPC who received chemotherapy with nab-paclitaxel/gemcitabine at two different European oncologic centers between January 2012 and November 2015. Variables assessed for prognostic correlations included age ≥ 66, sex, Karnofsky PS score, primary tumor site, baseline CA19.9 level ≥ 59xULN, 12-week decrease of the CA19.9 level ≥ 50% from baseline, basal bilirubin level, baseline NLR, biliary stent implantation, and liver metastasis. Survival analyses were generated according to the Kaplan-Meier method. Univariate and multivariate analyses were performed by a Cox proportional hazard model. *Results.* According to NLR values, the patients were divided into two groups: high and low. Low group patients showed a better median PFS (7 months versus 5 months) and median OS (13 months versus 7 months) in respect to high group patients. At multivariate analysis, Karnofsky PS < 80% (HR = 0.4; CI 0.2–1.2), liver metastases (HR = 0.4; CI 0.18–0.82), and NLR ≥ 5 (HR = 2.7; 95% CI 1.4–5.2) were predictors of poorer OS. Based on the presence of one or more independent prognostic factors, three risk categories were identified: good-risk, intermediate-risk and poor-risk. The median OS was 22, 10, and 7 months, respectively. *Conclusions.* Baseline NLR is an independent predictor of survival of patients with mPC receiving palliative chemotherapy and could be useful to develop a simple clinical score to identify a subgroup of patients with a low chance to benefit from chemotherapy.

1. Background

Pancreatic cancer is the ninth most common cancer and the forth cause of cancer-related mortality worldwide. Five-year overall survival (OS) does not exceed 5% due to the fact that more than 85% of patients are diagnosed with incurable locally advanced or metastatic disease [1, 2]. FOLFIRINOX (oxaliplatin, irinotecan, fluorouracil, and leucovorin) or gemcitabine plus albumin-bound paclitaxel is the current standard of care in the first-line setting for patients with metastatic disease [3, 4]. Despite these newer regimens have increased survival, it remains extremely poor still today. Therefore, it is important to clarify the biological mechanisms that contribute to tumor progression as well as to identify prognostic factors for stratify individual risk. During last years, tumor size, histologic grade, vascular invasion, perineural invasion, lymph node metastases, and distant metastases have been recognized as prognostic factors [5–7]. Recently, growing interest in the role of inflammatory response has emerged. Tumor microenvironment is known to have an important role in cancer development and progression and may be associated with systemic inflammation that could be a significant predictor of survival. Hypoalbuminemia, elevated C-reactive protein, increased levels of cytokines, and high leukocyte count and their subtypes are measurable parameters in blood that reflect the systemic inflammatory response [8–13]. Actually, several evidences suggesting that an elevated peripheral blood neutrophil to lymphocyte ratio (NLR) is related to a worse outcome in various types of cancer, including renal cell carcinoma, soft tissue sarcoma, nonsmall cell lung cancer (NSCLC), breast cancer, and colorectal cancer (CRC) [14–22]. We analyzed retrospectively the prognostic independent role of pretreatment NLR in a cohort of 70 metastatic pancreatic patients treated with gemcitabine plus nab-paclitaxel as first-line chemotherapy enrolled in two different European oncologic centers. In this study, we showed that NLR is an independent predictor of the prognosis for metastatic pancreatic cancer patients and that high NLR levels are associated with a short life expectancy.

2. Patients and Methods

70 patients were diagnosed with metastatic pancreatic cancer in the Department of Oncology at the Second University of Naples and in the Department of Oncology at the University Hospital in Valencia between January 2012 and December 2015. Written informed consent was obtained from each patient involved in the study, and the research was approved by the Ethic Committee of Second University of Naples. Patients with active infections, hematological disorders or malignancies, or autoimmune disorders, or treated with steroids were excluded from our analysis. Patients with prior adjuvant gemcitabine treatment were included in our analysis only if the treatment was completed at least 6 months before. Data were censored on December 2015. The characteristics of the series are summarized in Table 1. Neutrophil and lymphocyte counts were obtained in peripheral blood before starting chemotherapy and were calculated by dividing the absolute neutrophil count by the absolute lymphocyte count. The cut-off for the NLR was 5 on the basis literature results ($NLR < 5$, $NLR \geq 5$) [23–25]. All patients received first-line chemotherapy with nab-paclitaxel, 125 mg/m^2, followed by gemcitabine 1000 mg/m^2 administered intravenously (IV) on days 1, 8, and 15 every 4 weeks until disease progression or evidence of unacceptable toxicity. Recombinant human granulocyte colony-stimulating factor and erythropoietin were administered as needed. Dose reductions were applied in cases of grade III/IV toxicities.

Tumor assessment was performed every 12 weeks according to our clinical practice [26]. OS was defined as the interval between the start of nab-paclitaxel and gemcitabine first-line therapy to death or last follow-up visit. The progression-free survival (PFS) was defined as the interval between the start of nab-paclitaxel and gemcitabine therapy to clinical progression or death or last follow-up visit if not progressed. Variables assessed for prognostic correlations included age ≥ 66, sex, Karnofsky performance status (PS) score, primary tumor site, baseline CA19.9 level ≥ 59xULN, 12-week decrease of the CA19.9 level ≥ 50% from baseline, basal bilirubin level, baseline neutrophil to lymphocyte ratio (NLR), biliary stent implantation, and the presence of liver metastasis. Finally, a prognostic scoring index was planned using the independent prognostic factors identified at multivariate analysis.

Table 1

Characteristic	Nab-paclitaxel plus gemcitabine (range)
Age (range)	66 (41–77)
≥70	17 (24%)
Sex	
M	31 (44%)
F	39 (56%)
PS (Karnofsky)	
100%	24 (34%)
80–90%	37 (53%)
60–70%	9 (13%)
Pancreatic primary location	
Head	43 (61%)
Body/tail	27 (39%)
Site of metastasis	
Lung	14 (20%)
Node	7 (10%)
Liver	47 (67%)
Peritoneum	15 (21%)
Bone	3 (4%)
Brain	1 (1%)
Number of metastatic sites	
1	52 (74%)
≥2	17 (26%)
Biliary stent	16 (23%)
Median CA19.9	500 U/I (<1–61,564)
Previous surgery	16 (23%)
Previous adjuvant gemcitabine	10 (14%)

3. Statistical Analysis

The primary end-point of this analysis was to evaluate the role of prognostic factors on the median OS. Statistical analysis was performed using SPSS 21.0 statistical software. Associations between clinical and histopathological parameters with OS and PFS were investigated using Kaplan-Meier curves and compared by the log-rank test. The chi-square (χ^2) test was used to analyze the relationship between NLR and clinicopathological parameters. Cox regression was applied to multivariate survival analysis to

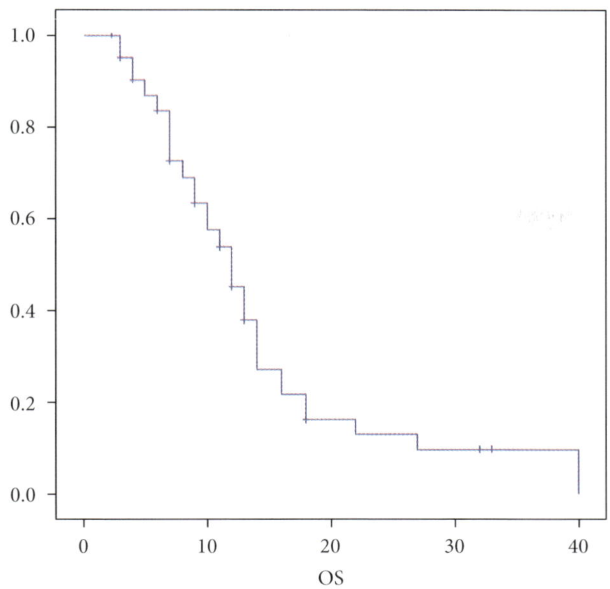

Figure 1: Median OS.

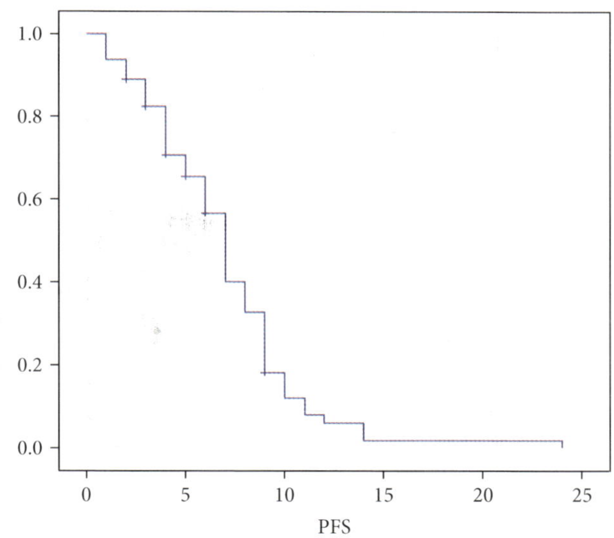

Figure 2: Median PFS.

determine effects of probable prognostic factors on PFS and OS. Survival distribution was estimated by the Kaplan-Meier method with 95% confidence interval (CI), and a significant difference was considered when $p < 0.05$ [27]. To adjust for selection bias, all available variables (age ≥ 66, sex, Karnofsky PS score, primary tumor site, baseline CA19.9 level ≥ 59xULN, 12-week decrease of the CA19.9 level ≥ 50% from baseline, basal bilirubin level, biliary stent implantation, and liver metastasis) were introduced in a multivariate logistic regression to calculate a propensity score for each patient with statistical analysis system software (STATA 11). The matching methods used in propensity score analysis are 1 : 1 matching.

4. Results

At the time of data censoring, 56 pts had progression of disease or died; median PFS was 7 months (95% CI 6.221–7.779), and median OS was 12 months (95% CI 9.926–14.074) with a 12-month OS rate of 34.3% (Figures 1 and 2). Three pts (4.3%) were still alive at 24 months after starting chemotherapy.

The patients were divided into two groups according to the cut-off of 5: high ($n = 49$) and low NLR ($n = 21$). With a median follow-up of 32 months, median OS of the high NLR groups and low NLR groups was 7 months and 13 months, respectively ($p = 0.003$) (Figure 3). Univariate analysis identified Karnofsky PS ($p = 0.005$), liver metastasis ($p = 0.01$), and NLR ≥ 5 ($p = 0.005$) as significant prognostic factors for poor OS. The Cox multivariate model showed NLR ≥ 5 as an independent prognostic factor (hazard ratio (HR) = 2.7; 95% CI 1.4–5.2; $p = 0.003$) together with Karnofsky PS (HR = 0.4; CI 0.2–1.2; $p = 0.04$) and liver metastasis (HR = 0.4; CI 0.18–0.82; $p = 0.01$) (Table 2).

To further confirm the results observed, a propensity score-matched analysis was performed. Twenty-eight couples were matched and were observed that the NLR ≥ 5 group

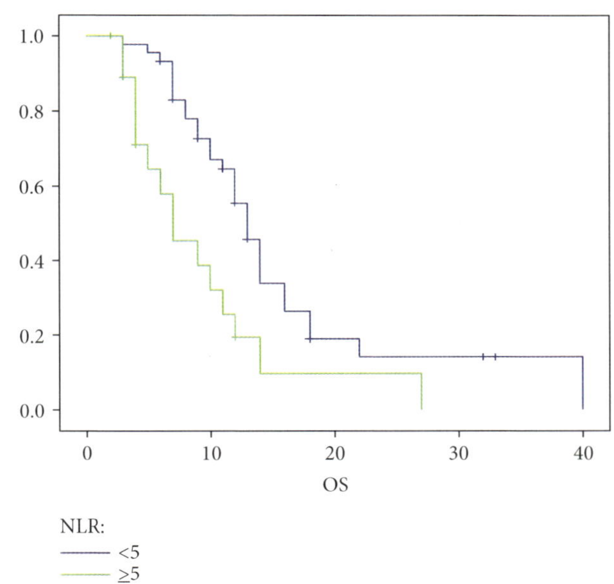

Figure 3: Median OS according to the NLR.

showed an increase death risk of 19% in respect to the NLR < 5 group ($p = 0.02$).

The PFS in the high NLR group was significantly shorter in respect to the low NLR group (5 versus 7 months; $p = 0.02$; Figure 4). Univariate analysis identified CA19.9 response, the presence of liver metastasis, Karnofsky performance status score, and NLR as significant prognostic factors for high PFS. In the multivariate regression analysis, CA19.9 response and NLR confirmed as independent prognostic factors for high PFS (Table 3).

Subsequently, we designed a prognostic model based on the independent prognostic factors related to OS: performance status, NLR, and liver metastasis. Based on these parameters, the study population was divided into three risk groups according to the number of independent prognostic factors involved: 0 factor → good prognosis; 1

Table 2: Univariate and multivariate analysis OS.

Variable	Univariate HR	Univariate 95% CI	Univariate p value	Multivariate HR	Multivariate 95% CI	Multivariate p value
Age (≥66 years versus <66 years)	0.7	0.4–1.3	0.27			
Gender (female versus male)	1.3	0.71–2.41	0.38			
Tumor location (nonhead versus head)	1.3	0.7–2.4	0.4			
Karnofsky performance status score (100–80% versus 70–60%)	0.3	0.12–0.69	**0.005**	0.4	0.2–1.2	0.04
CA19.9 basal (≥59 ULN versus <59 ULN)	1	0.5–2.2	0.8			
CA19.9 reduction (<50% versus ≥50%)	1.8	0.89–3.62	0.098			
Stent (yes versus no)	0.58	0.29–1.16	0.12			
N/L ratio (≥5 versus <5)	2.47	1.3–4.7	**0.005**	2.70	1.4–5.2	**0.003**
Liver metastasis	0.4	0.2–0.8	**0.01**	0.4	0.18–0.82	**0.01**

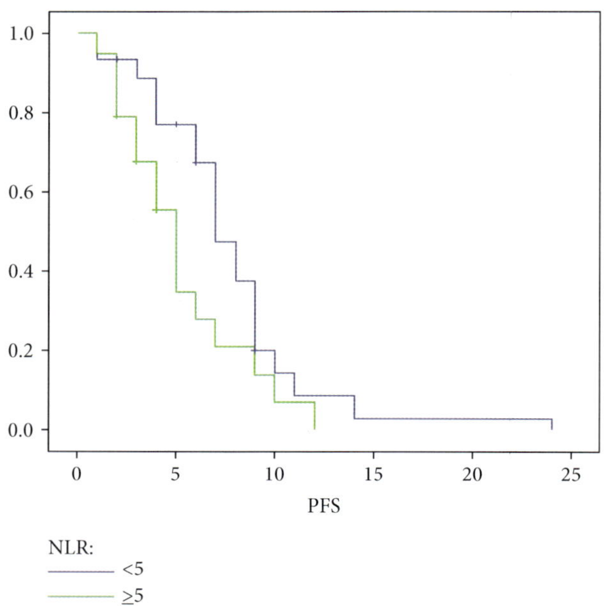

Figure 4: Median PFS according to the NLR.

factor → intermediate prognosis; and 2 factors → poor prognosis. The survival differed notably according to the risk stratification. Patients ($n = 22$) without risk factors (good prognosis) had a median OS of 22 months (95% CI: 8.8–35); patients ($n = 39$) with the presence of one factor (intermediate prognosis) had a median OS of 10 months (95% CI: 6.8–13), and patients ($n = 9$) with the presence of two or more factors (poor prognosis) had a median OS of 7 months (95% CI: 1–15) (Figure 5).

60%, 35.8%, and 22.2% of patients with good, intermediate, and poor prognosis were alive at 12 months, respectively. Furthermore, 20% of patients with good prognosis was alive at 24 months.

5. Discussion

Several studies have shown that elevated NLR is associated with worse prognosis in patients with different solid tumors. A recent meta-analysis showed that elevated NLR predicted a poor prognosis in patients with pancreatic cancer (28). These findings are consistent with our results. Using a NLR cut-off of 5, we found that elevated NLR was associated with decreased OS; indeed, patients with NLR ≥ 5 showed a median OS of 7 months compared to 12 months of patients with NLR < 5. Therefore, our results show that NLR ≥ 5 predicts a shorter OS, suggesting that elevated NLR could be a potential biomarker to identify patients with a poor outcome. The relation between NLR and worse prognosis is still unclear and under investigation. It is well known that inflammation contributes to cancer development and progression and that high neutrophil count is a hallmark of systemic inflammation. In particular, neutrophils secreting inflammatory cytokines such as interleukin-2 (IL-2), interleukin-6 (IL-6), interleukin-10 (IL-10), tumor necrosis factor α (TNF-α), and proangiogenic factors including vascular endothelial growth factor (VEGF) provide a favorable tumor microenvironment for cancer progression. Furthermore, the increased IL-10 and TNF-α levels lead to a decrease in the lymphocyte count, a crucial component of innate immunity and the adaptive immune response, with a relevant role in the immune surveillance process towards cancer cells. Therefore, a high NLR could indicate an increased neutrophil-dependent inflammatory response and a reduced lymphocyte-mediated antitumor immune response, in turn able to promote tumor invasiveness, thus resulting in tumor progression and poor outcome [9–11]. Furthermore, we carried out a propensity score matching to adjust for differences in baseline data; this analysis confirmed our results, thus excluding possible selection bias.

According to the results of the IMPACT study and the subsequent analyses [28], we confirm that in a population of metastatic pancreatic cancer patients treated with gemcitabine and nab-paclitaxel, Karnofsky performance status score, the presence of liver metastases, and baseline NLR were independent predictors of survival associated with an increased risk of death. Recently, Goldstein et al. showed that in advanced pancreatic cancer patients treated with FOLFOXIRI, ECOG PS, liver metastases, and NLR were the most important predictors of survival [29]. Furthermore, they categorized this series as good-risk (0 factors), intermediate-risk (1 factor), and poor-risk (≥2 factors), observing significant differences in terms of OS for these 3 groups. Using this prognostic score in a distinct population treated with a different

TABLE 3: Univariate and multivariate analysis PFS.

Variable	Univariate			Multivariate		
	HR	95% CI	p value	HR	95% CI	p value
Age (≥66 years versus <66 years)	0.86	0.5–1.5	0.58			
Gender (female versus male)	1.1	0.6–1.9	0.71			
Tumor location (nonhead versus head)	1.3	0.7–2.2	0.37			
Karnofsky performance status score (100–80% versus 70–60%)	0.5	0.2–1	0.08			
CA19.9 basal (≥59 ULN versus <59 ULN)	0.8	0.4–1.5	0.5			
CA19.9 reduction (<50% versus ≥50%)	2.44	1.3–4.6	**0.006**	3.22	1.6–6.4	**0.001**
Stent (yes versus no)	0.69	0.37–1.29	0.24			
N/L ratio (≥5 versus <5)	1.9	1.0–3.4	**0.036**	2.77	1.3–5.7	**0.006**
Liver metastasis	0.5	0.3–0.9	**0.038**	0.5	0.2–1.0	0.05

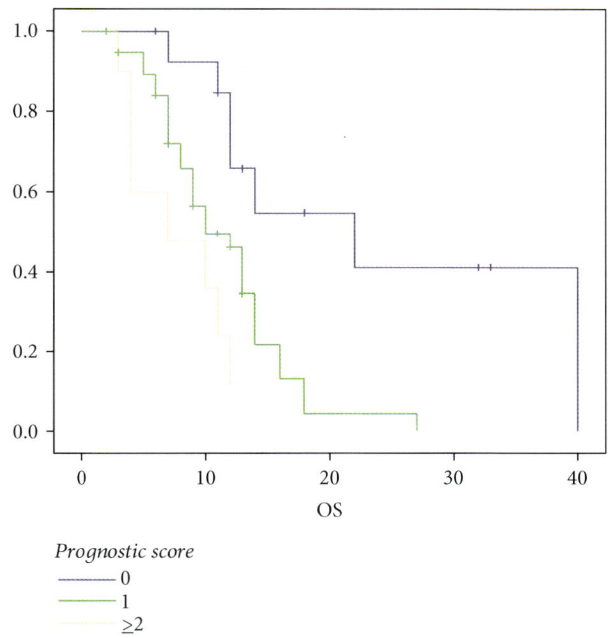

FIGURE 5: Median OS according to the prognostic score.

first-line regimen, we have confirmed its usefulness allowing the identification of a subgroup of patients with particularly poor outcome that does not seem to benefit from chemotherapy. Indeed, in our experience the poor-risk group exhibited a median OS of 7 months.

This study has several strengths: all patients presented metastatic disease and received the same chemotherapy regimen as first-line therapy; furthermore, the prognostic meaning of NLR was validated by a propensity score analysis to exclude potential selection bias. On the contrary, the main limitation was represented by the retrospective nature of the study with a small number of patients.

6. Conclusion

Our data confirm that elevated baseline NLR is associated with a poor prognosis in patients with metastatic pancreatic cancer treated with gemcitabine and nab-paclitaxel; in addition, the adopted prognostic scoring system might be useful to identify a subgroup of patients with poor prognosis who do not benefit from chemotherapy.

Abbreviations

mPC: Metastatic pancreatic cancer
NLR: Neutrophil to lymphocyte ratio
OS: Overall survival
NSCLC: Nonsmall cell lung cancer
CRC: Colorectal cancer
PFS: Progression-free survival
PS: Performance status
CI: Confidence interval
HR: Hazard ratio
IL-2: Interleukin-2
IL-6: Interleukin-6
IL-10: Interleukin-10
TNF-α: Tumor necrosis factor α
VEGF: Vascular endothelial growth factor.

Ethical Approval

The research was approved by the Ethic Committee of Second University of Naples and was performed, according to the Declaration of Helsinki.

Disclosure

All authors certify that they have no affiliations with or involvement in any organization or entity with any financial interest (such as honoraria; educational grants; participation in speakers' bureaus; membership, employment, consultancies, stock ownership, or other equity interest; and expert testimony or patent-licensing arrangements) or nonfinancial interest (such as personal or professional relationships, affiliations, knowledge, or beliefs) in the subject matter or materials discussed in this manuscript. Earlier version of this work was presented at "ESMO Congress," 2016.

Authors' Contributions

J. Ventriglia drafted the manuscript and performed the statistical analysis. A. Petrillo performed the statistical analysis; M. Orditura, A. Cervantes, and F. Ciardiello revised the article critically. F. De Vita revised the article critically for the important intellectual content and approved the final version to be published. M. Huerta Alváro, M. M. Laterza, B. Savastano, V. Gambardella, G. Tirino, L. Pompella, T. Troiani, E. Martinelli, F. Morgillo, and A. Diana participated in the acquisition and collection of data.

References

[1] R. L. Siegel, K. D. Miller, and A. Jemal, "Cancer statistics, 2016," *CA: A Cancer Journal for Clinicians*, vol. 66, no. 1, pp. 7–30, 2016.

[2] M. Sant, C. Allemani, M. Santaquilani et al., "EUROCARE-4. Survival of cancer patients diagnosed in 1995–1999. Results and commentary," *European Journal of Cancer*, vol. 45, no. 6, pp. 931–991, 2009.

[3] T. Conroy, F. Desseigne, M. Ychou et al., "FOLFIRINOX versus gemcitabine for metastatic pancreatic cancer," *The New England Journal of Medicine*, vol. 364, no. 19, pp. 1817–1825, 2011.

[4] D. D. Von Hoff, T. Ervin, F. P. Arena et al., "Increased survival in pancreatic cancer with nab-paclitaxel plus gemcitabine," *New England Journal of Medicine*, vol. 369, no. 18, pp. 1691–1703, 2013.

[5] A. Vincent, J. Herman, R. Schulick, R. H. Hruban, and M. Goggins, "Pancreatic cancer," *Lancet*, vol. 378, no. 9791, pp. 607–620, 2011.

[6] A. Bilici, "Prognostic factors related with survival in patients with pancreatic adenocarcinoma," *World Journal of Gastroenterology*, vol. 20, no. 31, pp. 10802–10812, 2014.

[7] J. Tabernero, E. G. Chiorean, J. R. Infante et al., "Prognostic factors of survival in a randomized phase III trial (MPACT) of weekly nab-paclitaxel plus gemcitabine versus gemcitabine alone in patients with metastatic pancreatic cancer," *The Oncologist*, vol. 20, no. 2, pp. 143–150, 2015.

[8] A. Mantovani, P. Allavena, A. Sica, and F. Balkwill, "Cancer-related inflammation," *Nature*, vol. 454, no. 7203, pp. 436–444, 2008.

[9] E. Elinav, R. Nowarski, C. A. Thaiss, B. Hu, C. Jin, and R. A. Flavell, "Inflammation-induced cancer: crosstalk between tumours, immune cells and microorganisms," *Nature Reviews Cancer*, vol. 13, no. 11, pp. 759–771, 2013.

[10] S. I. Grivennikov, F. R. Greten, and M. Karin, "Immunity, inflammation, and cancer," *Cell*, vol. 140, no. 6, pp. 883–899, 2010.

[11] D. S. O'Callaghan, D. O'Donnell, F. O'Connell, and K. J. O'Byrne, "The role of inflammation in the pathogenesis of non-small cell lung cancer," *Journal of Thoracic Oncology*, vol. 5, no. 12, pp. 2024–2036, 2010.

[12] Z. Mei, Y. Liu, C. Liu et al., "Tumour-infiltrating inflammation and prognosis in colorectal cancer: systematic review and meta-analysis," *British Journal of Cancer*, vol. 110, no. 6, pp. 1595–1605, 2014.

[13] G. Lin, Y. Liu, S. Li et al., "Elevated neutrophil-to-lymphocyte ratio is an independent poor prognostic factor in patients with intrahepatic cholangiocarcinoma," *Oncotarget*, vol. 7, no. 32, pp. 50963–50971, 2016.

[14] T. Sugiura, K. Uesaka, H. Kanemoto, T. Mizuno, and Y. Okamura, "Elevated preoperative neutrophil-to-lymphocyte ratio as a predictor of survival after gastroenterostomy in patients with advanced pancreatic adenocarcinoma," *Annals of Surgical Oncology*, vol. 20, no. 13, pp. 4330–4337, 2013.

[15] G. Garcea, N. Ladwa, C. P. Neal, M. S. Metcalfe, A. R. Dennison, and D. P. Berry, "Preoperative neutrophil-to-lymphocyte ratio (NLR) is associated with reduced disease-free survival following curative resection of pancreatic adenocarcinoma," *World Journal of Surgery*, vol. 35, no. 4, pp. 868–872, 2011.

[16] A. J. Templeton, M. G. McNamara, B. Šeruga et al., "Prognostic role of neutrophil-to-lymphocyte ratio in solid tumors: a systematic review and meta-analysis," *JNCI: Journal of the National Cancer Institute*, vol. 106, no. 6, 2014.

[17] G. J. K. Guthrie, K. A. Charles, C. S. D. Roxburgh, P. G. Horgan, D. C. McMillan, and S. J. Clarke, "The systemic inflammation-based neutrophil–lymphocyte ratio: experience in patients with cancer," *Critical Reviews in Oncology/Hematology*, vol. 88, no. 1, pp. 218–230, 2013.

[18] H. Shimada, N. Takiguchi, O. Kainuma et al., "High preoperative neutrophil–lymphocyte ratio predicts poor survival in patients with gastric cancer," *Gastric Cancer*, vol. 13, no. 3, pp. 170–176, 2010.

[19] M. Tomita, T. Shimizu, T. Ayabe, A. Yonei, and T. Onitsuka, "Preoperative neutrophil to lymphocyte ratio as a prognostic predictor after curative resection for non-small cell lung cancer," *Anticancer Research*, vol. 31, no. 9, pp. 2995–2998, 2011.

[20] Y. Ohno, J. Nakashima, M. Ohori, T. Gondo, T. Hatano, and M. Tachibana, "Followup of neutrophil-to-lymphocyte ratio and recurrence of clear cell renal cell carcinoma," *The Journal of Urology*, vol. 187, no. 2, pp. 411–417, 2012.

[21] J. Chen, Q. Deng, Y. Pan et al., "Prognostic value of neutrophil-to-lymphocyte ratio in breast cancer," *FEBS Open Bio*, vol. 5, no. 1, pp. 502–507, 2015.

[22] M. Orditura, G. Galizia, A. Diana et al., "Neutrophil to lymphocyte ratio (NLR) for prediction of distant metastasis-free survival (DMFS) in early breast cancer: a propensity score-matched analysis," *ESMO Open*, vol. 1, no. 2, article e000038, 2016.

[23] D. S. Wang, H. Y. Luo, M. Z. Qiu et al., "Comparison of the prognostic values of various inflammation based factors in patients with pancreatic cancer," *Medical Oncology*, vol. 29, no. 5, pp. 3092–3100, 2012.

[24] G. Luo, M. Guo, Z. Liu et al., "Blood neutrophil-lymphocyte ratio predicts survival in patients with advanced pancreatic cancer treated with chemotherapy," *Annals of Surgical Oncology*, vol. 22, no. 2, pp. 670–676, 2015.

[25] H. L. Martin, K. Ohara, A. Kiberu, T. Van Hagen, A. Davidson, and M. A. Khattak, "Prognostic value of systemic inflammation-based markers in advanced pancreatic cancer," *Internal Medicine Journal*, vol. 44, no. 7, pp. 676–682, 2014.

[26] J. Verweij, P. Therasse, E. Eisenhauer, and RECIST Working Group, "Cancer clinical trial outcomes: any progress in tumour-size assessment?," *European Journal of Cancer*, vol. 45, no. 2, pp. 225–227, 2009.

[27] E. L. Kaplan and P. Meier, "Nonparametric estimation from incomplete observations," *Journal of the American Statistical Association*, vol. 53, no. 282, pp. 457–481, 1958.

[28] J. J. Yang, Z. G. Hu, W. X. Shi, T. Deng, S. Q. He, and S. G. Yuan, "Prognostic significance of neutrophil to lymphocyte ratio in pancreatic cancer: a meta-analysis," *World Journal of Gastroenterology*, vol. 21, no. 9, pp. 2807–2815, 2015.

[29] D. Goldstein, R. H. El-Maraghi, P. Hammel et al., "Nab-paclitaxel plus gemcitabine for metastatic pancreatic cancer: long-term survival from a phase III trial," *JNCI Journal of the National Cancer Institute*, vol. 107, no. 2, article dju413, 2015.

29

Surgical Management of Gastric Gastrointestinal Stromal Tumours: Comparison of Outcomes for Local and Radical Resection

Anantha Madhavan,[1] Alexander W. Phillips,[1] Claire L. Donohoe,[1] Rebecca J. Willows,[1] Arul Immanuel,[1] Mark Verril,[2] and S. Michael Griffin[1]

[1]*Northern Oesophagogastric Cancer Unit, Royal Victoria Infirmary, Newcastle upon Tyne NE1 4LP, UK*
[2]*Northern Centre for Cancer Care, Freeman Hospital, Newcastle upon Tyne NE7 7DN, UK*

Correspondence should be addressed to S. Michael Griffin; mike.griffin@nuth.nhs.uk

Academic Editor: Alessandro Passardi

Gastrointestinal stromal tumours (GISTs) most commonly originate from the stomach. Their treatment is dependent on size and whether they are symptomatic. Curative treatment requires surgery, which may be preceded by neoadjuvant imatinib if it is felt that this will aid in achieving clear (R0) resection margins. The aim of this study was to evaluate outcomes from patients that underwent a "local" organ-preserving operation, with those that required a more radical resection, and the influences on selecting a more radical resection. A retrospective review of patients undergoing surgery for symptomatic gastric GISTs from a single institution over 9 years was carried out. Patients were divided into three cohorts dependent on whether they had a "local" resection, "anatomical" resection, or "extended" resection. 71 patients were included. Overall, 5-year survival was 92%. Operating time, blood loss, and length of stay were significantly lower in the group undergoing local resection ($p < 0.05$). Tumour size was also smaller in the local group (median 4 cm versus 5 cm $p < 0.05$). Tumour location also influenced the type of surgery performed, with tumours at the cardia, gastroesophageal junction, and antrum all having "anatomical" resections. Lymphadenectomy did not appear to impact on outcomes. These findings indicate that local excision, where possible, does not impair oncological outcomes.

1. Introduction

Gastrointestinal stromal tumours (GISTS) account for 1% of gastrointestinal malignancies [1]. They are mesenchymal in origin with the majority (60–70%) occurring in the stomach [2]. Presentation and management of gastric GISTs is dependent on the size, location, and presentation. Small GISTs, up to 2 cm in size, may be found incidentally and are frequently asymptomatic. They usually do not require surgical intervention, but rather surveillance to ensure they are not significantly enlarging [3]. Larger GISTs (greater than 5 cm) and those that are causing either obstructive symptoms or have bled require excision [4, 5].

The curative treatment of gastric GISTs involves surgical resection [3, 6, 7]. The aim of surgery is to achieve an R0 resection (no evidence of microscopic residual disease and negative margins) with an intact pseudocapsule [8]. The size of the tumour, location, and its proximity to adjacent intra-abdominal viscera may influence the surgical approach undertaken and the extent of stomach resected [7–10]. Whilst a localised surgical resection may be employed for some tumours, it may be preferable to perform a more conventionally "radical" approach including a lymphadenectomy for others. Current guidelines state that lymphadenectomy is "normally not required" but do not unequivocally state indications for lymphadenectomy [11]. In some instances, en bloc resection of adjacent organs may be required to obtain a clear resection margin [3]. In the last decade, imatinib has been used in the neoadjuvant setting to reduce the size of the primary tumour in order to improve

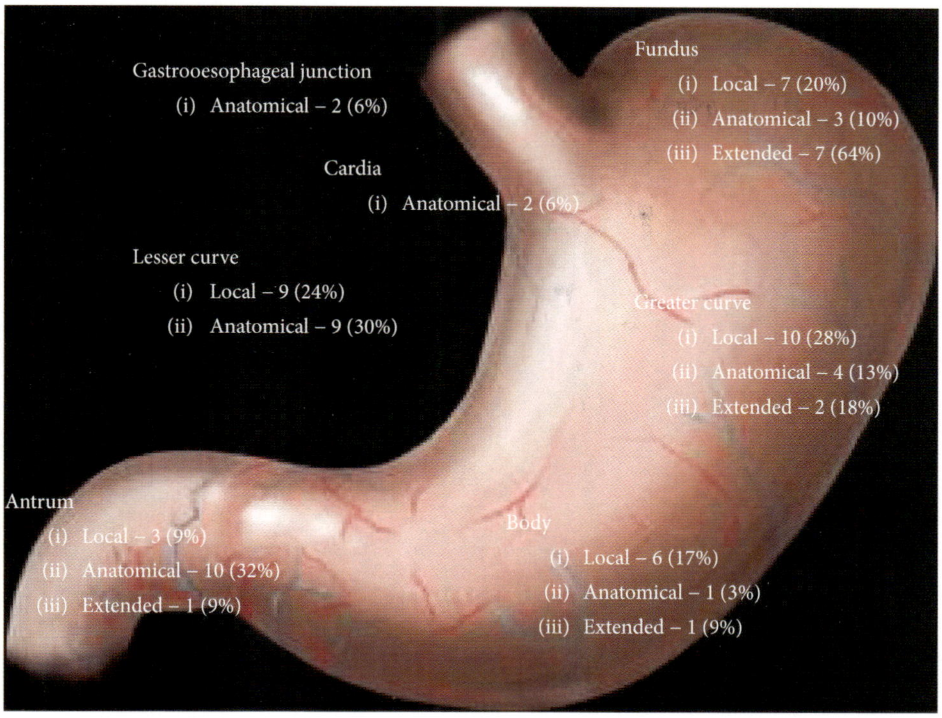

FIGURE 1: Distribution of gastrointestinal tumours in the anatomical, local, and extended resection cohort.

the success of obtaining a clear resection margin [12, 13]. Laparoscopic surgery is increasingly used to facilitate excision of small or medium sized GISTs below 5 cm in size; however, this can be challenging, and care is required when handling the tumour to try and minimise the risk of rupture which may compromise oncological outcomes [14, 15].

The aim of this study was to evaluate outcomes of patients requiring surgery for gastric GISTs from a single institution. Three cohorts that underwent either a "local" excision, anatomical resection, or an extended resection were compared, and factors influencing the extent of surgery were reviewed; role of lymphadenectomy and suitability of a local resection for those who received neoadjuvant imatinib were evaluated.

2. Method

2.1. Patient Population. A retrospective review of all patients undergoing curative surgery for a gastric GIST was performed. Patients were treated at a single centre (Northern Oesophagogastric Unit, Newcastle upon Tyne, UK) between January 2007 and January 2016. All patients underwent standard staging investigations which consisted of endoscopic assessment, endoscopic ultrasound, and CT, were then discussed in a multidisciplinary team meeting (MDM), and subsequently underwent either local resection (either open or laparoscopically), anatomical resection usually in the form of a total or subtotal gastrectomy, (with lymphadenectomy), or an extended anatomical or extended local resection (en bloc resection of all involved structures and lymphadenectomy). The principles of selection of a local operative approach included the ability to obtain an R0 resection margin and preservation of function where possible. In tumour encroaching on the cardia or the incisura or pylorus, a formal anatomical resection was performed (subtotal or total gastrectomy with Roux-en-Y reconstruction with lymphadenectomy or proximal partial gastrectomy with jejunal interposition reconstruction). Anatomical resection included at least a D1 lymphadenectomy as routine in those patients undergoing either a total or subtotal resection. Where tumours invaded surrounding structures, a resection was considered if R0 resection was possible with en bloc removal of invaded structures (distal pancreas, spleen, diaphragm, or colon) and classified as an extended resection.

Where a tumour was deemed not resectable without unacceptable morbidity, treatment with neoadjuvant imatinib was used at a starting dose of 400 mg/day. Treatment response was assessed by CT scan using the Choi criteria every 3 months [16]. The decision to proceed to surgery was when the tumour became resectable or if the tumour did not respond to the standard neoadjuvant treatment regimen. The algorithm for surgical decision-making is summarised in Figure 1.

2.2. Analysis. To assess the impact of operative approach on outcome, patients were divided into three cohorts: local excision, anatomical resection, and extended en bloc resection.

For analysis of impact of lymphadenectomy on outcome, patients were divided into three cohorts for analysis: those undergoing a resection where the underlying aim was to excise the tumour only, with adequate margins and no purposeful lymphadenectomy were regarded as "local excision"; and those where a conventional oncological resection was carried out were regarded as an "anatomical resection". This cohort included both patients who underwent a subtotal and total gastrectomy with either a D1 or D2 lymphadenectomy and patients who underwent a proximal partial gastrectomy with no formal lymphadenectomy. The third group was the extended resection cohort. In this cohort, extension of the tumours into adjacent abdominal viscera required an en bloc resection of the organ to achieve a clear resection margin. This was either combined with a local or anatomical resection.

Data were prospectively recorded using a standardised pro forma. Complications were assessed for twice daily and categorised using the Accordion classification system [17]. Pathological stage groups were assessed using the Miettinen and Lasota classification system [18].

2.3. Statistical Analysis. Statistical calculations were performed by SPSS software, version 22 (SPSS, Chicago, IL).

A Kruskal-Wallis test and Mann–Whitney U test were used to compare continuous variables, and categorical data were compared using a chi-squared/Fisher's exact test. A log-rank (Mantel-Cox) test was used to compare survival between groups. Survival statistics were calculated using Kaplan-Meier method, and the log-rank test was used to assess differences in survival between groups. Overall, survival rate was recorded for patients as well as time to recurrence for disease-free survival. Survival time was measured from the date of operation to the date of an event or last follow-up. All tests performed were two-tailed. p values less than 0.05 (2-sided) were considered statistically significant.

Table 1: Surgical procedures.

Procedure	Number
Local resections	
Open sleeve gastrectomy	3
Lap sleeve gastrectomy	2
Open wedge resection	13
Laparoscopic wedge resection	15
Anatomical resections	
Subtotal gastrectomy	16
Subtotal gastrectomy + D2 lymphadenectomy	4
Total gastrectomy	3
Proximal partial gastrectomy	2
Middle third gastrectomy	2
Oesophagogastrectomy	1
Proximal gastrectomy + jejunal interposition	2
Extended resections	
Open sleeve gastrectomy + distal pancreatectomy + splenectomy	2
Open sleeve gastrectomy + wedge resection diaphragm	1
Total gastrectomy + en bloc resection of diaphragm	1
Total gastrectomy + distal pancreatectomy + splenectomy	4
Partial gastrectomy + splenectomy	1
Wedge resection + splenectomy	1
Subtotal gastrectomy + transverse colon resection	1

3. Results

From January 2007 to January 2016, 76 patients underwent surgery for gastric GISTs. Operative mortality was 0%, and significant morbidity (classified as Accordion III or IV) was 5% with an overall recorded operative morbidity of 10.5%. The overall survival rates in the series at two and five years were 95% and 92%, respectively. Disease-free survival at two and five years was 95% and 92%, respectively.

3.1. Outcomes Based on the Extent of Surgical Resection. Patients were divided into three groups: local resection, anatomical resection, and extended resection. Surgeries carried out in each group are summarised in Table 1.

The baseline demographics (ASA, BMI, age, and gender) of those operated on were comparable between the groups, although those undergoing extended resection were more likely to be males (Table 2). The overall size of the tumour was smaller in the local excision cohort versus the anatomical and extended resection cohorts ($p = <0.05$).

Analysis of operative parameters revealed that there was significantly lower median operating time (100 minutes versus 180 minutes $p < 0.05$), blood loss (80 ml versus 255 ml $p < 0.05$), and length of stay (6 days versus 11 days $p < 0.05$) in the local excision cohort.

Most patients (70%) undergoing a local excision had their surgery performed laparoscopically. There was no significant difference in overall postoperative morbidity between the three cohorts. However, three (8.8%) patients in the local resection cohort had significant morbidity, classified as Accordion ≥ 3 compared to only one (3.3%) in the anatomical excision cohort. Pathological prognostic groups did not significantly differ between the groups (Table 2). R0 resection status was 97% in the local excision cohort and 97% in the anatomical resection group compared to 90% in the extended radical excision cohort ($p = 0.572$).

3.2. Impact of Location and Size on Surgery Performed. There was variation in the location of the tumours within the three cohorts. Tumours located within the cardia 2 (6%), gastrooesophageal junction 2 (6%), and antrum 10 (32%) underwent a formal anatomical resection. The choice of resection for tumours located within the lesser curve and fundus was influenced by the size.

For tumours located on the lesser curve, size appeared to influence whether a local resection or anatomical resection was performed. For those undergoing a local resection, median size was 4 cm (4–10 cm) versus 5 cm (5–15 cm) for those that underwent an anatomical resection ($p = 0.22$).

The median size of the tumour in the fundus in the local resection cohort was 4 cm (4–9 cm) versus 9 cm (8–10 cm) in the anatomical resection cohort ($p = 0.02$). There was a trend towards local resection for smaller tumours on the greater curve. The median tumour size in the local resection cohort was 4 cm (4-5 cm) versus 5 cm (5–10 cm) in the anatomical resection cohort but was not statistically significant ($p = 0.12$).

Extended resection was required to achieve a clear resection margin in tumours located in the fundus 7 (64%) and greater curve 2 (18%) due to extraluminal extension into adjacent viscera.

TABLE 2: Demographics.

	Local resection ($n = 35$)	Anatomical resection ($n = 30$)	Extended resection ($n = 11$)	p value
Age	64 (43–86)	68 (47–81)	58 (35–76)	0.03
BMI	28 (21–40)	25 (21–35)	26.5 (22–36)	0.403
Sex (M : F)	20 : 15	14 : 17	9 : 1	0.045
ASA				
1	3 (8.8%)	5 (16.7%)	1 (10%)	
2	25 (73.5%)	19 (63.3%)	7 (64%)	0.614
3	6 (17.6%)	5 (16.7%)	2 (18%)	
4	0	1 (3.3%)	1 (10%)	
Neoadjuvant treatment	1 (3%)	5 (16%)	7 (70%)	<0.001
Laparoscopic approach	19 (54.3%)	0	0	<0.001
Operating time (min)	90 (60–220)	180 (120–320)	170 (110–300)	<0.001
Blood loss (ml)	60 (50–80)	250 (50–1000)	550 (50–3800)	0.084
Length of stay (days)	6 (2–20)	10 (5–33)	10 (4–16)	<0.001
Postoperative complication	4 (15%)	2 (6.7%)	2 (18.2%)	0.465
Accordion > 3	3 (8.6%)	1 (3.3%)	0	0.34
Pathological size (cm)	3.5 (1.2–10.6)	5.0 (2.5–14.8)	7.0 (3.5–12.0)	0.021
Pathological risk group				
Very low	15 (42.9%)	8 (26.7%)	2 (18.2%)	
Low	11 (31.4%)	10 (33.3%)	5 (45.5%)	0.235
Medium	6 (17.1%)	5 (15.2%)	0	
High	3 (8.6%)	7 (23.3%)	4 (36.4%)	
Adjuvant treatment	1 (3%)	3 (10%)	3 (27%)	0.134
Lymph node yield	0 (0–19)	17 (0–54)	10 (0–48)	<0.001
Positive LN	0	1 (0-1)	0	
Resection margin				0.572
R0	34 (97.1%)	29 (96.7%)	10 (90.9%)	
R1	1 (2.9%)	1 (3.3%)	1 (9.1%)	

3.3. Role of Lymphadenectomy. In the anatomical and extended resection cohort, 30 patients had lymph nodes excised as part of their surgery. In the extended resection cohort, 9 patients (82%) had a lymphadenectomy with a median lymph node yield of 10 (6–48). In the anatomical resection cohort, 21 patients (70%) had lymphadenectomy with a median lymph node yield of 17 (4–54).

Only one patient had any positive nodes found at pathologic analysis. In this case, there was a single positive node out of twenty-four resected. This patient had undergone neoadjuvant imatinib for 12 months for a 10 cm fundal GIST invading the spleen and subsequently underwent a total gastrectomy with distal pancreatectomy and splenectomy. R0 resection margin was achieved, and the final pathology was low risk. After 12 months of adjuvant imatinib and follow-up of 24 months postoperatively, no disease recurrence was noted on surveillance CT.

3.4. Choice of Surgical Resection after Neoadjuvant Imatinib. Thirteen patients had neoadjuvant imatinib due the large size of the tumour and its close proximity to adjacent abdominal viscera, threatening the surgical resection margin. One patient underwent local excision, three patients underwent anatomical resection, and nine patients underwent extended resection due to extraluminal extension of the tumour into adjacent organs. The median duration of neoadjuvant treatment with imatinib was 12 months (range: 3–36 months) with a median percentage decrease in maximum diameter of −31.4% (range +10% to −67.3%).

Postoperative pathological risk of recurrence classification was found to be very low risk in 2, low in 5, intermediate in 1, and high in 5 patients. Two of the patients with low-risk tumours by size had no tumour cells at pathological analysis.

One patient had a palliative resection, as a peritoneal deposit was noted at the time of surgery and the resection margin was positive due to widespread extension of the primary tumour into adjacent organs. This patient died from metastatic disease at 11 months postoperatively despite treatment with adjuvant imatinib. Of the patients receiving neoadjuvant imatinib, six subsequently received adjuvant imatinib. Five out of the six patients had high-risk pathology, and one patient had intermediate risk.

Three patients developed recurrence in this cohort despite R0 resection, the median time to recurrence was 28 months (14–42). Two of the patients had high-risk pathology

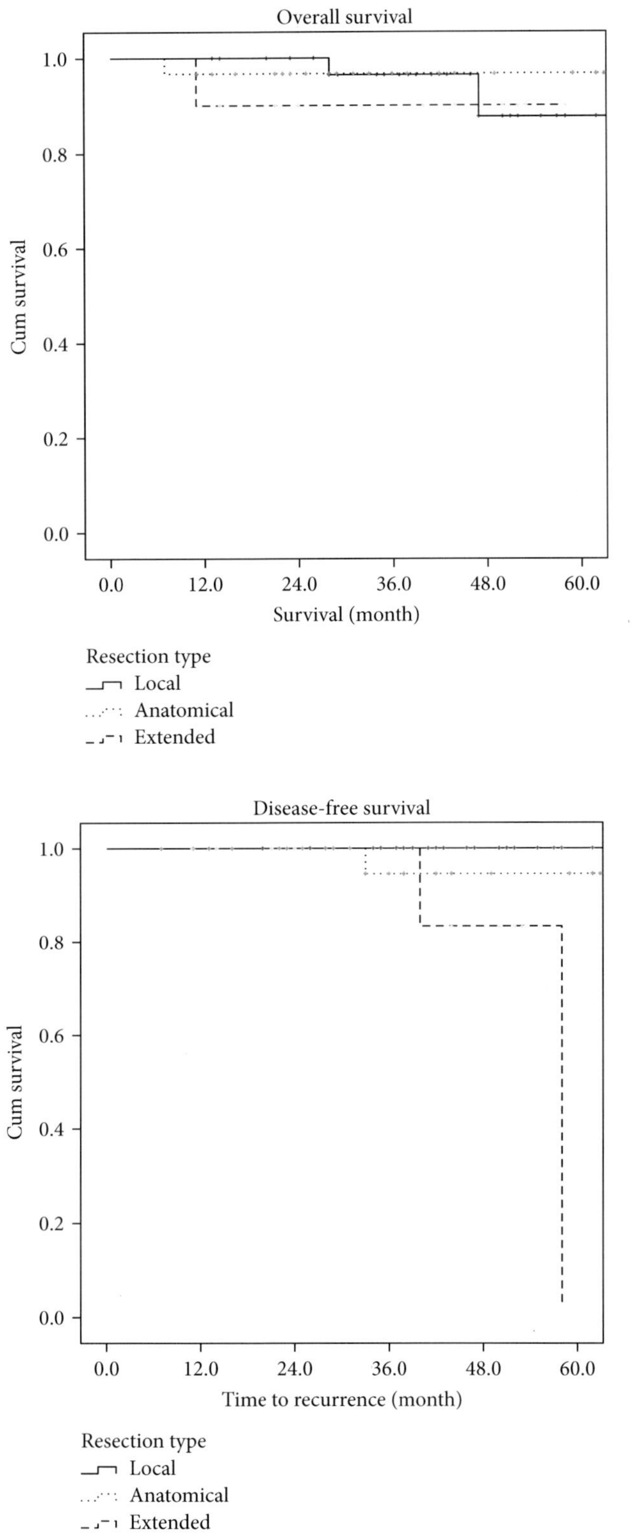

FIGURE 2: Overall survival and disease-free survival according to the surgery type.

and had adjuvant imatinib. The remaining patient had low-risk pathology and thus did not receive adjuvant imatinib. All the patients developed solitary metastases in the liver and underwent metastasectomy.

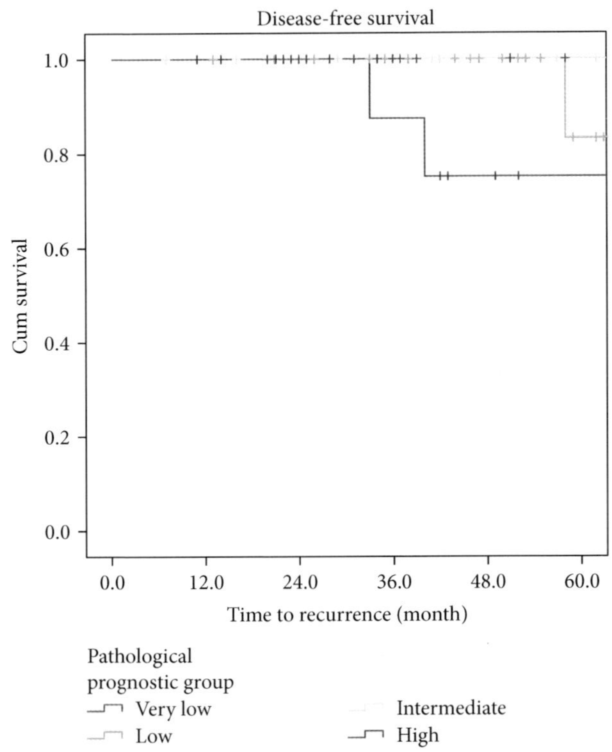

FIGURE 3: Survival according to the pathological prognostic group [18].

The overall five-year survival was 91%, and the 5-year disease-free survival rate was 77% in patients who underwent neoadjuvant imatinib and surgery.

3.5. Prognosis and Survival. Six patients (8%) had metastatic recurrence of the GISTs during the follow-up period. One patient in the local excision group following an R0 resection with low-risk pathology developed peritoneal and liver metastases 47 months after surgery. The patient subsequently died of metastatic disease despite adjuvant treatment with imatinib.

Of the remaining five patients, three underwent an anatomical resection and two underwent an extended resection. Three of the patients had postoperative high-risk pathology, of which two received adjuvant treatment. The other two patients had intermediate-risk and low-risk pathology, respectively. The median time to recurrence was 21 months (4–40). Four of these patients had concurrent solitary liver metastases and underwent metastasectomy. The remaining patient developed solitary metastases in the sacrum five months after surgery and was treated with adjuvant imatinib.

Only one patient had an incomplete resection (R1) in the local excision cohort. Postoperative pathology was low risk, and the patient remained tumour free over a 24-month surveillance period to date. Although tumour size and location influence the surgical approach taken in order to achieve an R0 resection status, none of the patients with R1 resection were found to have recurrence during surveillance. Overall survival did not significantly differ according to the operative approach with 5-year survival rates of 90%, 97%, and 90%, respectively ($p = 0.716$). The disease-free survival rate

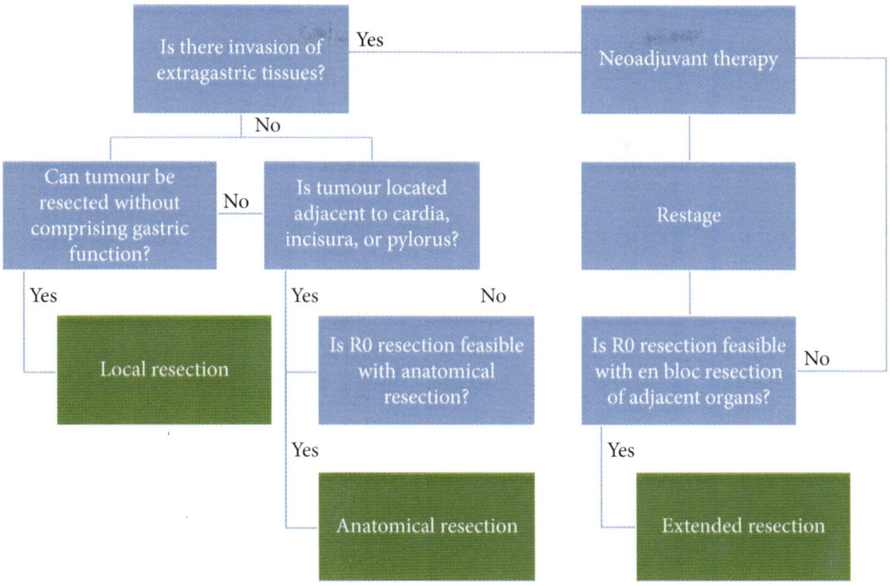

Figure 4: Algorithm for surgical decision-making for gastric GISTs.

was lower in patients undergoing anatomical (57%) or extended resection (45%) compared to local resection (100%) ($p = 0.012$) (Figure 2). Recurrence-free survival is closely correlated with the pathological prognostic group, although there was one patient with low-risk pathology with disease recurrence at 56 months postoperatively (Figure 3).

4. Discussion

The findings from this study demonstrate that patient outcomes are not compromised by performing a local resection provided that an R0 resection can be achieved. In this series, all patients were discussed within an MDM to ensure agreement that a local excision, where deemed surgically feasible, was also oncologically appropriate. In this study, those undergoing a local excision are more likely to have the procedure performed laparoscopically and have significantly less blood loss, a shorter operating time, and a shorter stay in hospital.

Within this study, tumour location appeared to have the most important impact on influencing whether or not local excision was performed. Tumours located in the cardia and gastrooesophageal junction required a formal anatomical resection to maintain the gastrointestinal function. For tumours located in the lesser curve and antrum, an additional consideration for the choice of resection was the size of the tumour. Larger tumours located in these regions required a formal anatomical resection compared to a local excision to achieve both an R0 resection and to provide an acceptable functional outcome. The majority of tumours (65%) located in the fundus, greater curve, and body were amenable to local excision. An extended resection was required if there was evidence of extraluminal extension into adjacent abdominal viscera to achieve a clear resection margin. However, the findings from this study demonstrate that curative resection can be achieved in patients with large extragastric GISTs with associated invasion of surrounding abdominal viscera provided that clear margins can be obtained. For those tumours confined to the gastric wall, without local invasion, systematic lymphadenectomy is not regarded as necessary as gastric GISTs rarely metastasise to lymph nodes [19]. We have developed an algorithm for surgical decision-making for gastric GISTs based on our experience (Figure 4). As demonstrated in this cohort, only one patient had a positive node following a total gastrectomy and D2 lymphadenectomy. It is thus difficult to determine whether lymphadenectomy has a prognostic influence in patients where nodal involvement may exists. However, this extremely low positive nodal yield indicates that radical lymphadenectomy is likely to be rarely important.

Laparoscopic gastric GIST resection was first described more than a quarter of a century ago [20]. Previous studies have shown that laparoscopic resection is associated with less postoperative pain, less morbidity, and shorter hospital stay [10, 21]. These results are corroborated by the findings from the present study. However, concerns over the appropriateness of laparoscopic resection exist with tumours greater than 5 cm in size. The most recent NCCN guidelines suggest that larger tumours may be resected laparoscopically or laparoscopically assisted with a hand port dependent on size and location of the tumour [8]. The findings from this study demonstrate that a local excision can be achieved with larger tumours. However, it should be noted that there was no significant increase in morbidity in resections that included a conventional oncological lymphadenectomy.

Ensuring that the whole tumour, where possible, is resected and that tumour rupture is avoided is of paramount importance in patients requiring gastric GIST resection. In this study, those undergoing a radical approach had larger tumours and as would be expected were associated with a more aggressive pathology. Despite this, five-year survival was comparable between cohorts; however, disease-free survival was lower at 76% in the radical cohort compared to that at 90% in the local group. This may reflect that a more radical operation provides good disease control in those with more aggressive tumours.

This series supports the work by Rutkowski et al., which highlights the role of neoadjuvant imatinib in downstaging patients with large gastrointestinal tumours. In this study, 92% R0 resection was achieved in patients undergoing neoadjuvant imatinib followed by surgery. The median tumour size was 11 cm (6–22). Three patients developed isolated liver metastases and underwent metastasectomy. Despite this, the overall five-year survival in the R0 resection cohort was 100%. The study is limited because of the focus primarily on patients who underwent surgery following neoadjuvant imatinib treatment. The outcomes of the patients who did not proceed to surgery following neoadjuvant imatinib were not evaluated. This was due to the progression of the disease during neoadjuvant treatment, which meant a curative R0 resection was not surgically achievable. Thus, response to neoadjuvant imatinib could be a prognostic factor in large gastrointestinal tumours of the stomach. However, this hypothesis requires further evaluation.

In conclusion, local resection, preserving the stomach, provides excellent outcomes for patients requiring excision of a GIST. In those patients with potentially more aggressive tumours, radical resection is not associated with significantly increased morbidity and may provide good long-term disease control. Further, prospective trials are required to fully establish any benefit from more radical resection.

References

[1] P. C. McGrath, J. P. Neifeld, W. Lawrence JR., S. Kay, J. S. Horsley III, and G. A. Parker, "Gastrointestinal sarcomas. Analysis of prognostic factors," *Annals of Surgery*, vol. 206, no. 6, pp. 706–710, 1987.

[2] H. Joensuu, P. Hohenberger, and C. L. Corless, "Gastrointestinal stromal tumour," *The Lancet*, vol. 382, no. 9896, pp. 973–983, 2013.

[3] I. Judson, R. Bulusu, B. Seddon, A. Dangoor, N. Wong, and S. Mudan, "UK clinical practice guidelines for the management of gastrointestinal stromal tumours (GIST)," *Clinical Sarcoma Research*, vol. 7, no. 1, p. 6, 2017.

[4] The ESMO/European Sarcoma Network Working Group, "Gastrointestinal stromal tumours: ESMO clinical practice guidelines for diagnosis, treatment and follow-up," *Annals of Oncology*, vol. 25, Supplement 3, pp. iii21–iii26, 2014.

[5] R. P. DeMatteo, J. J. Lewis, D. Leung, S. S. Mudan, J. M. Woodruff, and M. F. Brennan, "Two hundred gastrointestinal stromal tumors: recurrence patterns and prognostic factors for survival," *Annals of Surgery*, vol. 231, no. 1, pp. 51–58, 2000.

[6] J. D. Licht, L. B. Weissmann, and K. Antman, "Gastrointestinal sarcomas," *Seminars in Oncology*, vol. 15, no. 2, pp. 181–188, 1988.

[7] M. von Mehren, R. L. Randall, R. S. Benjamin et al., "Soft tissue sarcoma, version 2.2016, NCCN clinical practice guidelines in oncology," *Journal of the National Comprehensive Cancer Network*, vol. 14, no. 6, pp. 758–786, 2016.

[8] G. D. Demetri, M. von Mehren, C. R. Antonescu et al., "NCCN Task Force report: update on the management of patients with gastrointestinal stromal tumors," *Journal of the National Comprehensive Cancer Network*, vol. 8, Supplement 2, pp. S-1–S-41, 2010.

[9] K. Chen, Y. C. Zhou, Y. P. Mou, X. W. Xu, W. W. Jin, and H. Ajoodhea, "Systematic review and meta-analysis of safety and efficacy of laparoscopic resection for gastrointestinal stromal tumors of the stomach," *Surgical Endoscopy*, vol. 29, no. 2, pp. 355–367, 2015.

[10] Y. W. Novitsky, K. W. Kercher, R. F. Sing, and B. T. Heniford, "Long-term outcomes of laparoscopic resection of gastric gastrointestinal stromal tumors," *Annals of Surgery*, vol. 243, no. 6, pp. 738–747, 2006.

[11] R. P. Dematteo, M. C. Heinrich, W. M. El-Rifai, and G. Demetri, "Clinical management of gastrointestinal stromal tumors: before and after STI-571," *Human Pathology*, vol. 33, no. 5, pp. 466–477, 2002.

[12] P. Rutkowski, A. Gronchi, P. Hohenberger et al., "Neoadjuvant imatinib in locally advanced gastrointestinal stromal tumors (GIST): the EORTC STBSG experience," *Annals of Surgical Oncology*, vol. 20, no. 9, pp. 2937–2943, 2013.

[13] B. L. Eisenberg, J. Harris, C. D. Blanke et al., "Phase II trial of neoadjuvant/adjuvant imatinib mesylate (IM) for advanced primary and metastatic/recurrent operable gastrointestinal stromal tumor (GIST): early results of RTOG 0132/ACRIN 6665," *Journal of Surgical Oncology*, vol. 99, no. 1, pp. 42–47, 2009.

[14] J. Q. Cai, K. Chen, Y. P. Mou et al., "Laparoscopic versus open wedge resection for gastrointestinal stromal tumors of the stomach: a single-center 8-year retrospective cohort study of 156 patients with long-term follow-up," *BMC Surgery*, vol. 15, no. 1, p. 58, 2015.

[15] G. Piessen, J. H. Lefèvre, M. Cabau et al., "Laparoscopic versus open surgery for gastric gastrointestinal stromal tumors: what is the impact on postoperative outcome and oncologic results?," *Annals of Surgery*, vol. 262, no. 5, pp. 831–840, 2015.

[16] R. S. Benjamin, H. Choi, H. A. Macapinlac et al., "We should desist using RECIST, at least in GIST," *Journal of Clinical Oncology*, vol. 25, no. 13, pp. 1760–1764, 2007.

[17] S. M. Strasberg, D. C. Linehan, and W. G. Hawkins, "The accordion severity grading system of surgical complications," *Annals of Surgery*, vol. 250, no. 2, pp. 177–186, 2009.

[18] M. Miettinen and J. Lasota, "Gastrointestinal stromal tumors: pathology and prognosis at different sites," *Seminars in Diagnostic Pathology*, vol. 23, no. 2, pp. 70–83, 2006.

[19] I. Pidhorecky, R. T. Cheney, W. G. Kraybill, and J. F. Gibbs, "Gastrointestinal stromal tumors: current diagnosis, biologic behavior, and management," *Annals of Surgical Oncology*, vol. 7, no. 9, pp. 705–712, 2000.

[20] J. J. Lukaszczyk and R. J. Preletz Jr., "Laparoscopic resection of benign stromal tumor of the stomach," *Journal of Laparoendoscopic Surgery*, vol. 2, no. 6, pp. 331–334, 1992.

[21] J. Nishimura, K. Nakajima, T. Omori et al., "Surgical strategy for gastric gastrointestinal stromal tumors: laparoscopic vs. open resection," *Surgical Endoscopy*, vol. 21, no. 6, pp. 875–878, 2007.

Steatohepatitis Is Not Associated with an Increased Risk for Fibrosis Progression in Nonalcoholic Fatty Liver Disease

Hannes Hagström,[1,2] Olof Elfwén,[2] Rolf Hultcrantz,[1,2] and Per Stål[1,2]

[1]*Department of Upper GI, Unit of Liver Diseases, Karolinska University Hospital, Stockholm, Sweden*
[2]*Department of Medicine, Huddinge Karolinska Institutet, Stockholm, Sweden*

Correspondence should be addressed to Per Stål; per.stal@ki.se

Academic Editor: Mario Pirisi

Introduction. Nonalcoholic fatty liver disease (NAFLD) is the most common liver disease globally. The majority of NAFLD patients have fatty liver without inflammation (nonalcoholic fatty liver, NAFL), whereas a minority develop steatohepatitis (nonalcoholic steatohepatitis, NASH). Only NASH and not NAFL has been considered to increase the risk for fibrosis progression. The present study investigates risk factors for fibrosis progression in patients with NAFLD, and if fibrosis progression associates with subsequent mortality. *Material and Methods.* All patients with at least two liver biopsies more than a year apart at our hospital between 1971 and 2016 were identified. Data on plausible risk factors for fibrosis progression were collected. Biopsies were scored for the presence of NASH and fibrosis stage. Regression models were used to investigate the association between baseline NASH and fibrosis progression and fibrosis progression with future mortality. *Results.* 60 patients had undergone serial biopsies (median interval between biopsies 8.4 years, range 1–33 years), with 26 patients (43%) having fibrosis progression. We found no significant risk factors for progression of fibrosis except time between biopsies. Among patients with fibrosis progression, 54% had NAFL and 46% had NASH at baseline. There was a trend for an association between fibrosis progression per se and increased mortality (hazard ratio 2.83, 95% CI 1.0–8.1, $p = 0.05$). *Conclusions.* In this study on NAFLD, baseline steatohepatitis was not associated with an increased risk for fibrosis progression. NAFLD patients without steatohepatitis may develop progressive fibrosis, and those with progressive fibrosis appear to have a higher mortality risk irrespective of baseline NASH status.

1. Introduction

Nonalcoholic fatty liver disease (NAFLD) is the most common liver disease globally [1] and is projected to become the main indication for liver transplantation in the US in the coming decade [2] and also an increasing indication for liver transplantation in the Nordic countries [3]. Histologically, NAFLD is divided into two major subgroups, nonalcoholic fatty liver (NAFL) and nonalcoholic steatohepatitis (NASH). Approximately 10–20% of patients with NAFLD have NASH, whereas the majority have NAFL [4]. Some patients with NAFLD develop progressive fibrosis, which eventually may progress to cirrhosis. Fibrosis stage correlates well with clinical outcomes and is the strongest predictor for overall and liver-related mortality [5–7]. NAFL has generally been considered a benign condition, and it has been thought that only patients with NASH have a potential for fibrosis progression and cirrhosis development. However, this dogma has recently been challenged in several studies showing that fibrosis progression indeed can occur also in patients with NAFL [8, 9].

However, to date, no study has investigated the impact if fibrosis progression per se is associated with an increased risk of future mortality. We aimed to confirm recent findings from other studies, evaluate risk factors for fibrosis progression, and examine if fibrosis progression per se is associated with increased mortality in NAFLD.

2. Materials and Methods

We retrospectively included all patients with NAFLD who had undergone two or more liver biopsies at the Karolinska

University Hospital, Stockholm, Sweden in a cohort study. The methodology for the generation of the cohort and ascertainment of NAFLD has previously been described [5, 10]. Briefly, all liver biopsies performed between 1971 and 2009 with a histopathological finding of steatosis were identified, and the corresponding patient charts were examined to ascertain the NAFLD diagnosis. Furthermore, we used a local database created for financial registration based on ICD 10-codes, to identify additional cases that had undergone liver biopsy between 2009 and 2016. All charts were scrutinized from the earliest record, through the time of biopsies and to the death of the patient or to the end of the follow-up period (April 1st, 2016) to exclude liver diseases other than NAFLD. In total, 2176 patients were found to have evidence of fatty liver, with 510 cases being defined as NAFLD. The reason for the baseline liver biopsy was primarily persistent increased serum levels of ALT/AST or the finding of steatosis on a radiological exam. We excluded patients with a follow-up biopsy less than one year after the baseline biopsy or with insufficient clinical data. Likewise, we excluded all patients with any concurrent liver disease or evidence of excessive alcohol consumption, defined as more than 30 grams of alcohol per day in men and more than 20 grams in women.

The cohort was stratified on progression or no progression of fibrosis between the two biopsies. Progression of fibrosis was defined as an increase of at least one stage of fibrosis. In patients who underwent more than two biopsies ($n = 19$), the first and last biopsies were used.

Table 1: Clinical characteristics at baseline.

Parameter	*N* (%) or median	Range
Age (years)	46	19–70
Sex, male, *N* (%)	37 (62)	
BMI (kg/m^2)	26.4	21.2–38.7
Smoking, ever, *N* (%)	21 (37)	
T2DM, *N* (%)	10 (17)	
Hypertension, *N* (%)	14 (23)	
Platelets ($\times 1\bar{0}^9$/L)	256	56–347
ALT (IU/L)	88	10–307
AST (IU/L)	46	14–289
Ferritin (μg/L)	133	44–753
ALP (IU/L)	200	47–876
GGT (IU/L)	78	22–599
Bilirubin (mg/dL)	0.58	0.18–2.22
PK-INR	1	0.9–1.4
Albumin (g/dL)	4.4	3.2–5.3
AST/ALT ratio	0.7	0.4–4.5
CRP (mg/L)	10	1–26
Cholesterol (mg/dL)	221	77–402
Triglycerides (mg/dL)	186	44–460
Glucose (mg/dL)	95	67–305
NAS (0–8)	4	1–8
NASH *N* (%)	33 (61)	
Fibrosis stage		
0 *N* (%)	15 (25)	
1 *N* (%)	22 (37)	
2 *N* (%)	14 (23)	
3 *N* (%)	6 (10)	
4 *N* (%)	3 (5)	

Abbreviations: BMI: body mass index; DM2: diabetes mellitus type 2; ALT: alanine aminotransferase; AST: aspartate aminotransferase; ALP: alkaline phosphatase; GT: gamma glutamyltransferase; NAS: nonalcoholic fatty liver disease activity score.

2.1. Variables. Data from the time of the baseline and follow-up biopsies were collected from patient charts as per Table 1. Body mass index (BMI) was calculated as weight (kg) divided by height (m) squared. Type 2 diabetes mellitus (T2DM) and hypertension were defined as present if these diagnoses were stated in patient charts or if the patient was using antidiabetic or antihypertensive drugs. After the last biopsy, patients were followed until death of any cause occurred or until the end of the follow-up period (April 1st, 2016). We could ascertain mortality in all 60 patients.

2.2. Histological Assessment. Of the baseline biopsies, 54 were available, and for the follow-up biopsies, 41 were available for reevaluation including scoring of necroinflammatory changes and NASH. Available liver biopsies were reevaluated by two of the researchers (RH and HH), blinded to patient characteristics. The stage of fibrosis and the NAFLD activity score were determined according to Kleiner et al. [11]. The FLIP algorithm was used to define the presence of NASH [12]. For cases where the archival biopsy could not be retrieved, scoring of the fibrosis stage was obtained from the original pathology report, since the interagreement assessment regarding the fibrosis stage between the original report and the follow-up review was high (kappa 0.80). However, in these cases the original scoring of steatosis, lobular inflammation, and ballooning were not included in the analysis of data.

2.3. Statistical Analysis. Descriptive statistics for continuous variables are expressed as median (range), and categorical variables are presented as absolute numbers (percentages). Differences in continuous variables were analyzed using the Mann–Whitney *U* test and differences in categorical variables with Fisher's exact test. The median rate of fibrosis progression in patients with baseline NASH and NAFL, respectively, was calculated as the increase in fibrosis stages divided by time between biopsies, measured in years. A logistic regression model was used to identify factors at baseline and follow-up associated with progression of fibrosis. In multivariate modeling, we adjusted for a number of a priori defined possible confounders including sex, age, BMI, T2DM at baseline, and time between biopsies. A Cox regression model was used to investigate histological factors at baseline as well as fibrosis progression per se and their association with mortality after the second liver biopsy. These analyses were adjusted for the same confounders as in the logistic regression model.

As NASH might be more important in early stages of fibrosis, we performed sensitivity analyses excluding cases

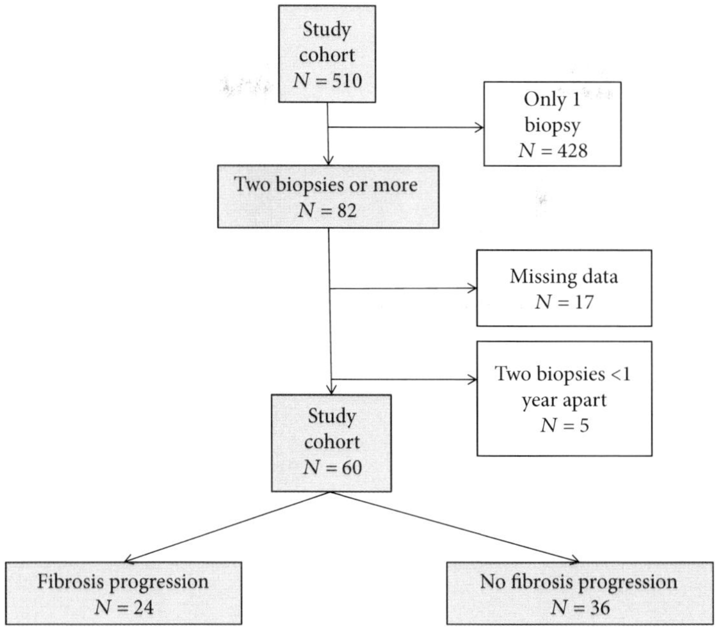

FIGURE 1: Flowchart for patient inclusion.

with advanced fibrosis (stages 3-4). All analyses were performed using STATA v 13.0 (StataCorp, College Station, Texas, USA). A two-tailed p value of <0.05 was considered as statistically significant.

2.4. Ethical Considerations. The study was conducted in accordance with the Helsinki Declaration of 1975, as revised in 1983, and approved by the Ethics Committee at Karolinska University Hospital, Stockholm, Sweden (Dnr: 2011/905-31/2 and 2015/1591-32).

3. Results

3.1. Study Population. Among the 510 patients with a histological diagnosis of NAFLD at baseline, 82 underwent a second biopsy. Of these, 17 patients were excluded due to missing clinical data from the time of the follow-up biopsy, and five patients were excluded because the second liver biopsy was performed within one year of the first, leaving 60 patients for analysis.

A flowchart for patient inclusion is presented in Figure 1. The main reasons for performing the follow-up biopsy were clinical follow-up of steatosis diagnosed at the first biopsy ($n = 28$), persistent high levels of ALT/AST ($n = 15$), while other causes included suspected cirrhosis on ultrasound, staging of fibrosis, or ruling out other suspected diseases ($n = 17$). The cohort was followed from the index biopsy to the death of the patient or until the end of the study period for a median time of 24.8 years (range 7.5–41.2). The median total follow-up time was similar in patients with (24.8 years) and without (25.3 years) fibrosis progression ($p = 0.85$).

3.2. Cohort Characteristics. Clinical, histological, and laboratory features of the cohort are summarized in Table 1. The median age of the cohort at baseline was 46 years (range 19–70 years). There were 62% male participants, and 17% had T2DM. Among the 54 patients with baseline biopsies available for reevaluation, 48% ($n = 26$) had NAS between 1 and 4 and 52% ($n = 28$) had NAS between 5 and 8. The median baseline NAS score was 5 (range 1–8), and NASH was present in 33 (61%) of patients.

Fibrosis staging at the baseline biopsy disclosed stage 0 in 15 (25.0%), stage 1 in 22 (36.7%), stage 2 in 14 (23.3%), stage 3 in 6 (10.0%), and stage 4 in 3 (5.0%) patients.

3.3. Histological Evolution of NAFLD during Follow-Up. The median follow-up interval between the first and second liver biopsies was 8.4 years (range 1–34 years). Twenty-seven patients (45%) had liver biopsies more than ten years apart. A total of 26 (43%) patients had fibrosis progression while 34 (57%) patients had stable or regression of fibrosis. Time between the index and the follow-up biopsy was significantly longer in the group with fibrosis progression (median 16.2 versus 5.5 years, $p = 0.01$). Differences at baseline and at follow-up between patients with and without fibrosis progression are presented in Table 2.

The distribution of fibrosis stages at the baseline and follow-up biopsies is shown in Table 3. Thirteen patients progressed by one stage, ten patients by two stages, two patients by three stages, and one patient progressed by four stages. At follow-up liver biopsy, 21 patients had advanced fibrosis of which 9 had stage 3 and 12 had stage 4 (cirrhosis).

Among the 41 patients with both baseline and follow-up biopsies available for scoring of steatosis, lobular inflammation and ballooning, 23 (62.1%) had NASH at baseline and 18 (48.7%) at follow-up. Of the 23 patients with baseline NASH, 10 (43.5%) experienced resolution of NASH, while 13 (56.5%) had NASH also at follow-up. Of the 14 patients

TABLE 2: Comparison of clinical characteristics at baseline and follow-up between patients with and without progression of fibrosis.

	No fibrosis progression N (%) or median ($N = 34$)	Range	Fibrosis progression N (%) or median ($N = 26$)	Range	p value
Baseline biopsy					
Sex, N male (%)	22 (65)		15 (58)		0.6
Age (years)	42.5	19–70	50	20–66	0.28
BMI (kg/m^2)	26.7	23.5–38.7	26.6	21.2–32.2	0.29
T2DM, N (%)	6 (18)		4 (15)		0.58
Hypertension, N (%)	7 (21)		7 (27)		0.4
Platelets ($\times 10^9$/L)	265	113–347	233	56–332	0.48
ALT (U/L)	92	22–307	86	10–264	0.53
AST (U/L)	49	29–135	46	14–288	0.64
Bilirubin (mg/dL)	0.58	0.35–2.22	0.53	0.16–1.29	0.65
Albumin (g/dL)	4.4	3.3–5.3	4.4	3.2–5.2	0.84
PK-INR	1.0	0.9–1.3	1.0	1.0–1.2	0.45
Total cholesterol (mg/dL)	232	77–402	189	127–340	0.09
NASH, yes (%)	19/30 (63)		14/24 (58)		0.71
Follow-up biopsy					
Years of follow-up	5.5	1.1–27.2	16.2	1.7–33.7	0.01
Age (years)	52	28–83	66	21–84	<0.01
BMI (kg/m^2)	27.8	24.7–38.7	27.1	21–35	0.3
Delta BMI	1.9	−7.5 to 6.4	0.8	−5.0 to 8.1	0.29
T2DM, N (%)	18 (53)		12 (46)		0.4
Hypertension, N (%)	13 (38)		11 (42)		0.48
Platelets ($\times 10^9$/L)	238	61–465	215	92–505	0.25
ALT (U/l)	59	11–343	64	17–604	0.62
AST (U/l)	41	13–238	53	19–299	0.04
Bilirubin (mg/dL)	0.58	0.23–1.87	0.79	0.23–5.73	0.22
Albumin (g/dL)	4.2	1.7–5.2	3.7	2.0–4.8	0.007
PK-INR	1.0	0.9–1.3	1.0	0.9–1.6	0.01
Total cholesterol (mg/dL)	208	93–347	178	131–290	0.17
NASH, yes (%)	10/24 (42)		9/17 (53)		0.54

Abbreviations: BMI: body mass index; DM2: diabetes mellitus type 2; ALT: alanine aminotransferase; AST: aspartate aminotransferase; ALP: alkaline phosphatase; GT: gamma glutamyltransferase; NAS: nonalcoholic fatty liver disease activity score.

TABLE 3: Distribution of the fibrosis stage at baseline and follow-up liver biopsies.

Baseline fibrosis stage	Follow-up fibrosis stage Stage 0	Stage 1	Stage 2	Stage 3	Stage 4	Total
Stage 0	6	**5**	**2**	**1**	**1**	15
Stage 1	2	13	**3**	**3**	**1**	22
Stage 2	1	3	3	**2**	**5**	14
Stage 3	0	1	0	2	**3**	6
Stage 4	0	0	0	1	2	3
Total	9	22	8	9	12	60

Cases with fibrosis progression are marked in bold.

without baseline NASH, five (35.7%) developed NASH while 9 (64.3%) did not.

The median rate of fibrosis progression was 0.15 stages/year (range 0.03–0.78) for patients with NASH at baseline and 0.11 stages/year (range 0.03–0.59) for patients with baseline NAFL ($p = 0.91$).

The presence of NASH at baseline was not associated with fibrosis progression in the multivariate logistic regression analysis (aOR 1.04, 95% CI 0.30–3.64, $p = 0.96$) (Table 4(a)). We found no parameter at baseline or follow-up that predicted fibrosis progression including NAS, baseline fibrosis stage, age, sex, BMI, T2DM, hypertension, or biochemical parameters (data not shown). As predicted, time between biopsies was significantly associated with fibrosis progression (aOR 1.08 for each year between biopsies, 95% CI 1.02–1.14, $p = 0.01$). Further adjusting the model for time between biopsies did not affect the estimates significantly (aOR for NASH at baseline 1.02, 95% CI 0.97–1.07, $p = 0.46$). Importantly, both patients with and without fibrosis progression had a similar development of BMI and type 2 diabetes during follow-up (Table 2). In patients with fibrosis progression, 9/26 (35%) had a reduction in BMI between the two biopsies while none had resolution of type 2 diabetes.

Table 4

(a) Steatohepatitis at baseline biopsy and association with fibrosis progression.

Parameter	OR	95% CI	*p* value	aOR[1]	95% CI	*p* value
NASH	0.81	0.27–2.43	0.71	0.97	0.25–3.69	0.96
NAS 5–8	0.88	0.30–2.56	0.81	0.74	0.21–2.62	0.65

[1]Adjusted for age at first biopsy, sex, BMI, type 2 diabetes, and time between biopsies. Abbreviations: OR: odds ratio; aOR: adjusted odds ratio; CI: confidence interval; NASH: nonalcoholic steatohepatitis; NAS: NAFLD activity score.

(b) The respective association between NASH at baseline, high NAS at baseline, and fibrosis progression per se, with mortality using Cox regression.

Parameter	HR	95% CI	*p* value	aHR[1]	95% CI	*p* value
NASH	1.43	0.55–3.69	0.46	0.97	0.20–4.67	0.97
NAS 5–8	1.02	0.41–2.54	0.97	0.46	0.12–1.69	0.24
Fibrosis progression	2.10	0.87–5.09	0.10	2.83	0.99–8.05	0.051

[1]Adjusted for sex, age, BMI, type 2 diabetes at first biopsy, and time between biopsies. Abbreviations: OR: odds ratio; aOR: adjusted odds ratio; CI: confidence interval; NASH: nonalcoholic steatohepatitis; NAS: NAFLD activity score.

Table 5: Histological disease activity at baseline and follow-up in patients with and without fibrosis progression. Fibrosis stage was determined in all biopsies.

Parameter	No fibrosis progression (mean)	SD	Fibrosis progression (mean)	SD	*p* value
*Baseline**					
Steatosis (1–3)	1.73	0.94	1.79	0.88	0.88
Lobular inflammation (0–3)	1.43	0.85	1.33	0.7	0.63
Ballooning (0–2)	0.97	0.85	0.88	0.85	0.69
NAS (0–8)	3.86	2.31	3.84	2.17	0.92
Fibrosis (0–4)	1.47	1.16	1.15	1.04	0.28
NASH (number of patients, %)	19/30	63%	14/24	58%	0.78
*Follow-up**					
Steatosis (1–3)	1.21	0.93	1.12	0.78	0.83
Lobular inflammation (0–3)	1.17	0.92	1.29	0.69	0.52
Ballooning (0–2)	0.54	0.78	0.94	0.83	0.11
NAS (0–8)	2.92	1.98	3.35	1.73	0.43
Fibrosis (0–4)	1.18	1.11	2.81	1.17	<0.001
NASH (number of patients, %)	10/24	42%	9/17	53%	0.54

*54 biopsies were available for scoring of NASH at baseline and 41 at follow-up. Abbreviations: NAS: NAFLD activity score; NASH: nonalcoholic steatohepatitis; SD: standard deviation.

3.4. Differences in Fibrosis Progression between NAFL and NASH. Among the 26 patients with fibrosis progression on the follow-up biopsy, 24 had biopsies available for baseline biopsy scoring. Of these, 10 (42%) had NAFL and 14 (58%) had NASH at the baseline biopsy. There were no significant differences at baseline concerning steatosis, lobular inflammation, ballooning, NAS, or fibrosis stage between patients with and without fibrosis progression (Table 5).

3.5. Mortality during Follow-Up. After the follow-up biopsy, patients were followed for a median of 6.7 years (range 0.1–34.0). During this time, 21 patients (35%) died, eight (25%) in the group without fibrosis progression and thirteen (50%) in the group with fibrosis progression ($p = 0.05$).

In the Cox regression model, only fibrosis progression was borderline associated with mortality (aHR 2.83, 95% CI 1.00–8.05, $p = 0.051$), while neither presence of NASH nor a high NAS (5–8) at baseline or follow-up showed any trend to an association with increased mortality (Table 4(b)).

3.6. Sensitivity Analysis. No association between baseline NASH and fibrosis progression or mortality was found when excluding cases with fibrosis stages 3-4 from the analysis (data not shown).

4. Discussion

In this retrospective cohort study of 60 NAFLD patients with sequential liver biopsies, a similar proportion of patients with NAFL and NASH had evidence of fibrosis progression. Thus, we confirm similar findings from other groups, which together strengthen the hypothesis that fibrosis progression also can occur in NAFLD patients without steatohepatitis at an initial baseline liver biopsy.

In addition, we found a trend towards increased mortality in patients with fibrosis progression, irrespective if NASH was present or not in the baseline liver biopsy and after adjustment for confounders. This finding is in line with results from previous studies implying that the fibrosis stage correlates with clinical outcomes and is the strongest predictor for overall and liver-related mortality [5–7]. However, due to the retrospective nature of this study, a risk of selection bias may be present. Cases with baseline NAFL and progressive fibrosis could have been selected for follow-up due to clinical events and suspicion of fibrosis progression. Nevertheless, it is obvious that some cases with NAFL without steatohepatitis have a risk for fibrosis progression, and future studies are needed to identify risk factors for fibrosis progression in larger cohorts of patients without NASH. Taken our data together with those from other groups [8, 13–15], it is clear that progression of liver fibrosis progress can occur in both NAFL and NASH.

The only significant risk factor for progression of fibrosis in the present study was the time between the two biopsies. In contrast, baseline T2DM and BMI were also associated with fibrosis progression in three recent studies with similar design as ours [8, 14, 15]. These studies differed from ours by having a greater proportion of patients with T2DM and also with a higher BMI at baseline. McPherson et al. included 108 patients who underwent two liver biopsies at least one year apart with a median follow-up interval of 6.6 years. In that cohort, T2DM was an independent predictor of fibrosis progression [8]. Forty-two percent of their patients had fibrosis progression, and 43% had advanced fibrosis in the follow-up biopsy. Our cohort had a longer follow-up interval (8.4 years), and 35% had advanced fibrosis on the follow-up biopsy. Since patients in our cohort had lower BMI (26.4 kg/m^2) and a lower prevalence of T2DM (17%), our cohort may possibly be more comparable to the general population. The prevalence of diabetes was 5% in the general Swedish population in 2012 [16], and the prevalence of obesity was 10% in a study from 2006 [17]. Nonetheless, the smaller fraction of patients with T2DM and a relatively low median BMI in our cohort limit our ability to assess the impact of diabetes and obesity on fibrosis progression. Therefore, we cannot exclude the possibility of a type 2 error in this respect.

4.1. Strengths and Limitations. The major strength of this study was the long follow-up duration. The follow-up interval between the first and second liver biopsies is the longest hitherto documented. A long enough follow-up time is essential when studying fibrosis progression in patients with NAFLD, since this is a slow process. In a recent meta-analysis, the rate of fibrosis progression was estimated to one stage per seven years in subjects with NASH and per 14 years in those with NAFL [13]. Furthermore, the access to highly valid outcome data on mortality after the second biopsy, with no missing data, is another strength. Also, the cohort was more comparable to the general population than those of previous studies regarding BMI and the presence of type 2 diabetes. The main indication for the first biopsy was elevated liver transaminases and not suspicion of cirrhosis, reflected by the low percentage of patients (15%) having advanced fibrosis at baseline, which suggests a low selection bias at the first biopsy in our study.

The primary limitation of this study is a possible selection bias at the second biopsy, since cases with progressive fibrosis are probably more likely to undergo repeat examination than cases without. However, liver biopsies were historically performed more frequently compared to today, due to a lack of other modalities. Eighty-three percent of patients in this study were originally investigated before year 2000, thus reducing (but not excluding) the risk of selection bias. Since the biopsies were not planned per a specific protocol, the follow-up interval varies to a wide extent. Longer follow-up intervals may have an overrepresentation of older patients with more severe liver disease. As seen in Table 3, the proportion of patients with advanced fibrosis (stages 3 and 4) more than doubled from the index to the follow-up biopsy. In the analysis, we therefore accounted for this by adjusting the statistical models for time between biopsies.

Other limitations include the small sample size, the lack of data on NASH at follow-up biopsy in 19 cases, and the absence of genetic status including *PNPLA3* polymorphisms due to lack of stored blood samples.

A major limitation of all paired biopsy studies in NAFLD, including ours, is the risk of residual confounding. Such confounding factors could comprise of lifestyle changes, including a change in alcohol consumption or medications during follow-up.

We did have access to data on development of BMI and type 2 diabetes, which were not associated with progression of fibrosis. Indeed, 35% of patients with fibrosis progression had a reduction in BMI during the follow-up period, suggesting that a reduction of BMI per se might not be enough to reduce the risk of fibrosis progression in some patients.

4.2. Implications for Clinical Practice and Future Research. The clinical impact of this study together with the conclusions from previous studies [8, 14, 15] is that progressive fibrosis can occur in both NAFL and NASH. This indicates that patients with steatosis but no inflammation on index liver biopsy should not be routinely excluded from clinical follow-up. The results do not help us to identify significant predictors of fibrosis progression, due to the limited size of the cohort, which thus must be a focus of future studies.

The rate of fibrosis progression was quite slow in this study but comparable to what has been found in a recent meta-analysis [13], indicating that repeat noninvasive measurements of fibrosis, such as transient elastography, could be performed with relatively long intervals.

Our study also demonstrates a trend towards higher mortality in patients with progressive fibrosis, which may have implications for selecting patients intended for more intense follow-up. This finding has to be confirmed in future studies on larger cohorts with a long enough follow-up time, which also should aim to find predictors for fibrosis progression.

The present study could possibly contribute to future meta-analyses on this topic.

5. Conclusions

Both NAFL and NASH can lead to progressive fibrosis, with a mean fibrosis progression rate in the present study from 0.11 to 0.15 stages per year. Baseline steatohepatitis was not associated with an increased risk for fibrosis progression. Patients with progressive fibrosis appear to have a higher risk for mortality, regardless if NASH is present or not at baseline. Larger studies are needed to identify which patients with NAFL are at an increased risk for fibrosis progression.

Authors' Contributions

Study conception and design were done by Hannes Hagström and Per Stål. Hannes Hagström, Olof Elfwén, and Rolf Hultcrantz were responsible for the acquisition of data. Statistical analysis was done by Hannes Hagström. Analysis and interpretation of data were done by Hannes Hagström, Olof Elfwén, Rolf Hultcrantz, Per Stål. Hannes Hagström, Olof Elfwén, and Per Stål did the drafting of the manuscript. Guarantors of the article are Hannes Hagström and Per Stål. All authors approved the final version of the article, including the authorship list. Hannes Hagström, Olof Elfwén, Rolf Hultcrantz, and Per Stål performed the critical revision of the manuscript.

Acknowledgments

Hannes Hagström was supported by grants from the Royal Swedish Academy of Sciences and the Swedish Gastroenterology Fund. Per Stål was supported by the Stiftelsen Tornspiran and the Stockholms Läns Landsting (ALF 20150403).

References

[1] R. Loomba and A. J. Sanyal, "The global NAFLD epidemic," *Nature Reviews Gastroenterology & Hepatology*, vol. 10, no. 11, pp. 686–690, 2013.

[2] Q. M. Anstee, G. Targher, and C. P. Day, "Progression of NAFLD to diabetes mellitus, cardiovascular disease or cirrhosis," *Nature Reviews Gastroenterology & Hepatology*, vol. 10, no. 6, pp. 330–344, 2013.

[3] M. Holmer, E. Melum, H. Isoniemi et al., "Nonalcoholic fatty liver disease is an increasing indication for liver transplantation in the Nordic countries," *Liver International*, 2018.

[4] N. M. W. de Alwis and C. P. Day, "Non-alcoholic fatty liver disease: the mist gradually clears," *Journal of Hepatology*, vol. 48, Supplement 1, pp. S104–S112, 2008.

[5] H. Hagström, P. Nasr, M. Ekstedt et al., "Fibrosis stage but not NASH predicts mortality and time to development of severe liver disease in biopsy-proven NAFLD," *Journal of Hepatology*, vol. 67, no. 6, pp. 1265–1273, 2017.

[6] M. Ekstedt, H. Hagström, P. Nasr et al., "Fibrosis stage is the strongest predictor for disease-specific mortality in NAFLD after up to 33 years of follow-up," *Hepatology*, vol. 61, no. 5, pp. 1547–1554, 2015.

[7] P. Angulo, D. E. Kleiner, S. Dam-Larsen et al., "Liver fibrosis, but no other histologic features, is associated with long-term outcomes of patients with nonalcoholic fatty liver disease," *Gastroenterology*, vol. 149, no. 2, pp. 389–397.e10, 2015.

[8] S. McPherson, T. Hardy, E. Henderson, A. D. Burt, C. P. Day, and Q. M. Anstee, "Evidence of NAFLD progression from steatosis to fibrosing-steatohepatitis using paired biopsies: implications for prognosis and clinical management," *Journal of Hepatology*, vol. 62, no. 5, pp. 1148–1155, 2015.

[9] S. Pelusi, S. Petta, C. Rosso et al., "Renin-angiotensin system inhibitors, type 2 diabetes and fibrosis progression: an observational study in patients with nonalcoholic fatty liver disease," *PLoS One*, vol. 11, no. 9, article e0163069, 2016.

[10] K. Bjorkstrom, P. Stal, R. Hultcrantz, and H. Hagstrom, "Histologic scores for fat and fibrosis associate with development of type 2 diabetes in patients with non-alcoholic fatty liver disease," *Clinical Gastroenterology and Hepatology*, vol. 15, no. 9, pp. 1461–1468, 2017.

[11] D. E. Kleiner, E. M. Brunt, M. van Natta et al., "Design and validation of a histological scoring system for nonalcoholic fatty liver disease," *Hepatology*, vol. 41, no. 6, pp. 1313–1321, 2005.

[12] P. Bedossa, "Current histological classification of NAFLD: strength and limitations," *Hepatology International*, vol. 7, Suppl 2, pp. 765–770, 2013.

[13] S. Singh, A. M. Allen, Z. Wang, L. J. Prokop, M. H. Murad, and R. Loomba, "Fibrosis progression in nonalcoholic fatty liver vs nonalcoholic steatohepatitis: a systematic review and meta-analysis of paired-biopsy studies," *Clinical Gastroenterology and Hepatology*, vol. 13, no. 4, pp. 643–654.e9, 2015, e649.

[14] L. A. Adams, S. Sanderson, K. D. Lindor, and P. Angulo, "The histological course of nonalcoholic fatty liver disease: a longitudinal study of 103 patients with sequential liver biopsies," *Journal of Hepatology*, vol. 42, no. 1, pp. 132–138, 2005.

[15] V. W. S. Wong, G. L. H. Wong, P. C. L. Choi et al., "Disease progression of non-alcoholic fatty liver disease: a prospective study with paired liver biopsies at 3 years," *Gut*, vol. 59, no. 7, pp. 969–974, 2010.

[16] S. P. O. Jansson, K. Fall, O. Brus et al., "Prevalence and incidence of diabetes mellitus: a nationwide population-based pharmaco-epidemiological study in Sweden," *Diabetic Medicine*, vol. 32, no. 10, pp. 1319–1328, 2015.

[17] J. S. de Munter, P. Tynelius, C. Magnusson, and F. Rasmussen, "Longitudinal analysis of lifestyle habits in relation to body mass index, onset of overweight and obesity: results from a large population-based cohort in Sweden," *Scandinavian Journal of Public Health*, vol. 43, no. 3, pp. 236–245, 2015.

31

Machine Learning Creates a Simple Endoscopic Classification System that Improves Dysplasia Detection in Barrett's Oesophagus amongst Non-expert Endoscopists

Vinay Sehgal,[1,2] Avi Rosenfeld,[3] David G. Graham,[1,2] Gideon Lipman,[1] Raf Bisschops,[4] Krish Ragunath,[5] Manuel Rodriguez-Justo,[6] Marco Novelli,[6] Matthew R. Banks,[1] Rehan J. Haidry,[1] and Laurence B. Lovat[1,2]

[1]*Department of Gastroenterology, University College London Hospitals NHS Foundation Trust, London, UK*
[2]*Research Department for Tissue & Energy, Division of Surgery & Interventional Science, University College London, London, UK*
[3]*Department of Industrial Engineering, Jerusalem College of Technology, Jerusalem, Israel*
[4]*Department of Gastroenterology, University Hospitals Leuven, Leuven, Belgium*
[5]*Department of Gastroenterology, Queen's Medical Centre, Nottingham, UK*
[6]*Department of Histopathology, University College London Hospitals NHS Foundation Trust, London, UK*

Correspondence should be addressed to Vinay Sehgal; v.sehgal@ucl.ac.uk

Academic Editor: Kazuhiko Uchiyama

Introduction. Barrett's oesophagus (BE) is a precursor to oesophageal adenocarcinoma (OAC). Endoscopic surveillance is performed to detect dysplasia arising in BE as it is likely to be amenable to curative treatment. At present, there are no guidelines on who should perform surveillance endoscopy in BE. Machine learning (ML) is a branch of artificial intelligence (AI) that generates simple rules, known as decision trees (DTs). We hypothesised that a DT generated from recognised expert endoscopists could be used to improve dysplasia detection in non-expert endoscopists. To our knowledge, ML has never been applied in this manner. *Methods.* Video recordings were collected from patients with non-dysplastic (ND-BE) and dysplastic Barrett's oesophagus (D-BE) undergoing high-definition endoscopy with *i-Scan* enhancement (PENTAX®). A strict protocol was used to record areas of interest after which a corresponding biopsy was taken to confirm the histological diagnosis. In a blinded manner, videos were shown to 3 experts who were asked to interpret them based on their mucosal and microvasculature patterns and presence of nodularity and ulceration as well as overall suspected diagnosis. Data generated were entered into the WEKA package to construct a DT for dysplasia prediction. Non-expert endoscopists (gastroenterology specialist registrars in training with variable experience and undergraduate medical students with no experience) were asked to score these same videos both before and after web-based training using the DT constructed from the expert opinion. Accuracy, sensitivity, and specificity values were calculated before and after training where $p < 0.05$ was statistically significant. *Results.* Videos from 40 patients were collected including 12 both before and after acetic acid (ACA) application. Experts' average accuracy for dysplasia prediction was 88%. When experts' answers were entered into a DT, the resultant decision model had a 92% accuracy with a mean sensitivity and specificity of 97% and 88%, respectively. Addition of ACA did not improve dysplasia detection. Untrained medical students tended to have a high sensitivity but poor specificity as they "overcalled" normal areas. Gastroenterology trainees did the opposite with overall low sensitivity but high specificity. Detection improved significantly and accuracy rose in both groups after formal web-based training although it did it reach the accuracy generated by experts. For trainees, sensitivity rose significantly from 71% to 83% with minimal loss of specificity. Specificity rose sharply in students from 31% to 49% with no loss of sensitivity. *Conclusion.* ML is able to define rules learnt from expert opinion. These generate a simple algorithm to accurately predict dysplasia. Once taught to non-experts, the algorithm significantly improves their rate of dysplasia detection. This opens the door to standardised training and assessment of competence for those who perform endoscopy in BE. It may shorten the learning curve and might also be used to compare competence of trainees with recognised experts as part of their accreditation process.

1. Introduction

Invasive oesophageal adenocarcinoma (OAC) is associated with a poor overall 5-year survival of 15% [1]. Barrett's oesophagus (BE) is the only identifiable premalignant lesion. Endoscopic surveillance of BE is performed to detect OAC at a pre-invasive stage that is likely to be amenable to curative treatment. Current surveillance strategies typically rely on white light endoscopy (WLE) to obtain random four-quadrant biopsies every 2 cm through the BE segment [2]. This approach samples less than 5% of the Barrett's epithelium and is therefore prone to missing early lesions [3].

A novel endoscopic image enhancement technology, *i-Scan* (PENTAX HOYA, Japan), has been developed to improve lesion recognition in the gastrointestinal tract. *i-Scan* utilises post processing light filtering technology to enhance different elements on the mucosa and microvasculature. We recently published the first formal classification system for *i-Scan* in the upper gastrointestinal tract [4]. There is also growing evidence to suggest increased accuracy of dysplasia detection using *i-Scan* in the assessment of colorectal polyps [5–7].

Machine learning (ML) is a branch of data mining that applies mathematical models to generate computerised algorithms. These can create novel prediction models. ML involves a computer "learning" important features of a dataset to enable predictions about other, unseen, data. A potential application would be to separate subjects into two (but sometimes more) categories based on the attributes measured. This could then be used to create predictive models about which subjects have a disease.

Over the past 10 years, ML has become increasingly used within the field of medicine. For instance, ML has already been applied to improve detection of ovarian and breast cancers using ultrasonography [8, 9]. Models use patient-specific information to predict a medical outcome or to help support doctors in making a diagnosis [10]. ML also has potential training applications. An example includes IBM's WatsonPaths project (IBM Research), which has been developed to improve training and diagnostic skills amongst medical students at the Cleveland Clinic (http://www.research.ibm.com). Other examples include ML to prognosticate in melanoma, predict susceptibility for cerebrovascular disease, risk of recurrence of breast cancer, and diagnosis of thyroid disease [11–13]. Interestingly, these systems often outperform the diagnostic abilities of specialists in each field.

Currently, there is no standardised method of assessing the competence of endoscopists who perform endoscopy in patients with BE. It is perhaps therefore not surprising that there is considerable variability in diagnostic competence amongst endoscopy trainees across Europe with almost one-third admitting to feeling uncertain when performing endoscopy in BE [14]. A training tool to improve endoscopic lesion recognition in BE is therefore desirable.

The aims of this study were:

(i) To evaluate the accuracy of expert endoscopists to detect dysplasia in patients with BE using *i-Scan*.

(ii) Using the data generated by expert endoscopists to generate a simple automatic machine-based algorithm to help detect dysplasia in patients with BE.

(iii) To assess if training non-expert endoscopists using this algorithm could improve their detection of dysplasia.

2. Methods

2.1. i-Scan Technology. i-Scan is a novel endoscopic post processing light filtering technology (PENTAX HOYA Corporation). Software algorithms with real-time image mapping technology are embedded with an EPKi processor. The EPKi processor enables resolution above high-definition television (HDTV) standard with a resolution of approximately 1.25 megapixels per image. Using distinct digital filters, i-Scan offers post processing of images to allow the endoscopist to make additional analyses. There are three image enhancement modes, which are controlled by pressing a button on the endoscope handpiece (Figure 1):

i. Surface enhancement (i-Scan 1): enhancement of the structure through recognition of the edges.

ii. Contrast enhancement (i-Scan 2): enhancement of depressed areas and differences in structure through the presentation of low-density areas.

iii. Surface and tone enhancement (i-Scan 3): enhancement tailored to individual organs through modification of the combination of red, green and blue (RGB) light components for each pixel.

2.2. Classification System. Classification systems using narrow band imaging (NBI, Olympus®) in patients with BE have already been published [15–19]. Broadly speaking, these take into account mucosal and microvascular patterns to predict dysplasia in BE [20]. A recent multi-national consortium of NBI experts (BING consortium) developed a consensus-driven NBI classification system based on 60 NBI magnification images with encouraging results [21]. In this study, the mucosa was classified as normal (circular, ridged, or tubular pattern) or abnormal (absent or irregular patterns) and the vascular pattern as normal (regular vessels with normal or long branching patterns) or abnormal (focally or diffusely distributed vessels following abnormal mucosal architecture). Dysplasia detection was achieved with an accuracy of 85%, (sensitivity 80%, specificity 88%) with substantial interobserver agreement ($\kappa = 0.681$).

Acetic acid (ACA) chromoendoscopy is increasingly being used to enhance the endoscopic detection of Barrett's dysplasia [22]. When sprayed onto Barrett's mucosa, an acetowhitening reaction occurs such that areas of dysplasia lose their acetowhitening effect faster than areas without dysplasia. This phenomenon helps facilitate targeted biopsies of the Barrett' mucosa. We previously used data from the BING consortium to validate a classification system using i-Scan magnification endoscopy and ACA chromoendoscopy reporting similar outcomes (accuracy 83%) with

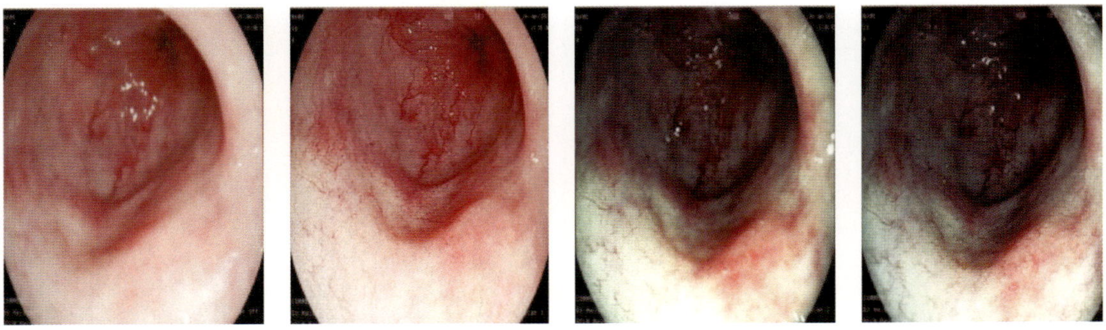

Figure 1: Endoscopic appearances of a flat segment of nondysplastic Barrett's in each separate i-Scan mode. (a) - WLE, (a) i-Scan 1, (c) i-Scan 2, and (d) i-Scan 3.

substantial interobserver agreement ($\kappa = 0.69$) [4]. We graded lesions based on mucosal (M) and vascular (V) patterns as follows:

i. M1: regular circular or villous pits.

ii. M2: distorted or irregular pits or featureless mucosa.

iii. V1: regular and uniform vessels.

iv. V2: irregular, dilated tortuous vessels.

Expert endoscopists used the same classifications in the current study. We also took into consideration the presence of nodularity and ulceration (Figure 2). We believed this to be important as both of these features are associated with higher rates of dysplasia in patients with BE and can be easily recognised at endoscopy [23].

2.3. Data Mining and Machine Learning. Data mining is the process of selecting, exploring, and modelling large amounts of data in order to discover unknown patterns or relationships [24].

Several types of data classification algorithms exist to classify data into two or more categories. We used decision trees as they output rules that are easily understood by doctors. We entered the endoscopic assessments of three expert endoscopists (Matthew R. Banks, Raf Bisschops, and Rehan J. Haidry) into the "WEKA" ML package to help construct the predictive model [25].

2.4. Patients. This study was a UK Health Regulatory Agency (HRA) approved national clinical trial (REC reference 08/H0808/8, study number 08/0018). Patients undergoing surveillance endoscopy for BE were invited to participate. All provided written informed consent. They were asked to stop any anticoagulant therapy for 7 days before endoscopy. Patients in whom acquisition of oesophageal biopsies was contraindicated (coagulopathy, inability to stop anticoagulants, or oesophageal varices) were excluded.

2.5. Endoscopy and Recording. High-definition (HD) video recordings were collected from 40 patients at University College London Hospital over an 18-month period. All patients were taking proton pump inhibitors.

Endoscopy was performed using a PENTAX EG-2990i or EG29-i10 HD video gastroscope (PENTAX HOYA, Japan). All procedures were performed by one of three endoscopists with a specialist interest in BE (Laurence B. Lovat, Matthew R. Banks, Rehan J. Haidry). Patients were given conscious sedation using intravenous midazolam and fentanyl. In cases of excessive oesophageal peristalsis, an antispasmodic agent such as hyoscine-*N*-butylbromide (Buscopan) was administered intravenously.

Once the endoscopist had selected an area of interest, the area was cleaned with sterile water. A mucolytic agent such as "N-acetylcysteiene" was used to improve mucosal clarity. The endoscopist switched between white light endoscopy and each separate "i-Scan" mode ensuring each was recorded for 10 seconds. A corresponding biopsy was then taken from all recorded areas to confirm the histological diagnosis. In 12 cases, 3% (ACA) was also applied to the BE segment prior to biopsy. In these cases, the same protocol for recording was used both before and after the application of ACA. ACA was applied at the discretion of the endoscopist. The endoscopist did not classify recordings in real time. Once complete, patients continued to routine endoscopy including acquisition of further biopsies for clinical purposes if relevant.

2.6. Histology. All biopsy specimens were reviewed by one of two expert gastrointestinal pathologists (Manuel Rodriguez-Justo and Marco Novelli) who were blinded to endoscopists' interpretations. All biopsies were reported according to the revised Vienna classification [26]. Cases of suspected dysplasia were reviewed by both pathologists in line with current recommendations [27].

2.7. Postendoscopy Assessment. Recordings were downloaded to a secure memory drive after the procedure. Recordings were edited using iMovie (Apple Inc.®) to construct individual video files lasting up to 60 seconds that included recordings of each separate "i-Scan" mode. Once the corresponding histology had been reviewed, information was anonymised and entered into a structured database. Later, all videos were transferred to an encrypted memory stick for each expert to review.

2.8. Expert Review and Interpretation of Videos. All videos were reviewed blindly by three expert endoscopists (Matthew

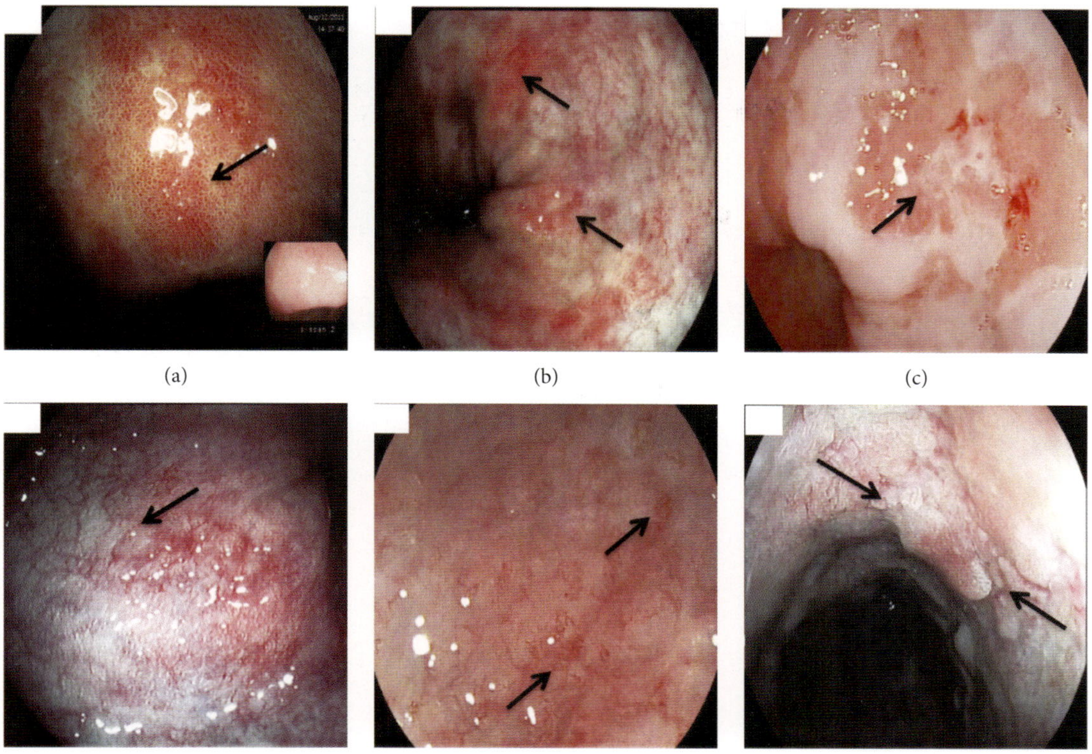

(a) (b) (c) (d) (e) (f)

FIGURE 2: Endoscopic appearances of different mucosal, microvascular patterns, and architecture of Barrett's segment using i-Scan. Arrows denote particular areas of interest. (a) M1: regular circular, oval pits; (b) M1: villous/gyrus ridged pits; (c) M2: distorted, featureless mucosa with surface ulceration; (d) V1: regular uniform vessels; (e) V2: irregular, "corkscrew-like" vessels; (f) nodularity with surrounding distortion of the normal mucosal surface pattern.

R. Banks, Raf Bisschops, and Rehan J. Haidry). All were part of the group that developed our i-Scan classification system for dysplasia detection in BE [4]. They were required to provide the following information for each video: M and V scores, presence of nodularity, and ulceration and prediction of histological diagnosis (ND-BE or D-BE). They were also asked to score how certain they were of the diagnosis on a scale of 1–6 (1 completely uncertain, 6 completely certain).

2.9. Construction of a Decision Tree for Dysplasia Prediction. Data generated was entered into the WEKA package. This was then used to construct the simplest DT for dysplasia prediction that gave a high accuracy but which was also easy enough to teach to non-expert endoscopists.

2.10. Non-expert Review and Interpretation of Videos. Two groups of non-expert endoscopists took part in the study. The first group comprised specialist registrars (SpRs) in gastroenterology who had varying levels of experience in endoscopy and BE assessment. The second group was final year medical students who had no prior experience in either endoscopy or BE.

Both groups were invited to visit a website that hosted all the videos, which were presented in a random fashion. When scoring videos before training, both groups were only asked to record their overall suspected diagnosis and how certain they were of this. Each individual scorer had their own unique access to the website and was unaware of the scoring given by other participants. Once all videos had been scored, individuals were given online access to a 4-minute training presentation. This presentation used a different set of endoscopic videos to highlight the different mucosal and vascular patterns seen both with and without ACA. At the end of this video, the decision tree for dysplasia prediction constructed from expert opinion was presented. The training presentation could be repeated as many times as individuals wished. After training, both groups then scored the original 40 videos. In addition to the suspected diagnosis and certainty, both groups were also asked to record their interpretation of the M and V scores as well as the presence of nodularity or ulceration.

2.11. Statistical Analysis. Accuracy, sensitivity, and specificity values were calculated before and after training. Student's paired t-test was used to assess differences, and $p < 0.05$ was considered to be statistically significant.

3. Results

Video recordings from 40 patients were collected. Twelve had an endoscopy performed using ACA with recordings collected both before and after. Biopsy samples obtained from 23 cases revealed ND-BE and 17 showed D-BE (low-grade dysplasia, 4; high-grade dysplasia, 12; intramucosal cancer, 1). In the cases in which ACA was used, 5 had

Table 1: Comparison of sensitivity and specificity between cases before and after acetic acid for all 3 experts. ND-BE: no dysplasia; D-BE: dysplasia.

	Expert 1 (%)	Expert 2 (%)	Expert 3 (%)	Total (%)
Before acetic acid				
Sensitivity, % (95% C.I.)	94 (71–99)	76 (50–93)	94 (71–99)	88 (76–96)
Specificity, % (95% C.I.)	87 (66–97)	87 (66–97)	83 (61–95)	86 (75–93)
Negative predictive value, %	99.6	98.5	99.6	86 (75–93)
After acetic acid				
Sensitivity, % (95% C.I.)	100 (48–100)	80 (28–99)	100 (48–100)	93 (68–99)
Specificity, % (95% C.I.)	71 (29–96)	85 (42–99)	57 (18–90)	71 (47–89)
Negative predictive value, %	100	98.8	100	71 (47–89)

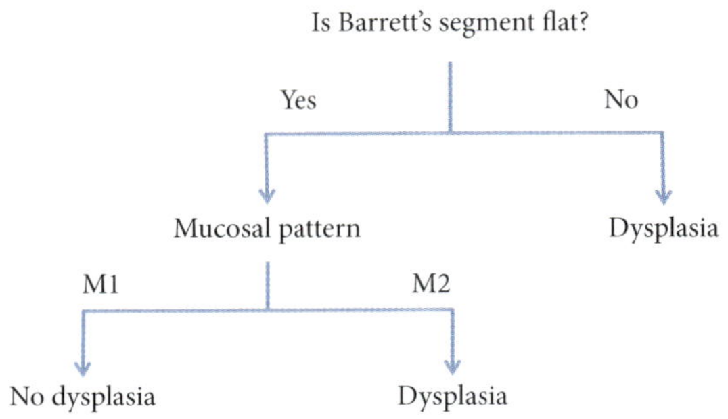

Figure 3: Decision tree constructed from expert opinion that was used to train non-expert endoscopists. M1: regular circular (oval) or villous/gyrus ridged pits; M2: distorted irregular pits or featureless mucosa. Flat means absence of endoscopically visible nodularity or ulceration.

D-BE (low-grade dysplasia, 1; high-grade dysplasia, 3; intramucosal cancer, 1) and 7 had ND-BE.

3.1. Dysplasia Prediction amongst Experts. The mean sensitivity and specificity of dysplasia prediction amongst experts were 88% and 86%, respectively (Table 1). The mean sensitivity of detecting D-BE increased to 93% in the 12 patients who also underwent ACA chromoendoscopy, but this difference was not statistically significant ($p = 0.5$). Negative predictive values (NPV) were calculated for a hypothetical endoscopic surveillance population in which dysplasia is present in 5% of attendees.

3.2. Construction of a Decision Tree for Dysplasia Prediction. Addition of ACA chromoendoscopy did not lead to a significant difference in dysplasia prediction. The decision tree was therefore constructed without considering experts' answers after ACA was used. As each expert interpreted videos differently, we hypothesised that a model that aggregated their opinions would be helpful. The decision tree was based on aggregated data from all 3 experts equally. Thus, all the information for all dysplastic lesions was aggregated and the machine identified the simplest way to classify based on combining all possible information. The same process was used for all nondysplastic lesions. This is a validated approach in data mining [28]. The final DT is shown in Figure 3.

Table 2: Accuracy, sensitivity, and specificity amongst both groups on non-experts before and after web-based training.

	Registrars ($n = 13$)	Medical students ($n = 9$)	Both groups ($n = 22$)
Accuracy			
Before training (%)	65	53	60
After training (%)	68	63	66
p value	0.07	<0.001	<0.001
Sensitivity			
Before training	71	83	76
After training	83	84	83
p value	<0.0001	0.44	<0.001
Specificity			
Before training	60	31	48
After training	57	49	54
p value	0.20	<0.0001	0.02

According to this tree, the most important attribute (i.e. the root of the tree) was the presence or absence of nodularity or ulceration. If there is nodularity or ulceration, according to our proposed DT, the lesion in question is dysplastic. If, however, the Barrett's segment is flat, only then should the assessment of the mucosal pattern be made. When normal (M1), there is no dysplasia, but when abnormal (M2), the lesion in question should be considered dysplastic. This DT, which combined all the experts' assessments led to an overall accuracy for dysplasia prediction of 92%, sensitivity 97%, and specificity of 88%. This was higher than the accuracy of any individual expert.

3.3. Dysplasia Prediction amongst Non-experts. In total, 13 SpRs and 9 medical students analysed all 40 videos both before and after training (Table 2). Mean and standard deviation for the accuracy of dysplasia prediction before training in each group was $65\% \pm 9.5\%$ and $53\% \pm 7.5\%$, respectively. After training, the mean accuracy amongst SpRs increased to $68\% \pm 9.0\%$ ($p = 0.07$) and for medical students to $63\% \pm 8.9\%$ ($p = 0.0005$). When analysed together, the average accuracy amongst both groups before and after training increased significantly from 60% to 66% ($p = 0.0005$).

The sensitivity of dysplasia prediction amongst SpRs significantly increased after training from 71% ± 13.1% to 83% ± 12.0% ($p < 0.0001$). In contrast, the sensitivity of dysplasia prediction amongst medical students did not increase significantly after training (83% before training, 84% after training; $p = 0.44$).

There was no change in specificity of dysplasia prediction amongst SpRs after training (60% before training versus 57% after, $p = 0.2$). In contrast, the specificity of dysplasia prediction improved dramatically after medical student training from 31% to 49% ($p < 0.0001$).

4. Discussion

By using data from three expert endoscopists, a simple classification system derived from machine learning technologies predicted D-BE correctly in 96% of cases with a mean sensitivity and specificity of 93% and 99%. This is better than any single expert's analysis. Although data mining techniques have been used to predict medical outcomes [29] and have also been proposed to help train doctors [30], to our knowledge, machine learning has never been actually applied to medical student teaching and certainly not to improve the endoscopic detection of pre-malignant lesions in the gastrointestinal tract. The only reference in world literature in using machine learning in this way that we could find was to train helicopter pilots [31].

The accuracy of the classification system generated from this small dataset is comparable to select published data using NBI which demonstrated a sensitivity of dysplasia/early cancer detection of 87% both with and without ACA [32].

In contrast to existing classification systems, which are often complex, our proposed algorithm, which was entirely machine generated, is relatively simple [15–19]. The first question is whether the BE segment is flat. Only if nodularity or ulceration is not seen does the system require the user to interpret mucosal architecture. Microvascular patterns can be completely ignored. This is potentially useful, as during the development of our i-Scan classification system of BE dysplasia, we found that experts usually found interpretation of different microvascular patterns more difficult than mucosal surface patterns [4]. The simple machine learning-derived algorithm therefore lends itself well to training.

For non-expert endoscopists, high sensitivity of dysplasia detection is crucial, to ensure adequately targeted biopsies. Before training, medical students, who had no previous experience, had a higher sensitivity of dysplasia detection (83%) than SpRs with varying levels of experience (71%). However, specificity amongst medical students was considerably lower than SpRs (31% versus 60%). This is probably because students were more likely to "overcall" normal areas whereas SpRs did the opposite. Interestingly, after web-based training, specificity rose significantly amongst medical students without loss of sensitivity and significant improvement in overall detection. In contrast, specificity amongst SpRs fell slightly after training (57%) but sensitivity improved significantly (83%) as did the overall accuracy of dysplasia detection albeit the difference reached was not statistically significant. From this, we can conclude that after training, students were more confident in making a diagnosis of ND-BE without loss of sensitivity at detecting D-BE whist for SpRs, the sensitivity at detecting D-BE improved significantly without loss of specificity. However, neither group was able to reach the accuracy of the experts. Reassuringly, when both groups of non-experts were combined, the diagnostic accuracy, sensitivity, and specificity improved significantly after training.

Preservation and incorporation of valuable endoscopic innovations (PIVI) define thresholds that are used to direct endoscopic technology development towards resolving important clinical issues in endoscopy. In response to the limitations of endoscopic surveillance of BE that are currently practiced, the American Society for Gastrointestinal Endoscopy (ASGE) published a PIVI to address real-time imaging of BE [33]. They concluded that to eliminate the need for random mucosal biopsies in BE, any imaging technology with targeted biopsies should have a sensitivity of 90% or greater, a specificity of 80%, and a negative predictive value of at least 98%. Expert assessment did reach the PIVI, but despite improvement in sensitivity and specificity when non-experts used the DT, it did not reach the PIVI standards. It may be useful to expand the current dataset and number of non-experts to evaluate this further.

A similar web-based educational tool to improve the detection and delineation of Barrett's oesophagus-related neoplasia (BORN) has also been published in abstract format [34]. In this study, endoscopy recordings from patients with BORN and non-dysplastic BE were shown to 3 expert endoscopists. After experts had used specialist software to delineate BORN lesions, 68 assessors from the USA and Europe (trainee, junior, and senior gastroenterologists) were asked to detect and delineate these in 4 sets of 20 videos (48 BORN, 32 non-dysplastic) with online training and tailored feedback after each set. Detection and delineation scores significantly increased over the 4 sets (detection score increase: 11%, median delineation score increase: 52%; $p < 0.0001$) with no significant difference between trainees, juniors, and seniors. After removal of 55 videos that were classed as being either "too easy" or "too difficult," the study was repeated for a new group of 121 assessors across the USA, Canada, and Europe with similar outcomes across all levels of seniority (detection score increase: 26%, median delineation score increase: 77%; $p < 0.0001$). Although the results of this study are not directly comparable with ours, its findings are strengthened by the considerably greater number of videos and assessors with varying levels of experience across multiple centres worldwide that were studied. Until the methods and results of this study are fully published, it remains unclear what exact training was delivered after consecutive video sets and if a classification system was presented to assessors or not.

The novelty of this study from a data mining perspective is that our DT, which was based on expert knowledge, is being used not to improve diagnosis but as an aid to training. To date, DT algorithms have been used as diagnostic support tools as experts can typically easily understand the simple rules generated [10]. In contrast, the approach here is to use DT's to create a logical process that doctors in training can use to assess a new clinical scenario, in this case, unfamiliar endoscopic findings. The reason that DT's are so suited to this purpose is that they are generated to identify the most important features first. Accuracy of diagnosis could be improved in our dataset by using more complex trees. This would defeat the purpose of creating a simple tool which can be used to rapidly train junior doctors. Clearly, this brief training does not elevate the trainees to the level of expert, but it does significantly enhance competence. It is interesting to speculate as to whether higher detection rates after this training might be associated with greater competence when fully trained as it does in other areas of endoscopy [35].

Despite the encouraging data that we have presented, there are some limitations when using ML in this setting. The software that is used to derive machine-based algorithms can sometimes be prone to "overfitting" or being specific to only the specific data analysed. Another problem of many of these methods is that they are often prone to finding spurious associations [36]. This means that although they perform well when applied to the original training set, they are not useful when applied to new data. Practically, this could be evaluated by expanding the current dataset to include new videos for external validation through asking users to score new lesions using our proposed decision tree. Lastly, all of the videos used in the study were taken from patients having an endoscopy performed using i-Scan image enhancement technology (PENTAX). This is still a relatively emerging technology compared to, for instance, NBI (Olympus) that is used in most endoscopy units. Therefore, unless the current training set is expanded to include videos of patients having endoscopy for BE with NBI (Olympus), the application of our algorithm to most hospitals would remain limited.

Although our algorithm appears to be more accurate than current classification systems, data for the two are not entirely comparable. Whereas existing classification systems only include patients with "flat" BE, high-definition endoscopy now allows the endoscopist to appreciate that many of these areas have subtle nodularity or ulceration [4, 37, 38]. We therefore also included patients with these lesions. We already know that the latter is more likely to harbour dysplasia or cancer and skew opinion. One could argue, however, that the inclusion of patients with "non-flat" BE is likely to be more representative of what is seen in day-to-day clinical practice.

Our classification system did not consider findings using ACA chromoendoscopy as no benefit was found when this was used. This is despite larger studies having demonstrated that the diagnostic accuracy is higher with targeted biopsies taken after ACA compared to a standard biopsy protocol [22]. More recently a two-staged training module was developed to evaluate the use of ACA for the detection of Barrett's neoplasia [39]. In this study, initial online training significantly improved the sensitivity of dysplasia detection from 83% to 95%. In contrast to our study, they then invited individuals to a one-day interactive seminar including live cases which further increased sensitivity of dysplasia detection to 98%. Furthermore, this group used 40 images and 20 videos to develop their training module compared to only 12 video cases of ACA in our study (although no difference in assessment between images and videos was observed). Based on these data, it would not be unreasonable to speculate that had a larger cohort of ACA data been used in our study, there is a greater likelihood that ACA would have been incorporated into a decision tree for dysplasia prediction.

5. Conclusion

ML is able to define rules learned from expert opinion. These generate a simple algorithm to accurately predict dysplasia. Once taught to non-experts, the algorithm significantly improves dysplasia detection rates. This opens the door to standardised training and assessment of competence for those who perform endoscopy in BE. It may shorten the learning curve and might also be used to compare competence of trainees with recognised experts for accreditation purposes.

Abbreviations

OAC: Oesophageal adenocarcinoma
BE: Barrett's oesophagus
WLE: White light endoscopy
ML: Machine learning
HD: High definition
ACA: Acetic acid
ND-BE: Nondysplastic Barrett's oesophagus
D-BE: Dysplastic Barrett's oesophagus
SpRs: Specialist Registrars.

Disclosure

This work has been presented in abstract format at the British Society of Gastroenterology Annual Meeting in Liverpool in June 2016. The views expressed in this publication are those of the authors and not necessarily those of the Department of Health NIHR Biomedical Research Centres.

Authors' Contributions

Vinay Sehgal, Avi Rosenfeld, David G. Graham, Rehan J. Haidry, and Laurence B. Lovat were involved in the study concept and design. Vinay Sehgal, Avi Rosenfeld, and Laurence B. Lovat were involved in the statistical analysis and interpretation of data. All authors were involved in the acquisition of data and approved the final manuscript.

Acknowledgments

This work was undertaken at UCLH/UCL, which received a proportion of funding from the Department of Health's

NIHR Biomedical Research Centres funding scheme. The work was also supported by the CRUK UCL Early Cancer Medicine Centre.

References

[1] Cancer Research UK, *Cancer Statistics*, 2014.

[2] K. K. Wang and R. E. Sampliner, "Updated guidelines 2008 for the diagnosis, surveillance and therapy of Barrett's esophagus," *The American Journal of Gastroenterology*, vol. 103, no. 3, pp. 788–797, 2008.

[3] P. Sharma, K. McQuaid, J. Dent et al., "A critical review of the diagnosis and management of Barrett's esophagus: the AGA Chicago workshop," *Gastroenterology*, vol. 127, no. 1, pp. 310–330, 2004.

[4] G. Lipman, R. Bisschops, V. Sehgal et al., "Systematic assessment with I-SCAN magnification endoscopy and acetic acid improves dysplasia detection in patients with Barrett's esophagus," *Endoscopy*, vol. 49, no. 12, pp. 1219–1228, 2017.

[5] M. R. Banks, R. Haidry, M. A. Butt et al., "High resolution colonoscopy in a bowel cancer screening program improves polyp detection," *World Journal of Gastroenterology*, vol. 17, no. 38, pp. 4308–4313, 2011.

[6] A. Hoffman, F. Sar, M. Goetz et al., "High definition colonoscopy combined with i-scan is superior in the detection of colorectal neoplasias compared with standard video colonoscopy: a prospective randomized controlled trial," *Endoscopy*, vol. 42, no. 10, pp. 827–833, 2010.

[7] F. Pigò, H. Bertani, M. Manno et al., "*i*-Scan high-definition white light endoscopy and colorectal polyps: prediction of histology, interobserver and intraobserver agreement," *International Journal of Colorectal Disease*, vol. 28, no. 3, pp. 399–406, 2013.

[8] W. J. Kuo, R. F. Chang, D. R. Chen, and C. C. Lee, "Data mining with decision trees for diagnosis of breast tumor in medical ultrasonic images," *Breast Cancer Research*, vol. 66, no. 1, pp. 51–57, 2001.

[9] A. Vlahou, J. O. Schorge, B. W. Gregory, and R. L. Coleman, "Diagnosis of ovarian cancer using decision tree classification of mass spectral data," *Journal of Biomedicine & Biotechnology*, vol. 2003, no. 5, 314 pages, 2003.

[10] R. Bellazzi and B. Zupan, "Predictive data mining in clinical medicine: current issues and guidelines," *International Journal of Medical Informatics*, vol. 77, no. 2, pp. 81–97, 2008.

[11] B. Sierra and P. Larranaga, "Predicting survival in malignant skin melanoma using Bayesian networks automatically induced by genetic algorithms. An empirical comparison between different approaches," *Artificial Intelligence in Medicine*, vol. 14, no. 1-2, pp. 215–230, 1998.

[12] D.-Y. Yeh, C.-H. Cheng, and Y.-W. Chen, "A predictive model for cerebrovascular disease using data mining," *Expert Systems with Applications*, vol. 38, no. 7, pp. 8970–8977, 2011.

[13] I. Kononenko, "Inductive and Bayesian learning in medical diagnosis," *Applied Artificial Intelligence*, vol. 7, no. 4, pp. 317–337, 1993.

[14] R. Bisschops, A. Wilmer, and J. Tack, "A survey on gastroenterology training in Europe," *Gut*, vol. 50, no. 5, pp. 724–729, 2002.

[15] L. A. Herrero, W. L. Curvers, A. Bansal et al., "Zooming in on Barrett oesophagus using narrow-band imaging: an international observer agreement study," *European Journal of Gastroenterology & Hepatology*, vol. 21, no. 9, pp. 1068–1075, 2009.

[16] G. K. Anagnostopoulos, K. Yao, P. Kaye, C. J. Hawkey, and K. Ragunath, "Novel endoscopic observation in Barrett's oesophagus using high resolution magnification endoscopy and narrow band imaging," *Alimentary Pharmacology & Therapeutics*, vol. 26, no. 3, pp. 501–507, 2007.

[17] M. A. Kara, M. Ennahachi, P. Fockens, F. J. W. ten Kate, and J. J. G. H. M. Bergman, "Detection and classification of the mucosal and vascular patterns (mucosal morphology) in Barrett's esophagus by using narrow band imaging," *Gastrointestinal Endoscopy*, vol. 64, no. 2, pp. 155–166, 2006.

[18] P. Sharma, A. Bansal, S. Mathur et al., "The utility of a novel narrow band imaging endoscopy system in patients with Barrett's esophagus," *Gastrointestinal Endoscopy*, vol. 64, no. 2, pp. 167–175, 2006.

[19] M. Singh, A. Bansal, W. L. Curvers et al., "Observer agreement in the assessment of narrowband imaging system surface patterns in Barrett's esophagus: a multicenter study," *Endoscopy*, vol. 43, no. 9, pp. 745–751, 2011.

[20] V. Sehgal, D. Graham, M. Banks et al., "A novel endoscopic classification system using i-scan improves dysplasia detection in Barrett's oesophagus," *United European Gastroenterology Journal*, vol. 2, Supplement 1, 2014.

[21] P. Sharma, J. J. G. H. M. Bergman, K. Goda et al., "Development and validation of a classification system to identify high-grade dysplasia and esophageal adenocarcinoma in Barrett's esophagus using narrow-band imaging," *Gastroenterology*, vol. 150, no. 3, pp. 591–598, 2016.

[22] S. Tholoor, R. Bhattacharyya, O. Tsagkournis, G. Longcroft-Wheaton, and P. Bhandari, "Acetic acid chromoendoscopy in Barrett's esophagus surveillance is superior to the standardized random biopsy protocol: results from a large cohort study (with video)," *Gastrointestinal Endoscopy*, vol. 80, no. 3, pp. 417–424, 2014.

[23] R. C. Fitzgerald, M. di Pietro, K. Ragunath et al., "British Society of Gastroenterology guidelines on the diagnosis and management of Barrett's oesophagus," *Gut*, vol. 63, no. 1, pp. 7–42, 2014.

[24] P. Giudici, *Applied Data Mining Statistical Methods for Business and Industry*, Wiley Sons, 2003.

[25] I. H. Witten and E. Frank, *Data Mining: Practical Machine Learning Tools and Technqiues (Morgan Kaufmann Series in Data Management Systems).*, Morgan Kaufmann, 2005.

[26] R. J. Schlemper, R. H. Riddell, Y. Kato et al., "The Vienna classification of gastrointestinal epithelial neoplasia," *Gut*, vol. 47, no. 2, pp. 251–255, 2000.

[27] C. Bennett, N. Vakil, J. Bergman et al., "Consensus statements for management of Barrett's dysplasia and early-stage esophageal adenocarcinoma, based on a Delphi process," *Gastroenterology*, vol. 143, no. 2, pp. 336–346, 2012.

[28] L. Rokach and O. Maimon, *Data Mining with Decision Trees. Vol. 69*, Series in Machine Perception and Artificial Intelligence, Series in Machine Perception and Artificial Intelligence, 2007.

[29] S. Palanippan and R. Awang, "Intelligent heart disease prediction system using data mining techniques," in *2008 IEEE/ACS International Conference Computer Systems and Applications*, vol. 8, no. 8, pp. 343–350, Doha, Qatar, 2008.

[30] O. Wegwarth, W. Gaissmaier, and G. Gigerenzer, "Smart strategies for doctors and doctors-in-training: heuristics in medicine," *Medical Education*, vol. 43, no. 8, pp. 721–728, 2009.

[31] R. A. Richards, "Principle hierarchy based intelligent tutoring system for common cockpit helicopter training," *Intelligent Tutoring Systems*, vol. 2363, pp. 473–483, 2002.

[32] J. Pohl, A. May, T. Rabenstein et al., "Comparison of computed virtual chromoendoscopy and conventional chromoendoscopy with acetic acid for detection of neoplasia in Barrett's esophagus," *Endoscopy*, vol. 39, no. 7, pp. 594–598, 2007.

[33] P. Sharma, T. J. Savides, M. I. Canto et al., "The American Society for Gastrointestinal Endoscopy PIVI (preservation and incorporation of valuable endoscopic innovations) on imaging in Barrett's esophagus," *Gastrointestinal Endoscopy*, vol. 76, no. 2, pp. 252–254, 2012.

[34] J. Bergman, O. Pech, K. Ragunath et al., "A novel, interactive web-based educational tool improves detection and delineation of Barrett's oesophagus related neoplasia (BORN): the born project," *Gastrointestinal Endoscopy*, vol. 85, no. 5, article AB48, 2017.

[35] P. D. James, L. Antonova, M. Martel, and A. Barkun, "Measures of trainee performance in advanced endoscopy: a systematic review," *Best Practice & Research Clinical Gastroenterology*, vol. 30, no. 3, pp. 421–452, 2016.

[36] D. I. Broadhurst and D. B. Kell, "Statistical strategies for avoiding false discoveries in metabolomics and related experiments," *Metabolomics*, vol. 2, no. 4, pp. 171–196, 2007.

[37] S. S. Sami, V. Subramanian, W. M. Butt et al., "High definition versus standard definition white light endoscopy for detecting dysplasia in patients with Barrett's esophagus," *Diseases of the Esophagus*, vol. 28, no. 8, pp. 742–749, 2015.

[38] A. Espino, M. Cirocco, R. Dacosta, and N. Marcon, "Advanced imaging technologies for the detection of dysplasia and early cancer in Barrett esophagus," *Clinical Endoscopy*, vol. 47, no. 1, pp. 47–54, 2014.

[39] F. J. Q. Chedgy, K. Kandiah, H. Barr et al., "Development and validation of a training module on the use of acetic acid for the detection of Barrett's neoplasia," *Endoscopy*, vol. 49, no. 2, pp. 121–129, 2017.

Permissions

All chapters in this book were first published in GRP, by Hindawi Publishing Corporation; hereby published with permission under the Creative Commons Attribution License or equivalent. Every chapter published in this book has been scrutinized by our experts. Their significance has been extensively debated. The topics covered herein carry significant findings which will fuel the growth of the discipline. They may even be implemented as practical applications or may be referred to as a beginning point for another development.

The contributors of this book come from diverse backgrounds, making this book a truly international effort. This book will bring forth new frontiers with its revolutionizing research information and detailed analysis of the nascent developments around the world.

We would like to thank all the contributing authors for lending their expertise to make the book truly unique. They have played a crucial role in the development of this book. Without their invaluable contributions this book wouldn't have been possible. They have made vital efforts to compile up to date information on the varied aspects of this subject to make this book a valuable addition to the collection of many professionals and students.

This book was conceptualized with the vision of imparting up-to-date information and advanced data in this field. To ensure the same, a matchless editorial board was set up. Every individual on the board went through rigorous rounds of assessment to prove their worth. After which they invested a large part of their time researching and compiling the most relevant data for our readers.

The editorial board has been involved in producing this book since its inception. They have spent rigorous hours researching and exploring the diverse topics which have resulted in the successful publishing of this book. They have passed on their knowledge of decades through this book. To expedite this challenging task, the publisher supported the team at every step. A small team of assistant editors was also appointed to further simplify the editing procedure and attain best results for the readers.

Apart from the editorial board, the designing team has also invested a significant amount of their time in understanding the subject and creating the most relevant covers. They scrutinized every image to scout for the most suitable representation of the subject and create an appropriate cover for the book.

The publishing team has been an ardent support to the editorial, designing and production team. Their endless efforts to recruit the best for this project, has resulted in the accomplishment of this book. They are a veteran in the field of academics and their pool of knowledge is as vast as their experience in printing. Their expertise and guidance has proved useful at every step. Their uncompromising quality standards have made this book an exceptional effort. Their encouragement from time to time has been an inspiration for everyone.

The publisher and the editorial board hope that this book will prove to be a valuable piece of knowledge for researchers, students, practitioners and scholars across the globe.

List of Contributors

Xingchen Cai
Department of General Surgery, Jinling Hospital, Nanjing Medical University, Nanjing, China

Weisong Shen, Zhen Guo, Yi Li, Lei Cao, Jianfeng Gong and Weiming Zhu
Department of General Surgery, Jinling Hospital, Medical School of Nanjing University, Nanjing, China

Tong Li, Qi Wang, Juanjuan Li, Yuting Qian, Lumin Wei, Mingping Xie, Xu Liu, Ying Zhu and Lifu Wang
Department of Gastroenterology, Ruijin Hospital Affiliated to Shanghai Jiao Tong University School of Medicine, Shanghai 200025, China

Yi Zang
Department of Gastroenterology, Ruijin Hospital Affiliated to Shanghai Jiao Tong University School of Medicine, Shanghai 200025, China
Department of Gastroenterology, Changzheng Hospital, Second Military Medical University, Shanghai 200003, China

Wen-Hao Tang
Department of General Surgery, Huadong Hospital Affiliated to Fudan University, Shanghai 200040, China

Lei Zhu
Department of General Surgery, Huadong Hospital Affiliated to Fudan University, Shanghai 200040, ChinaDepartment of Surgery, Yancheng No. 1 People's Hospital, Yancheng, Jiangsu 224005, China

Jun Lu, Long-long Cao, Ping Li, Jian-wei Xie, Jia-bin Wang, Jian-xian Lin, Qi-yue Chen, Mi Lin, Ru-hong Tu, Chang-ming Huang and Chao-hui Zheng
Department of Gastric Surgery, Fujian Medical University Union Hospital, Fuzhou, China
Department of General Surgery, Fujian Medical University Union Hospital, Fuzhou, China
Key Laboratory of Ministry of Education of Gastrointestinal Cancer, Fujian Medical University, Fuzhou, China
Fujian Key Laboratory of Tumor Microbiology, Fujian Medical University, Fuzhou, China

Rani Berry
Department of Internal Medicine, Ronald Reagan UCLA Medical Center, Los Angeles, CA, USA

James Han
Department of Internal Medicine, University of California, Irvine, CA, USA

Mohit Girotra
Division of Gastroenterology, University of Miami, Miller School of Medicine, Miami, FL, USA

James H. Tabibian
Division of Gastroenterology, Department of Medicine, Olive View-UCLA Medical Center, Sylmar, CA, USA

Lin Gao, Jingzhu Zhang, Kun Gao, Jing Zhou, Weiqin Li and Zhihui Tong
Surgical Intensive Care Unit (SICU), Department of General Surgery, Jinling Hospital, Medical School of Nanjing University, No. 305 Zhongshan East Road, Nanjing, 210002 Jiangsu, China

Guotao Lu
Surgical Intensive Care Unit (SICU), Department of General Surgery, Jinling Hospital, Medical School of Nanjing University, No. 305 Zhongshan East Road, Nanjing, 210002 Jiangsu, China
Department of Gastroenterology, Affiliated Hospital of Yangzhou University, No. 386 Hanjiang Media Road, Yangzhou, 225000 Jiangsu, China

Yiyuan Pan
Department of Intensive Care Unit, Suzhou Hospital Affiliated to Nanjing Medical University, No. 16 Baita West Road, Suzhou, 215002 Jiangsu, China

Xiaotao Qin and Jie Zhang
Hope Assist Medical Assistance Service Company, No. 1111 Tower A, Chaoyang SOHO, Beijing 100020, China

N. Inayet, J. O. Hayat and A. Poullis
Department of Gastroenterology, St. George's Hospital, London, UK

A. Kaul
Department of Rheumatology, St. George's Hospital, London, UK

M. Tome and A. Child
Department of Cardiology, St. George's Hospital, London, UK

Naohisa Yoshida, Ritsu Yasuda, Takaaki Murakami, Ryohei Hirose, Ken Inoue, Osamu Dohi, Yuji Naito and Yoshito Itoh
Department of Molecular Gastroenterology and Hepatology, Kyoto Prefectural University of Medicine, Graduate School of Medical Science, Kyoto, Japan

Yutaka Inada
Department of Gastroenterology, Fukuchiyama City Hospital, Kyoto, Japan

Kiyoshi Ogiso
Department of Gastroenterology, Osaka General Hospital of West Japan Railway Company, Osaka, Japan

Yukiko Morinaga, Mitsuo Kishimoto and Eiichi Konishi
Department of Surgical Pathology, Kyoto Prefectural University of Medicine, Graduate School of Medical Science, Kyoto, Japan

Qian Chen, Li Cao, Guang-Quan Liao, Qiao-Zhen Guo and Qi Zhou
Endoscopic Unit, Department of Gastroenterology and Hepatology at Tongji Hospital, Tongji Medical College, Huazhong University of Science and Technology (HUST), Wuhan, China

Heng-Hui Cheng and Dong Kuang
Department of Pathology at Tongji Hospital, Tongji Medical College, HUST, Wuhan, China

Shuang Deng
Tongji Medical College, HUST, Wuhan, China

Chang Shu
Department of Epidemiology and Biostatistics, School of Public Health, Tongji Medical College, HUST, Wuhan, China

Diletta Cozzi, Chiara Moroni, Gloria Addeo, Ginevra Danti, Monica Marina Lanzetta, Edoardo Cavigli and Vittorio Miele
Department of Radiology, Careggi University Hospital, Florence, Italy

Massimo Falchini
Department of Experimental and Clinical Biomedical Sciences, Radiodiagnostic Unit No. 2, University of Florence-Careggi University Hospital, Florence, Italy

Fabio Marra
Department of Clinical and Experimental Medicine, Internal Medicine and Hepatology, University of Florence, Florence, Italy

Claudia Lucia Piccolo and Luca Brunese
Department of Medicine and Health Sciences, University of Molise, Campobasso, Italy

Iatagan R. Josino, Antônio C. Madruga-Neto, Igor B. Ribeiro, Hugo G. Guedes, Vitor O. Brunaldi, Diogo T. H. de Moura, Wanderley M. Bernardo and Eduardo G. H. de Moura
Gastrointestinal Endoscopy Unit, University of São Paulo Medical School, Dr. Arnaldo Av 455, São Paulo 01246-903, Brazil

Cristiano Pagnini
Digestive and Liver Disease Department, S. Andrea Hospital, Rome, Italy

Spyros I. Siakavellas
Academic Department of Gastroenterology, Laiko General Hospital, University of Athens Medical School, Athens, Greece

Giorgos Bamias
Gastroenterology Unit, Third Depatment of Internal Medicine, Sotiria General Hospital, University of Athens Medical School, Athens, Greece

Zubair Khan, Yaseen Alastal, Mohammad Saud Khan, Basmah Khalil and Ali Nawras
Division of Gastroenterology and Hepatology, University of Toledo Medical Center, Toledo, OH, USA

Muhammad Ali Khan, Shreesh Shrestha, Faisal Kamal and Colin W. Howden
Division of Gastroenterology and Hepatology, The University of Tennessee Health Science Center, Memphis, TN, USA

Tao Li, Jun Wen, Like Bie and Biao Gong
Digestive Endoscopy Center, Department of Gastroenterology, Ruijin Hospital, Affiliated to Shanghai Jiao Tong University School of Medicine, Shanghai, China

Neeraj Narula and Brandon McGuinness
Department of Medicine (Division of Gastroenterology) and Farncombe Family Digestive Health Research Institute, McMaster University, Hamilton, ON, Canada

Sameer Masood and Saama Sabeti
Harvard TH Chan School of Public Health, Boston, MA, USA

Samira Shojaee
Department of Medicine (Division of Pulmonary and Critical Care Medicine), Virginia Commonwealth University, Richmond, VA, USA

Arianne Buchan
Department of Medicine, The Ottawa Hospital, Ottawa, ON, Canada

Rose-Marie Satherley
School of Populations Sciences and Health Services Research, Guy's Campus, King's College London, 5th Floor Addison House, London SE1 1UL, UK

Ruth Howard and Suzanne Higgs
School of Psychology, University of Birmingham, 52 Pritchatts Road, Edgbaston, Birmingham B15 2SB, UK

Siyan "Stewart" Cao
Department of Medicine, University of California, San Francisco, San Francisco, CA 94143, USA

Katarzyna Neubauer
Department of Gastroenterology and Hepatology, Wroclaw Medical University, 50-556 Wroclaw, Poland

Malgorzata Matusiewicz, Iwona Bednarz-Misa and Malgorzata Krzystek-Korpacka
Department of Medical Biochemistry, Wroclaw Medical University, 50-368 Wroclaw, Poland

Andrzej Gamian
Department of Medical Biochemistry, Wroclaw Medical University, 50-368 Wroclaw, Poland
Laboratory of Medical Microbiology, Ludwik Hirszfeld Institute of Immunology and Experimental Therapy, Polish Academy of Sciences, 53-114 Wroclaw, Poland

Sabina Gorska
Laboratory of Medical Microbiology, Ludwik Hirszfeld Institute of Immunology and Experimental Therapy, Polish Academy of Sciences, 53-114 Wroclaw, Poland

Aruchuna Ruban, Hutan Ashrafian and Julian P. Teare
Department of Surgery and Cancer, Imperial College, London, UK

Patrick L. Stoner, Fares Ayoub, Sarah C. Glover and Ellen M. Zimmer
Department of Medicine, Division of Gastroenterology, University of Florida, 2000 SW Archer Rd, Gainesville, FL 32610, USA

Amir Kamel
Department of Pharmacotherapy, College of Pharmacy, University of Florida, 2000 SW Archer Rd, Gainesville, FL 32610, USA

Sanda Tan and Atif Iqbal
Department of Surgery, Division of Colorectal Surgery, College of Medicine, University of Florida, 2000 SW Archer Rd, Gainesville, FL 32610, USA

Sung Hoo Kim, Byung Kyu Ahn and Kang Hong Lee
Department of Surgery, Hanyang University College of Medicine, Seoul, Republic of Korea

Seung Sam Paik
Department of Pathology, Hanyang University College of Medicine, Seoul, Republic of Korea

Thomas M. Diehl
McGill University, Faculty of Medicine, Montreal, QC, Canada H3G 2M1

Daniel J. Adams
Department of Pediatrics, Naval Medical Center Portsmouth, Portsmouth, VA 23708, USA

Cade M. Nylund
Department of Pediatrics, F. Edward Hébert School of Medicine, Uniformed Services University of the Health Sciences, Bethesda, MD 20814, USA

Fumio Omata, Yasutoshi Shiratori, Daiki Kobayashi and Hiroko Arioka
Department of Internal Medicine, St. Luke's International University, 9-1 Akashi-cho, Chuo-ku, Tokyo 104-8560, Japan

Toshihiko Komai
Department of Internal Medicine, St. Luke's International University, 9-1 Akashi-cho, Chuo-ku, Tokyo 104-8560, Japan
Department of Allergy and Rheumatology, Graduate School of Medicine, The University of Tokyo, 7-3-1 Hongo, Bunkyo-ku, Tokyo 113-8655, Japan

Grace H. Elta and Sheryl Korsnes
Division of Gastroenterology, University of Michigan Health System, Ann Arbor, MI, USA

Stacy B. Menees
Division of Gastroenterology, University of Michigan Health System, Ann Arbor, MI, USA
Division of Gastroenterology, Ann Arbor Veterans' Administration Health Care System, Ann Arbor, MI, USA

H. Myra Kim
Division of Gastroenterology, Ann Arbor Veterans' Administration Health Care System, Ann Arbor, MI, USA

Philip Schoenfeld
John D. Dingell VA Medical Center, Detroit, MI, USA

Lan-Lan Geng, Cui-Ping Liang, Pei-Yu Chen, Qiang Wu, Min Yang, Hui-Wen Li, Zhao-Hui Xu, Lu Ren, Hong-Li Wang, Shunxian Cheng, Wan-Fu Xu, Yang Chen, Chao Zhang, Li-Ying Liu and Si-Tang Gong
Department of Gastroenterology, Guangzhou Women and Children's Medical Center, 9 Jinsui Road, Guangzhou 510623, China

Ding-You Li
Division of Gastroenterology, Children's Mercy Hospital, 2401 Gillham Road, Kansas City, MO 64108, USA

Zibo Meng, Feiyang Wang, Yushun Zhang and Heshui Wu
Department of Pancreatic Surgery, Union Hospital, Tongji Medical College, Huazhong University of Science and Technology, Wuhan 430022, China

Mingsi Cao
Institute of Cardiology, Union Hospital, Tongji Medical College, Huazhong University of Science and Technology, Wuhan 430022, China

Ferial El-Kalla, Loai Mansour, Abdelrahman Kobtan, Asmaa Elzeftawy, Lobna Abo Ali, Sherief Abd-Elsalam, Sahar Elyamani, Mohamed Yousef and Mohamed Elhendawy
Tropical Medicine and Infectious Diseases Department, Faculty of Medicine, Tanta University, Tanta, Egypt

I. Amer
Hepatology and Gastroenterology Department, Faculty of Medicine, Kafrelsheikh University, Kafr Elsheikh, Egypt

H. Mourad
Clinical Pathology Department, Faculty of Medicine, Tanta University, Tanta, Egypt

Jun Woo Bong, Seok-Byung Lim, Jong Lyul Lee, Chan Wook Kim, Yong Sik Yoon, In Ja Park, Chang Sik Yu and Jin Cheon Kim
Department of Surgery, Asan Medical Center, University of Ulsan College of Medicine, 88 Olympic-ro 43-gil, Songpa-gu, Seoul 05505, Republic of Korea

J. Ventriglia
Uro-Gynaecological Department, INT G. Pascale, Via Mariano Semmola, 80131 Naples, Italy

A. Petrillo, M. M. Laterza, G. Tirino, L. Pompella, A. Diana, T. Troiani, E. Martinelli, F. Morgillo, M. Orditura, F. Ciardiello and F. De Vita
U.O.C. Medical Oncology, School of Medicine, Università della Campania L. Vanvitelli, c/o II Policlinico, Via Pansini 5, 80131 Naples, Italy

M. Huerta Alváro, V. Gambardella and A. Cervantes
Department Hematology and Medical Oncology, INCLIVA Biomedical Research Institute, University of Valencia, Blasco Ibáñez 17, 46010 Valencia, Spain

B. Savastano
Breast Department, INT G. Pascale, Via Mariano Semmola, 80131 Naples, Italy

Iovino
Department of Cardiothoracic and Respiratory Sciences, School of Medicine, Università della Campania L. Vanvitelli, c/o II Policlinico, Via Pansini 5, 80131 Naples, Italy

Anantha Madhavan, Alexander W. Phillips, Claire L. Donohoe, Rebecca J. Willows, Arul Immanuel and S. Michael Griffin
Northern Oesophagogastric Cancer Unit, Royal Victoria Infirmary, Newcastle upon Tyne NE1 4LP, UK

Mark Verril
Northern Centre for Cancer Care, Freeman Hospital, Newcastle upon Tyne NE7 7DN, UK

Hannes Hagström, Rolf Hultcrantz and Per Stål
Department of Upper GI, Unit of Liver Diseases, Karolinska University Hospital, Stockholm, Sweden
Department of Medicine, Huddinge Karolinska Institutet, Stockholm, Sweden

Olof Elfwén
Department of Medicine, Huddinge Karolinska Institutet, Stockholm, Sweden

Gideon Lipman, Matthew R. Banks and Rehan J. Haidry
Department of Gastroenterology, University College London Hospitals NHS Foundation Trust, London, UK

Vinay Sehgal, David G. Graham and Laurence B. Lovat
Department of Gastroenterology, University College London Hospitals NHS Foundation Trust, London, UK
Research Department for Tissue and Energy, Division of Surgery and Interventional Science, University College London, London, UK

Avi Rosenfeld
Department of Industrial Engineering, Jerusalem College of Technology, Jerusalem, Israel

Raf Bisschops
Department of Gastroenterology, University Hospitals Leuven, Leuven, Belgium

Krish Ragunath
Department of Gastroenterology, Queen's Medical Centre, Nottingham, UK

Manuel Rodriguez-Justo and Marco Novelli
Department of Histopathology, University College London Hospitals NHS Foundation Trust, London, UK

Index